Cutaneous Laser Surgery

The Art and Science of Selective Photothermolysis

Second edition

Cutaneous Laser Surgery

The Art and Science of Selective Photothermolysis

mitchel p. **Goldman, MD**

Associate Clinical Professor
Department of Medicine
Division of Dermatology
University of California, San Diego
San Diego, California

richard e. **Fitzpatrick, MD**

Associate Clinical Professor
Department of Medicine
Division of Dermatology
University of California, San Diego
San Diego, California

Second edition

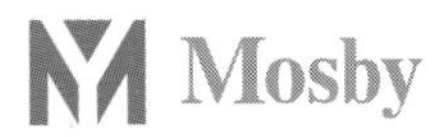

St. Louis Baltimore Boston Carlsbad
Chicago Minneapolis New York Philadelphia Portland
London Milan Sydney Tokyo Toronto

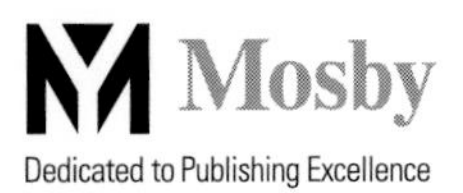

A Times Mirror
Company

Publisher: Laura DeYoung
Editor: Gina Almond
Developmental Editor: Ellen Baker Geisel
Project Manager: Carol Sullivan Weis
Manuscript Editor: Roger McWilliams
Senior Production Editor: Florence Achenbach
Designer: Jen Marmarinos
Manufacturing Manager: Dave Graybill

Second edition

Printed in the United States of America
Composition by Graphic World
Lithography/color film by Graphic World
Printing/binding by Walsworth

Mosby Inc.
11830 Westline Industrial Drive
St. Louis, Missouri 63146

Library of Congress Cataloging-in-Publication Data
Goldman, Mitchel P.
Cutaneous laser surgery : the art and science of selective photothermolysis / Mitchel P. Goldman, Richard E. Fitzpatrick.—2nd ed.
p. cm.
Includes bibliographical references and index.
ISBN 0-8151-3610-2
1. Skin—Laser surgery. I. Fitzpatrick, Richard E. II. Title.
[DNLM: 1. Laser Surgery—methods. 2. Skin—surgery. 3. Skin—radiation effects. 4. Lasers—therapeutic use. WR 650 G619c 1998]
RL 120.L37G65 1998
617.4'77059—dc21
DNLM/DLC
for Library of Congress 98-31526
CIP

International Standard Book Number 0-8151-3610-2
99 00 01 02 / 9 8 7 6 5 4 3 2 1

Contributor List

R. Rox Anderson, M.D.
Associate Professor of Dermatology
Harvard Medical School
Research Director
Massachusetts General Hospital Laser Center
Boston, Massachusetts

Robert Bissonnette, M.D., MS.C., F.R.C.P.C.
Clinical Research Fellow
Division of Dermatology
University of British Columbia
Vancouver Hospital and Health Sciences Centre
Vancouver, British Columbia, Canada

Richard W. Cunningham, M.D.
Private Practice
San Diego, California

Richard E. Fitzpatrick, M.D.
Associate Clinical Professor
Department of Medicine
Division of Dermatology
University of California, San Diego
San Diego, California

Mitchel P. Goldman, M.D.
Associate Clinical Professor
Department of Medicine
Division of Dermatology
University of California, San Diego
San Diego, California

Melanie C. Grossman, M.D.
Instructor, Department of Dermatology
Cornell University
Columbia Presbyterian Hospital
New York, New York

Suzanne Linsmeier Kilmer, M.D.
Assistant Clinical Professor
Department of Dermatology
University of California, Davis Medical School
Director, Laser and Skin Surgery Center of Northern California
Sacramento, California

Harvey Lui, M.D., F.R.C.P.C.
Assistant Professor
Division of Dermatology
University of British Columbia
Active Staff
Division of Dermatology
Vancouver Hospital and Health Sciences Centre
Vancouver, British Columbia
Canada

John A. Parrish, M.D.
Professor and Chairman
Department of Dermatology
Harvard Medical School
Chief, Dermatology Service
Director, Wellman Laboratories of Photomedicine
Massachusetts General Hospital
Boston, Massachusetts

Danielle M. Reicher, M.D.
Chief of Anesthesia
Scripps Memorial Hospital
Encinitas, California

Penny J. Smalley, R.N.
President, Technology Concepts International
Chicago, Illinois

Bradley G. Williams, M.D.
Anesthesia Service Medical Group
San Diego, California
Staff Anesthesiologist
Scripps Memorial Hospital
La Jolla, California

To our families, both personal and professional

Acknowledgments

To Ann-Marie Andrews and Susan Alexander, our secretaries "extraordinaire," whose ability to translate hieroglyphics enabled them to put together a cohesive document. They somehow knew what we were trying to say when we wondered.

To the partners and staff of Dermatology Associates of San Diego County, Inc., who not only put up with our multiple laser purchases but also our piles of charts and photos meticulously stacked in strategic places throughout the office. We thank you for your patience in assisting multiple, frantic, last-minute searches for the missing pieces of data.

To our colleagues and mentors, who provided us with inspiration, encouragement, enlightenment at times, and support: Rox Anderson, John Parrish, Jerry Garden, Ron Wheeland, Roy Geronemus, Gary Lask, Larry David, David Goldberg, Randy Roenigk, David Apfelberg, Ken Arndt, Gary Brauner, Billie Aronoff, Stuart Nelson, Alan Schliftman, Robert Weiss, Tina Alster, Martin Van Gemert, Gerry Goldberg, Bill Hanke, Suzanne Kilmer, Joop Grevelink, Roy Grekin, Jeff Dover, Milt Waner, Sue McCoy, Paul Thibault, Richard Gregory, Tom McMeeken, Nick Lowe, and the many others we failed to include because of space limitations.

To the memory of Leon Goldman and Larry Shoenrock, friends, mentors, and colleagues of all laser surgeons.

Finally,

we would like to acknowledge the technical support and theoretical assistance provided by Dale Koop of Coherent Medical Group, and Shimon Eckhouse and Hillel Bachrach of Energy Systems Corporation.

Foreword

John A Parrish

Lasers have come to occupy unique and important roles in the diagnostic and therapeutic armament of medicine. Lasers, brightest known sources of light (man-made or natural), can have extremely powerful effects on biological systems. The uniqueness of lasers derives from a number of special properties, that is, high intensity, coherence (which permits focusing on a spot size of one micrometer or less), collimation, extreme monochromaticity, and the ability to be delivered in very brief pulses. Lasers are to other sources of light as music is to noise.

The collective properties of lasers can cause unique alterations of biological materials. And the ability to launch high optical power into single optical fibers extends enormously the clinical applications of lasers. This capability permist remote (endoscopic, intravascular, intracavitary, interstitial) delivery of precisely controlled energy to tissue deep within the body with minimal damage to intervening structures. The precision in wavelength (monochromaticity) and the capability for control of the spatial and temporal output of lasers also make a number of diagnostic applications possible.

Cutaneous Laser Surgery focuses primarily on dermatologic applications of lasers. There is a growing number of skin lesions that are usually best treated by lasers. Examples include many port-wine stains, certain forms of facial telangiectasias (Chapter 2), many decorative and accidental tattoos (Chapter 4), and certain congenital, dermal-pigmented lesions such as nevus of Ota (Chapter 3).

Dermatology has played an important role in laser medicine. Skin is an obvious, highly accessible target organ for diagnostic and therapeutic uses of lasers. Dermatologist investigators and physicians have contributed fundamental new knowledge, concepts, and ideas useful in other organ systems. The well-informed practicing dermatologist using lasers with skill and good judgment can help solidify the image and substance of laser medicine and dermatology. In doing so, he or she can also take better care of the patients. This book, with Drs. Goldman and Fitzpatrick as editors, is one attempt to further these goals.

Research continues and new developments in laser surgery will allow us to improve patient care. We hope this text will serve as a stimulus to further the development of this exciting field of medicine. We are fortunate to be a part of its expansion.

Preface

Since the publication of the first edition four years ago, there has been an exponential increase in both the development as well as application of new laser technologies to cutaneous laser surgery. This necessitated the task of producing this *second edition.*

Specifically, laser resurfacing through use of the theory of *"Selective Photothermolysis"* and the development of multiple forms of both carbon dioxide as well as erbium:YAG lasers, alone and in combination, has opened up a new field which crosses specialty boundaries to encompass all surgeons who work with rejuvenation techniques. The popularity of this technique is directly related to advancement in both laser technology as well as treatment techniques. In addition, the continuing development of new laser technologies to treat benign vascular lesions has led to the development of both new technologies as well as treatment parameters. Finally, again using the theory of *"Selective Photothermolysis,"* it is now possible to remove and possibly permanently eradicate unwanted body hair. Various flash lamp, as well as pulsed laser systems, have been developed towards this end.

Therefore, this second edition represents an enhanced viewpoint of Cutaneous Laser Surgery. Towards this end, we have enlisted the expertise of Melanie Grossman, M.D. who has trained extensively at the Wellman Laboratories and is now continuing her research as well as private practice in New York City. Dr. Grossman has compiled an outstanding summary of the present state of technology regarding Laser Hair Removal.

We have also enlisted the support of another Wellman trained laser expert, Dr. Suzanne Kilmer, who now maintains an active research and private practice in Sacramento, California. Dr. Kilmer has added extensive sections to the chapters on Treatment of Pigmented Lesions and Tattoo Removal.

Doctors Harvey Lui and Robert Bissonnette have added a much needed chapter on photodynamic therapy. This treatment modality has tremendous potential to enhance our ability to treat both benign and malignant cutaneous lesions.

Because of the evolving increase in technology in anesthesia, we have enlisted the support of Dr. Bradley Williams who was instrumental in updating the chapter on Anesthesia for Cutaneous Laser Surgery. The chapter on Laser Safety Regulations was updated and expanded by Dr. Penny Smalley and Dr. Mitchel Goldman. Dr. Richard Fitzpatrick, with his colleague Dr. Mitchel Goldman, have extensively revised the CO_2 Laser Surgery chapter as well as an additional chapter on Cosmetic Applications of the CO_2 Laser, including a section on the newly developed and utilized erbium:YAG Laser. Finally, both Dr. Goldman and Dr. Fitzpatrick have revised the chapter on Laser Treatment of Cutaneous Vascular Lesions to more accurately reflect the present state of knowledge with multiple new technological advancements. Indeed, this chapter, which has now doubled in size, could comprise its own separate textbook.

We have tried, once again, to put the majority of the available research and information on Cutaneous Laser Surgery into one text. It is our hope that this text will serve as a stimulus to further the development of this exciting field of medicine. We thank our colleagues for their contribution to this field of medicine and especially thank the new co-authors represented in this text for helping to simplify this rapidly expanding field in a text format. We are fortunate to be a part of this age of minimally invasive surgery and be part of its continuing evolution.

Mitchel P. Goldman, MD

Richard E. Fitzpatrick, MD

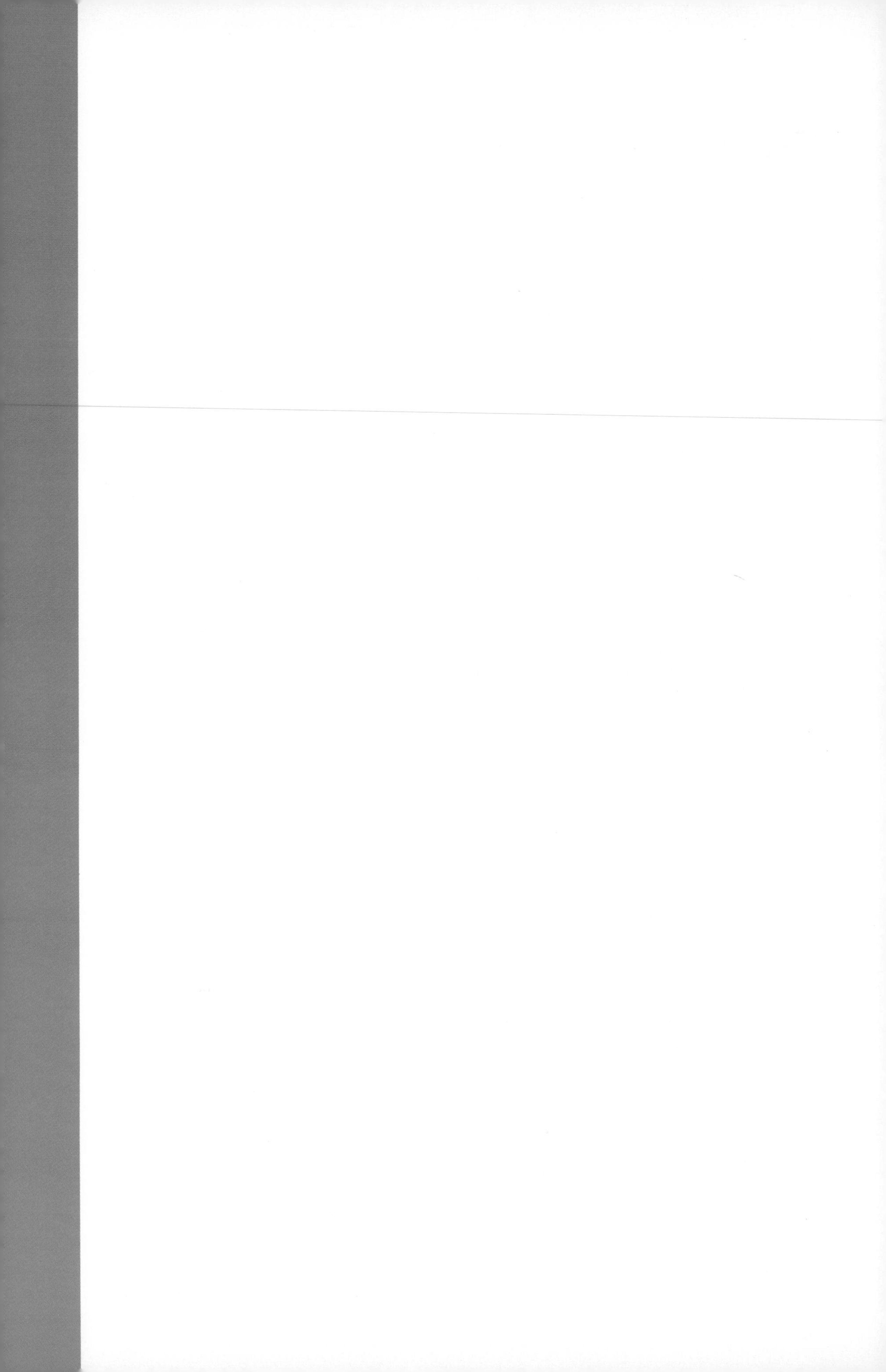

Contents

Appendices

Detailed Contents

Appendixes 493

Cutaneous Laser Surgery

The Art and Science of Selective Photothermolysis

CHAPTER one

Laser-Tissue Interactions

R. Rox Anderson

OVERVIEW

Electromagnetic Radiation

All the effects of light, including laser light on skin, begin with the absorption of electromagnetic radiation (EMR). EMR is a fundamental form of energy that exhibits *wave* properties, because of an alternating electric and magnetic field, and *particle* properties, because the energy is carried in quanta known as *photons.* Long-wavelength photons carry less energy than short-wavelength photons, according to Planck's law. Starting on the long-wavelength, low-photon energy end of the spectrum, EMR includes radio waves, microwaves, infrared (IR) radiation, visible light, ultraviolet (UV) radiation, and x-rays. EMR is absorbed by matter through interactions with charged particles such as electrons or the partial separation of charges in molecules called *dipoles.* Whenever a photon is absorbed, some movement or separation of charged matter occurs, and the energy carried by the photon is invested in this excitation. Absorption and excitation are necessary for all photobiologic effects and laser-tissue interactions.

The units in which EMR is measured form an important part of understanding laser-tissue interactions. Energy is measured in *joules* (J). The amount of energy delivered per unit area is the *fluence,* sometimes called the *dose,* usually given in J/cm^2. The rate at which energy is delivered is called *power,* measured in watts (W). By definition, one watt is one joule per second (W = J/sec). The power delivered per unit area is therefore the rate of energy delivery per amount of skin surface, called the *irradiance,* usually given in W/cm^2. Laser exposure duration, called *pulse width* for pulsed lasers, is extremely important because this sets the time over which energy is delivered. Dermatology uses laser exposures ranging from seconds to nanoseconds. The fluence delivered is equal to the irradiance times the exposure duration. Other important factors are the laser exposure spot size, which greatly affects intensity inside the skin; whether the incident light is convergent, divergent, or diffuse; and the uniformity of irradiance over the exposure area.

Photochemistry

Visible and UV light occupy the portion of the EMR spectrum for which photon energy corresponds to the transitions of electrons between orbitals in many different molecules. Thus UV and visible light can promote specific chemical reactions by activation of electrons that account for chemical bonding. Phenomena such as life on Earth, most skin cancer, vitamin D production, and vision are impossible without photochemistry. Dermatology traditionally used photochemistry: UV phototherapy, the use of photosensitizers such as psoralens, and photodermatoses such as porphyria are classic examples.

Recently, long-wavelength (red and near-IR) photosensitizers activated by deeply penetrating laser light have been developed for photodynamic therapy of tumors.[1] These potent new drugs and prodrugs hold great potential for treatment of skin diseases.[2] Although lasers have been used lately as sources for photodynamic therapy, they apparently are not essential, especially for dermatologic uses. The emphasis is on drugs, with different tissue localization, routes of administration, and photochemical mechanisms. Photodynamic therapy drugs being tested include porphyrin derivatives, porphyrin precursors (aminolevulinic acid [ALA]), phthalocyanines, and chlorines, all of which are oxygen-dependent photosensitizers and most of which are lipophilic. Their primary mechanism of action is by energy transfer to molecular oxygen, which produces singlet oxygen, a potent oxidizer. These drugs probably will have broader use in dermatology than initially anticipated. Intravenous porphyrin derivatives produce a necrotizing photosensitivity of blood vessels and are being tested for treatment of port-wine stains.[3] ALA is effective for treating actinic keratoses.[4] Other potential dermatologic applications include psoriasis, condyloma, and mycosis fungoides.

Heat

By far, the majority of laser applications in dermatology use laser-induced heating. In contrast to photochemistry, heating does not require any particular photon energy. Therefore absorption of any wavelength of EMR can and does cause heating.

Temperature is directly related to the average kinetic excitation of molecules, that is, amount of movement, vibration, rotation, and other molecular motion. As temperature is raised, the large, specially configured molecules necessary for life are shaken open. Most proteins, deoxyribonucleic acid (DNA), ribonucleic acid (RNA), membranes, and their integral structures begin to unwind or melt at temperatures of 40° to 100° C. Because molecular configuration is necessary for biologic activity, the result is *denaturation,* meaning loss of function. At the high concentrations of macromolecules present in tissue, the unfolded molecules also become entangled with each other, and the tissue becomes coagulated. A familiar example of denaturation and coagulation is the cooking of an egg white. Thermal denaturation is temperature and time dependent, yet it has a thresholdlike behavior. For a given heating time there is usually a narrow temperature region above which wholesale denaturation occurs. For denaturation of most proteins, one must increase the temperature by about 10° C for every decade of decrease in the heating time to achieve the same amount of thermal coagulation.

In laser-tissue interactions, thermal coagulation causes cell necrosis, hemostasis, welding, and gross alteration of the extracellular matrix at specific temperature–heating time combinations. Thermal coagulation is also a burn, and it is well worth remembering that laser surgery consists mainly of controlling where and how much heat injury occurs. The relatively low-power continuous lasers such as carbon dioxide (CO_2) and argon-ion, and the quasi-continuous (rapid-pulsed) lasers, such as copper vapor and potassium titanyl phosphate (KTP), usually cause a well-controlled superficial partial-thickness burn. In contrast, pulsed yellow dye lasers designed for selective photothermolysis of microvascular lesions cause selective burns of microvessels.

Selective photothermolysis uses selective absorption of light pulses by pigmented targets such as blood vessels, pigmented cells, and tattoo ink particles to achieve selective thermally mediated injury.[5] Short pulses are necessary to deposit energy in the targets before they can cool off, thus achieving extreme, localized heating. Thermal coagulation and thermally mediated mechanical damage are involved, depending on the rate of energy deposition in the targets. In the past 15 years, selective photothermolysis has largely transformed dermatologic laser surgery and is discussed in detail throughout this text.

Mechanical injury, sometimes misnamed photoacoustic injury, occurs from rapid heating by high-energy, short-pulse lasers. The rate of local heating can be so severe that structures are torn apart by shock waves (highly destructive, supersonic pressure waves), cavitation (sudden expansion and collapse of a steam bubble), or rapid thermal expansion. Mechanical damage has an important role in selective photothermolysis with high-energy, submicrosecond lasers for tattoo and pigmented lesion removal.

Before discussion of laser-tissue interactions in more detail, the optics of human skin is reviewed because it determines the penetration, absorption, and internal dosimetry of laser light in skin.

SKIN OPTICS

Two fundamental processes govern all interactions of light with matter: absorption and scattering. When *absorption* occurs, the photon surrenders its energy to an atom or molecule, known as a *chromophore*. On absorption the photon ceases to exist, and the chromophore becomes excited; it may undergo photochemistry or may dissipate the energy as heat or reemission of light (e.g., fluorescence). The probability that absorption will occur depends on specific transitions between allowed electron orbitals or molecular vibration modes. Thus chromophore molecules exhibit characteristic bands of absorption around certain wavelengths.

The absorption spectra of major skin chromophores dominate most laser-tissue interactions in dermatology. The *absorption coefficient* is the probability per unit path length that a photon at a particular wavelength will be absorbed. It is therefore measured in units of 1/distance and is typically designated μa, given as cm^{-1}. The absorption coefficient depends on the concentration of chromophores present. Skin is replete with interesting pigments and distinct microscopic structures that have different absorption spectra.[6,7] This heterogeneity is what allows selective photothermolysis to work. Figure 1-1 shows the absorption coefficients for major skin

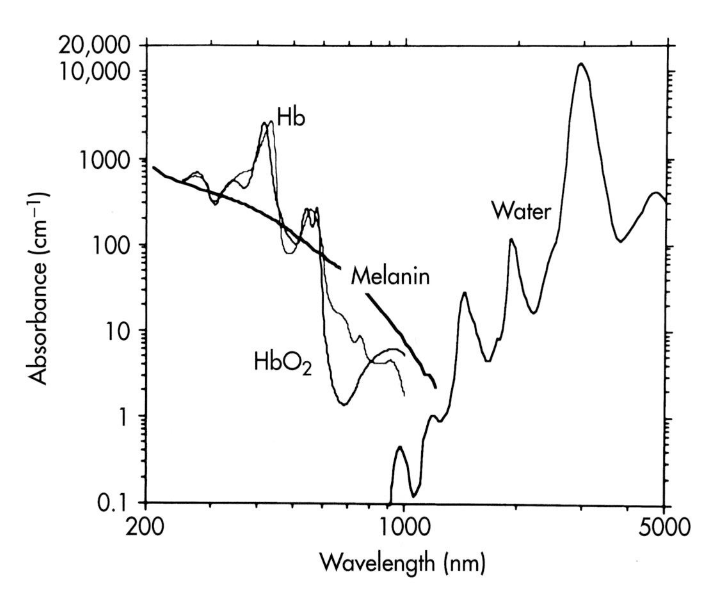

Figure 1-1 Absorption spectra of major skin pigments at concentrations for which they typically occur. Values shown are absorption coefficients (μa) for pure water, human hemoglobins at 11 g/dl, and dihydroxyphenylalanine (DOPA)-melanin, which has an absorption spectrum very similar to pigmented epidermis, at 15-mg/dl concentration in water. DOPA-melanin concentration shown is approximately equivalent to heavily pigmented human epidermis. Absorption coefficient of single melanosomes is unknown. *Hb*, Hemoglobin; *HbO_2*, oxyhemoglobin. (Courtesy S. Prahl; from Anderson RR: Optics of the skin. In HW Lim, NA Soter, editors: *Clinical photomedicine*, New York, 1993, Marcel Dekker.)

chromophores at typical concentrations as they appear in skin structures. Ironically, the curve for melanin is least well known, although melanin is probably the only major skin chromophore that functions mainly as a pigment.

Note that melanin, which occurs normally only in epidermis and hair follicles, absorbs broadly across the optical spectrum. In contrast, blood absorption is dominated by absorption of oxyhemoglobin and reduced hemoglobin, which exhibits strong bands in the UV, blue, green, and yellow bands. The 577-nm (yellow) absorption band of oxyhemoglobin was chosen for targeting superficial microvessels by selective photothermolysis,[8] but this is certainly not the only band possible for this application.[9] Despite high absorption by blood in the blue band (420 nm), limited penetration and interference by melanin absorption make this region less desirable. However, it is theoretically possible that near-IR pulses within the broad oxyhemoglobin band beyond 900 nm would work well and provide much greater depth of penetration.

Scattering occurs when the photon changes its direction of propagation. A small momentum is imparted by scattering, but the photon continues along its way in a different direction. All light returning from skin is scattered light. As light strikes the skin surface, about 5% is reflected because of the sudden change in refractive index between air (n = 1.0) and stratum corneum (n = 1.55) (regular reflectance). Once inside skin, the remaining 95% of the light can be either absorbed or scattered by molecules, particles, and structures in the tissue. Scattering by large particles is rather wavelength independent, such as the white and gray seen in clouds. For particles smaller than the wavelength of light (i.e., below a few hundred nanometers in size), scattering is much stronger for shorter wavelengths. For example, the sky is blue because molecular scattering is stronger at shorter wavelengths.

In the normal epidermis, absorption is the dominant process over most of the optical spectrum. In the UV wavelengths below 300 nm, strong absorption by proteins, melanin, urocanic acid, and DNA occurs. For wavelengths of 320 to 1200 nm, absorption by melanin dominates epidermal optical properties, depending on skin type. The transmission of white epidermis increases steadily from about 50% at 400 nm (blue) to 90% at 1200 nm, with only a minor decrease at the 950-nm water absorption band. In contrast, dark black epidermis transmits less than 20% throughout the visible spectrum but rises to 90% by 1200 nm.[10] Melanin in the epidermis (as in café-au-lait macules and lentigines) and the dermis (as in nevus of Ota) is an important target chromophore for laser selective photothermolysis. In the IR region beyond 1200 nm, no skin types exist, and epidermal transmission depends on thickness and water content but not pigmentation.

In the dermis, strong wavelength-dependent scattering by collagen fibers occurs. Optical penetration into dermis is largely dominated by this scattering, which varies inversely with wavelength (Table 1-1). The absorption coefficient of dermis other than its blood vessels is very low throughout the visible and near-IR spectrum. Dermal μa is less than about 1 cm^{-1} in the visible region and falls to less than 0.1 cm^{-1} in the near-IR region between water absorption bands. In contrast, blood has extremely strong absorption in the blue, green, and yellow wavelengths of the visible spectrum and a weak but significant absorption band in the 800- to 1000-nm region (see Figure 1-1).

Optical penetration into skin is governed by a combination of absorption and scattering. From the UV through the near-IR spectrum, both tend to be stronger at shorter wavelengths. However, the absorption bands of hemoglobin are such that 532-nm radiation penetrates dermis deeper than 577-nm radiation. In general, however, a gradual increase occurs in the depth of penetration into skin at longer wavelengths over a very broad spectrum. The most penetrating wavelengths are in the 650 to 1200 nm, red and near-IR region, for which photodynamic therapy drugs are being developed for cancer treatment. The least penetrating wavelengths are in

Table 1-1
Approximate optical penetration in normal fair white skin*

Wavelength (nm)	Laser	Depth at 50% Penetration (μm)	Skin Chromophores
193	Excimer	0.5	Protein
355	Tripled Nd	80	Melanin
488	Argon ion	200	Melanin, blood
514	Argon ion, dye	300	Melanin, blood
532	Doubled Nd	400	Melanin, blood
577	Pulsed dye	400	Blood, melanin
585	Pulsed dye	600	Blood, melanin
694	Ruby	1200	Melanin
760	Alexandrite	1300	Melanin
1060	Nd:YAG	1600	Melanin, blood
2100	Holmium	200	Water
2940	Erbium	1	Water
10,600	CO_2	20	Water

Nd, Neodymium; *YAG,* yttrium-aluminum-garnet.
*Compiled from in vivo and in vitro data for a wide incident beam. When the beam radius is less than or approximately equal to the penetration depth listed in the table, intensity within the skin decreases much more rapidly with depth, because of beam broadening from optical scattering to the sides. Normal skin is rarely treated and optical penetration is frequently less in vascular or pigmented skin lesions.

the far-UV (protein absorption) and far-IR (water absorption) regions. For example, the 193-nm excimer laser radiation penetrates only a fraction of a micrometer into the stratum corneum. The surgically popular CO_2 laser at 10.6 μm wavelength (10,600 nm) penetrates only about 20 μm into water and is therefore excellent for vaporization and cutting. Table 1-1 gives approximate optical penetration depths in white (fair) skin for many laser wavelengths of current interest in dermatology, along with the dominant skin chromophores at each laser wavelength.

The exposure spot size also affects the loss of intensity with depth into skin (see Table 1-1 footnote) in a wavelength-dependent manner. For example, one would expect spot sizes (diameters) of about 3 mm or less to suffer significant loss at 1064 nm. In essence, spot size affects optical penetration when the exposure spot radius is equal to or less than the distance for which light is free to diffuse within the tissue. However, another factor is the forward-directed nature of scattering in dermis, which is also wavelength dependent. Accurate, direct measurements of fluence or irradiance profiles inside skin are essentially lacking for any spot size.

THERMAL INTERACTIONS

Thermal Injury to Cells

Most human cells can withstand prolonged exposure to 40° C. At 45° C, cultured human fibroblasts die after about 20 minutes. However, the same cells can withstand more than 100° C if present for only 10^{-3} seconds.[11] Thus it is not temperature per se but a combination of temperature and time that governs coagulative thermal damage. This is because thermal denaturation is a rate process: heat increases the rate at which molecules denature, depending on the specific molecule. For most cells the critical temperature for necrosis increases by approximately 10° to 20° C for each decade of decrease in the heating time. This behavior is important for cell injury in the setting of selective photothermolysis, during which extreme temperatures are present in target sites of the skin for very short duration.

Some biomolecules are heat stable. Interestingly, very little is known about the primary sites or macromolecules involved in thermal killing of mammalian cells over any range of temperatures and times. Nature provides an intriguing example of maximal thermal adaptation in that some thermophilic bacteria can survive and reproduce at 80° to 90° C. These organisms possess specialized proteins, and some have unique monolayer cell membrane structures. It is known that thermal cell killing involves irreversible denaturation. All cells have mechanisms for removing denatured proteins, provided the cell is still viable. The induction of *heat shock proteins* (HSPs) is a ubiquitous phenomenon in diploid cells, which confers resistance to further thermal injury.[12] The mechanism for induced thermotolerance remains obscure and may be a combination of many effects of the family of HSPs. HSPs are induced by laser exposures, and heat shock response has been shown to protect human fibroblasts to a modest degree against CO_2 laser–induced thermal injury.[11]

Thermal denaturation and coagulation

About 50 years ago, Henriques[13] determined the time-temperature behavior for coagulation necrosis of animal epidermis, which was described by an Arrhenius integral model. This appears to hold well for laser-induced thermal injury in skin and retinal coagulation.[14] The *Arrhenius model* states that the rate of denaturation is exponentially related to temperature. Therefore the accumulation of denaturated material rises exponentially with temperature and proportionally to time. As a consequence, thermal coagulation of tissue has a sharp, thresholdlike character. As a critical temperature is reached, coagulation occurs. This accounts for the well-defined histologic boundaries of dermal coagulation in laser and other burn injuries.

In contrast to the epidermis, connective tissue such as the dermis contains a large amount of extracellular matrix dominated by structural proteins such as collagen and elastin. *Elastin* is incredibly thermally stable, surviving boiling for hours with no apparent change. However, *type I collagen,* which is the major type in dermis, has a sharp melting transition for the fibrillar form between 60° and 70° C. This transition appears to present an absolute limitation for the bulk dermal temperature, beyond which scarring is highly likely. If the entire collagen-based scaffolding of the dermis is destroyed, it is likely that nothing short of complete tissue remodeling will allow healing. In contrast to diffuse coagulation injury, selective photothermolysis can achieve high temperatures at structures or individual cells with little risk of scarring because gross dermal heating is minimized.

Vaporization, tissue ablation, and charring

The vaporization (boiling) temperature of water at 1 atmosphere pressure is 100° C. However, lasers or electrosurgical tools usually vaporize tissue above this temperature because (1) higher pressures are present, especially with pulsed lasers and almost all electrodesiccators; (2) superheating of water occurs before it is vaporized; and (3) with continuous-wave (CW) lasers the surface layer becomes desiccated and charred (carbonized), reaching temperatures of at least several hundred degrees Celsius.

High-energy pulsed versus CW lasers can differ greatly in their tissue ablation and residual thermal damage. For example, CO_2 lasers are available in continuous and so-called superpulsed modes. When they are used in typical CW mode at modest powers for vaporization, the skin surface temperature fluctuates in cycles between about 120° and 200° C during ablation, and charring occurs. Thermal coagulation injury occurs to a depth of about 1 mm because of heat conduction, despite the 20 μm shallow penetration depth of CO_2 laser radiation. The charring occurs because of extreme heating of desiccated tissue, which carbonizes. Thus the tissue bed remaining after CW CO_2 laser vaporization is typically coagulated to a depth of about 1 mm, desiccated, and charred. In contrast, appropriately short (less than 10^{-3} second), energetic (greater than 5 J/cm^2) pulses of CO_2 laser radiation remove tissue with greater efficiency, less thermal damage (about 50-100 μm residual denaturation), and no charring[15] (see Chapter 6).

These two basically different modes of tissue ablation are easily demonstrated by comparing CW with pulsed modes of operation, but they are not unique to either. Indeed, a tightly focused CW CO_2 or other laser being scanned rapidly enough along the tissue can produce the intense, short–exposure time conditions needed for pulsed laser ablation effects. Conversely, a short-pulse CO_2 laser, when operated at a subablative pulse fluence (e.g., less than about 1 J/cm^2 per pulse) at repetition rates less than about 100 Hz, will produce the deeper injury and charring associated with CW effects. Despite the convenience of labeling pulsed versus CW laser vaporization, a more precise understanding is clearly necessary. The following discussion attempts to provide this.

Tissue is removed with minimal thermal injury and no charring when the entire energy needed for vaporization (about 2500 J/cm^3) *is delivered into the most superficial layer possible* (i.e., the layer about equal to the optical penetration depth) *during a time equal to or less than the thermal relaxation time for this superficial heated layer.* Thus the thinnest layer possible (for a given wavelength) is endowed with all the energy it needs to vaporize before much heat transfer to the underlying tissue can occur. Under these conditions the layer suddenly vaporizes away, leaving a residual thermally injured layer about two to four times the optical penetration depth. Because the laser energy is turned off before desiccation occurs, there is no charring. In contrast, if energy is delivered for a much longer time, thermal conduction increases the depth of injury, decreases ablation efficiency, and allows desiccation during the laser exposure, and charring may occur.

These principles can be illustrated in the important practical example of the CO_2 laser just given. The *laser energy* deposited per unit volume is equal to:

(EQ. 1)

$$Ev = E\mu a$$

where E is the local fluence (J/cm^2), and μa is the absorption coefficient defined earlier (cm^{-1}). Setting Ev = 2500 J/cm^{-1}, about the heat of vaporization for water, closely approximates the requirement for removal of tissue. Solving for E, the applied fluence needs to be at least $E = 2500/\mu a$, in units of J/cm^2. The value of μa at the well-absorbed CO_2 laser wavelength of 10,600 nm is about 500 cm^{-1}, which gives E = 5 J/cm^2 as the necessary pulse fluence to achieve pulsed laser ablation of skin tissue.

The next issue is, how quickly does this 5 J/cm^2 have to be delivered to limit thermal injury? The answer: before the superficially heated layer has time to cool. The penetration depth of CO_2 laser radiation (see Table 1-1) is about d = 20 μm. Note that this penetration depth is equal to $1/\mu a$ because absorption dominates the CO_2 laser wavelength's penetration into tissue. The *thermal relaxation time* (time for significant cooling) for a layer of thickness d is about:

(EQ. 2)

$$tr = d^2(4k)$$

where k is thermal diffusivity (1.3×10^{-3} cm^2). Thus the thermal relaxation time for our pulsed CO_2 laser–heated, 20 μm superficial layer is about $tr = (2 \times 10^{-3}\ cm^2)/(4 \times 1.3 \times 10^{-3}\ cm^2/sec) = 0.8 \times 10^{-3}$ sec. In effect, for the CO_2 laser wavelength, one must deliver the necessary 5 J/cm^2 in, at most, 0.8 msec, preferably less, if one expects to minimize injury to the underlying tissue. When this is done, one can expect each exposure pulse to remove about one optical penetration depth (20 μm) of tissue and to leave two to four times the optical penetration depth (i.e., about 40-80 μm) of residual thermally damaged tissue. This layer of thermally damaged tissue is responsible for hemostasis, or the lack thereof, and also for effects on wound healing.[16]

It is easy to see from this information that the fluence needed for ablation and the depth of residual injury depend on the penetration depth ($1/\mu a$). This holds true for other IR lasers and governs the development and also the utility of new IR lasers in medicine. The holmium laser output near 2000 nm, with $\mu a = 50$ cm^{-1} and penetration depth of about 200 μm, requires a fluence of about 50 J/cm^2 (10 times that of the CO_2 laser, because μa is 10 times less), removes about 200 μm per pulse, and leaves behind about 400 to 800 μm of thermally coagulated tissue when delivered in less than about 80 msec. The holmium laser is being developed mainly because it is fiberoptic compatible for endoscopic applications and produces excellent hemostasis. For tasks requiring extremely high-precision, low-injury ablation, however, the holmium laser is generally a poor choice.

In the other direction, the IR erbium laser, operating at 2940 nm, is very strongly absorbed by water and is capable of high-precision, superficial ablation. With μa of about 10,000 cm^{-1} in skin, a mere 0.25 J/cm^2 is therefore required for tissue removal (1/20 that of the CO_2 laser), but it must be delivered in a few microseconds or less to achieve removal of just 1 μm of tissue per pulse, leaving the minuscule residual injury depth of only 2 to 4 μm. Short-pulse erbium lasers are therefore capable of ablating only one or two cell layers at a time, with very minimal residual injury. This is excellent for extremely fine ablation but a poor choice when hemostasis is needed. However, if one operates the erbium laser with longer pulses, hemostasis can be achieved (and thermal injury increased intentionally) by allowing more thermal conduction to occur.

Excimer laser pulses at 193 nm have been shown to remove tissue by a combination of thermal and photochemical ablation.[17] At 193 nm, μa is about 12,000 cm^{-1} in skin, similar to the erbium laser wavelength. However, the photon energy is sufficient to break chemical bonds in polymers, such that tissue is removed by heat vaporization of tissue water and also by volatilization of large macromolecules. To date there have been no dermatologic uses of excimer laser ablation other than experimental removal of stratum corneum.[18] However, precise excimer laser ablation of the cornea is a promising method being developed for correction of visual refraction.[19] Excimer laser ablation of skin of 193 nm produces shock waves that cause cell disruption and injury well into the epidermis and upper dermis.[20]

Selective Photothermolysis

This approach changed the scope of lasers in dermatology over the 15 years since its formulation. The term *selective photothermolysis* was coined to describe site-specific, thermally mediated injury of microscopic, pigmented tissue targets by selectively absorbed pulses of radiation.[5] It is by far the most precise use of heat in all of medicine.

Light deposits energy only at sites of absorption. At wavelengths that penetrate into skin and are preferentially absorbed by chromophoric structures such as blood vessels or melanin-containing cells, heat is created in these targets. As soon as heat is created, however, it begins to dissipate by conduction and radiative transfer. Thus a competition between active heating and passive cooling determines how hot the targets become. The most selective target heating is achieved when the energy is deposited at a rate faster than the rate for cooling of the target structures.

Three basic elements are necessary to achieve selective photothermolysis: (1) a wavelength that reaches and is preferentially absorbed by the desired target structures; (2) an exposure duration less than or equal to the time necessary for cooling of the target structures; and (3) sufficient fluence to reach a damaging temperature in the targets. When these criteria are met, exquisitely selective injury occurs in thousands of microscopic targets, without the need to aim the laser at each one. The effect is equivalent to the legendary "magic bullets," which seek only the desired target. A variety of thermally mediated damage mechanisms are possible in selective photothermolysis, including thermal denaturation, mechanical damage from rapid thermal expansion or phase changes *(cavitation)*, and changes in primary chemical structure *(pyrolysis)*.

Exposure duration and thermal relaxation

A sometimes difficult concept underlying selective photothermolysis is the relationship between exposure duration and confinement of heat and thus extent of thermal injury. A useful construct is the so-called thermal relaxation time alluded to in equation 2, that is, the time required for significant cooling of a small target structure. When the laser exposure is less than the thermal relaxation time, maximal thermal confinement will occur. Many processes are involved in cooling, including convection, radiation, and conduction. Of these, thermal conduction dominates the cooling of microscopic structures in skin. However, microscale radiational cooling in tissue has never been thoroughly examined and in theory may be important for very small targets at high temperatures, such as tattoo ink particles or melanin granules.

It is common experience that smaller objects cool more quickly than larger objects. For example, a cup of tea cools faster than a hot bath, even though both are hot water in a porcelain container. More precisely, the thermal relaxation time for heat conduction is proportional to the square of size (see equation 2). For any given material and shape, an object half the size will cool in one fourth the time, and an object one tenth the size will cool in one hundredth the time. This behavior is important in optimizing pulse duration or exposure duration for selective photothermolysis of blood vessels. Blood vessels vary from capillaries, which have thermal relaxation times of tens of microseconds, to venules and arterioles, which have thermal relaxation times of hundreds of microseconds, to the larger venules of adult port-wine stains (PWSs), which have thermal relaxation times up to tens of milliseconds. Therefore, in a typical PWS, vessels are present with thermal relaxation times ranging over three orders of magnitude, and it is ludicrous to define a single thermal relaxation time for vessels.

Target size selectivity is also possible in selective photothermolysis by picking the pulse or exposure duration appropriately. In PWSs the large ectatic vessels are the targets, and it is their thermal relaxation time that should not be exceeded (e.g., up to about 5 msec). When the pulse duration exceeds a target's thermal relaxation time, heating of the target becomes inefficient. Therefore selectivity for larger-vessel damage is possible by choosing laser exposures that exceed thermal relaxation times of capillaries yet are less than thermal relaxation times for the target PWS vessels. Capillaries are relatively spared by pulses of at least several hundred microseconds because they cool significantly during the laser energy delivery. This concept has not yet been explored or exploited in laser dermatology (see Chapter 2).

Thermal relaxation time is also related to shape, reflecting differences in volume and surface area of the targets. For a given thickness, spheres cool faster than cylinders, which cool faster than planes. All three are relevant to dermatology: melanosomes are elliptic, vessels are cylindric, and tissue layers are planar. A material property called the *thermal diffusivity (k)* expresses the ability of heat to diffuse and is equal to the square root of the ratio between heat conductivity and specific heat capacity. Thermal properties for soft tissues other than fat are dominated by the high water content. The value of $k = 1.3 \times 10^{-3}$ cm^2/sec for water is approximately equal to that of most soft tissues, as used in the earlier examples describing pulsed laser tissue vaporization. However, thermal diffusivity of native melanosomes is unknown.

For most tissue targets a simple rule of thumb can be used: *the thermal relaxation time in seconds is about equal to the square of the target dimension in millimeters.* Thus a 0.5-μm melanosome (5×10^{-4} mm) should cool in about 25×10^{-8} sec, or 250 nsec, whereas a 0.1-mm PWS vessel should cool in about 10^{-2} sec, or 10 msec. The natural variation of target sizes in tissue leads to an even greater variation in thermal relaxation times, such that much more precise calculations, although certainly possible, are probably unnecessary.

Microvascular interactions

Many details of laser-tissue interaction during selective photothermolysis in dermatology are poorly understood, but a good conceptual basis exists for understanding the observations to date. The best studied example is that of visible laser pulse effects on microvessels, done to develop the present pulsed yellow dye lasers used for treating PWSs in children. Indeed, the histology of pediatric PWSs was used to define the task of this laser,[8,21] for which it works very well. The same laser can be used for adult PWSs, telangiectasias, and other microvascular lesions, but different laser parameters may be better for some of these lesions, as discussed next.

In general, ideal laser parameters are not the only ones that can be used effectively. An experienced laser surgeon can often achieve good results with a less-than-ideal tool, and poor results are certainly possible even with an ideal laser. Selective photothermolysis with a long-pulse (300-500 μsec) flashlamp-pumped tunable dye laser near 585 nm is now a strongly preferred method for treating PWSs because of a very low risk of scarring when used in single pulses at 6 to 8 J/cm^2 fluence.[22] The present generation of these lasers is still far from ideal, however, both in interactions with skin vessels and in their clinical use. This chapter does not present clinical data but summarizes what is known about the laser-tissue interactions involved (see Chapter 2).

In the first theoretic formulation of selective photothermolysis,[8] a 1-msec, 577-nm pulse of at least 2 J/cm^2, was predicted on theoretic grounds to be ideal. Initially, however, such long pulses were not available at this wavelength. A 1 μsec pulsed dye laser (1/1000 the ideal pulse duration) was tested at 577 nm in normal human and animal skin, which was noted to cause histologically selective injury to dermal vessels with extensive hemorrhage.[23,24] The temperature dependence and fluences needed for this damage, seen grossly as purpura, were consistent with mechanical rupture of vessels from vaporization of blood.[25] In an attempt to minimize vaporization injury and maximize thermal coagulation of vessels, the pulse duration was lengthened. As pulse duration increased beyond 20 μsec, hemorrhage was significantly less in normal human skin, and the fluence required for vascular damage increased in accordance with theory.[26]

Therefore a 400-μsec, 577-nm pulsed dye laser was constructed, tested clinically on PWSs, and noted to work well[27] with a low risk of scarring, even in children.[28] A longer wavelength, approximately twice as penetrating, was shown to offer similar vascular selectivity but greater depth of effect,[29] and 585 nm was subsequently used clinically.[30] The present standard is a 585-nm, 400-μsec pulsed dye laser delivered at 6 to 8 J/cm^2 fluence in single nonoverlapping pulses, in 5-mm-diameter exposure spots. Histologically this long-pulse yellow dye laser produces selective intravascular and perivascular coagulation necrosis, with epidermal injury to the basal cell layer in darker skin types.[31] Hypopigmentation is a frequent and usually transient side effect, as is postinflammatory hyperpigmentation.[32] This laser produces transiently disfiguring purpura from hemorrhage and a delayed vasculitis, presumably because of its still shorter-than-ideal pulse duration. In addition, for unknown reasons, six or more treatments are usually needed to remove PWSs.

An "ideal" set of laser pulse parameters for PWS treatment has never been tested. The present pulsed dye lasers fail to extend beyond 1 msec. The best pulse duration for PWSs in children is probably in the region of 1 to 5 msec and may be longer for adult PWSs, which in general contain larger vessels.

With regard to wavelength, the apparent improvement in optical penetration depth between 577 and 585 nm could almost certainly be improved further by using even longer wavelengths. Although the study leading to the choice of 585 nm[29] was well performed, it was intrinsically flawed. Fixed fluences at various wavelengths were compared with regard to histologic depth of injury in dermal vessels in an animal model. However, as the absorption coefficient of blood decreases with increasing wavelength beyond 577 nm, greater local fluence is required to achieve the same thermal excitation at any given vessel site. By comparing a limited and fixed fluence range, the ability to damage vessels selectively seemed simply to disappear at longer wavelengths. The inappropriate conclusion was therefore reached that longer wavelengths were ineffective for causing highly selective microvascular injury.

With higher incident fluences, selective microvascular injury can be obtained well into the penetrating red visible wavelengths of 600 nm and beyond; the action spectrum for purpura in white skin tracks the absorption spectrum of venous blood well out to at least 630 nm.[33] Vascular-selective injury is not lost until the absorption coefficient of blood approaches that of the surrounding dermis. The absorption coefficient of bloodless dermis is only 0.1 to 0.3 cm^{-1} throughout the red wavelength region, which is not approached by blood absorption until 700 nm (Figure 1-1). The most fundamental limitation of using red laser pulses for PWS treatment is therefore absorption by epidermal melanin. Indeed, the 694-nm Q-switched ruby laser is highly selective for damage to melanized cells alone.[34] Despite this, long-pulse, higher fluence, red (e.g., 590-610 nm) laser pulses appear to work well for treating PWSs or telangiectasias. At the longer pulse durations appropriate to PWS treatment, pigment cell injury is minimized.[35] Epidermal injury tends to heal well without scarring and is already produced by 585-nm pulses. In a small comparative clinical trial, 600-nm pulsed dye laser pulses were reported to work better than 585-nm pulses for treating adult PWSs.[36]

Another significant issue is the number of pulses delivered to a single skin site. With each laser pulse the pigmented target sites experience a thermal cycle of heating and cooling. When hemorrhage is caused by the first laser pulse for treatment of microvessels, subsequent laser pulses can cause widespread dermal injury simply because the target chromophore is no longer confined to blood vessels. However, the Arrhenius model suggests that thermal injury is cumulative over time; therefore, in theory, multiple lower fluence pulses that do not cause hemorrhage might be used to accumulate selective, gentler, and more complete damage to microvessels. This is clearly the case and offers a wholly new approach to delivering selective photothermolysis.

Trocolli and colleagues[37] reported a study of microvessel injury by multiple, 585-nm, 160-μsec dye laser pulses delivered at 0.5 Hz. For 50-μm-diameter hamster cheek pouch venules, the threshold fluence for hemorrhage was 6 J/cm^2, at which only half the vessels were closed (thrombosed). In contrast, using 10 to 100 pulses at fluences of 2 to 4 J/cm^2, vessel closure was achieved consistently without hemorrhage. This study suggests that one reason PWSs require so many treatments is that the probability for irreversible vessel damage is far less than unity for single-pulse exposures within the tolerated fluence range. PWSs should respond more rapidly to multiple, lower fluence pulses delivered at an average irradiance (pulse fluence times repetition rate) that does not cause gross thermal injury.

Pigmented lesion removal

Melanin is normally present only in the epidermis and hair follicles, which are impressively capable of regeneration. Therefore almost any laser with sufficient power can be used skillfully to remove benign pigmented lesions of the epidermis, including CO_2 lasers, which heat the skin nonselectively through absorption by water.[38] Indeed, almost every dermatologic laser on the market has been shown to remove lentigines effectively, without scarring. However, a more precise interaction occurs with selective photothermolysis. The selective rupture of skin melanosomes was first noted by electron microscopy in 1983, after 351 nm, submicrosecond excimer laser pulses of only about 0.1 J/cm^2.[5] At fluences damaging melanocytes and pigmented keratinocytes, epidermal Langerhans cells apparently escape injury[39] (see Chapter 3).

Melanosomes are the fundamental site for melanin synthesis and occur as 0.5 to 1 μm oblong organelles. In melanocytes they exist in various stages of pigmentation and are bound to cytoskeletal proteins in the cytoplasm. On transfer to keratinocytes, melanosomes appear in membrane-limited phagosomes. In white skin the melanosomes are smaller and are packaged in groups within keratinocyte phagosomes.[40] As discussed earlier, the thermal relaxation time of melanosomes is unknown but probably lies in the region of 250 to 1000 nsec, depending on size. With regard to wavelength, absorption by melanin extends from the deep UV through visible and well into the near IR (see Fig. 1-1). Across this broad spectrum, optical penetration into skin increases from several micrometers to several millimeters. One would therefore expect melanosomes and the pigmented cells containing them to be affected at different depths across this broad spectrum.

Melanosome rupture behaves in a manner remarkably consistent with the basic theory of selective photothermolysis. The calculated thermal relaxation time for melanosomes is approximately 250 to 1000 nsec. The rupture of melanosomes is independent of pulse duration below 100 nsec, including even psec (10^{-12} second) and even fsec domain (10^{-15} second) pulses[35] (Fig. 1-2). This suggests that optical absorption by melanin is not saturable; that is, even terawatt/cm^2 intensities are absorbed the same as lower intensity pulses, which is highly unusual for organic chromophores. The wavelength dependence for melanosome rupture in guinea pig epidermis is also quantitatively consistent with the absorption spectrum of melanin.[41-44] For 10- to 40-nsec pulses the threshold fluence for rupture of melanosomes in guinea pig epidermis is 0.11, 0.20, 0.30, and 1.0 J/cm^2 for 355, 532, 694, and 1064 nm, respectively. At longer wavelengths, leukotrichia was observed after hair regrowth in pigmented guinea pigs following Q-switched laser pulses, which is consistent with the increased penetration depth of red and near-IR radiation compared with green or UVA laser pulses,[41] and melanocytes are permanently absent from depigmented hair follicles after Q-switched ruby laser irradiation of guinea pig skin.[42] However, leukotrichia has not been reported in

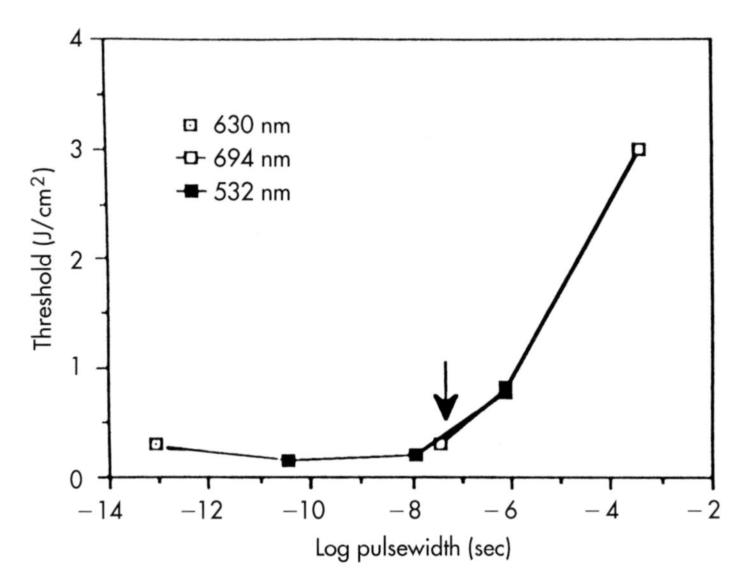

Figure 1-2 Pulse-duration dependence for intracellular rupture of melanosomes in guinea pig skin. (From Watanabe S, Anderson RR, Brorson S et al: *Photochem Photobiol* 53:757, 1991.)

human skin despite thousands of high-fluence treatments with this laser system to remove tattoos (see Chapter 4).

The rupture of melanosomes is a submicroscopic, largely mechanical form of damage. Local pressure waves and deformations beyond the elastic limits probably account for pigmented cell killing.[43] At sublethal fluences, pulses appear to cause stimulation of melanogenesis by unknown mechanisms. Shorter wavelength pulses well below the threshold for melanosome rupture appear to cause melanocyte stimulation, histologically apparent days after exposure in guinea pigs.[44]

Grossly, the immediate effect of submicrosecond near-UV, visible, or near-IR laser pulses in pigmented skin is immediate whitening. This response correlates very well with melanosome rupture seen by electron microscopy[35] and is therefore presumably a direct consequence of melanosome rupture. A nearly identical but deeper whitening occurs with Q-switched laser exposure of tattoos, which, as with melanosomes, consist of insoluble, submicrometer, intracellular pigmented granules. Although the exact cause of immediate whitening is unknown, it is almost certainly related to the formation of gas bubbles that intensely scatter light. Over several to tens of minutes, these bubbles dissolve, causing the skin color to return to normal or nearly normal. A common misconception is that these bubbles are steam. Although vaporization of water to form steam may create transient vapor cavities, these must collapse to zero volume within microseconds if they truly contain only steam (water vapor). The residual gas bubbles must therefore contain some other gas. Several possibilities exist. A process called *rectified diffusion* may occur, in which dissolved nitrogen diffuses into the transient steam vapor cavity, leaving a small residual bubble on collapse of the cavity. This process accounts for the ability of high-intensity ultrasound to remove dissolved gases from liquids. Alternatively or in addition, pyrolysis may occur at the extreme temperatures reached within melanosomes or tattoo ink particles, directly releasing gases locally. Regardless of its cause, immediate whitening offers a clinically useful immediate endpoint that apparently relates directly to melanosome or tattoo ink rupture.

Trains of low-fluence, submicrosecond laser pulses may cause even more exquisitely selective injury to pigmented cells by limiting mechanical damage modes. In a recent study, retinal pigment epithelial cells (a specialized neuroocular melanocyte) were targeted in vivo without damage to the delicate, immediately adjacent Bruch membrane using multiple, microsecond pulse trains from a modulated argon ion laser.[45] The use of pulse trains specifically designed to affect pigmented cells selectively in skin has not yet been tested.

Clinically, selective photothermolysis has not been effective for dermal melasma, postinflammatory hyperpigmentation, or drug-induced hyperpigmentation.[46] However, it is highly useful for epidermal and dermal lesions in which cellular pigmentation itself is the cause. These include lentigines, café-au-lait macules (which exhibit a high rate of recurrence), nevi spilus, Becker nevi, blue nevi, and nevi of Ota. Probably the best combination of selectivity, depth of penetration, and broadest effectiveness for pigmented lesions is achieved at present by the Q-switched ruby laser at 694 nm, or the essentially similar Q-switched alexandrite laser at 760 nm. However, two commercial green short-pulsed lasers are also effective for epidermal lesions: a 510-nm, 300-nsec green pulsed dye laser and the 532 nm, Q-switched, frequency-doubled (fd) neodymium:yttrium-aluminum-garnet (Nd:YAG) laser.

Tattoo removal

Remarkably little is known about selective photothermolysis for tattoo removal, aside from "it works." Tattoos consist of mainly intracellular, submicrometer-size, insoluble ink particles that have been ingested by phagocytic skin cells after intradermal injection. The stability and longevity of most tattoos show that many phagocytic skin cells do not traffic or migrate widely, although tattoos do become less distinct over decades. A great variety of inks are used in professional tattoos, which consist mainly of insoluble metal salts, oxides, or organic complexes. Amateur tattoos are almost always carbon in some form: india ink (amorphous carbon), graphite, or ash. Conventional tattoo treatments are grossly destructive, including surgical excision, dermabrasion, salabrasion, and CO_2 laser vaporization.

Goldman and colleagues[47] first noted that tattoos were responsive to pulsed laser treatment, using normal-mode ruby laser pulses, which were later used widely in Japan. Successful treatment of tattoos without tissue removal was reported 15 and 30 years ago using Q-switched ruby laser pulses.[48,49] A dose-response and histologic study was subsequently performed, which led to widespread interest in Q-switched ruby lasers in the United States,[50] followed by further ultrastructural studies of response.[51] It is now apparent that the Q-switched ruby laser is a generally effective and relatively well tolerated means for treatment of black, blue-black, and green tattoos. Multiple treatments are required at fluences ranging from 4 to 10 J/cm^2, depending on skin type and response. Typically, four to six treatments given at 1-month intervals are needed for amateur tattoos, and six to eight such treatments are needed for professional tattoos, although individual response is extremely variable. The risk of scarring is about 5% to 10% for the series of treatments,[52] although more than 25% of patients have transient textural changes.[53] The Q-switched ruby laser causes blistering and hypopigmentation in most patients and permanent depigmentation in about 1% to 3%.[53]

The mechanisms involved in tattoo removal are largely unknown. Clearly much of the ink, although apparently removed from the skin, is not removed from the body. All persons with tattoos have tattoo ink pigmentation of the lymph nodes draining the tattooed skin, and this is likely the fate of most of the ink after laser treatment. Lightening of the tattoo occurs gradually about 1 week after each treatment and may continue for months. Occasionally, ink clearly is present in the scale crust that forms following epidermal injury and sheds 1 to 2 weeks after treatment, but it is equally apparent that tattoos are removed in cases where no scale crust is formed. Before treatment, ink particles are contained in phagolysosomes in fibroblasts, macrophages, and mast cells. After treatment by Q-switched ruby laser, electron microscopy suggests that the average ink particle is fractured into 10 to 100 smaller fragments, which are extracellular, presumably released by rupture of the phagocytic cells. Local collagen denaturation marking thermal coagulation injury is occasionally seen but does not appear to be central to ink removal. Rephagocytosed laser-altered ink particles can be found weeks after treatment and are occasionally obvious histologically despite nearly complete removal of the tattoo clinically.

These observations[50,51] strongly suggest but do not prove that the primary effects on tattoo ink are (1) fragmentation of ink particles, (2) release into the extracellular dermal space, (3) partial elimination of ink in a scale crust if present, (4) probably greater elimination into lymphatics, and (5) rephagocytosis of laser-altered residual tattoo ink particles.

Irreversible laser-induced photochemical changes can occur in tattoo inks, especially those used in cosmetic skin-colored tattoos.[54] Photochemical changes may conceivably affect tattoo ink removal for some kinds of ink. All the pulsed lasers used for tattoo removal occasionally cause irreversible immediate darkening of these tattoos, which may be temporarily obscured in part by the immediate whitening reaction, as discussed earlier. It is therefore prudent to perform a small test exposure of cosmetic, red, or white tattoos to see whether immediate darkening occurs. In some cases the darkened ink cannot be removed by subsequent laser treatments and adds to the disfigurement. The mechanism of tattoo ink darkening is not known but probably involves reduction of ferric oxide (rust color) to ferrous oxide (black). Pure ferric oxide is easily converted in this manner by Q-switched laser pulses in vitro and is present in many cosmetic tattoos. However, titanium oxides and other compounds are also present and appear to darken as well.

A side-by-side comparison study of Q-switched ruby (694 nm, 40 nsec) and Q-switched Nd:YAG (1064 nm, 30 nsec) laser pulses at equal fluences (2-6 J/cm^2) and equal exposure spot sizes (5 mm) was reported by DeCoste and Anderson,[55] who noted equal efficacy for black ink removal at equal fluences and a significant dose-response relationship. In contrast to the Q-switched ruby laser, the Q-switched Nd:YAG laser was incapable of lightening green ink tattoos but produced no blistering, hypopigmentation, or textural changes. The commercial Q-switched ruby and Nd:YAG lasers operate at shorter pulse durations (26 and 12 nsec, respectively) than those reported by DeCoste and Anderson, and the Q-switched Nd:YAG laser is typically used with a smaller (2 or 3 mm) exposure spot diameter because of its limited pulse energy. Levine and Geronemus[56] made side-by-side comparison of these commercial lasers that favored the Q-switched ruby laser for black ink lightening and also noted a lower incidence of textural change with the ruby laser.[56] In this study, higher fluences and smaller exposure spot diameters were used with the Nd:YAG laser; thus different wavelengths, spot sizes, fluences, and pulse durations were simultaneously compared, and it is unclear which factors are most important. Taken together with DeCoste and Anderson's study,[55] however, it appears that exposure spot size is a very important factor. This is consistent with skin optics behavior (see Table 1-1) for red and near-IR wavelength pulses, especially when the target is deep within the dermis.

Other lasers available and known to work for selective photothermolysis of tattoos are a 760-nm, 75- to 100-nsec Q-switched alexandrite laser; a 532-nm, 10-nsec fd Q-switched Nd:YAG laser; and a 510-nm, 300-nsec short-pulse dye laser. In general, results clearly are better for colored tattoos when the laser wavelength is well absorbed by the particular ink. For example, the alexandrite, ruby, and IR Nd:YAG lasers only occasionally remove bright-red inks, which can be subsequently removed in only a few treatments with either of the green lasers.

Physicians interested in providing this form of treatment may be understandably confused. There has been an impressive rush to the marketplace by laser companies, resulting in a range of wavelengths and pulse durations chosen by "well-educated guesses" and sometimes promoted on the same basis. Controlled studies to understand and optimize tattoo removal are essentially lacking. Of major importance, the pulse-width dependence is unknown; strong arguments can be made for radically shortening the pulse width, if mechanical fracture of the ink particles is the goal. Somewhat analogous to the concept of thermal confinement, inertial confinement can be achieved when the laser pulse is delivered within the time for which pressure can be relieved from the ink particles. The *inertial confinement time* is simply the particle diameter divided by the speed of sound, which for tattoo ink particles equals about 1 nsec. Therefore all the laser pulses being used now may be too long.

Significant details of wavelength-dependent effects are unknown. The chemical identity of most tattoo inks and how they are affected by high-intensity laser pulses are unknown. The physical mechanisms underlying ink particle and phagocyte cell rupture are unknown and, more important, have never been linked with clinical response. Is a laser-induced plasma involved? Must the ink particles be fractured? Is it the ink or the cells containing it that are the targets? How is the ink removed, and where does it go? What role might phagocytosis by different cell types play in the retention of ink after treatment, and how can this be optimized? A chapter on this topic in 5 years might be more informative than this one.

SUMMARY

The use of lasers in dermatology grows at a steady pace, based largely on a better understanding and manipulation of the underlying laser-tissue interactions. This trend will increase, as will the options for other high technology integrated with lasers, including sources replacing lasers but using similar principles. Leon Goldman, who first used a laser as a surgical tool and has been doing so ever since, kindly warns, "If you don't need a laser, don't use one." This timeless advice emphasizes that a practical understanding of laser-tissue interactions is more important than the instruments themselves, no matter how fancy.

REFERENCES

1. Henderson BW, Dougherty TJ, editors: *Photodynamic therapy: basic principles and clinical applications,* New York, 1992, Marcel Dekker.
2. Lui H, Anderson RR: Photodynamic therapy in dermatology: recent developments, *Dermatol Clin* 11:1, 1993.
3. Orenstein A, Nelson JS, Liaw OL et al: Photochemotherapy of hypervascular dermal lesions: a possible alternative to photothermal therapy? *Lasers Surg Med* 10:334, 1990.
4. Kennedy JC, Pottier RH, Pross DC: Photodynamic therapy with endogenous protoporphyrin IX. Basic principles and present clinical experience, *J Photochem Photobiol* 6:143, 1990.
5. Anderson RR, Parrish JA: Selective photothermolysis: precise microsurgery by selective absorption of pulsed radiation, *Science* 220:524, 1983.
6. Anderson RR, Parrish JA: The optics of human skin, *J Invest Dermatol* 77:13, 1981.
7. van Gemert JMC, Jacques SL, Stereborg HJCM et al: Skin optics, *IEEE Trans Biomed Eng* 36:1146, 1990.
8. Anderson RR, Parrish JA: Microvasculature can be selectively damaged using dye lasers: a basic theory and experimental evidence in human skin, *Lasers Surg Med* 1:263, 1981.
9. van Gemert JMC, Henning JPC: A model approach to laser coagulation of dermal vascular lesions, *Arch Dermatol Res* 270:429, 1981.
10. Everett MA, Yeargers E, Sayre RM et al: Penetration of epidermis by ultraviolet rays, *Photochem Photobiol* 5:533, 1966.
11. Polla BS, Anderson RR: Thermal injury by laser pulses: protection by heat shock despite failure to induce heat-shock response, *Lasers Surg Med* 7:398, 1987.
12. Subjeck JR, Shyy TT: Stress protein system of mammalian cells, *Am J Physiol* 250:C1, 1986.
13. Henriques FC: Studies of thermal injury, *Arch Pathol* 43:489, 1947.
14. Welch AJ: The thermal response of laser irradiated tissue, *IEEE J Quant Electron* QE-20:1471, 1984.
15. Walsh JT Jr, Flotte TH, Anderson RR et al: Pulsed CO_2 laser tissue ablation: effect of tissue type and pulse duration on thermal damage, *Lasers Surg Med* 8:108, 1988.
16. Green HA, Burd E, Nishioka N et al: Skin graft take and healing after continuous wave CO_2, pulsed CO_2, 193 nm excimer, and holmium laser ablation of graft beds, *J Invest Dermatol* 92:436, 1989 (abstract).
17. Srinivasan R: Ablation of polymers and biological tissue by ultraviolet lasers, *Science* 234:559, 1986.
18. Jacques SL, McAuliffe DJ, Blank IH et al: Controlled removal of human stratum corneum by pulsed laser, *J Invest Dermatol* 88:88, 1987.
19. Trokel SL, Srinivasan R, Braren B: Excimer laser surgery of the cornea, *Am J Ophthalmol* 96:710, 1983.
20. Watanabe S, Flotte TJ, McAuliffe DJ et al: Putative photoacoustic damage in skin induced by pulsed ArF excimer laser, *J Invest Dermatol* 90:761, 1988.
21. Barsky SH, Rosen S, Geer DE et al: The nature and evolution of port wine stains: a computer-assisted study, *J Invest Dermatol* 74:154, 1976.
22. Garden JM, Polla LL, Tan OT: The treatment of port wine stains by the pulsed dye laser: analysis of pulse duration and long-term therapy, *Arch Dermatol* 124:889, 1990.
23. Greenwald J, Rosen S, Anderson RR et al: Comparative histologic studies of the tunable dye (at 577 nm) laser and argon laser: the specific vascular effects of the dye laser, *J Invest Dermatol* 77:305, 1981.
24. Anderson RR, Jaenicke KF, Parrish JA: Mechanisms of selective vascular changes caused by dye lasers, *Lasers Surg Med* 3:211, 1983.
25. Paul BS, Anderson RR, Jarve J et al: The effect of temperature and other factors on selective microvascular damage caused by pulsed dye laser, *J Invest Dermatol* 81:333, 1983.

26. Garden JM, Tan OT, Kershmann R et al: Effect of dye laser pulse duration on selective cutaneous vascular injury, *J Invest Dermatol* 87:653, 1986.
27. Morelli JG, Tan OT, Garden J et al: Tunable dye laser (577 nm) treatment of port wine stains, *Lasers Surg Med* 6:94, 1986.
28. Tan OT, Sherwood K, Gilchrest BA: Treatment of children with port-wine stains using the flashlamp-pulsed tunable dye laser, *N Engl J Med* 320:416, 1989.
29. Tan OT, Murray S, Kurban AK: Action spectrum of vascular specific injury using pulsed irradiation, *J Invest Dermatol* 92:868, 1989.
30. Tan OT, Morrison P, Kurban AK: 585 nm for the treatment of port-wine stains, *Plast Reconstr Surg* 86:1112, 1990.
31. Tong AKF, Tan OT, Boll J et al: Ultrastructure: effects of melanin pigment on target specificity using a pulsed dye laser (577 nm), *J Invest Dermatol* 88:747, 1987.
32. Reyes BA, Geronemus R: Treatment of port-wine stains during childhood with the flashlamp pumped pulsed dye laser, *J Am Acad Dermatol* 23:1142, 1990.
33. Levins PC, Grevelink JM, Anderson RR: Action spectrum of immediate and delayed purpura in human skin using a tunable pulsed dye laser, *J Invest Dermatol* 96:588, 1991 (abstract).
34. Polla LL, Margolis RJ, Dover JS et al: Melanosomes are a primary target of Q-switched ruby laser irradiation in guinea pig skin, *J Invest Dermatol* 89:281, 1987.
35. Watanabe S, Anderson RR, Brorson S et al: Comparative studies of femtosecond to microsecond laser pulses on selective pigmented cell injury in skin, *Photochem Photobiol* 53:757, 1991.
36. Rispler J, Neister SE: Coaxial flashlamp dye laser in clinical use, *Lasers Surg Med Suppl* 3:281, 1991 (abstract).
37. Troccoli J, Roider J, Anderson RR: Multiple-pulse photocoagulation of blood vessels with a 585 nm tunable dye laser, *Lasers Surg Med Suppl* 4:3, 1992 (abstract).
38. Dover JS, Smaoller BR, Stern RS et al: Low-fluence carbon dioxide laser irradiation of lentigines, *Arch Dermatol* 124:1219, 1988.
39. Murphy GF, Shepard RS, Paul BS et al: Organelle-specific injury to melanin-containing cells in human skin by pulsed laser irradiation, *Lab Invest* 49:680, 1983.
40. Szabo G et al: Racial differences in the fate of melanosomes in human epidermis, *Nature* 222:1081, 1969.
41. Anderson RR, Margolis RJ, Watanabe S et al: Selective photothermolysis of cutaneous pigmentation by Q-switched Nd:YAG laser pulses at 1064, 532, and 355 nm, *J Invest Dermatol* 93:28, 1989.
42. Dover JS, Margolis RJ, Polla LL et al: Pigmented guinea pig skin irradiated with Q-switched ruby laser pulses: morphologic and histologic findings, *Arch Dermatol* 125:43, 1989.
43. Ara G, Anderson RR, Mandel KG et al: Irradiation of pigmented melanoma cells with high intensity pulsed radiation generates acoustic waves and kills cells, *Lasers Surg Med* 10:52, 1990.
44. Margolis RJ, Dover JS, Polla LL et al: Visible action spectrum for melanin-specific selective photothermolysis, *Lasers Surg Med* 9:389, 1989.
45. Roider J, Birngruber R: Spatial confinement of photocoagulation effects using high repetition rate laser pulses, *Conference on Lasers and Electro-optics Technical Digest Series,* vol 7, Washington, DC, 1990, Optical Society of America.
46. Taylor CR, Flotte T, Michaud N et al: Q-switched ruby laser (QSRL) irradiation of benign pigmented lesions: dermal vs. epidermal, *Lasers Surg Med Suppl* 3:65, 1991 (abstract).
47. Goldman L, Blaney DJ, Kindel DJ et al: Pathology of the effect of the laser beam on the skin, *Nature* 197:912, 1963.
48. Laub DR, Yules RB, Arras M et al: Preliminary histopathological observation of Q-switched ruby laser radiation on dermal tattoo pigment in man, *J Surg Res* 5:220, 1968.
49. Reid WH, McLeod PJ, Ritchie A et al: Q-switched ruby laser treatment of black tattoos, *Br J Plast Surg* 36:455, 1983.
50. Taylor CR, Gange RW, Dover JS et al: Treatment of tattoos by Q-switched ruby laser: a dose response study, *Arch Dermatol* 126:893, 1990.
51. Taylor CR, Anderson RR, Gange RW et al: Light and electron microscopic analysis of tattoos treated by Q-switched ruby laser, *J Invest Dermatol* 97:131, 1991.
52. Levins PC, Grevelink JM, Anderson RR: Q-switched ruby laser treatment of tattoos, *Lasers Surg Med Suppl* 3:63, 1991 (abstract).

53. Grevelink JM, Casparian JM, Gonzalez E et al: Undesirable effects associated with treatment of tattoos and pigmented lesions with the Q-switched lasers at 1064 nm and 694 nm: the MGH experience, *Lasers Surg Med Suppl* 5:270, 1993 (abstract).
54. Anderson RR, Geronemus R, Kilmer SL et al: Cosmetic tattoo ink darkening: a complication of Q-switched and pulsed laser treatment, *Arch Dermatol* 129:1010, 1993.
55. DeCoste SD, Anderson RR: Comparison of Q-switched ruby and Q-switched Nd:YAG laser treatment of tattoos, *Lasers Surg Med Suppl* 3:64, 1991 (abstract).
56. Levine V, Geronemus R: Tattoo removal with the Q-switched ruby laser and the Nd:YAG laser: a comparative study, *Lasers Surg Med Suppl* 5:260, 1993 (abstract).

CHAPTER two

Laser Treatment of Cutaneous Vascular Lesions

Mitchel P. Goldman and Richard E. Fitzpatrick

Dr. Leon Goldman was a driving force behind the development of laser medicine and surgery. In 1963 his Laser Laboratory at Children's Hospital Research Foundation in Cincinnati, Ohio, began investigating treatment of port-wine stain (PWS) and cavernous hemangioma using ruby, neodymium:yttrium-aluminum-garnent (Nd:YAG), and argon lasers. His initial report of 45 patients treated with these three lasers appeared in 1968 and stimulated great interest in this new treatment modality.[1] Beginning in 1970, early pioneering work in argon laser surgery was accomplished at the Palo Alto Medical Clinic by Apfelberg, Maser, and Lash[2] for treatment of cutaneous vascular lesions. By 1984 the argon laser was generally accepted as the treatment of choice for PWS.[3] Indeed, before the development of the argon laser, no effective form of treatment could be recommended to patients.

During the early years of laser medicine and surgery, considerable interest surrounded the carbon dioxide (CO_2) laser for the treatment of superficial telangiectasias,[4] hemangiomas,[5] and PWSs.[6] As discussed in Chapter 6, this laser's nonspecific interaction with tissue made it less desirable as a treatment for vascular lesions. The CO_2 laser has been used successfully in treatment of PWSs, but the epidermis and superficial papillary dermis must be vaporized to reach the vessels to be eliminated by laser interaction. This results in a wound with a much higher risk of adverse healing than wounds from treatment with lasers that interact more specifically with the vessels.

TYPES OF LASERS

Argon Laser

The argon laser emits light at six different wavelengths from 458 to 514 nm, with 80% of its emission at 488 nm and 514.5 nm. The laser is used with shuttered pulse durations of 50 msec to 0.3 sec at an energy of 0.8 to 2.9 watts (W) through spot sizes of 0.1 to 1.0 mm with or without a scanning device to produce the endpoint of tissue blanching. Although 75% of patients could expect good to excellent results using the argon laser for PWS (lightening of color by more than 50%),[7-9] the two primary problems of treatment were the risk of hypertrophic scarring, especially in children (4% to 23%),[7,8,10-13] and persistence of the lesion (95% or more of patients treated).[7,8,13] Persistence was related to destruction of blood vessels in the superficial papillary dermis, leaving ectatic middle and deep reticular dermal vessels intact.[14]

In an effort to avoid scarring and pigmentary changes, other treatment methods were developed but have shown variable efficacy. They included treatment of small areas only,[15] treatment in alternating stripes,[16,17] chilling of the lesion before therapy,[18] careful selection of patients and lesions to treat,[10,19,20] low-dose therapy,[13,21] mechanical scanning devices,[22] and meticulous tracing of vessels with a very-small-diameter beam.[23] By using a combination of these techniques, the incidence of hypertrophic scarring was reduced but still occurred in 87% of questioned patients.[24]

Treatment of children with the argon laser, particularly infants, remained a problem and was ill-advised because hypertrophic scarring was reported in as many as 38% of patients under the age of 12.[25] Because of this high rate of hypertrophic scarring, treatment of patients less than 17 years of age was not recommended.[10,20]

The difficulty in treating PWS with the argon laser is a result of three factors: short wavelengths, high energy fluences with small spot sizes, and long pulse durations. The *shorter wavelengths* of this laser (488 and 514 nm) are absorbed more heavily in the epidermis and superficial dermis by melanin, with the absorbed heat causing nonvascular damage. Deeper vascular damage is achieved by increasing the wavelength from 514 to 585 so that fluences 64 to 186 times lower can be equally effective[26] (Figure 2-1).

A *small spot size* is the second factor limiting penetration. A large spot size effectively increases penetration because of heavier scattering in the epidermis and superficial dermis. As a comparison, the 5 mm spot size of a flashlamp-pumped pulsed dye laser (FLPDL) penetrates substantially deeper than a 0.1- to 1.0-mm spot size of the argon laser at identical power densities.

Although a decrease in spot size results in an increase in laser fluence, and vice versa, for a spot size greater than 3 mm, mechanisms responsible for clinical effects are more complex. Tan et al[27] found that a 1-mm-diameter spot size (with the FLPDL) affected blood vessels only in the most superficial vascular plexus (0.2 mm from the dermal-epidermal junction), even though extremely high fluences (27 J/cm^2) were needed to produce purpura. Here, purpura resolved quickly because only superficial damage occurred. The authors hypothesize that a 1 mm spot size alters dermal components, changing the refraction of tissue, which alters distribution and scattering of laser fluence. Although a 1-mm-diameter spot could affect deeper dermal vessels, extensive nonspecific damage occurred as compared with 3- and 5-mm-diameter spot sizes. Clearly, nonlinear changes in the optical behavior of tissue occurs through manipulation of laser scatter[28] (Figures 2-2 to 2-4).

Er:YAG 2,940nm
CO_2 10,600nm
PLDL 510nm
Argon 514nm
KTP 532nm
Krypton 568nm
CV/CB 578nm
FLPDL 585-600nm
Ruby 694nm
Alex 755nm
Nd: YAG 1060nm

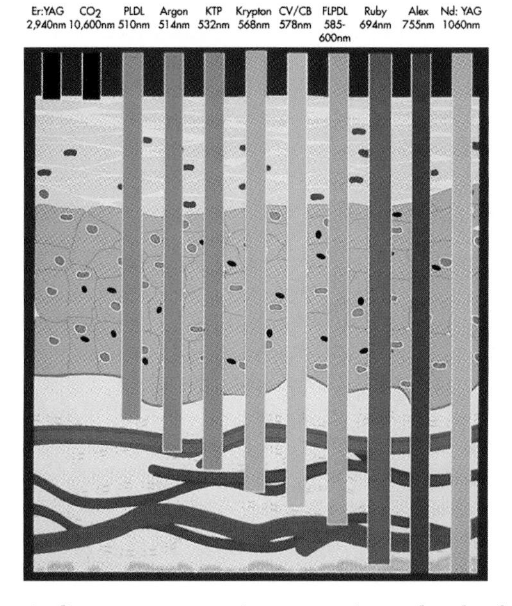

Figure 2-1 Schematic diagram representing approximate levels of penetration for various lasers. *Er:YAG,* Erbium:yttrium-aluminum-garnet; *CO_2,* carbon dioxide; *PLDL,* Candela pigment lesion dye laser; *KTP,* potassium titanyl phosphate; *CV/CB,* copper vapor/copper bromide; *FLPDL,* flashlamp-pumped pulsed dye laser; *Alex,* alexandrite; *Nd,* neodymium.

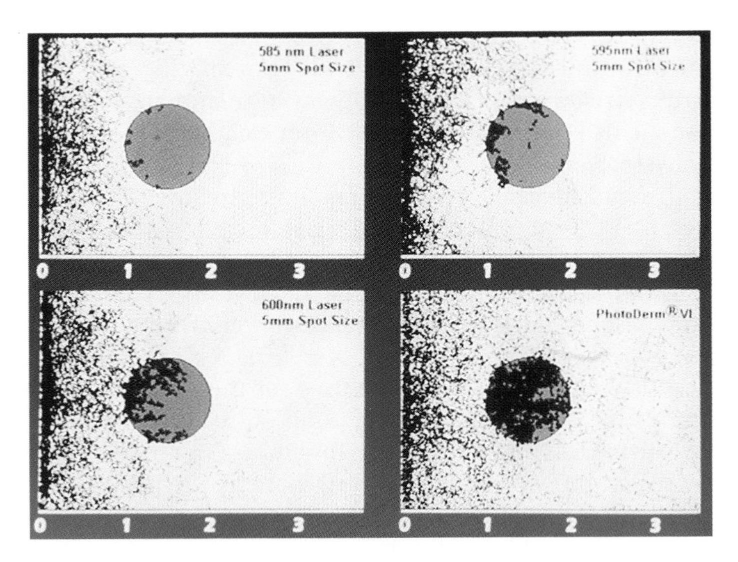

Figure 2-2 Mathematic representation of distribution of photons into skin as a function of spot size diameter and wavelength. (Courtesy ESC Medical, Inc.)

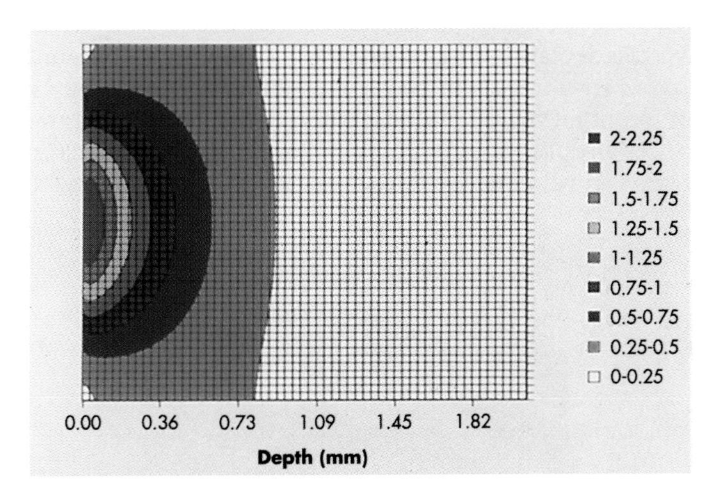

Figure 2-3 Computer-generated distribution of light into skin based on mathematic formula. (Courtesy ESC Medical, Inc.)

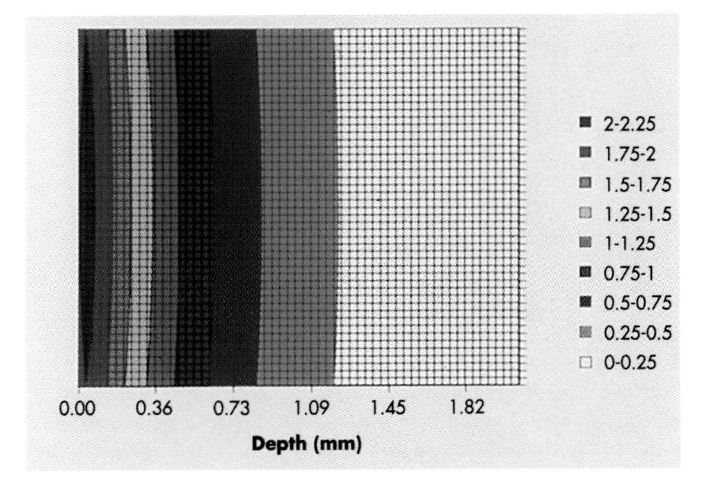

Figure 2-4 Computer-generated distribution of light into skin based on mathematic formula. (Courtesy ESC Medical, Inc.)

Third, *long pulse durations* with essentially continuous operation of the laser forces the physician to control the fluence manually to a specific area of the skin. The physician therefore relies on a clinical endpoint in treatment, which can vary with different lesions. This limits reproducibility from treatment to treatment and from physician to physician.

Therefore, to avoid adverse effects and maximize treatment efficacy, when using the argon laser, it is critical to perform a test patch on a section of the PWS. A test patch will help determine the optimal energy fluence and pulse duration to maximize a successful outcome. However, even a patch test may not predict treatment efficacy because different locations on the face and elsewhere respond in a unique manner.[29]

Nevertheless, if the argon laser is to be used for the treatment of PWS, our recommendation is to use minimal power and pulsed delivery as described by Cosman[13] and Fitzpatrick and Feinberg.[21] In short, a 1-mm-diameter spot size is pulsed at 0.05 sec and moved across the birthmark as the power is increased from 0.4 W until minimal blanching occurs, usually between 0.6 and 1.2 W. This becomes the median parameter for the test patch, which should include laser powers 0.4 W above and below this median. (This technique results in a minimal and often clinically insignificant, nonspecific dermal-epidermal burn [Figure 2-5] because visible blanching as an endpoint denotes protein denaturization.) Our favorable clinical experience with short exposure times of 0.05 sec has been confirmed by others, who noted less hypopigmentation and atrophy.[30,31] Computerized scanners (described later) may also improve treatment efficacy by minimizing operator variability.[32,33]

In addition to optimizing energy fluences, attempts are being made to increase wavelength selectivity for vascular lesions. Exogenous chromophores introduced into blood vessels may also increase the specificity of the argon laser.[34] A large num-

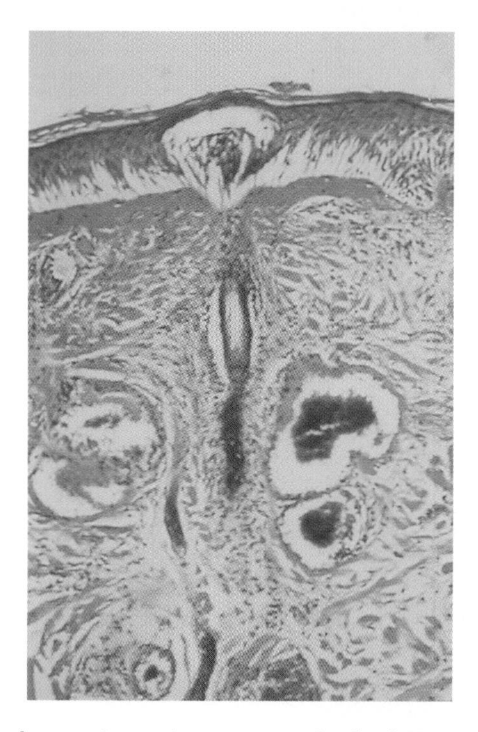

Figure 2-5 Biopsy of port-wine stain (PWS) on cheek of 40-year-old man immediately after argon laser treatment at 15 J/cm^2, 1-mm spot diameter, which produced clinical epidermal whitening. Note coagulation of ectatic vessels in middle and deep dermis with some smudging of perivascular collagen. Overlying epidermis shows marked thermal effects with streaming of epidermal cells and coagulation necrosis of superficial papillary dermis. (Hematoxylin-eosin; ×200.)

ber of dyes that absorb at 488 and 514 nm exist. If these dyes were selectively absorbed by target tissue (blood vessels), the argon (or other laser wavelengths) should achieve the vascular specificity of tunable dye lasers at 577 to 585 nm. Even with increased targeting specificity, however, the shorter wavelength and smaller spot size prevent the necessary energy fluence from reaching deeper vascular structures.

Flashlamp-pumped Pulsed Dye Lasers

Because of the limitations inherent with the argon laser, attention was focused on developing lasers with more specific absorption characteristics for intravascular oxyhemoglobin (HbO_2), the treatment target. Experimental, in vitro studies have demonstrated HbO_2 in red blood cells (RBCs) to be the absorbed target at 577 nm in 50-μm vessels 1 mm below the epidermal granular layer.[35] Endothelial cells are also damaged at this wavelength independent of RBC absorption, but in the presence of HbO_2, this effect is minimal. This led to the development of lasers having a wavelength of 577 nm, which corresponds to one of the absorption peaks of hemoglobin (Hb) associated with relatively lower melanin absorption[15,36] (Figure 2-6).

In addition to observing wavelength specificity, ideally one should limit energy absorption to the target tissue. This concept is the premise of Anderson and Parrish's theory of selective photothermolysis (described later).[37,38] This theory focused attention not only on the wavelength, but also on the pulse duration and the need to limit thermal diffusion by keeping the laser pulse shorter than the time necessary to allow heat to spread from the treated target (for PWS, RBCs within vessels) to surrounding tissue, or the thermal relaxation time (Table 2-1). This theory led to the development for medical use of flashlamp-pumped pulsed dye lasers (FLPDLs), which have been very successful in treating small blood vessels in the variety of clinical conditions described in this chapter.

Tan et al's successful treatment of children with PWSs established the safety and efficacy of the FLPDL.[39] Garden and others[40-42] further refined the treatment parameters and expanded the use to lesions in adults. This clinical efficacy has been confirmed by other authors,[35,43-47] and the use has been expanded to include the early treatment of capillary hemangiomas as well as many different cutaneous lesions that have a vascular component.[48-50]

Two manufacturers produce this type of laser. Candela Corporation (Wayland, Mass) manufactures the SPTL line of machines, which originally emitted a wavelength of 585 nm and now can emit wavelengths of 590, 595, and 600 nm. The original pulse duration was 450 μsec and now can be increased to 1500 μsec. The beam profile can be circular at 2, 3, 5, 7, and 10 mm in diameter or elliptic at 2 × 7 mm. The pulse rate is either 1 Hz or 0.5 Hz, and maximal energy fluences of 10 or 20 J/cm^2 are available. The other FLPDL is the PhotoGenica V manufactured by Cynosure, Inc.

Table 2-1
Approximate thermal relaxation time (*Tr*) for vessels of different diameters

Diameter (μm)	*Tr* (msec)
10	0.048
20	0.19
50	1.2
100	4.8
200	19.0
300	42.6

Data from Anderson RR, Parrish JA: *Lasers Surg Med* 121:217, 1981.

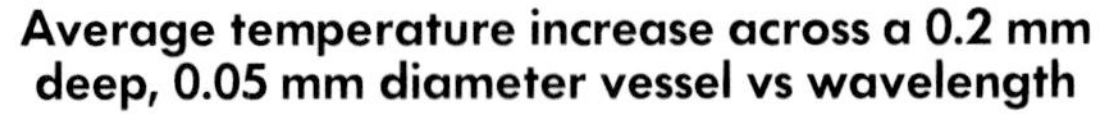

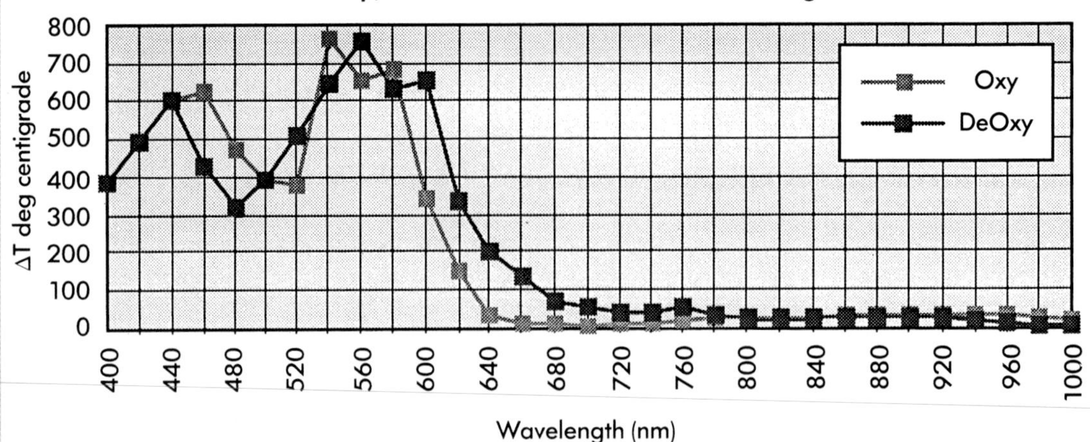

Average temperature increase across a 2 mm deep, 1 mm diameter vessel vs wavelength

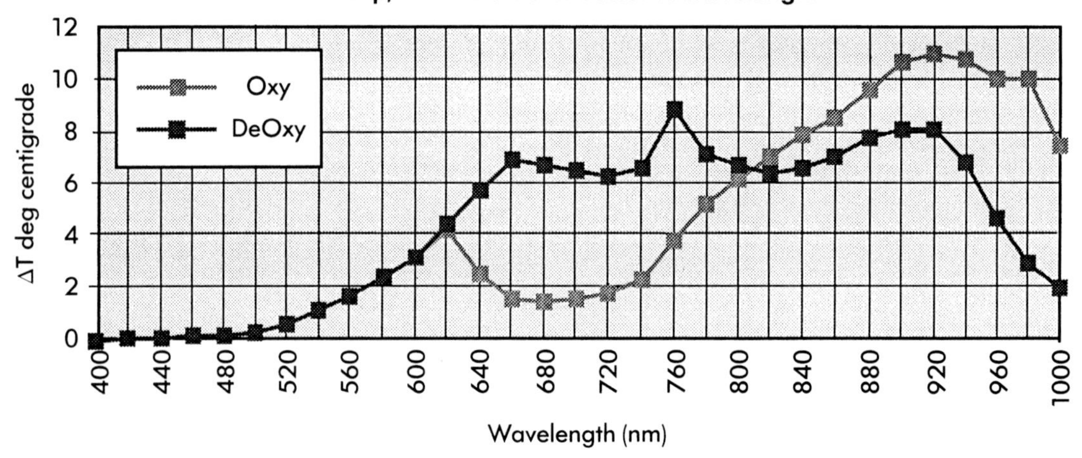

Figure 2-6 Average temperature increase across a cutaneous vessel as a function of wavelength for two extreme cases: shallow capillary vessel and deeper (2-mm depth) larger-diameter (1 mm) vessel. Calculation is done assuming that main light-absorbing chromophore in blood is either oxyhemoglobin (Oxy) or deoxyhemoglobin (DeOxy). Calculation is carried out for a 10 J/cm^2 fluence and does not take into account cooling by heat conductivity. Note dramatic shift in optional wavelength as a function of vessel depth and diameter. Also note difference between oxygenated and deoxygenated vessels. Absorption coefficients for dermis and two main blood chromophores are a function of wavelength. Dermis values are for fair white skin. (Courtesy Shimon Eckhouse, PhD.)

(Bedford, Mass; Millennium VLS Dual Pulse). The advantage of the longer wavelengths and longer pulse durations are discussed in separate sections later.

The one difference between the two lasers is the beam profile. With the Candela FLPDL a 10% to 20% overlapping spot provides for an even distribution of energy fluence. This is because of the gaussian distribution of beam output. An 18% overlap has been found to cover the largest surface area with the least overlap.[51] In contrast, the Cynosure FLPDL has a "top hat" distribution of energy fluence (Figures 2-7 and 2-8).[52] In addition, when the 5-mm–diameter spot size of the two lasers were tested, the Candela laser spot size was up to 35% larger than 5 mm while the Cynosure laser was up to 8% smaller. Therefore it is prudent to check the diameter of the spot with burn paper before switching from one FLPDL machine to another.

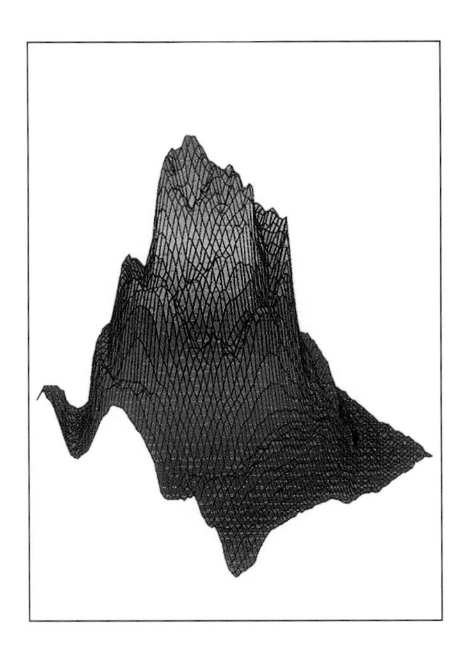

Figure 2-7 Beam profile of Candela SPTL-1 from laser head. It exhibits gaussian-like distribution of energy with some irregularities. (From Jackson BA, Arndt KA, Dover JS: *J Am Acad Dermatol* 34:1000, 1996.)

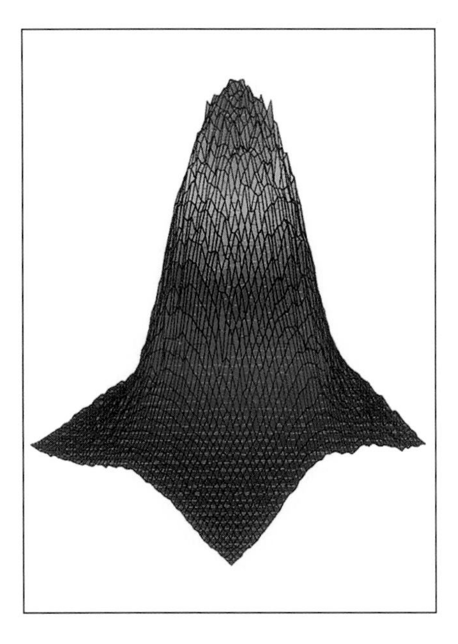

Figure 2-8 Cynosure PhotoGenica V laser from laser head. As with Candela SPTL-1, it exhibits gaussian energy distribution with irregularities. (From Jackson BA, Arndt KA, Dover JS: *J Am Acad Dermatol* 34:1000, 1996.)

Although the wavelengths of the Candela and Cynosure FLPDLs are both reported to be 585 nm in the standard machines, the spatial profiles of the two machines are somewhat different when measured. The Candela SPTL-1 has a central wavelength of 587 nm and a bandwidth of approximately 4 nm. The Cynosure PhotoGenica has a central wavelength of 581 nm and a bandwidth of 3 nm.[53] The wavelengths also show different temporal profiles during each pulse. In the SPTL-1 the longer wavelengths are dominant in the first part of the pulse. The clinical significance of these measurements has not been evaluated.

There appears to be an advantage when treating PWS with a 7-mm-diameter spot size compared with a 5-mm-diameter spot size. Fourteen patients treated with either a 5- or 7-mm-diameter spot size at equal energy fluences were evaluated clinically and histologically.[54] The number of pulses required to treat the clinical area was 35% lower with the 7-mm spot, which caused more purpura and crusting, but with an equal incidence of hyperpigmentation. Histologic evaluation showed coagulation of slightly deeper and slightly larger-diameter vessels with the 7-mm spot. The increased crusting and purpura are probably secondary to a more pronounced, wider gaussian curve with the 7-mm spot, which thus gives a higher energy fluence in the middle of the beam compared with the 5-mm spot. We recommend decreasing the energy fluence 0.5 to 1.0 J/cm^2 when switching from a 5- to a 7-mm-diameter spot size.

Tunable Dye Lasers, 577 to 585 nm

Another approach to treatment of vascular lesions has been the meticulous tracing of vessels using a 100 μ spot size at 577 nm wavelength generated by an argon-pumped tunable dye laser. This laser is manufactured by Coherent-Lihtan (Palo Alto, Calif) and produces wavelengths of 488 and 514 nm and continuously tunable wavelengths from 577 to 638 nm. This is a continuous-wave (CW) laser. The beam is delivered through a fiberoptic handpiece. It also may be used with a robotic scanner or mechanical shutter.

A study on 100 patients treated to minimal blanching with a 2 mm diameter spot size, 0.2- to 2-sec pulse duration, and energy fluence of 10 to 32 J/cm^2 demonstrated good results in two thirds of patients, with hypopigmentation occurring in 15%, hypertrophic scarring in 5%, and atrophic scarring in 15% of patients.[55] In contrast, Scheibner and Wheeland[56] have found this technique to be very safe and effective in adults and children.[23]

Dover et al[57] compared the effects of the same wavelength of light with a Hexascan scanning device and the FLPDL. They used the FLPDL at 6.0 to 7.5 J/cm^2 and the dye laser at 16 to 24 J/cm^2 to obtain an equal threshold of graying for laser impacts. Patients were evaluated at 6 weeks and found to have better clearing on average with the FLPDL. Hyperpigmentation and hypopigmentation occurred more frequently with the Hexascan.

Copper Vapor and Copper Bromide Lasers

The copper vapor and copper bromide lasers (CVL, CBL) have also been promoted for treatment of telangiectasia and PWS in adults.[58-60] These lasers are produced by Innovative Health Concepts and CJ Lasers (CVL) and Continuum Biomedical, Inc. (Livermore, Calif)(CBL). The CVL or CBL with a wavelength of 511 nm and/or 578 nm, pulsed at 20 nsec and repetition rate of 15,000 Hz, has an appropriate wavelength to treat vascular lesions selectively (578 nm). However, each 20-nsec pulse is far short of the thermal relaxation time of even the smallest vascular ectasia and as a single pulse does not deliver enough energy to heat a vascular lesion to a temperature required to produce injury (2.4 mJ/pulse compared with 0.5 to 2.0 J/pulse with the FLPDL). It therefore must be used in a train of pulses to coagulate vascular lesions[61] (Figure 2-9). The train of pulses at 15,000 Hz is additive and reacts in tissue as if it were a continuous beam. Furthermore, because the peak power within each pulse is very high, this laser may cause rupture rather than coagulation of smaller vessels. The net tissue effect of this laser is very similar to that of the argon-pumped dye laser. The train of pulses is released in 20- to 40-nsec pulses at a frequency of 10 to 15 kHz. This chain can be electronically broken into short series of pulses of 0.075 to 0.3 sec in duration. It is usually used at an average power of 0.35 to 0.55 W delivered in 0.2-sec pulses.

Using a laser with a wavelength greater than the argon laser should have therapeutic advantages by bypassing epidermal melanocytes and penetrating deeper into the skin. An evaluation of 21 patients with telangiectasia or PWS previously treated with the argon laser who underwent CVL treatment showed that about half had better results, with the other half having similar results.[62] However, seven patients developed hyperpigmentation and mild scarring (three with hypertrophic and three with depressed atrophy) after CVL treatment, given with a power output of 1.5 W, a "pulse duration" of 50 msec, and a calculated energy fluence of 7.9 to 9.6 J/cm^2 to produce minimal blanching of the lesion.

To provide a larger safety margin, a mechanical shuttered pulse or a mechanical scanner is necessary to prevent unwanted thermal diffusion. However, nonspecific epidermal and dermal damage does occur with this laser. Best results are reported when a Hexascan delivery system is used with the CVL. With this scanner, a pulse width of 155 msec and mean skin surface fluence of 26 J/cm^2 have been shown to produce minimal blanching with marked fading.[63] In a study of 31 patients, this system resulted in temporary hyperpigmentation in one patient and slight textural change in another. A second study with the CVL Hexascan system by the same group was performed with a mean pulse width of 50 msec and fluence of 18 J/cm^2 in 43 patients with PWS.[64] They compared this modality to the FLPDL used with a 5-mm-diameter spot size at 6.5 J/cm^2. They found better fading of macular, blanchable PWS in the FLPDL-treated patients without a significant difference in adverse sequelae.

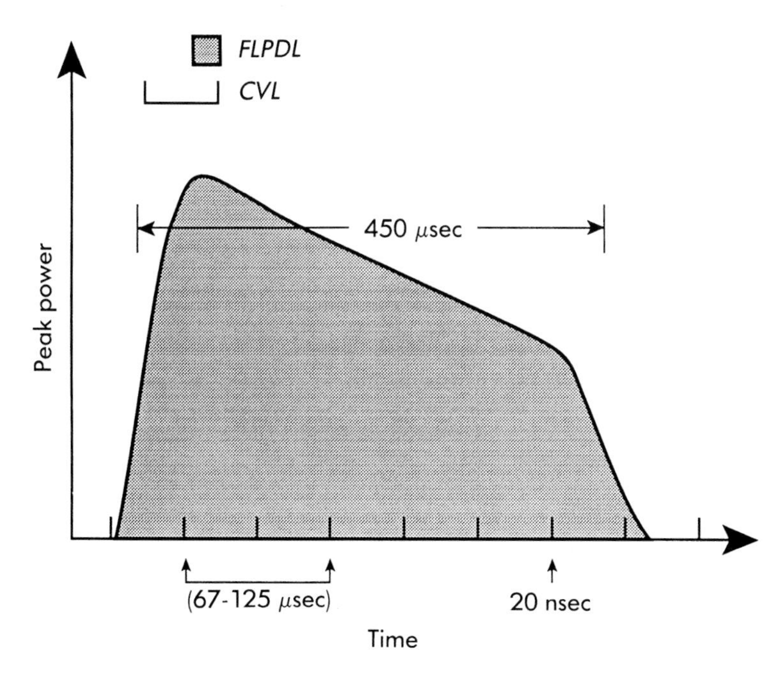

Figure 2-9 Graphic comparison of peak power output from flashlamp-pumped pulsed dye laser (*FLPDL*) and copper vapor laser (*CVL*).

Although the CVL wavelength of 578 nm is selective for oxygenated and deoxygenated Hb in ectatic blood vessels, significant epidermal melanin absorption occurs when used at an energy fluence necessary to thermocoagulate these vessels. In a study on Korean skin with PWS treated with the CVL, vascular selectivity without epidermal damages could not be achieved with a 50-msec exposure at energy densities greater than 6 J/cm^2.[65] The energy density for clinically minimal whitening was 6 to 8 J/cm^2, with a maximum penetration depth of 0.4 mm (Figure 2-10). Korean skin looks brownish and is usually classified into Fitzpatrick types III, IV, and V. Thus the CVL, as with the argon and FLPD lasers, is not suitable for treating PWS in non-Caucasian skin.

A study of Caucasian Fitzpatrick types I to V skin treated with the CVL through a Hexascan delivery system at pulse durations of 200 msec and fluences of 14.1,17.8, 20.2, 25.5, 26.2, and 33.1 J/cm^2 confirmed the nonspecific damage on epidermal melanocytes seen in non-Korean skin.[66,67] A person with pretreatment skin pigmentation of 17% measured by skin reflectance has a 5% risk of scarring and 50% risk of pigmentary changes after laser treatment at 20.2 J/cm^2, whereas a pale person with pretreatment pigmentation of 10% has a 10% risk of pigmentary changes with virtually no risk of scarring.[67] The authors therefore recommend that pretreatment skin reflectance measurements be used to select appropriate patients for CVL treatment.

A

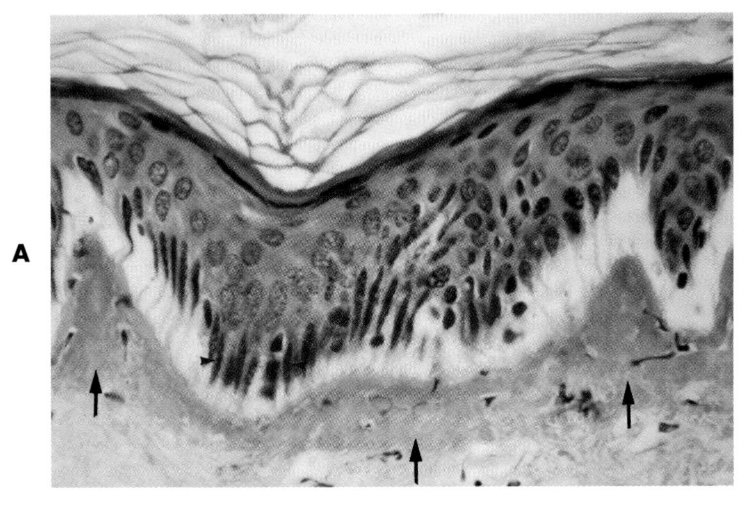

B

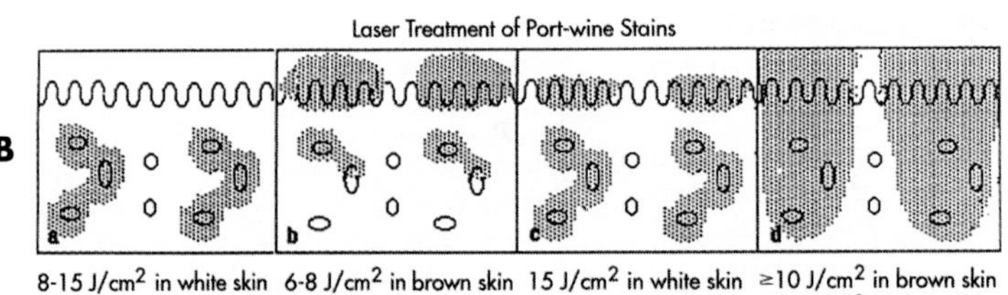

Figure 2-10 **A,** CVL treatment at 8 J/cm^2. Diffuse morphologic changes in epidermis with elongation and vesiculation of nuclei and separation of dermoepidermal junction. Note basophilic degeneration of papillary dermis (*arrows*). Epidermal melanin pigments (*arrowheads*) are abundant in basal layer. (Hematoxylin and eosin; bar = 50 μm.) **B,** Comparison of epidermal and dermal damage (*shading*), in PWS after CVL (578 nm) treatment. Selective damage to dermal vessels and perivascular tissue (*a*), viable connective tissue between epidermis and vessels (*b* and *c*), and nonspecific diffuse necrosis (*d*). (From Chung JH, Koh WS, Youn JI: *Lasers Surg Med* 18:358, 1996.)

Neodymium:Yttrium-Aluminum-Garnet Laser

The Nd:YAG laser (1064 nm) has also been reported to have benefit in the treatment of selected hemangiomas of the head and neck.[68] However, because of nonspecific blood/tissue interaction at this wavelength in either the continuous or Q-switched (4-7 nsec) mode, the depth of thermal injury is 5 to 8 mm.[69] Its usefulness is therefore limited to those lesions having a thick, bulky mass.[70] This laser has also been used for treatment of PWSs[69] but has too wide a field of thermal necrosis and a substantial risk of scarring to be useful for these lesions.[71]

A comparative study of the Nd:YAG laser with the argon laser found that similar efficacy occurred, with a greater incidence of scarring with the Nd:YAG.[72] All treatments were performed with immediate minimal blanching parameters. Histologic assessment showed no significant difference in depth or degree of damage, but scarring occurred in 50% to 100% of Nd:YAG-treated patients.

A more recent development, which doubles the frequency and halves the wavelength to 532 nm, has made the Nd:YAG laser more potentially useful in the management of vascular lesions. This laser is produced by Continuum (CB Diode/532), Candela (Derma-Lase), Coherent (Versapulse), and other laser companies. The beam is delivered through an articulated arm. In this modified laser system the 1064-nm light is passed through an optical crystal composed of potassium titanyl phosphate (KTP), which converts the wavelength to 532 nm.[73] The lasers use a krypton arc lamp, which runs at a constant current to excite the Nd:YAG crystal. This produces a quasi-continuous output that is composed of 0.8-μsec pulse duration pulses 40 μsec apart. Because these systems are Q-switched, they have high peak energies (50 times the laser's average power) and short pulse durations (4-7 nsec). Although the peak power of each Q-switched pulse is high (1000 W), the low energy of each Q-switched pulse and the high Q-switched rate cause tissue effects similar to those produced by true continuous lasers of the same wavelength and average power. Minimal thermal damage to nonvascular tissue occurs because the usual pulse energy used is less than 1 J.

The frequency-doubled (fd) Nd:YAG laser (532 nm) is used with nanosecond pulses to treat vascular lesions. The 532-nm wavelength is at one of the hemoglobin peaks for 50-μm superficial blood vessels. This allows some selectivity in treating vascular lesions. However, its shorter wavelength does not allow deep penetration. A preliminary study using the Con-Bio Laser (Continuum) at fluences ranging from 1 to 6 J/cm^2 (maximum 10 nsec, 150 mJ) in mice and rabbit ear veins showed a depth of coagulation of 0.73 $\pm$ 0.44 mm and hemorrhage of 0.68 $\pm$ 0.41 mm. In addition, edema (blistering) was observed at all fluences tested with mild subcutaneous fibrosis and epidermal hypertrophy. Therefore this laser can produce vascular injury, but because of its interaction with epidermal melanin, it is relatively nonselective.

The CB Diode/532 has exposure durations varying from 1 to 100 msec with pulse repetition rates of 1, 5, and 10 Hz. Fluences of 0.3 to 240 J/cm^2 are capable of being delivered through spot sizes of 0.04, 0.8, and 1.2 mm.

A "long-pulse" variant of the KTP has been developed by Coherent (Versapulse). This laser delivers a 532-nm pulse width in 2 to 10 msec at energy fluences (depending on spot size) to 15 J/cm^2 (3-mm diameter) with available spot sizes of 2, 3, and 4 mm. The maximum energy per pulse is 1750 mJ. The repetition rate can be varied from 1, 2, 3, 6 Hz. The laser beam can be delivered through a 4° or 7° C cooled sapphire contact chamber placed on the skin overlying the lesion, that protects the epidermis from the nonspecific thermal effects of this wavelength.

Potassium titanyl phosphate laser

Although also an fd Nd:YAG laser, the novelty of the KTP laser system is in its ability to lengthen the pulse from the nanosecond time of other lasers at 532 nm. LaserScope (San Jose, Calif) has developed a modulated KTP laser (Starpulse, Orion, and Auratm lasers) that uses an arc lamp running at a constant current pulsed to a much higher current than the lamp can tolerate under current operation. This produces an average power up to 160 W packaged into a single pulse that can be adjusted to pulse durations of 1 to 50 msec at pulse rates that are adjustable from one to ten pulses per second. Ten watts of power are available, with peak power of up to 60 W for pulse widths of 1 to 50 msec. The fluence is delivered through a bare fiber 0.2 to 2 mm in diameter, which can be connected to various scanning delivery systems. The KTP laser is reported to be equivalent to the CVL or 577 CW dye laser for the treatment of vascular lesions.[74,75]

The KTP lasers are used in three modes when treating vascular lesions. In one mode the laser is used with the Dermastat (LaserScope), which applies a spot size to the skin varying in size from 0.1 to 2.0 mm in diameter. This fully integrated microprocessor-controlled scanning device is 30 times faster than the Hexascan. The maximum average laser power is 5 W, and the pulse duration can be varied in the range of 0.1 to 1.0 sec. The 1-mm spot size at 5 W with a pulse duration of 0.2 sec generates a fluence of 127 J/cm^2 on the skin. Higher fluences can be selected by using longer pulse durations or smaller spot sizes. These high energies may not be appropriate for treating PWS in children or pink superficial lesions.

When treating PWS, the KTP laser has been used with a "Hexascanner delivery system" at fluences between 10 and 20 J/cm^2. The recommended pulse width ranges from 3 to 5 msec. For facial telangiectasia, 0.15- to 2-mm spot sizes are used at fluences of 12 to 70 J/cm^2, depending on the diameter used, with pulse widths of 10 to 20 msec at one to five pulses per second. Cherry angiomas are treated with a 1- to 2-mm spot size at 8 to 20 J/cm^2 with a 15-msec pulse duration. These recommended parameters are derived from reports to LaserScope.

Krypton Laser

The krypton laser produces wavelengths of 520, 532, and 568 nm. When used in treating vascular lesions, the two green bands are filtered out, yielding a beam of pure yellow light (568 nm). This energy can then be delivered in a manner identical to the argon dye, copper vapor, and Nd:YAG lasers using a tracing technique or a robotic scanner.

The HGM Digital Spectrum K1 system (HGM, Inc., Salt Lake City) has exposure intervals of 0.2 to 10 sec with exposure times of 0.05, 0.1, 0.2, 0.5, 1.0, 2.0, and 5.0 sec. Treatment power is 1 W at 568 nm and 2 W at 521 and 532 nm. Three handpieces of 1 mm, 2 mm and 100 μm are available. The 100-μm handpiece is used at 0.4 to 0.6 W with a 0.2-sec pulse. The 1-mm-diameter handpiece is used at 0.7 to 0.9 W with a 2-sec pulse. Lesional blanching is the treatment endpoint.

For treating telangiectasia, a 1-mm-diameter handpiece is usually used at a setting of 0.5 to 0.75 W, 0.2-sec pulse duration, and 0.2-sec pulse intervals at the 568-nm setting. The vessel is traced until blanching occurs. With these parameters, 75% of patients tolerate the procedure without requiring any topical anesthesia. An ice pack is usually applied for a few minutes after therapy. Many patients require multiple treatments because vessels tend to recur after a few weeks. In fact, many vessels that are not apparent while the patient is lying down become apparent when the patient sits up. Treatment sessions are recommended after 2 to 3 weeks.

Table 2-2 compares the various lasers used to treat vascular lesions.

DYE-ENHANCED LASER THERAPY

Increased epidermal pigment competes with laser penetration and limits the effect on erythrocytes and vessels.[76-78] Therefore patients with light skin color, types I and

II, respond better than those with more deeply pigmented skin. It has been theorized that if an exogenous intravascular dye in the spectral region near or beyond 1100 nm is used to create an intravascular laser target that is beyond the absorption spectrum of melanin, selective photothermolysis of vessels without melanin interaction and interference is possible.[77] In addition, a wavelength of 900 to 1000 nm penetrates more deeply in tissue and therefore will also be absorbed by deeper blood vessels (Figure 2-6).

An experimental study in rabbits using the ruby laser with a pulse duration of 283 μsec and Prussian blue solution demonstrated vascular coagulation to an average of 2.33 mm.[79] This was significantly deeper than with the FLPDL, which had an average depth of coagulation of 1.45 mm in this animal model.

INTENSE PULSED NONCOHERENT LIGHT

The PhotoDerm VL is an intense pulsed light source emitting a continuous light spectrum with most of its energy fluence between 515 and 1000 nm. The pulse durations can be adjusted from 2 to 25 msec/pulse given as a single, double, or triple pulse with delays between pulses of 2 to 100 msec. The total energy fluence emitted can range from 3 to 90 J/cm^2. The fluence is delivered through a quartz light guide with a spot size/surface area of 8 × 35 mm (Figures 2-11 to 2-13). This spot size can be minimized by covering the surface area with any opaque covering, such as white paper. The intense pulse light source produces incoherent light whose spectrum can be cut off through the use of colored filters. Filters in standard use are 515, 550, 570, 595, 610, 645, and 695 nm. This filters out the shorter wavelengths, allowing the energy fluence to be concentrated up to 1000 nm with resulting deeper penetration of the high-intensity pulsed light (Figure 2-14). All settings are computer controlled to deliver the desired energy to a flashlamp. The physics dictating the wavelength output of the flashlamp can be modified to deliver fluence in a longer portion of the wavelength by switching to a "longpulse" mode. The exact wavelength spectral output is proprietary.

The ability to pulse the intense light rapidly within the thermal relaxation time of the target vessel allows an accumulation of heat to occur within the

Table 2-2
Lasers for vascular lesions

Laser	Wavelength (nm)	Color	Type
Argon	488-514	Blue-green	Continuous
Argon dye	577-630	Yellow-red	Continuous
Potassium titanyl phosphate (KTP)	532	Green	Pulse train
Q-switched Nd:YAG (frequency doubled)	532	Green	20-nsec pulse
Nd:YAG (frequency doubled)	532	Green	1-15 msec
Krypton	521-532-568	Yellow	Continuous
Copper vapor, copper bromide	578	Yellow	Pulse train
Flashlamp-pumped pulsed dye (FLPD)	577-600	Yellow	450-μsec pulse 1.5-msec pulse

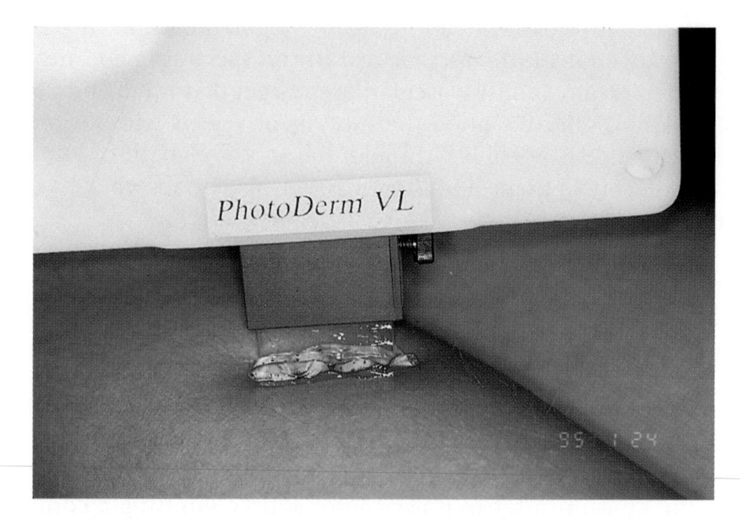

Figure 2-11 Application of treatment head of Photoderm VL on skin. Pulsed light passes through quartz crystal light guide and layer of clear coupling gel before going into skin.

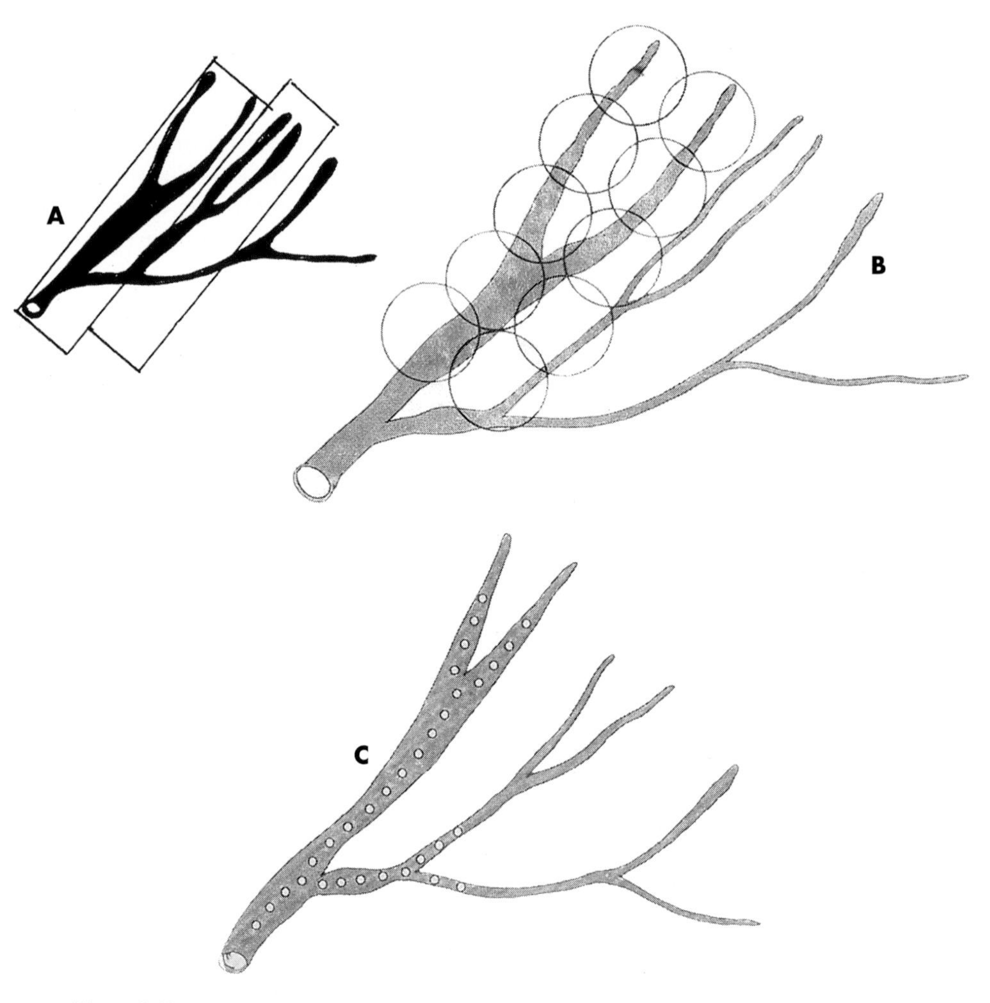

Figure 2-12 **A,** Footprint of the PhotoDerm VL. **B,** Footprint of 5-mm-diameter FLPDL. **C,** Footprint of typical CVL. (Courtesy ESC Medical, Inc.)

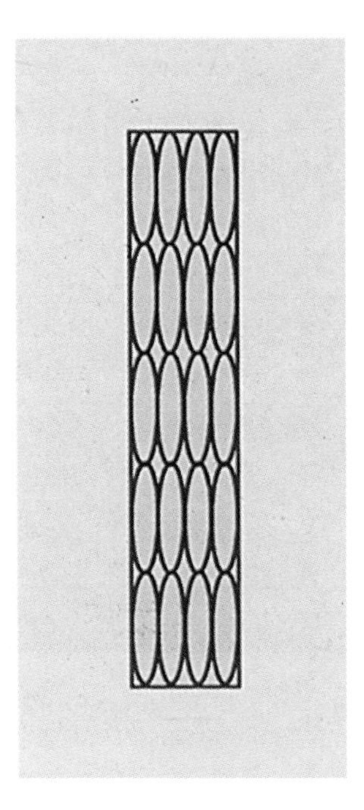

Figure 2-13 Footprint of elliptic FLPDL compared with PhotoDerm VL footprint. (Courtesy ESC Medical, Inc.)

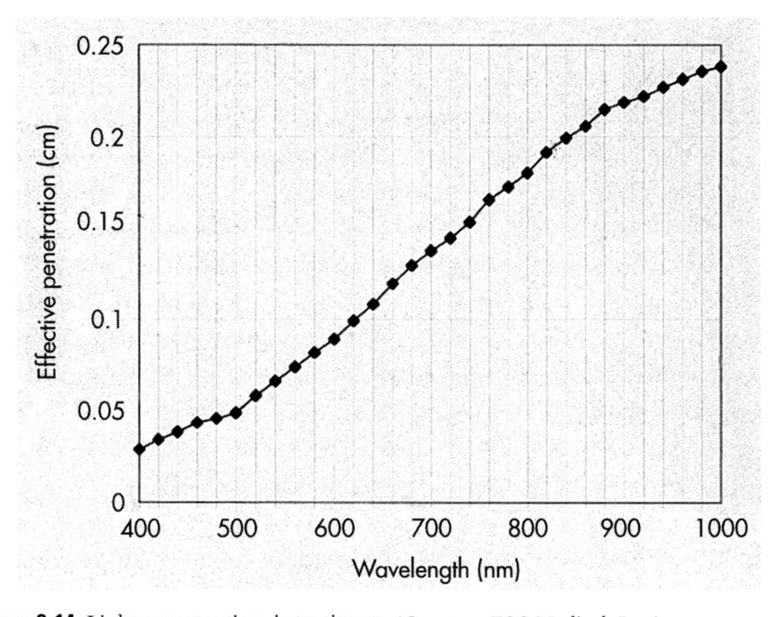

Figure 2-14 Light penetration into tissue. (Courtesy ESC Medical, Inc.)

target vessel with dissipation of heat within the epidermis (Figures 2-15 and 2-16). The use of a cool gel on the skin surface further enhances epidermal cooling (Figures 2-12, *A*, and 2-17). The ability of the epidermis to cool more quickly than the target vessel is a function of the vessel size (Table 2-1 and Figure 2-18) When one combines the longer wavelength, longer pulse duration, larger spot size, and ability to deliver multiple pulses within the thermal relaxation time of the target vessel, treatment efficacy is enhanced (Figures 2-19 and 2-20). This

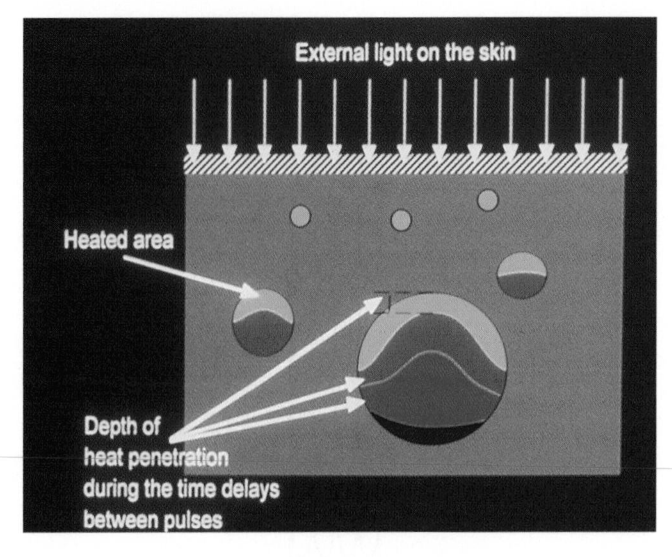

Figure 2-15 Diagram of effect of repetitive pulses of PhotoDerm VL on 2-mm vessel, 1 mm below epidermis. (Courtesy ESC Medical, Inc.)

advantage results from the average temperature increase being related to the wavelength delivered and the diameter of the target vessel (Figures 2-21 and 2-22).

Mechanized Scanning Devices

Because of the need to control thermal damage and scarring from continuous-output lasers, mechanized scanning devices have been developed to deliver the beam in patterned shuttered pulses or a patterned continuous beam. Laser pulses are placed in a pattern designed to minimize unwanted thermal damage.[32] Scanning devices can be used with the argon, copper vapor, tunable dye, or krypton lasers[33,80-82] (Figure 2-23). Another advantage of the scanner is minimizing the tedious performance of the tracing technique.

The computer-controlled programs are designed to deliver pulses automatically in precise geometric patterns. There are currently three models of scanners, the Scanall, Autolase, and Multiscan, and two models of automated handpieces, the Hexascan and CC-Scan. These systems have adjustable pulse durations that vary from 30 to 990 msec with a pulse interval of 50 msec. They deliver a 1-mm beam of light in geometric patterns that vary in size from 1 to 13 mm in dimension.

The most common of these systems (Hexascan) uses a 1-mm beam of light; an adjustable pulse duration of 30 to 990 msec, which varies according to the selected energy fluence; a pause interval of 100 msec; and different sizes of hexagonal grids 1, 3, 5, 9, 11, and 13 mm in diameter. The total time required to treat a 13-cm-diameter hexagon using 127 1-mm-diameter pulses is 20 seconds. The first model available was the Mark I. The newer Mark II releases laser light at 50 to 75 msec.

Metalaser Technologies (Pleasanton, Calif) manufactures the Autolase for use with its CVL. This scanner produces a hexagonal pattern 10 mm in diameter. Individual pulses are 400 μm in size and can be placed at three densities: 500, 750, or 1000 μm (between each spot). The largest grid accommodates 397 spots without overlapping. The scanning pattern is a linear raster (row-by-row) pattern with pulse durations varying from 50 to 500 msec in 10-msec increments and 8-msec pause

A

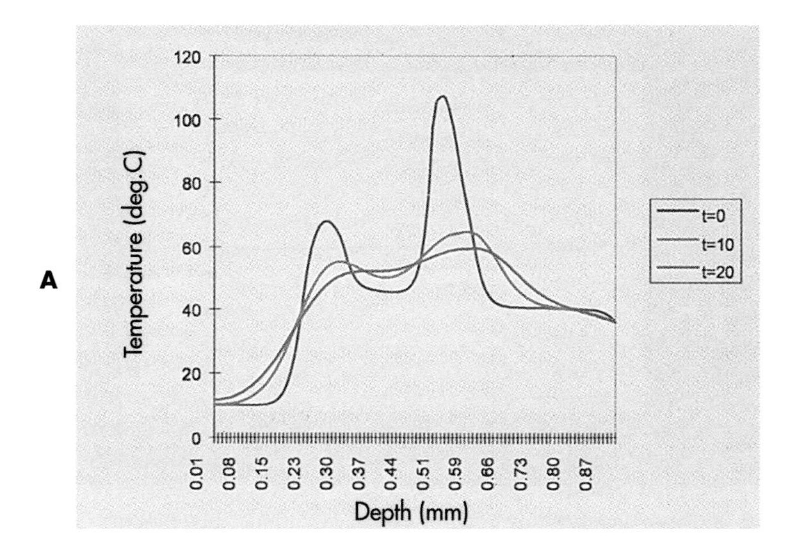

B

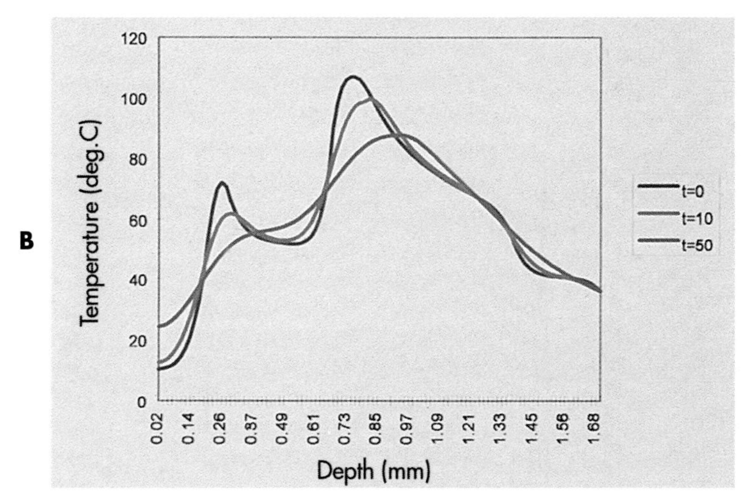

Figure 2-16 **A,** Vessel size is 0.2 mm in diameter. Double pulse with 550-nm cutoff filter is used with energy of 35 J/cm^2 given in 2.4-msec pulses. **B,** Vessel size is 1 mm in diameter. Double pulse is given with 590-nm cutoff filter and energy of 40 J/cm^2 given in 2.4- and 4.0-msec pulses. (Courtesy ESC Medical, Inc.)

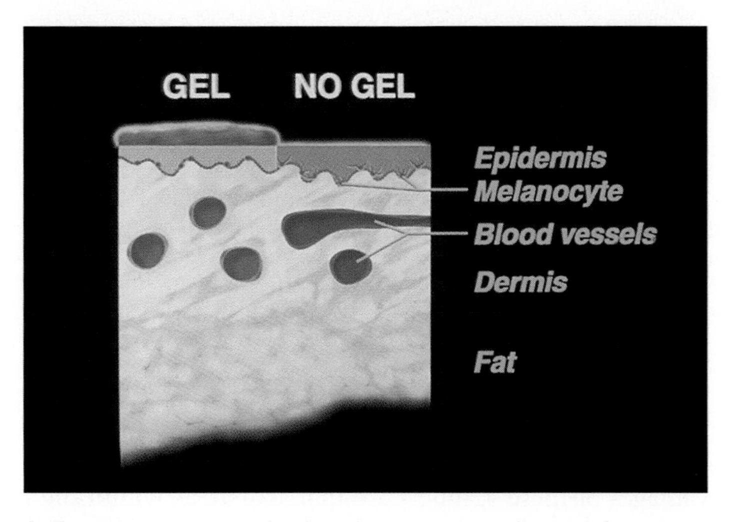

Figure 2-17 Application of cool gel to skin minimizes thermal damage and allows thermocoagulation to occur in vessel. Without gel, skin is thermally damaged before underlying vessel is thermocoagulated.

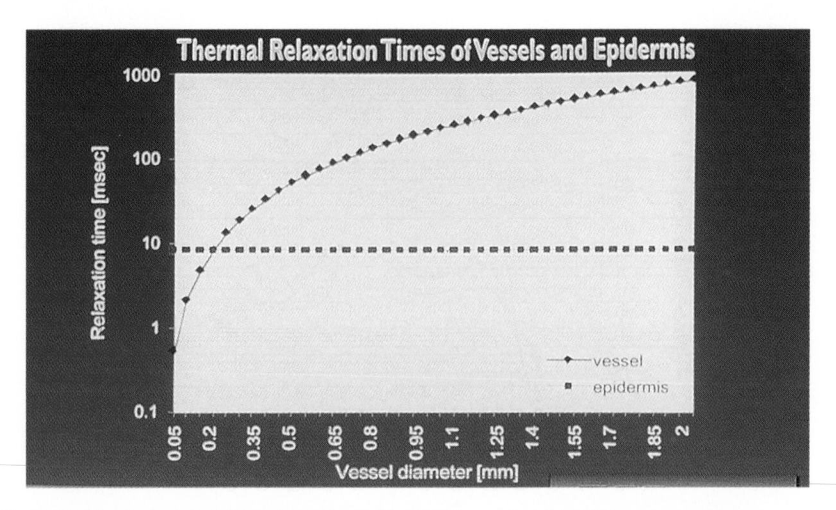

Figure 2-18 Thermal relaxation time of vessels and epidermis. (Courtesy ESC Medical, Inc.)

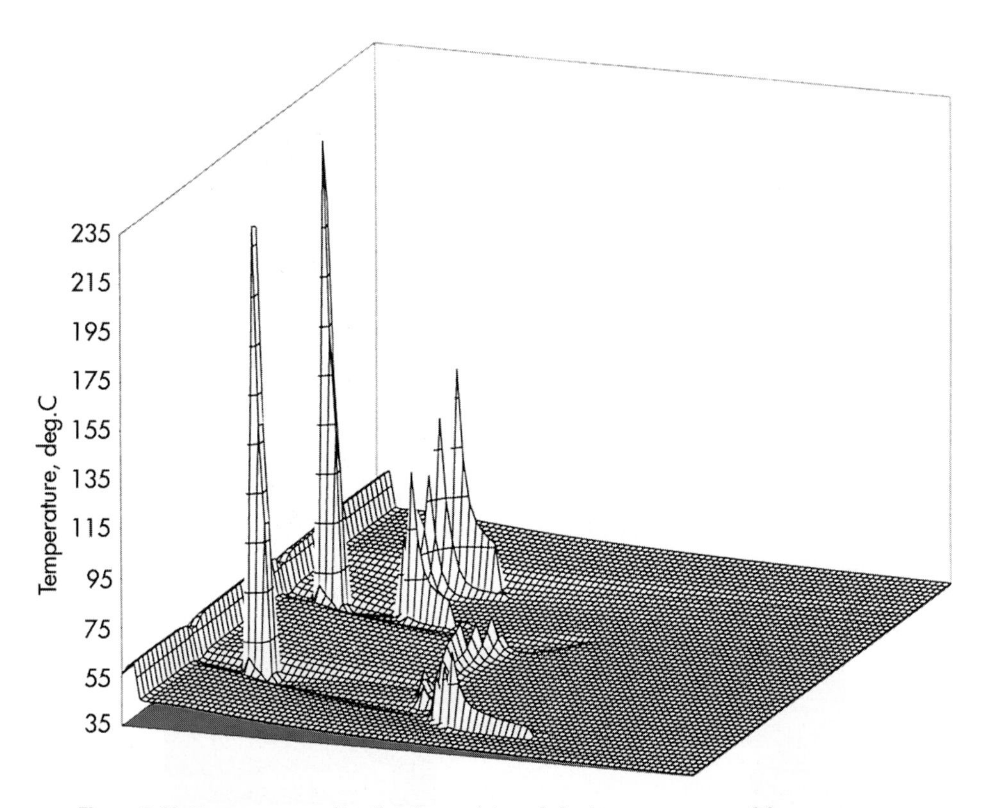

Figure 2-19 Temperature distribution achieved during treatment of four different-size vessels with FLPDL. Two 0.05-mm-diameter vessels are located at 0.4- and 0.5-mm depths. Large 1-mm-diameter vessel is located at depth of 1.1 mm. Medium 0.4-mm-diameter vessel is located at depth of 0.6 mm. Treatment conditions: 585-nm wavelength, 6-mm-diameter spot size, 10-J/cm^2 fluence. (From Goldman MP, Eckhouse S et al: *Dermatol Surg* 22:323, 1996.)

between each pulse. Three sizes of grids are available: 4, 7, or 10 mm. The most rapid time for maximally dense packing of the 10-mm grid is 23 sec.[83]

The disadvantages of these scanners are that skip areas within the grid pattern occur because of the limited gaussian curve of delivered laser fluence within the small spot size of the scan pulses. This is clinically apparent and requires retreatment

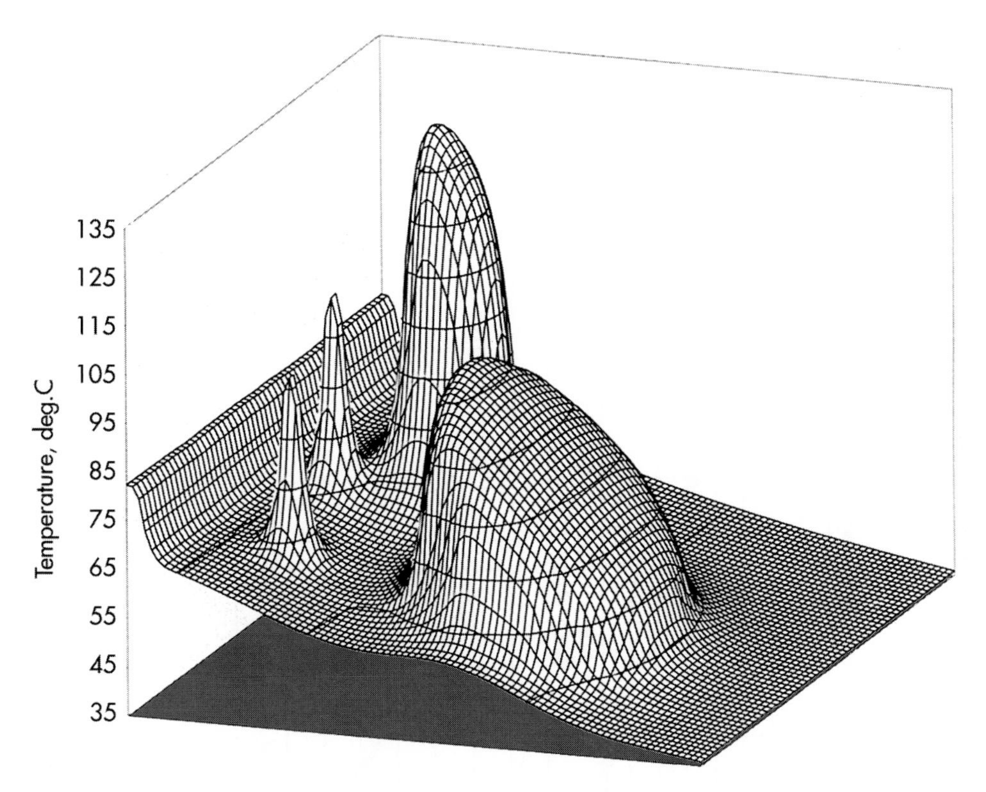

Figure 2-20 Temperature distribution achieved during treatment of four different-size vessels with FLPDL. Two 0.05-mm-diameter vessels are located at 0.4- and 0.5-mm depths. Large 1-mm-diameter vessel is located at depth of 1.1 mm. Medium 0.4-mm-diameter vessel is located at depth of 0.6 mm. Treatment conditions: 590-nm cutoff filter, double pulse of 5 and 10 msec, 150-msec delay between pulses, irradiance of 55 J/cm^2. (From Goldman MP, Eckhouse S et al: *Dermatol Surg* 22:323, 1996.)

of the same grid at another time with a slightly offset application. The edges of the grids are also difficult to overlap so that "freehand" tracing is necessary to fill in the gaps of persistent lesions. Finally, irregular lesions and borders of lesions require either treatment of normal skin or shielding of normal skin with wet gauze or laser-blocking material, which causes the "burst count" to be inaccurate.

LASER THEORY: SELECTIVE PHOTOTHERMOLYSIS

Histologic studies of PWSs have shown these lesions to have a characteristic architecture: generally 40% or more of the lesion is present in the upper 0.6 mm of the dermis. Vessel number is highest just beneath the epidermis, dropping quickly in number as depth increases[19] (Figure 2-24).

The argon laser, which has emission peaks at 488.8 and 512.5 nm, is thought to be effective in treating PWS because of selective absorption by the intravascular HbO_2 molecule (absorption peaks of 425, 542, and 577 nm), with conversion to heat. However, although the argon laser absorption in blood is about ten times greater than that of the surrounding dermis, the epidermis is by no means untouched by the argon laser. At this wavelength, epidermal melanin has an absorption coefficient only two times smaller than Hb. The addition of backscattering further increases epidermal absorption.[15] Therefore, at high energy densities, the argon laser is relatively nonspecific, resulting in coagulation necrosis of the epidermis and dermis to a depth of 0.4 ± 0.1 mm, which heals with dense fibrosis of the upper

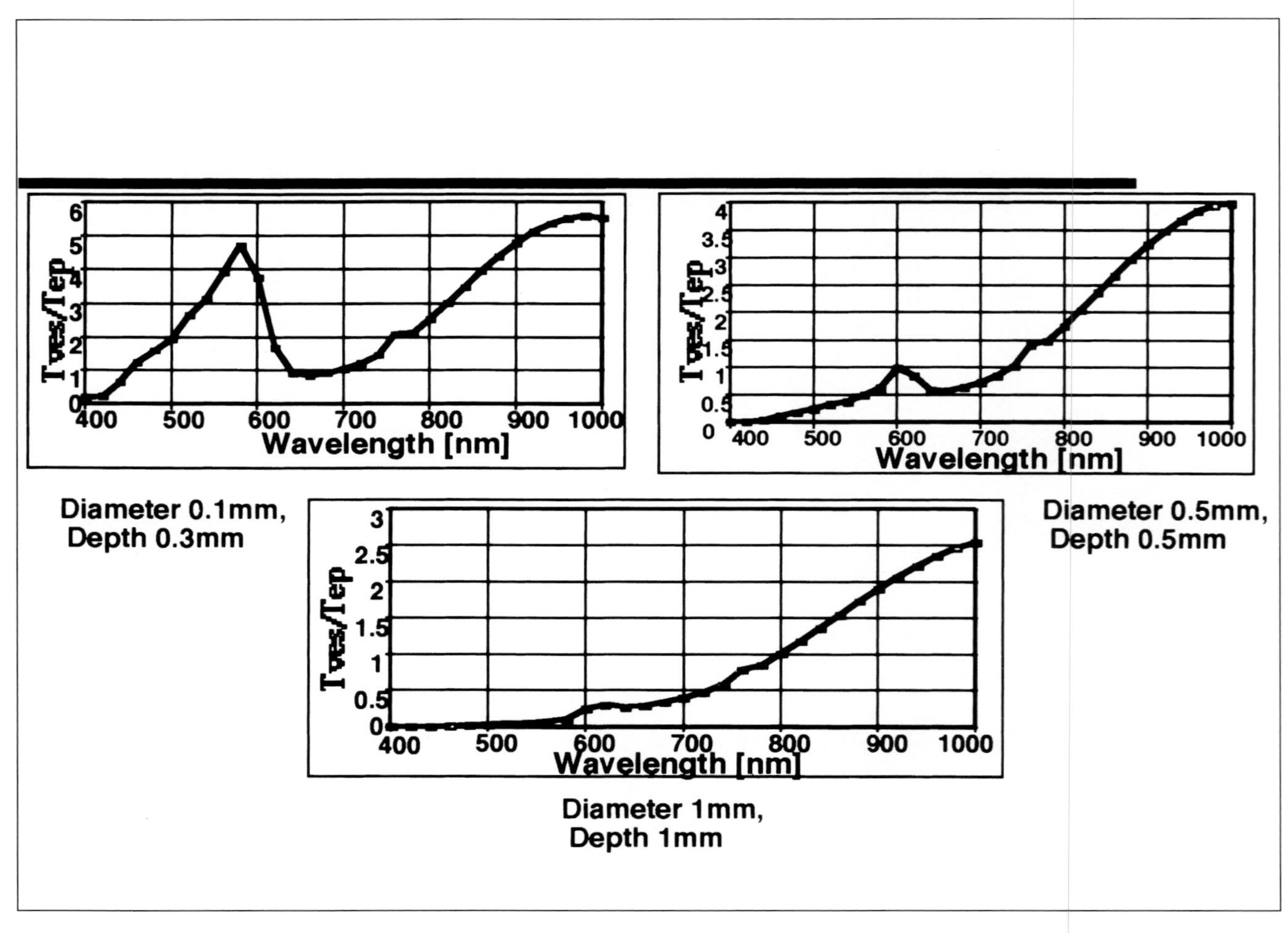

Figure 2-21 Ratio of vessel temperature to epidermis temperature versus wavelength, for three different depths and diameters. (Courtesy ESC Medical, Inc.)

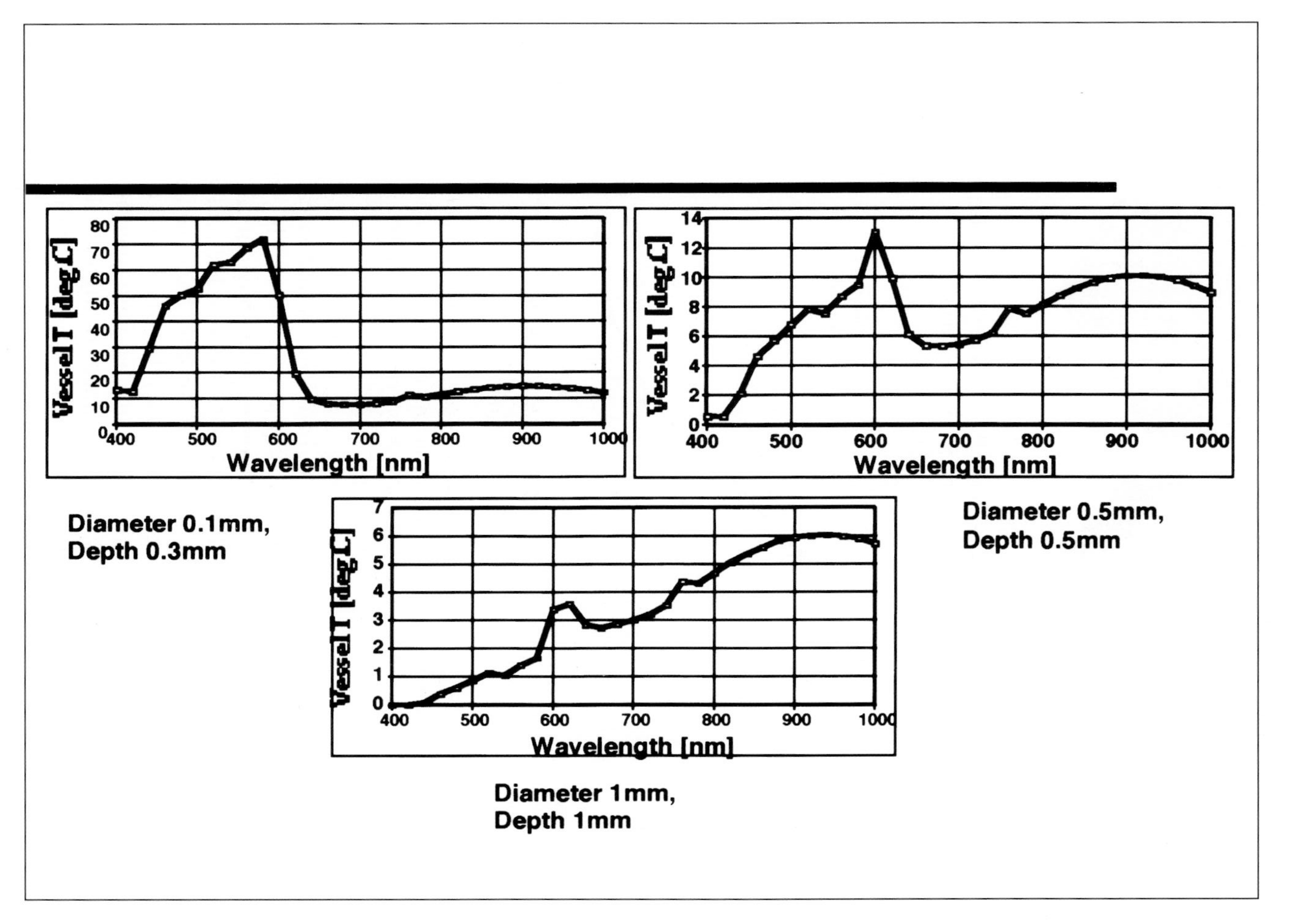

Figure 2-22 Average vessel temperature increase versus wavelength for three different depths and diameters at 10-J/cm² fluence. (Courtesy ESC Medical, Inc.)

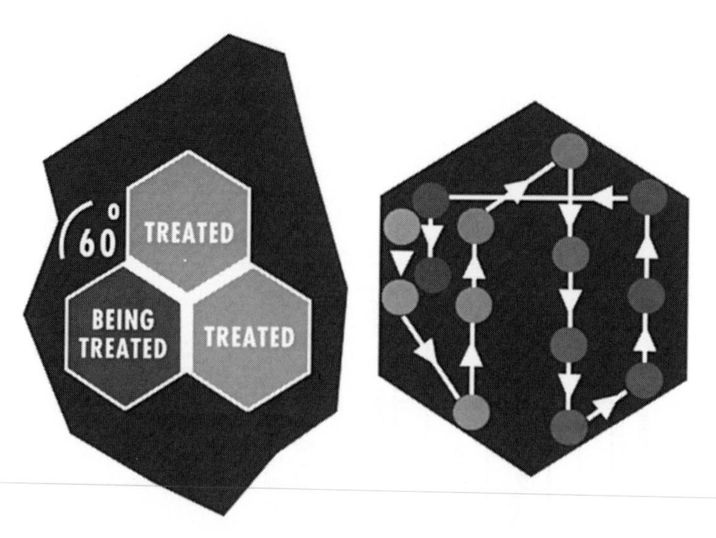

Figure 2-23 Diagram of scanning action of Hexascan device showing pulsing method. (Courtesy Lihtan Technologies, Inc, San Rafael, Calif.)

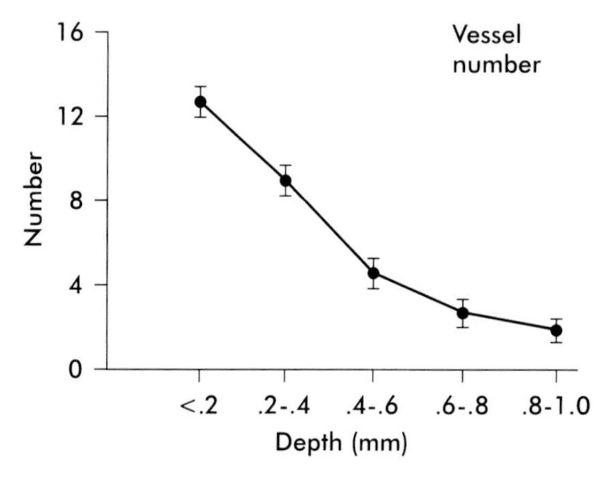

Figure 2-24 Correlation between number of vessels and dermal depth. In PWSs, vessel number is highest just beneath epidermis and decreases rapidly into dermis. (From Barsky S, Rosen S, Geer D et al: *J Invest Dermatol* 74:154, 1980.)

dermis.[15,36,84,85] Skin appendages, such as hair follicles and sweat and sebaceous glands, are relatively less damaged and help to reconstitute the epidermis, which may minimize scarring[86] (Figure 2-25). One study has shown more selective vascular photocoagulation at treatment fluences of 15 J/cm^2 or less and nonspecific thermal changes occurring at 45 J/cm^2 or more.[87] Another study confirms the relative vascular selectivity of the argon laser and suggests that in addition to the major nonspecific component of argon laser therapy, a smaller, more specific zone of damage exists where the vascular target is the determinant of injury.[88] However, a typical 0.2-sec exposure of 1.0 W with a spot size of 1 mm (2.5 J/cm^2) causes extensive thermal damage to the epidermis and dermis that may lead to disturbed wound healing and scarring.[89] Vessel-specific thermal damage has also been demonstrated with histologic activity of cellular enzyme activity.[90] Finally, vessels larger than 0.5 mm in diameter and those located deeper than 1.0 to 1.5 mm in the dermis are not photocoagulated by this laser unless very high fluences are used that would nonselectively destroy the overlying epidermis and perivascular tissues.[86,91]

In summary, the nonspecific damage from argon laser treatment is a consequence of two factors: direct and undesired absorption by other chromophores, pri-

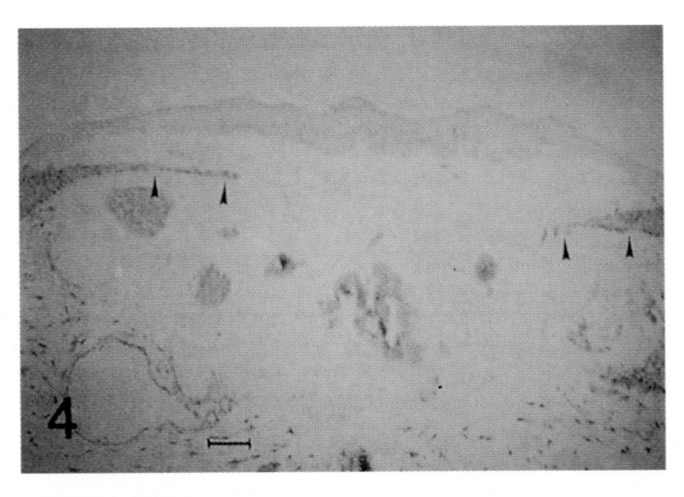

Figure 2-25 PWS 10 minutes after argon laser treatment. Arc-shaped, unstained, Nitroblue tetrazolium chloride–negative area of coagulation necrosis is present. Thermal damage is sharply demarcated from viable (blue-stained) surrounding tissues. This border runs straight through all dermal structures. (Bar = 100 μm.) (From Neumann RA, Knobler RM, Pieczkowski F et al: *J Am Acad Dermatol* 25:991, 1991.)

marily melanin, and diffusion of heat from the absorbing chromophore, HbO_2, to the surrounding dermis. The use of a more selective wavelength (577 nm) solves only one of these problems. The second problem of thermal diffusion is related to pulse duration and accumulation of undesired heat during the laser pulse.

Importance of Pulse Duration

To limit thermal damage to the intended target, the pulse duration must be shorter than the thermal relaxation time of the target tissue (Tables 2-1 and 2-3). The *thermal relaxation time* of tissue is defined as the time necessary for target tissue to cool down by 50% through transfer of its heat to surrounding tissue through thermal diffusion. If a targeted tissue can be heated sufficiently to affect it irreversibly before its surrounding tissue is damaged by thermal diffusion, selective photocoagulation occurs.[37,38]

For vascular lesions, the exposure time should be long enough to conduct heat from the RBC-filled lumen to the entire blood vessel wall (Figure 2-26). An additional consideration occurs with treating venulectases. Merely coagulating the endothelium is insufficient because a direct correlation exists between permanent eradication of a vein and depth of vessel wall injury. Greater success is expected as the depth of mural damage progresses from the endothelial cell layer, intima, and media to the adventitia.[92-95] Pickering et al[96] have demonstrated that exposure times of 0.1 to 0.3 msec are necessary to damage irreversibly 100-μm-diameter vessels with a wall thickness of 3 to 6 μm. The thermal relaxation time of vessels 10 to 50 μm in diameter is 0.1 to 10 msec, averaging 1.2 msec.[37,38] However, pulse durations less than 20 μsec result in vessel rupture and hemorrhage secondary to RBC explosion.[97] This will lead to hemosiderin pigmentation. Therefore, with single laser pulses, the therapeutic window is small. This argues for the development of a wider single pulse or a multipulsed laser that is able to transfer absorbed heat to the endothelium without causing its rupture (Figure 2-20). In addition, multiple pulses should result in uniform heat transfer around the entire vessel diameter (top and bottom), enhancing therapeutic efficacy (Figure 2-15).

Increasing the pulse duration of the standard FLPDL from 450 to 750 μsec to 1.5 msec initially produced conflicting results. Garden et al[98] reported insignificant

Table 2-3
Thermal relaxation time *(Tr)* of laser targets

Target	Diameter (μm, approx)	*Tr*
Epidermis	60	2 msec
Basal layer	20	400 μsec
Melanosome	1	0.2 μsec
Erythrocyte	5	5 μsec

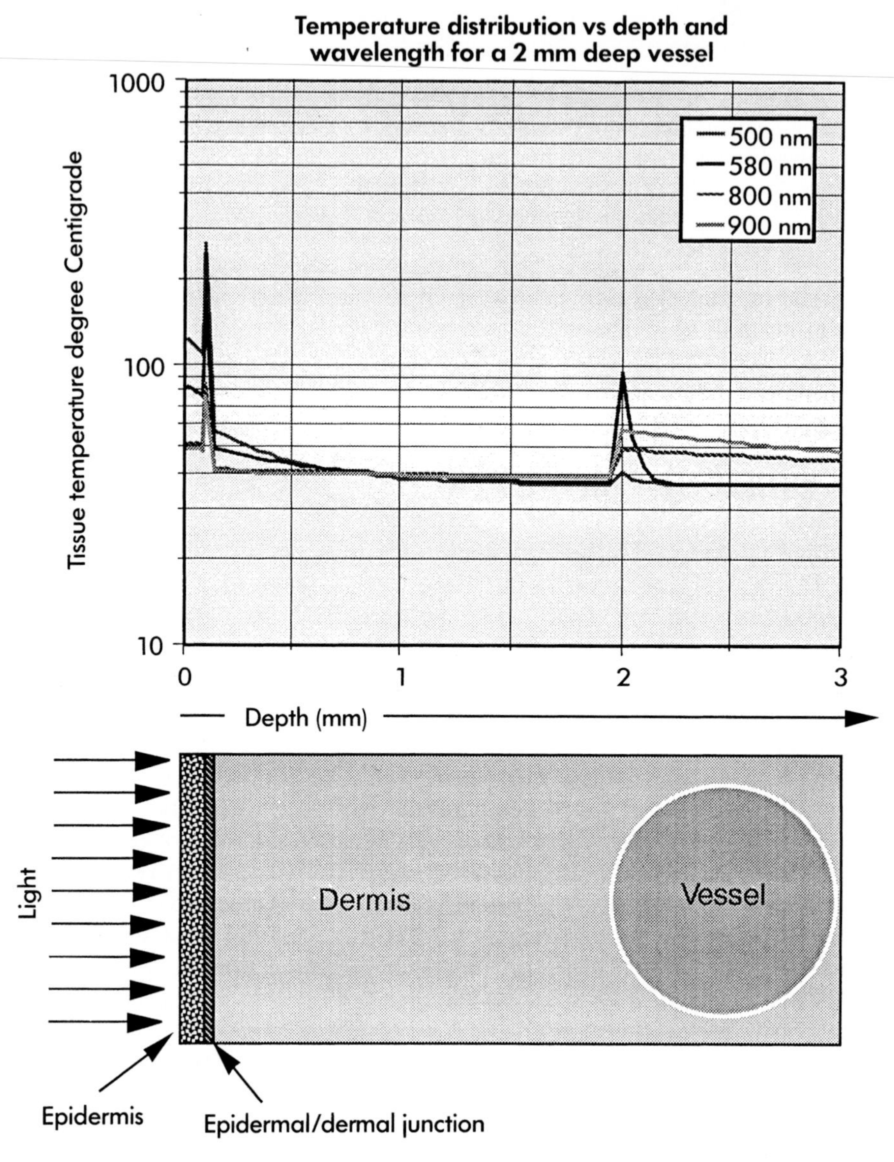

Figure 2-26 Temperature distribution across skin and blood vessel, assuming 2-mm-deep, 1-mm-diameter vessel and 10-J/cm² fluence at four different wavelengths. Calculation takes into account scattering effects in epidermis and dermis and fluence enhancement from scattering. Note very high temperature on skin surface and at epidermal/dermal junction for shorter wavelengths. Note also very shallow depth of penetration in vessel at 500-nm and 580-nm wavelengths. (Courtesy Shimon Eckhouse, PhD, Newton, Mass.)

differences in clearance in 30 patients with PWS treated at 585 nm with a 450-μsec versus a 750-μsec pulse. When they compared the pulse duration in 26 patients, the difference between 750 μsec and 1.5 msec was insignificant. However, Kauvar[99] using an FLPDL with both a longer pulse width (1.5 msec) and a higher wavelength and (595 nm) in the treatment of 15 PWSs, found enhanced efficacy with these parameters. An additional variable in Kauvar's study was the change in spot size diameter between the long and short pulses. Kauvar compared treatment with a standard FLPDL at 5 J/cm^2 using a 10-mm-diameter spot size to a 1.5-msec FLPDL at 595 nm with a 7-mm-diameter spot size at 8 to 10 J/cm^2. Kauvar found decreased purpura and a 10% to 40% increase in fading for all lesions except those on the legs, which did not respond. Pain increased with the latter parameters, and crusting, edema, vesiculation, hyperpigmentation, and hypopigmentation occurred when fluences of 12 to 14 J/cm^2 were used. These adverse effects decreased with a fluence of 8 to 10 J/cm^2. Kauvar also found that all adverse events were increased when a 600-nm wavelength was used and speculated that backscattering into the epidermis resulting from less efficient absorption by vascular targets at this increased wavelength was the cause. Kauvar[99] therefore recommends that all adult PWSs be treated with the 1.5-msec, 595-nm FLPDL with a 7-mm-diameter spot size at fluences of 8 to 10 J/cm^2.

Importance of Wavelength

The theory of selective photothermolysis is the basis for the FLPDL with a wavelength of 585 nm and a pulse duration of 450 μsec. Initial studies on normal skin confirmed the validity of this theory and stressed the importance of pulse duration. Subsequent clinical studies confirmed the efficacy of this laser for treatment of both children and adults. Although the original FLPDL wavelength was set at 577 nm, it was later changed to 585 nm to increase penetration into the dermis without loss of vascular specificity.[100] Although blood absorbs 585-nm light about one-half as efficiently as it absorbs 577-nm light,[101] 585-nm light will coagulate larger vessels better than 577-nm light at a given depth because of deeper penetration of laser energy. In addition, deeper vessels absorb laser energy at longer wavelengths[102] (Figure 2-22). Blood composes approximately 5% to 10% by volume of an average PWS.[103] This explains the superiority of 585 nm over 577 nm in the treatment of PWSs.

Tan et al[104] cleared PWSs in nine adults previously treated without clearance at 577 nm when the FLPDL wavelength was increased to 585 nm.[135] Histologic examination demonstrated laser penetration into the subcutaneous fat at 585 nm, which implied that irreversible vascular damage must occur to a depth greater than 1 mm to treat the PWS fully. This clinicohistologic determination correlates with mathematic models.[105]

The tissue depth to which a given fluence will coagulate the target vessel depends largely on the blood volume of vessels above the target vessels. Superficial vessels containing blood will absorb laser light before it reaches deeper target vessels. This explains why multiple treatments are necessary for complete PWS resolution. Ideally the first treatment should be at 577 nm to produce the most specific fluence absorption by HbO_2. Additional treatments could then be at higher wavelengths so that deeper penetration of laser energy would occur without reduction of fluence by the already coagulated, more superficially located ectatic vessels. Pickering and van Gemert[102] have found that 590 nm produces deeper vascular damage than 577 nm in PWSs with more than 10% dermal blood volume. However, Garden and Bakus[106] found no statistical difference in treating 30 PWS patients with wavelengths varying among 577, 583, 588, and 593 nm. Some patients responded best to one wavelength and some to other wavelengths. This variable effect may be caused by the nonuniformity of PWSs. As previously mentioned, increasing both the wavelength and the pulse duration has been shown to result in increased efficacy.

The FLPDL effect at 577 or 585 nm is unique because it selectively destroys ectatic PWS vessels. With time, histologically normal-appearing dermal capillary blood vessels grow into the area of the destroyed lesion.[107] Elimination of abnormal ectatic vessels may also promote normalization of other dermal cells, such as mast cells and perivascular neurons.

As mentioned previously, because blood also has an absorption peak at 532 nm, the fd Nd:YAG lasers are also effective in treating superficial vascular lesions. However, to obtain a degree of selectivity over the high melanin absorption at 532 nm and to penetrate to clinically useful depths, cooling the overlying epidermis is important.

Effect of Epidermal Cooling

Cooling the epidermis has been previously shown with the argon laser to increase the depth of penetration of effective thermocoagulation.[108,109] Cooling the epidermis overlying a leg telangiectasia with an ice water–cooled device through which an argon or argon dye, 577-nm or 585-nm laser is used also has been shown to enhance therapeutic success, with a decreased incidence of nonspecific adverse sequelae.[110] This same effect has also been demonstrated with the FLPDL.[111] Reasons for the increased efficacy and decreased incidence of adverse sequelae have been presumed to be secondary to decreased epidermal heating not only from the initial impact of laser fluence, but also from the backscattered light, which is also absorbed.

Adrian[112] has demonstrated marked improvement in 7 of 10 patients with PWS treated with ice cooling of the epidermis for 30 sec before FLPDL treatment. These patients had been previously treated 7 to 47 times with the FLPDL without further improvement. Addition of the pretreatment epidermal cooling allowed for treatment to occur at higher energy fluences (9-10 J/cm² versus 6-7 J/cm² without cooling) without increasing the incidence of scarring or pigmentary changes.

The Beckman Laser Institute has developed a method of delivering a cryogen spurt of tetrafluorethane (boiling point −26.2° C) just before laser impact. Skin surface temperature was reduced by as much as 40° C with a 20- to 80-msec cryogen spurt after FLPDL exposure. This allows for fluences of 10 J/cm² to be delivered without adverse epidermal effect. This has been demonstrated to increase efficacy, allow deeper laser penetration, and minimize treatment pain.[111, 113]

Ideally the duration of the cryogen spurt should be determined for each patient based on the PWS vessel depth distribution. The time for the cold front produced by the cryogen spray to reach the most superficial layer of blood vessels is about 100 msec. Therefore cryogen spurt durations of 40 msec were demonstrated to permit selective photothermolysis of these ectatic vessels.

Precooling the skin should also offset the absorption of laser energy, with resulting skin heating in darkly pigmented races. In one study, patients with skin types III and IV had improvement in pain ratings when cooling was used compared with the FLPDL alone.[114]

As of 1998, the cryogen spray cooling device is only approved by the U.S. Food and Drug Administration (FDA) for pain relief. This has been the only clearly established benefit. Timing the spray so that the dermal vessels are not cooled as well has proved to be difficult. When cooling at this level is achieved, a higher fluence is needed to produce the same clinical effect as that produced without cooling. Thus improved efficacy has not been clearly established.

The effect of epidermal cooling to enhance clinical efficacy has been shared by other therapeutic modalities, particularly the pulsed-light PhotoDerm VL, Versapulse 532-nm long-pulsed Nd:YAG system described later in this chapter, and the Epilyte hair removal systems (ESC Medical, Inc., Needham, Mass), as well as long-pulsed ruby laser hair removal systems described in later chapters.

Adverse Effects of Flashlamp-pumped Pulsed Dye Laser

Although the superiority of the FLPDL over CO_2 and argon lasers is clearly established with respect to safety and efficacy in treating vascular lesions, adverse effects can occur. Hypopigmentation can occur in treated areas in dark-skinned patients and was found in 3.2% of patients in one study, who were Hispanic or Middle Eastern.[115] Persistent hypopigmentation is more common on the neck, legs, and chest (Figure 2-27). Persistent hyperpigmentation may also occur with premature sun exposure on facial areas and after treatment of vascular lesions on the leg.

Although rare, hypertrophic scarring has been reported with high laser fluences and when treating lesions on the neck, arms, or shoulder.[35,115] Another report described "isolated, superficial, depressed scars" in 2 of 35 children treated, reportedly in areas traumatized within 24 hours after laser treatment.[39] Two of 92 adults with facial telangiectasia developed dermal atrophy with normal skin texture on the nose, nasolabial folds, and malar regions that lasted at least 6 months. These areas were treated with a 1-mm spot diameter at a fluence of 7 J/cm^2.[116] A persistent hypertrophic scar was also reported in a 27-year-old man with a PWS of the anterior chest at a fluence of 7 J/cm^2.[117] There was no history of trauma or laser malfunction. We have seen two patients with localized hypertrophic scars treated at 7.5 to 8.0 J/cm^2 on the anterior chest and shoulder (Figure 2-28). The patient with the shoulder lesion reported trauma to the treated area within 24 hours of treatment. Laser fluence, lesion location, and posttreatment care are important factors that may contribute to the risk of scarring when using the FLPDL.

Two cases of transient cutaneous pustulosis have been reported to develop after treatment with the FLPDL. No predisposing factors existed to explain this development. Energy fluences were within standard protocols (6.5-7.0 J/cm^2). All cultures for bacteria, fungi, and mycobacteria were negative. Biopsy demonstrated epidermal necrosis with a perivascular lymphohistiocytic infiltrate. The pustules appeared after each of three treatments.[118] The authors suspected excessive epidermal burning from overlapping of pulses or a heightened sensitivity of the patient's skin to thermal injury.

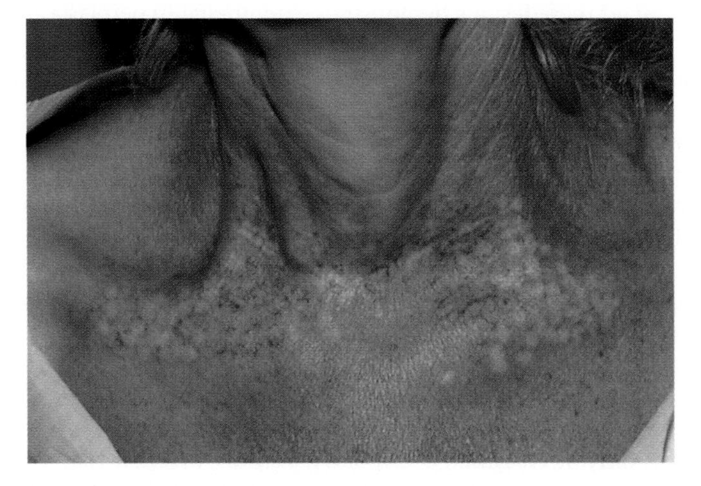

Figure 2-27 A 48-year-old woman 20 years after radiation therapy for thyroid tumor with development of telangiectasia. Clinical appearance 6 months after treatment with FLPDL at 7 J/cm^2. Hypopigmented macules took approximately 18 months for complete resolution.

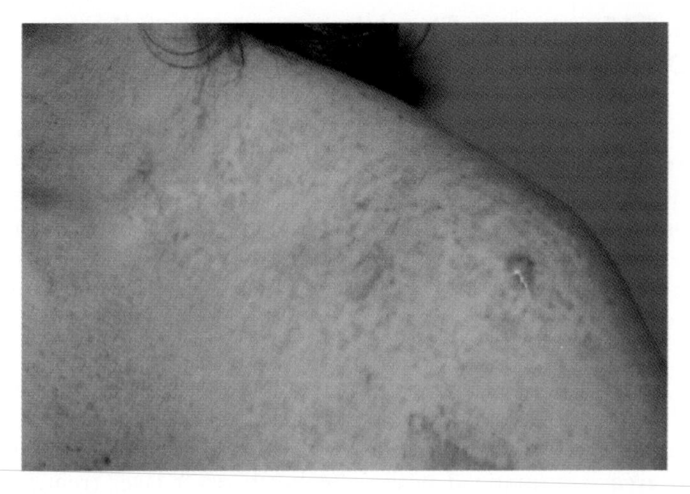

Figure 2-28 A 28-year-old woman with extensive PWSs over left side of body. Clinical appearance of hypertrophic scar on left deltoid area appearing 8 weeks after third treatment with FLPDL at energy of 7.5 J/cm². Patient reported that area blistered and scabbed from trauma approximately 2 days after laser treatment.

CLASSIFICATION OF VASCULAR LESIONS

As emphasized by Mulliken,[119] much confusion and inconsistency surround the terminology of vascular lesions. Many descriptive terms, such as "strawberry patch," "port-wine stain," "salmon patch," and "cherry angioma," are used and are random vernacular terms that defy classification. In addition, the same terms are often used to describe two very different lesions, such as "strawberry hemangioma" and "port-wine hemangioma." Adding to the confusion are hybrid words, such as "lymphangiohemangioma," and Latin terminology, such as "naevus maternus."[119] Often the same name is given to different lesions by different specialties, thereby confusing both interspecialty communication and analysis of reports on pathophysiology and treatment.

Mulliken[119] has proposed a standardized terminology and classification based on cell kinetics, with the following three major categories of lesions:

1. Hemangiomas: all these lesions demonstrate endothelial hyperplasia.
2. Malformations: all these lesions demonstrate normal endothelial turnover.
3. Ectasias: all these lesions have normal endothelial turnover but also vascular dilatation.

Hemangiomas are vascular neoplasms that enlarge by rapid cellular proliferation. They have a proliferative phase and an involutional phase, during which the lesion shrinks and vascular parenchyma is replaced with fibrous tissue. Hemangiomas may be superficial (capillary), deep (cavernous, venous), or both superficial and deep (capillary-cavernous). Whether superficial or deep, the histologic appearance is consistent throughout, and involution proceeds at the same rate throughout. The clinical appearance (color and texture) reflects the depth of the lesion and the degree of proliferation or involution.

A *pyogenic granuloma* is an acquired vascular neoplasm with a proliferative endothelium. These lesions are thought to be reactive in nature.

Malformations may be classified as capillary, venous, arterial, lymphatic, or a combination thereof, according to the type of vessels involved (Box 2-1). They represent an abnormality of morphogenesis comprised of vascular channel abnormalities. These lesions are present at birth and grow commensurate with the child. Certain types, although congenital, may not become visible or symptomatic until adoles-

Box 2-1 Classification of vascular malformations

Capillary Malformation (CM)
Port-wine stain
  Sturge-Weber syndrome
Telangiectasia

Lymphatic Malformation (LM)
Localized
Diffuse

Venous Malformation (VM)
Localized
Diffuse

Arterial Malformation (AM)
Bonnet-Dechaume-Blanc syndrome
Cobb syndrome

Complex-Combined Malformation
Capillary-lymphatic malformation (CLM)
  Circumscribed
  Angiokeratomas
Regional
  Klippel-Trenaunay syndrome (CLM, VM)
  Parkes-Weber syndrome (CLM, VM, AM)
Diffuse
  Maffucci syndrome (LM, VM, enchondromas)
  Solomon syndrome (CM, VM, intracranial AM, epidermal nevi, osseous defects, tumors)
  Riley-Smith syndrome (LM, VM, macrocephaly, pseudopapilledema)
  Bannayan syndrome (AM, LM, VM, macrocephaly, lipomas)
  Proteus syndrome (CM, VM, macrodactyly, hemihypertrophy, lipomas, pigmented nevi, scoliosis)

Modified from Mulliken JB: The classification of vascular birthmarks. In Tan OT, editor: *Management and treatment of benign cutaneous lesions,* Philadelphia, 1992, Lea & Febiger.

cence or adulthood. Therefore, in this situation they may appear to be "acquired."[120] The capillary and venous malformations are low-flow lesions, whereas lymphatic and arterial lesions are high-flow lesions. A port-wine stain is more properly called a *capillary malformation.* These lesions are stable in size, but their natural history is to thicken gradually and develop nodularity from progressive vessel ectasia in the third to fourth decades of life.[119]

Of the *ectasias,* the most common lesions are those now called "cherry angioma," "spider angioma," and "angioma serpiginosum." These lesions are not tumors but rather vascular anomalies.

PORT-WINE STAIN (CAPILLARY MALFORMATION)

Port-wine stains (PWSs) occur in 0.3% to 0.5% of newborns[121,122] and represent a congenital malformation of the superficial dermal capillaries. They should not be confused with the common pink patches known as "nevus flammeus neonatorum," "angel's kiss," "stork bite," or "salmon patch." These "stains" fade within the first year of life in 50% of patients. A midline PWS-appearing lesion may represent a capillary malformation that clears quickly with one or two treatments and thus is not typical of the more ectatic and venular PWS (Figure 2-29). These midline lesions may represent a maturation delay in autonomic innervation because up to 60% of lesions resolve spontaneously.[123] A butterfly-shaped mark that occurs on the sacrum is less common than a facial or nuchal nevus flammeus and tends to resolve more slowly. These lesions are not associated with vascular malformations.[124]

PWSs can be differentiated by their large size and appearance beyond the glabellar area or nape of the neck. Most PWSs are superficial, with a mean vessel depth of 0.46 mm.[19] The lesion is first present as a relatively sharply marginated pink patch, most often involving the head and neck in 90% of patients, especially in the areas of the first and second trigeminal nerves.[121,122]

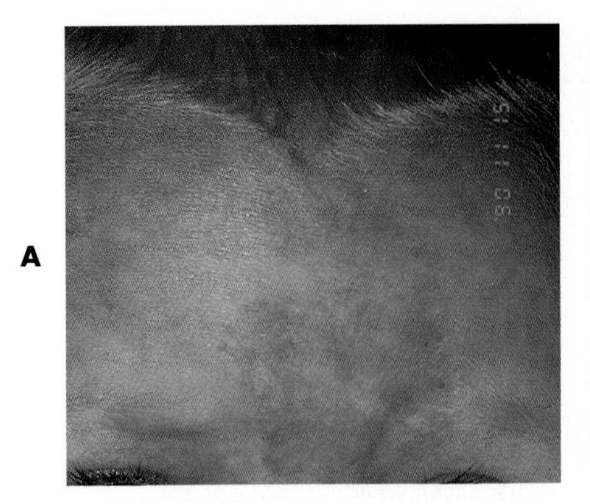

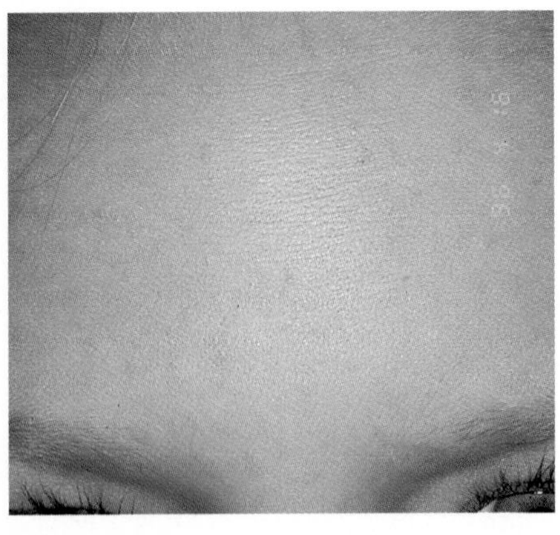

Figure 2-29 **A,** Four-month-old girl with urticaria pigmentosa and midline PWS before treatment. **B,** Six and one-half years after single treatment with FLPDL at 5.5 J/cm² using 5-mm-diameter spot size, lesions show 100% clearance without adverse sequelae and no evidence of recurrence.

Videomicroscopy has demonstrated two patterns of vascular abnormality: *type 1* consists of tortuous, superficial, dilated capillary loops (blobs), and *type 2* consists of dilated ectatic vessels in the superficial horizontal vascular plexus (rings)[125] (Figures 2-30 and 2-31). Two groups of PWS patients, 15 before treatment and 13 who had a poor response to FLPDL treatment, were evaluated with transcutaneous videomicroscopy. All patients with type 1 vascularity demonstrated excellent response to FLPDL treatment. Patients who were poor responders to FLPDL treatment had type 2 vascularity. Therefore, because type 2 PWS lesions are more deeply situated and consist of freely anastomosing dilated vessels of the superficial horizontal vascular plexus, they respond poorly to lasers, which only thermocoagulate superficial small vessels. Videomicroscopy may allow the physician to choose the most appropriate laser or pulsed light source for treatment of PWS.

Adverse Medical Effects

In addition to their abnormal cosmetic appearance, PWSs may be associated with medical problem, the most common and serious being glaucoma and less common and serious being inflammation. Glaucoma occurs in approximately 45% of patients with a PWS involving both the ophthalmic (V_1) and maxillary (V_2) divisions of the trigeminal nerve.[126] The most well-known condition is the *Sturge-Weber syndrome,* which consists of a PWS involving the first branch of the trigeminal nerve, a high incidence of glaucoma of the ipsilateral eye (especially if the upper lid is involved), angioma of the lids, choroidal hemangiomas (in up to 40% of patients),[127] calcification and vascular anomalies of the brain with associated seizure disorders, and in some cases mental retardation.[126,128,129] In 70% to 80% of patients with glaucoma,

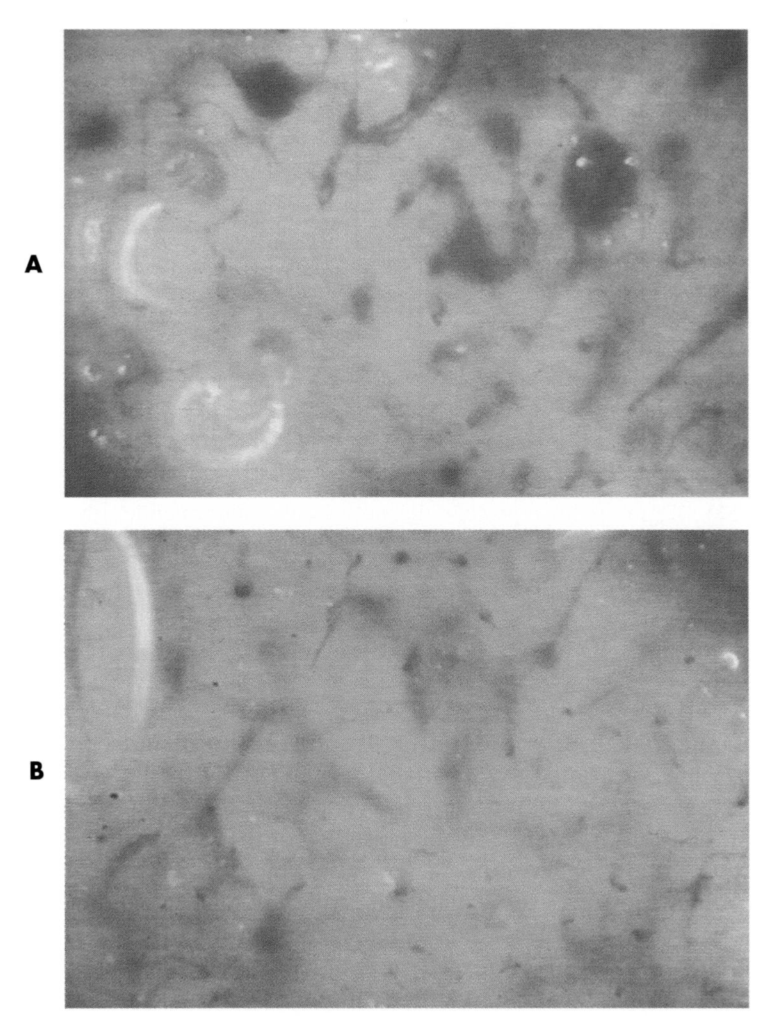

Figure 2-30 A, Results of transcutaneous videomicroscopy of patient with PWS showing type 1 blob abnormalities. (×200.) **B,** Results of transcutaneous videomicroscopy of patient with PWS showing type 2 ring abnormalities. Note small, fine capillary dots that are capillary loops in normal dermal papillae. Dilated vessels of horizontal plexus lie in a deeper plane. (×200.) (From Motley RJ, Lanigan SW, Katugampola GA: *Arch Dermatol* 133:921, 1997.)

Sturge-Weber syndrome presents as *buphthalmos,* a grossly enlarged eye soon after birth. The remaining patients develop glaucoma in childhood, with 44% diagnosed after 4 years of age.[130] Therefore repeated intraocular pressures should be taken every 3 to 4 months if glaucoma is not present initially.

The extent of the PWS does not usually correlate with neurologic disease.[131] However patients with bilateral PWS have a greater likelihood of neurologic involvement with an earlier onset of seizures.[128,132] Epileptic seizures occur in 72% of SturgeWeber patients with unilateral lesions and 93% of patients with bihemispheric involvement.[127,128] Mental retardation occurs in up to 30% of Sturge-Weber patients, with a 92% incidence of retardation in patients with bilateral lesions.[128] Recommended neurologic tests include electroencephalography and functional testing with positron emission tomography (PET), single-photon emission computed tomography (SPECT), computed tomography (CT) of cranium, or magnetic resonance imaging (MRI).[133]

Other congenital syndromes include the Klippel-Trenaunay and Klippel-Trenaunay-Weber syndromes (PWS with associated varicose vein and hypertrophy

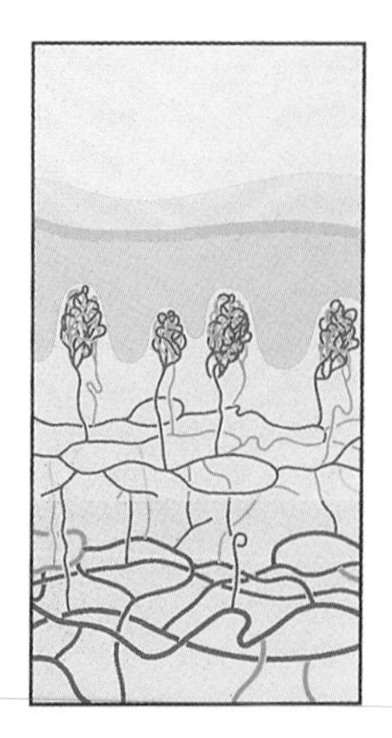
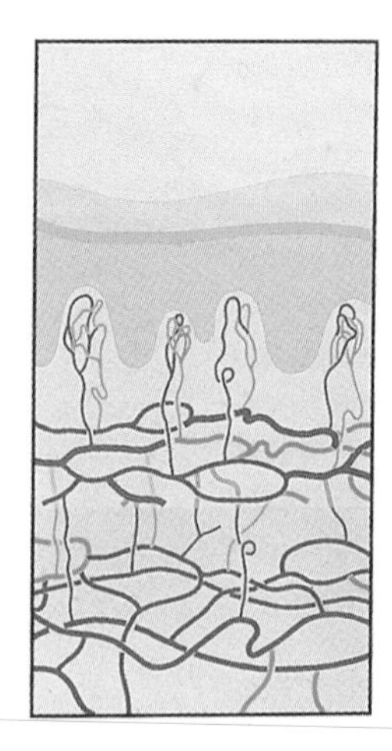

Figure 2-31 Diagrammatic representations of vascular abnormalities found with videomicroscopy. *Left,* Tortuous, dilated papillary tip vessels. *Right,* Dilated vessels of superficial horizontal vascular plexus. Note that type 1 abnormality (*left*) presents a superficial target with limited blood supply. Type 2 abnormality (*right*) is more deeply situated, and vessels anastomose freely. (From Motley RJ, Lanigan SW, Katugampola GA: *Arch Dermatol* 133:921, 1997.)

of skeletal tissue[134] with or without arteriovenous malformations [AVMs], respectively) and Cobb syndrome (PWS with underlying AVM of the spinal cord).[135] A PWS may be associated with an underlying venous malformation or occasionally an arterial malformation or AVM,[119] so the existence of these associated lesions should not cause confusion in diagnosis.

Various support groups are available for children with congenital vascular abnormalities and their families. The Sturge-Weber Foundation (PO Box 460931, Aurora, CO 80046) publishes an excellent booklet for children that clearly explains the syndrome as well as multiple treatment options. The Klippel-Trenaunay Support Group (4610 Wooddale Ave., Edina, MN 55424) publishes a useful quarterly newsletter and holds support group and educational meetings for the public. The National Congenital Port-Wine Stain Foundation (125 E. 63rd St., New York, NY 10021) also provides information and support to patients and families of children with PWSs. Patients and parents should be encouraged to use these resources.

PWSs can also present with an inflammatory component consisting of scaling, excoriations, oozing, and crusting, resembling a dermatitis.[136] PWS with this secondary inflammation has been reported in lesions on the nuchal and occipital areas. Treatment with topical steroids helps decrease the inflammation, but the FLPDL is curative after one treatment.

The natural history of a PWS is that the vessels become progressively ectatic over time.[10,19] This results in gradual darkening, thickening, and development of nodularity (Figure 2-32). One study found that two thirds of patients develop hypertrophy and nodularity by age 46, with a mean age of 37 years for hypertrophy.[137] Rarely, spontaneous improvement may occur,[138] possibly during the first 3 years of life.

Giant proliferative hemangiomas may also arise in PWSs and can develop without any prior history of trauma.[139]

Psychologic Impact

In addition to lesion characteristics that may cause bleeding and produce physical deformity, a PWS carries a definite risk for lasting detrimental effects on a child's psychologic, social, interpersonal, and cognitive development.[140-142] The exact age

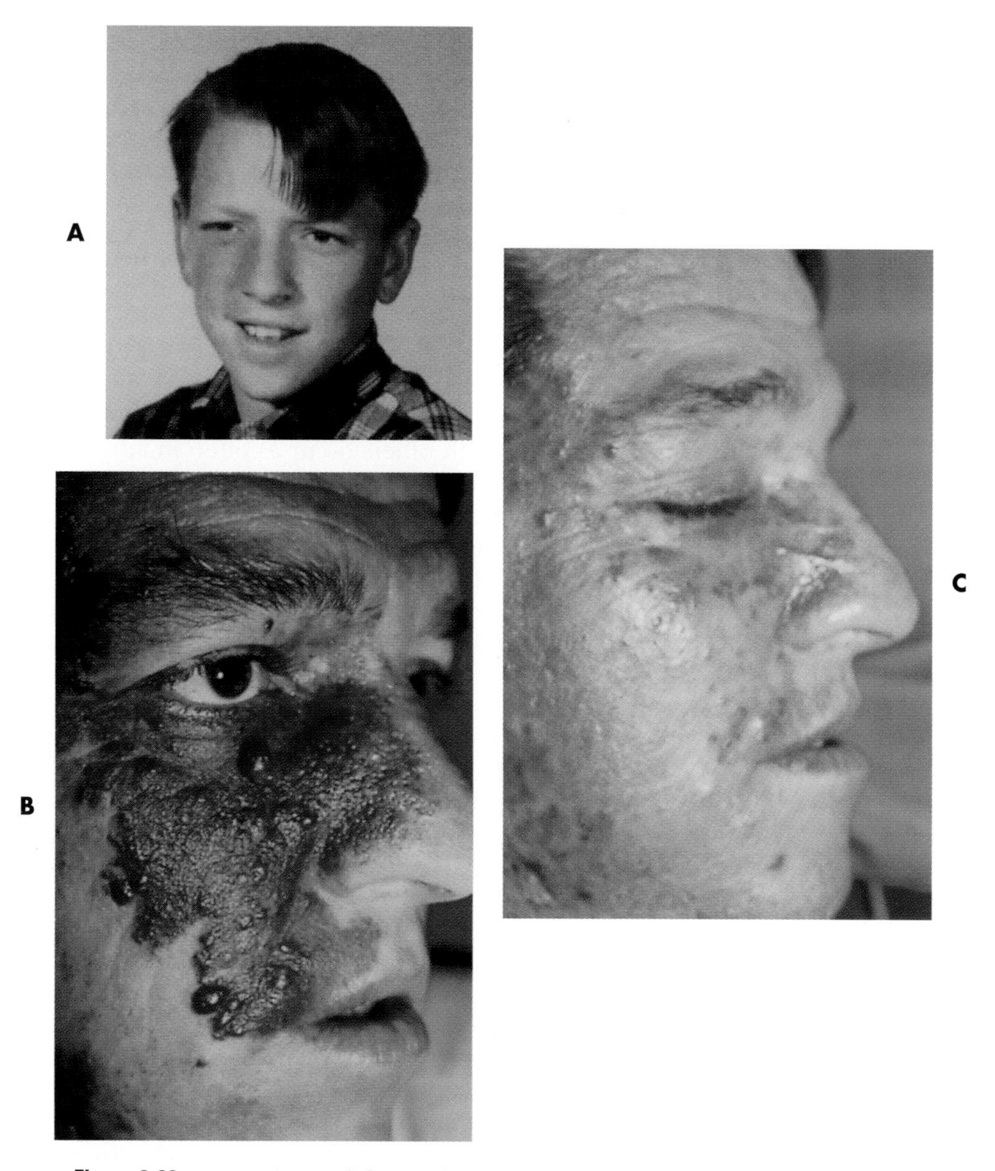

Figure 2-32 Progressive nodularity of PWS is noted with aging. **A,** Patient, age 15, has light-pink PWS on right cheek. **B,** Patient, age 35, has marked nodularity and darkening of PWS. **C,** Clinical appearance after 12 separate treatments with FLPDL at average fluence of 7.0 to 7.5 J/cm^2. Each treatment averaged 600 5-mm impacts. (Courtesy Gerald Goldberg, MD.)

when psychosocial development is affected is speculative. A psychiatric study of 19 children 3 to 5 years old with face, head, or neck hemangiomas found no association with major problems in psychosocial development.[143] However, early treatment improves the responsiveness, decreases the number of treatments, and reduces the likelihood of permanent adverse sequelae.[39,45-47,144] Therefore we recommend that treatment be started at the earliest possible age.

A common misperception regarding PWS in adults is that if one has reached adulthood without psychologic damage from a cosmetic deformity, one does not require treatment. Former Soviet president Mikail Gorbachev is an example of successful "coping" with a cosmetic handicap. (Interestingly, the Soviet news agency, Tass, airbrushed out Gorbachev's PWS from published photographs until "perestroika.") However, such presumptions are often incorrect. More often the misperception of treatment complications along with cost considerations are the primary reasons for avoiding treatment. These misconceptions are often used by insurance companies to deny coverage and save money. Unfortunately, cosmetic considerations are not the only reasons PWS should be treated in adults. Hypertrophy, hemorrhage, and infection are the medical reasons for treatment.

Adult PWS can also have an adverse impact on social relationships. A questionnaire given to 186 patients who sought treatment for their PWS found that 29% thought the PWS was disadvantageous in forming interpersonal relationships with members of the opposite sex.[145] Half rated their PWS as unattractive, although only 33% thought that other people perceived their PWS to be moderately to very unattractive. The true incidence of psychologic problems from PWS may be higher or lower because this study was obviously skewed to patients who were actively seeking treatment. Nevertheless, the survey does show that a significant number of adults with PWS would benefit psychologically from treatment.

Psychologic difficulties in interactions with others occur as often in adults as in children. An experiment during the 1989 annual meeting of the American Academy of Dermatology dramatically demonstrates this point. A model had a PWS painted on her face and then feigned an illness that led to unconsciousness on a public bus. Not one passenger came to her aid. When the same model feigned the same illness on a bus without the facial PWS, all those present eagerly came to her aid. Pena Clementina Masclarelli,[146] a senior occupational therapist who also has an extensive PWS, wrote a poignant chapter about her interactions with others that should be required reading for all physicians.

Personal perceptions are also noted to change dramatically in our treated patients. A 12-year-old girl first sought treatment in our practice for a PWS on the right cheek. Initially, although of above-average intelligence, she was introverted and interacted sparingly with her classmates. After three treatment sessions, resulting in 75% clearance, she began dating, joined the school band, and excelled academically (Figure 2-33). These are the observations so gratifying to the physician and medical staff involved in laser treatment.

Despite the psychologic and medical complications of PWS, insurance coverage for laser treatment of PWS varies from state to state. A study by McClean and Hanke[147] of insurance reimbursement in 18 states found that determination for approval of treatment was made on a case-by-case basis, with the majority requiring preauthorization. The percentage of requests approved for coverage varied from 50% to 100% without apparent reason. Some insurance carriers would only approve treatment if functional impairment existed and some only if the patient was less than 1 year of age. Only Minnesota has a law requiring all health insurance to cover the elimination or maximum feasible treatment of PWS.

Treatment

Many therapeutic methods have been attempted to treat PWSs. These include surgery (excision, grafts, flaps, dermabrasion),[126,148,149] radium implants,[150] x-ray therapy,[126] cryosurgery,[151] electrocautery,[41] sclerotherapy,[144] tattooing,[152,153] and cosmetic camouflage.[154] These methods all have limited and unpredictable results as well as potentially serious complications.[144] In addition to currently recommended laser treatments, the CO_2 laser,[6,155-157] Nd:YAG laser,[69] CVL,[158,159] and argon laser[10,25,160-162] have previously been used to treat PWS in children. As previously discussed, cosmetic results with these lasers have been poor in children, with the risk of scarring unacceptably high.

Childhood port-wine stains

The FLPDL was specifically designed to treat the small vessels found in childhood PWSs.[39,41] The first published reports noted complete clearing of pink-to-red macular PWSs in 35 children less than 14 years old (mean age 7 years 2 months) with an

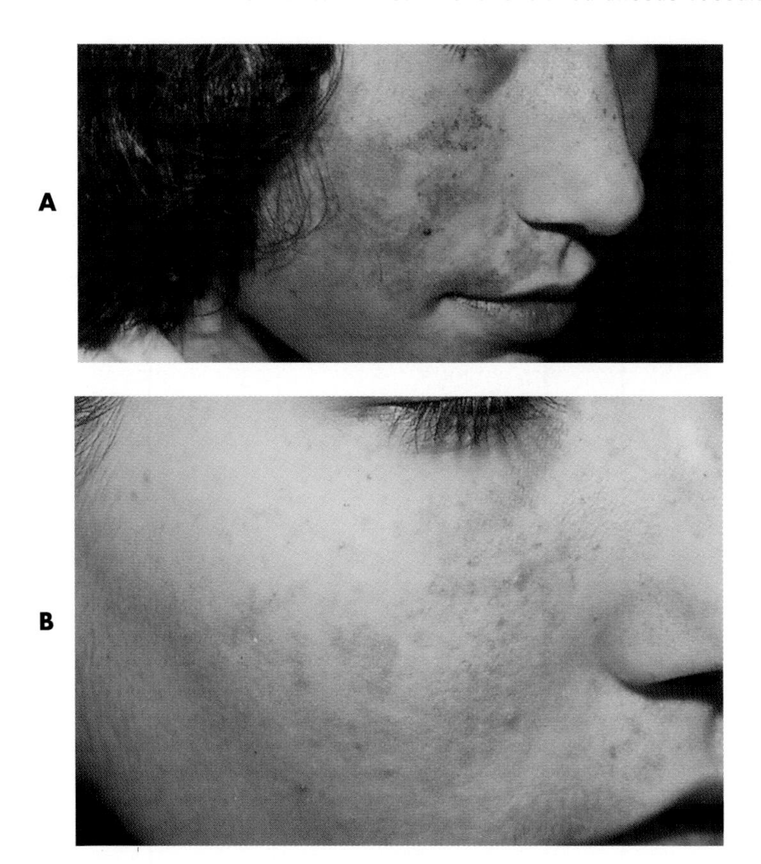

Figure 2-33 **A,** Twelve-year-old girl with congenital PWS on right cheek. **B,** After third treatment with FLPDL. First treatment used a fluence of 7.25 J/cm² with 213 5-mm pulses, second treatment 7.5 J/cm² with 109 5-mm pulses, and third treatment 7.5 J/cm² with 40 5-mm pulses. Patient and parents noted 90% resolution of entire lesion. (From Goldman MP, Fitzpatrick RE, Ruiz-Esparza J: *J Pediatr* 122:71, 1993.)

average of 6.5 treatments.[39] Subsequent clinical studies demonstrated notable efficacy and defined more reasonable expectations. Reyes and Geronemus[45] successfully treated 73 patients between age 3 months and 14 years. The overall average lightening after one treatment was 53%, and the percentage of lightening increased with subsequent treatments. More than 75% lightening was achieved with an average of 2.5 treatments in 33 patients.

Morelli and Weston[163] advocate beginning treatment as early as 7 to 14 days of age so that three treatments can be done before the infant reaches 6 months of age. They noted a 50% resolution with this protocol by the third treatment. In their population of 132 patients, complete clearance was obtained in 25% of PWSs when treatment was begun before 18 months of age (average 7.8 treatment sessions) versus 7% to 10% having total clearance when treatment was begun between ages 1½ and 18 years (average 7.0 treatment sessions). A follow-up evaluation of this patient population confirmed the authors' initial observations with 83 children: 32% of children who began treatment before 1 year of age had complete clearing of their PWS compared with 18% of children treated after 1 year of age.[164] In this later study, 32% of patients with PWS less than 20 cm² in size completely cleared compared with an 8% complete clearance rate in patients with larger PWSs.

Our studies on the treatment of 43 children between ages 2 weeks and 14 years with 49 lesions of capillary malformation confirm these results.[47] Lesions treated in children under age 4 had greater overall improvement with less treatment sessions compared with those in children over age 4½ years (Table 2-4). In general, improvement and clearance were gradual and required 5 to 10 treatments. However,

Table 2-4
Childhood port-wine stains: treatment response by age

No. of Patients	No. of Lesions	Average Range	Agerage Age	Average Treatments	Average Improvement	Median Improvement	95% Improvement	
							No. of Lesions	Average Treatments
Age 0-4 yr								
21	25	2 wk-4 yr	2.15 yr	3.4	70%	75%	5 (20%)	3.8
Age 4.5-14 yr								
22	24	6-14 yr	10.3 yr	4.0	68%	75%	3 (12.5%)	6.5
Total 0-14 yr								
43	49	2 wk-14 yr	6.2 yr	3.7	69%	75%	8 (16.3%)	4.8

From Goldman MP, Fitzpatrick RE, Ruiz-Esparza J: *J Pediatr* 122:71, 1993.

very superficial lesions cleared more quickly, with four lesions reaching a level of 95% clearing in one or two treatments (Table 2-5).

An additional study of 12 children 6 to 30 weeks of age confirmed that treatment of infants only a few weeks old can be undertaken safely and with an accelerated response: 45% demonstrated 75% or more lightening of their lesions after a mean of 3.8 treatments.[144] Alster and Wilson[165] reported an 87% clearance rate in patients less than 2 years of age, 78% clearance in patients ages 3 to 8, and 73% clearance rate in patients 16 years and older. All these studies demonstrate a better treatment outcome with younger patients.

Only one study of 23 facial PWS lesions in patients up to age 17 showed no difference among different ages in the average number of treatments to obtain maximum lesion lightening.[166] However, this study only evaluated four lesions in children less than 1 year of age and eight lesions in those 1 to 7 years of age.

Although treatment is efficacious and most laser surgeons recommend treatment at the earliest sign of a lesion, photothermolysis of blood vessels does result in the release of free Hb into the circulation. Hemoglobinemia may theoretically lead to renal impairment in a young patient. Therefore a study of 15 patients under age 5 treated with the FLPDL tested serum haptoglobin and urine hemosiderin postoperatively.[167] Even though patients had a treatment region more than 3% of total body surface area and received more than 1500 5-mm-diameter pulses in some cases, the authors found no evidence of urine hemoglobin and reported normal levels of serum haptoglobin levels.

Therefore the advantages of early treatment are (1) quicker resolution requiring fewer treatments, (2) fewer laser pulses because of smaller size (children triple in size from birth to age 2 and further double in size from ages 2 to 8), and (3) less need for anesthesia.

Unfortunately, pediatricians and family practitioners are reluctant to refer their patients for treatment. This is most likely a result of too few reports in all but the most recent pediatric literature and thus lack of knowledge. Second, older physicians may remember the failures of the argon laser in treating these lesions and equate all laser treatment with the argon laser. Third, treatment is usually painful to the child.

In our experience, treatment is considerably eased with topical anesthetic creams, cooling the epidermis with cryogen spray or ice, or conscious sedation administered by a pediatric anesthesiologist, but necessary only in children 8 years old or younger. Fortunately, earliest childhood memories usually occur after 2 or 3 years of age.[168] Thus treatments given before this time should not have long-term psychologic effects. We have been treating infants with the FLPDL since 1985 and have yet to observe adverse psychologic effects in our patients with continuing

Table 2-5
Childhood port-wine stains: response per number of treatments

		Improvement				Improvement of Nonclear Lesions		
No. of Treatments	No. of Lesions	Average Treatment Energy (J)	Mean (%)	Median (%)	No. of Lesions >95% Clear	Percent	Mean (%)	Median (%)
1	10	6.73	51	50	1	10	46	40
2	12	6.96	70.4	72	3	25	61	50
3	5	6.55	62	60	0	0	62	60
4	4	6.86	70	70	0	0	70	70
5	10	7.05	77.5	80	2	20	72.5	77
6-11	8	6.50	85	90	3	37.5	78	80

From Goldman MP, Fitzpatrick RE, Ruiz-Esparza J: *J Pediatr* 122:71, 1993.

long-term follow-up. Some of our initial patients, treated in the first few months of life with continued treatment at 4- to 6-month intervals, are now 8 to 10 years old and continue to receive treatment without apparent psychologic trauma.

For children less than age 12 years, we recommend laser fluences between 5.75 and 7.75 J/cm^2 with a 5-mm-diameter spot size (mean 7.0 J/cm^2). An improved response appears to occur in those lesions treated with energies greater than 6.0 J/cm^2, because 23% completely cleared as opposed to none of those treated with 5.75 J/cm^2. As described later, if a 7-mm-diameter spot size is used, recommended laser fluence is 5 to 6 J/cm^2. If a 10-mm-diameter spot size is used, an energy fluence of 4 to 5 J/cm^2 is recommended. The initial treatment session usually results in an average improvement of approximately 50%. Each subsequent treatment provides an additional increment of approximately 10% improvement. After six treatments, 40% of our patients completely clear, and those who are not clear have an average improvement of approximately 80% (Figures 2-33 and 2-34). We have not had patients with scarring or persistent pigmentary changes despite rare episodes of

A

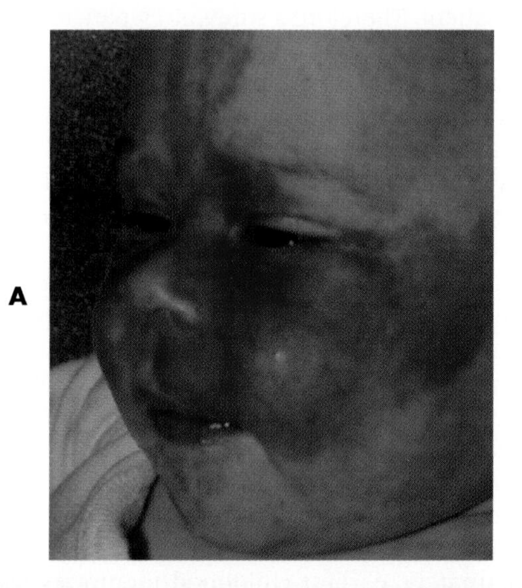

B

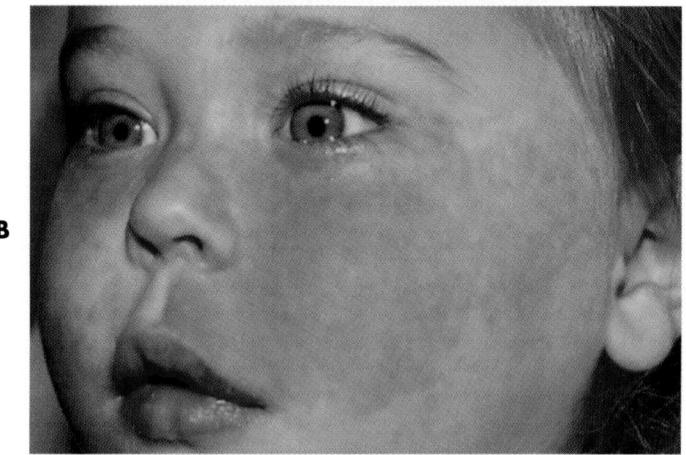

Figure 2-34 **A,** Initial appearance of extensive PWS on 10-week-old girl. Evaluation by pediatric neurologist was entirely within normal limits. **B,** Same patient, 4 months after her fourth treatment with the FLPDL. First and second treatments were performed at an energy of 6 J/cm^2 and third and fourth treatments at 6.25 J/cm^2. Total of 400 pulses were given to entire PWS during each treatment visit. Parents and physician noted almost 90% resolution of PWS. (From Goldman MP, Fitzpatrick RE, Ruiz-Esparza J: *J Pediatr* 122:71, 1993.)

vesiculation and crusting after treatment. Skin type (I-III) also does not appear to influence the ultimate treatment outcome, but darker skin requires more treatment sessions to achieve the same degree of clearing as in PWSs of fair-skinned patients. Lesions on distal limbs respond with less fading than lesions elsewhere, such as on the neck and torso (Table 2-6). The diminished response of PWS on the limbs has been reported by others.[169,170]

Fortunately, treatment of PWS in childhood and infancy not only has been very efficacious with the FLPDL, but also has proved to be safe. Swelling and erythema are frequently present immediately after treatment, especially around the eyes, but resolve within 24 to 48 hours. Hyperpigmentation of the treated site occurs in 25% to 30% of patients but is temporary and resolves over 2 to 3 months. Hypopigmentation occurs infrequently and resolves spontaneously over 3 to 6 months. Cutaneous depressions or atrophic scars have occurred in isolated laser impact sites and have been associated with excessive delivery of energy, excessive spot overlap, or posttreatment trauma to the site. Almost all reported cases have resolved spontaneously within 1 year[41,45,47] (Figure 2-35).

Adult port-wine stains

The treatment of PWS in adults has been as equally gratifying as our experience in children (Figure 2-36). The FLPDL is used in the same manner as with children except that fluences are usually increased to 6.0 to 8.5 J/cm^2 depending on the lesion's color and thickness. A 5- or 7-mm-diameter spot size is used per patient tolerance. A 7-mm-diameter spot size is preferred because of its deeper penetration, and when used, fluence is usually lowered 0.5 J/cm^2 from the fluence used with a 5-mm-diameter spot size. Fluence is decreased because the laser beam with a 7-mm spot size delivers a higher fluence in the central portion of the beam than at its periphery. We recommend beginning with a fluence of 5.0 to 5.5 J/cm^2 with a 7-mm-diameter spot size and increasing by 0.5 J/cm^2 with each subsequent treatment at 3- to 4-month intervals.

PhotoDerm VL

The PhotoDerm VL has also been used to treat PWS (see later discussion for treatment parameters). This high-intensity flashlamp can be used in a number of different settings to effect vascular-specific thermocoagulation. Different settings are used with each treatment, which can be given at monthly intervals. We usually increase the fluence with each subsequent treatment as well as the pulse duration, cutoff filter, and number of simultaneous pulses (Figure 2-37). The following settings are effective for initial and subsequent treatments:

- 515-nm or 550-nm cutoff filter, single pulse at 2 to 5 msec with 20 to 25 J/cm^2
- 550-nm cutoff filter, double-pulsed at 2.4 msec with 10-msec delay, 4.0 msec with 35 to 42 J/cm^2

Table 2-6
Childhood port-wine stains: treatment response by location

Location	No. of Lesions	Average Treatments	Average Improvement	>95% clear		
				No. of Lesions	Percent	Average Treatments
Face	33	3.5	65%	4	12	4.0
Neck	4	5.3	90%	2	50	4.5
Torso	6	3.0	85%	3	50	3.0
Hand and arm	6	3.7	63%	0	—	0

From Goldman MP, Fitzpatrick RE, Ruiz-Esparza J: *J Pediatr* 122:71, 1993.

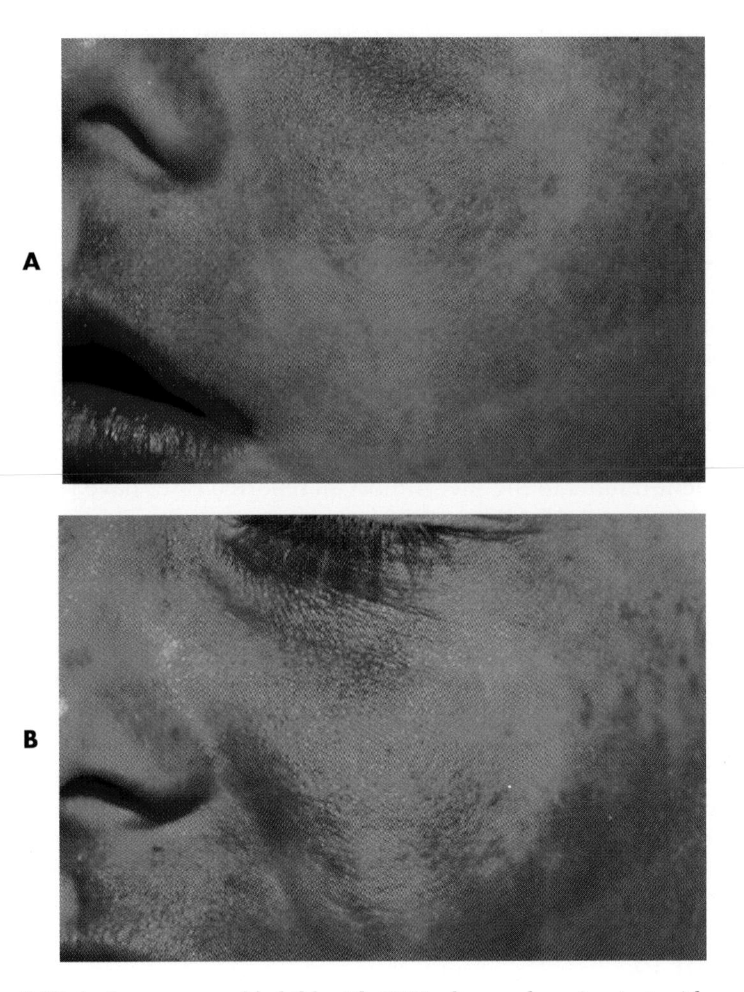

Figure 2-35 **A,** Seven-year-old child with PWS after undergoing test with various laser fluences. Patient was treated with the FLPDL at a fluence of 7 J/cm^2 for a total of 43 5-mm impacts on left cheek. Patient was seen 6 weeks later, and atrophic circular depression was noted in treated area. Parents did not remark on any scabbing or trauma to the area. Further treatments were performed at a fluence of 6.75 J/cm^2. **B,** After 18 months there is complete resolution of atrophic scar. (Because of financial considerations, patient has had only two treatments for the PWS.)

- 570-nm cutoff filter, double-pulsed at 3.0 msec with 20-msec delay, 6 msec with 40 to 45 J/cm^2
- 590-nm cutoff filter, triple-pulsed at 3 msec with 30-msec delay, 4.5 msec with 30-msec delay, 7 msec with 30-msec delay at 50 to 60 J/cm^2

As with other lesions, patients with more darkly pigmented skin are treated with higher cutoff filters to circumvent melanin absorption and longer delay times between double and triple pulses because epidermal heat is higher in these patients. Icecold coupling gel is always used.

One advantage when using the PhotoDerm VL is the minimization of purpura after treatment (Figure 2-38). Other advantages are described later.

Complications and adverse sequelae

Complications and adverse sequelae when treating vascular lesions with the FLPDL as described previously are rare. Adverse sequelae are usually temporary and limited to purpura and epidermal crusting. In almost every patient, *purpura* occurs im-

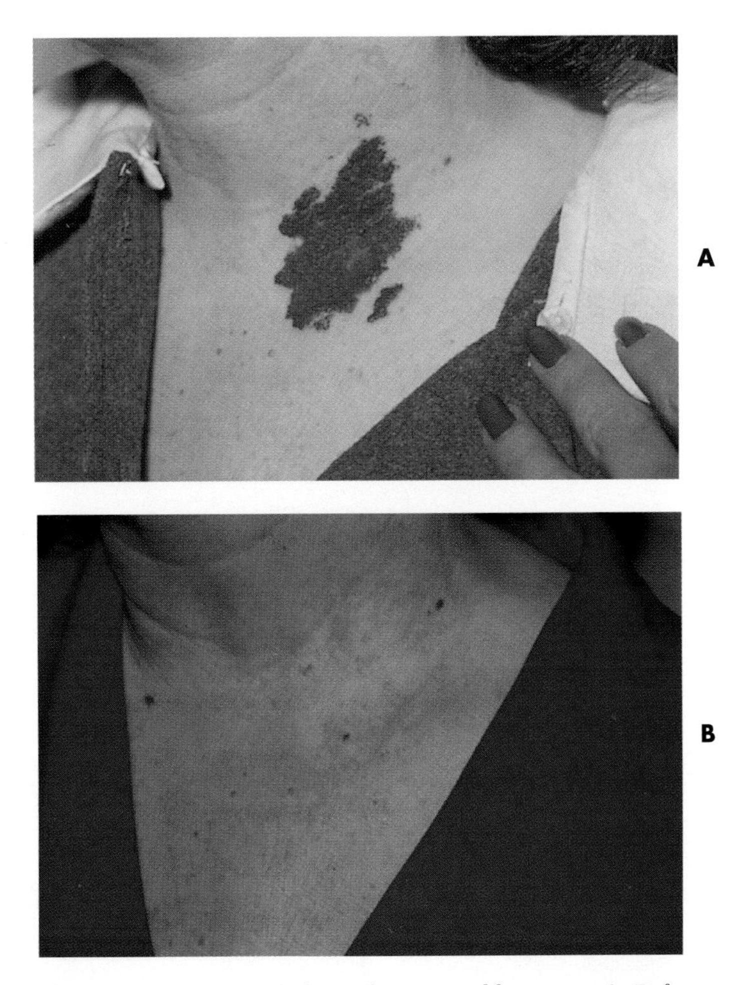

Figure 2-36 PWS on left anterior chest of 44-year-old woman. **A,** Before treatment. **B,** Near 100% resolution after six treatments. Each treatment used a fluence of 7.25 J/cm^2 with FLPDL. First treatment used 136 5-mm impacts, second treatment 175 5-mm impacts, third treatment 117 5-mm impacts, fourth treatment 87 5-mm impacts, fifth treatment 77 5-mm impacts, and sixth treatment 37 5-mm impacts. (From Fitzpatrick RE: *Am J Cosmetic Surg* 9:107, 1992.)

mediately after treatment and may be persistent for 1 to 2 weeks. When high fluences are used (>8 J/cm^2), temporary crusting may occur (Figure 2-39).

The most common longterm adverse sequelae are *pigmentary changes.* Because melanin also absorbs light at 585 nm, patients with Fitzpatrick type III skin or greater may develop hypopigmentation, especially when tanned. Alternatively, postinflammatory melanocytic hyperpigmentation may occur. At times this may appear as a "checkerboard" pigmentation (Figure 2-40). When this occurs, additional treatments are usually necessary to even out the skin color. One can use the FLPDL at an energy fluence 1 J/cm^2 less than the treatment fluence with the largest spot size available (7- or 10-mm diameter) or back off on the spot size to beyond the focal length to create a "fuzzy spot." Alternatively, we advise switching to the PhotoDerm VL, which with its larger spot size evens out the dyspigmentation in addition to the nontreated areas (discussed later). In addition, the use of depigmenting agents such as hydroxyquinone, alpha-hydroxy acids, azelaic acid, and kojic acid alone or in combination with retinoic acid both before and after treatment is helpful. Fortunately, permanent scars or pigmentary changes are very rare.

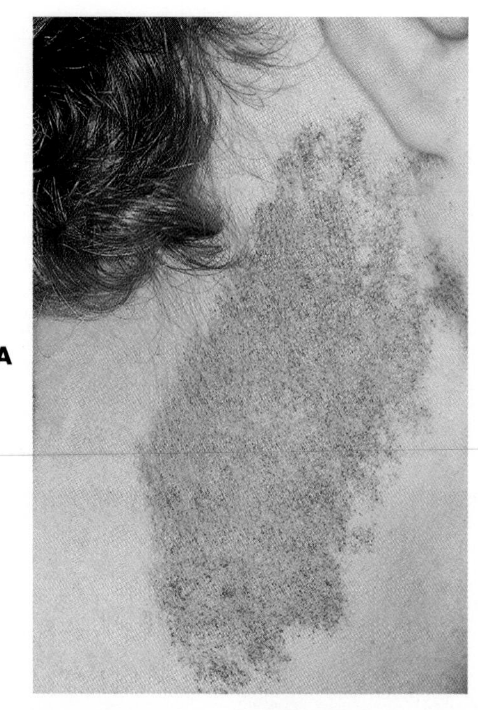

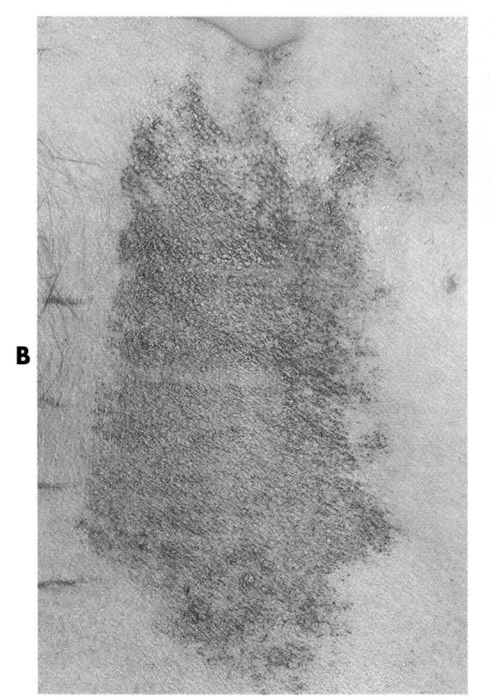

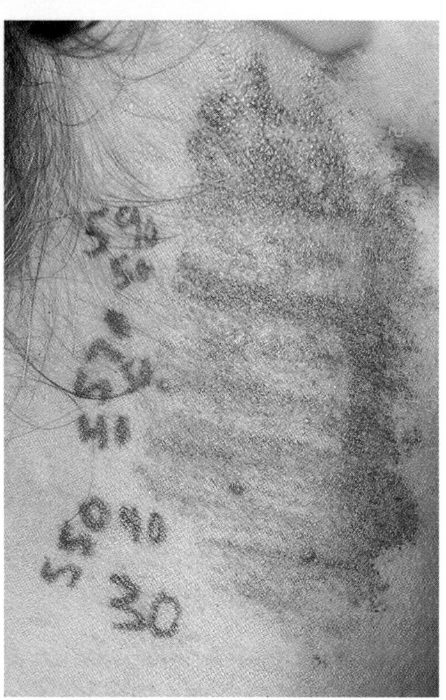

Figure 2-37 **A,** PWS on 24-year-old male before treatment. **B,** Immediately after treatment with PhotoDerm VL. Note purpuric response to treated areas **C,** One month after treatment. Note resolution at various treatment parameters, all given in single pulses. *Top* to *bottom,* 590-nm cutoff filter at 50 J/cm^2, 570-nm cutoff filter at 40 J/cm^2, 550-nm cutoff filter at 30 J/cm^2.

More serious potential adverse events include *atrophic and hypertrophic scarring* and *keloid formation.* The formation of keloids may be enhanced when the patient is also taking isotretinoin. Multiple case reports of the development of keloid formation in patients receiving isotretinoin have been reported with argon laser and dermabrasion treatment.[171,172] A single case report of this occurrence with FLPDL treat-

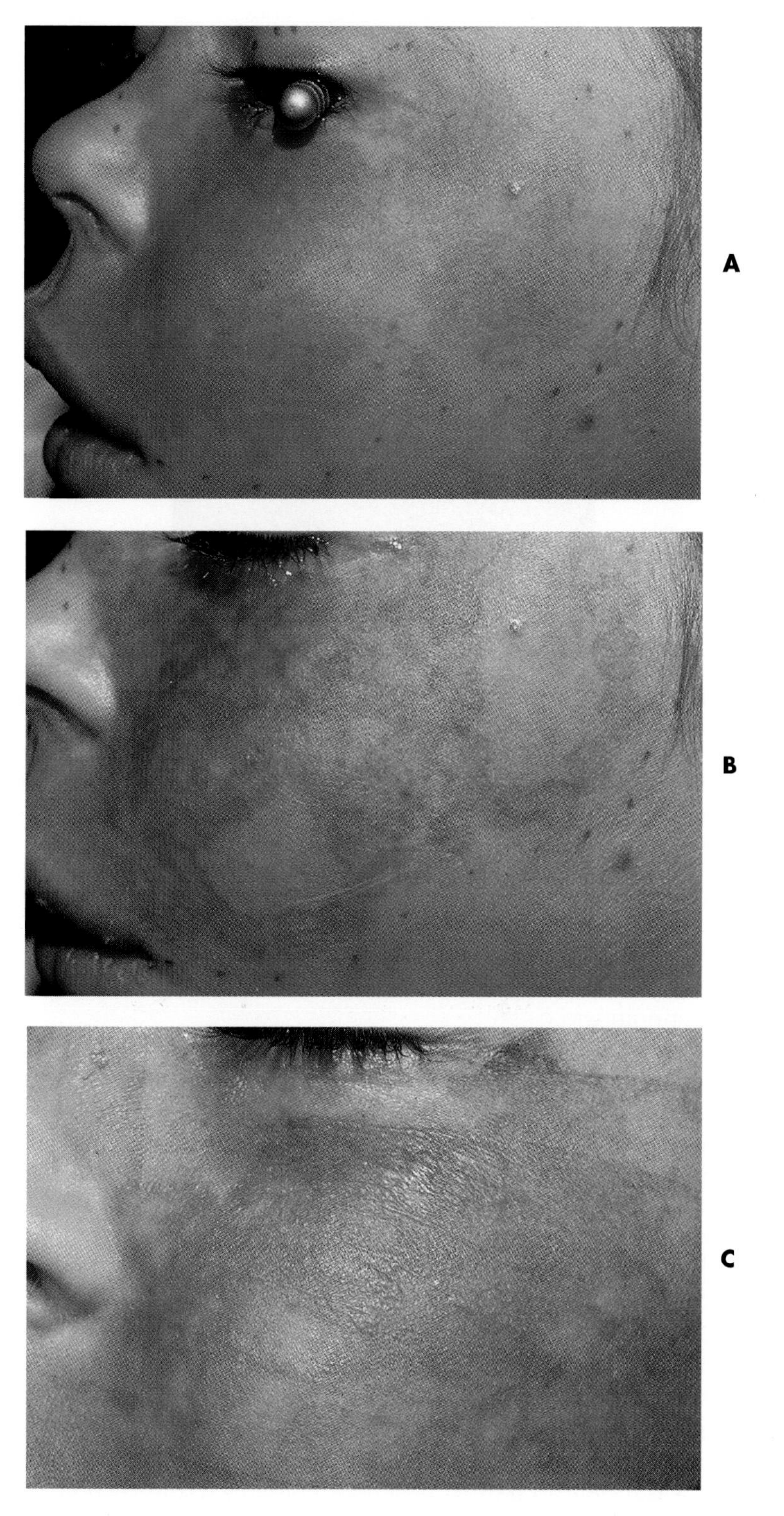

Figure 2-38 **A,** PWS on cheek of 4-year-old girl immediately before treatment. **B,** Purpuric response immediately after treatment with FLPDL at 7.0 J/cm^2 delivered through 7-mm-diameter spot size. **C,** Opposite cheek with identical PWS immediately after treatment with PhotoDerm VL with 570-nm cutoff filter at 40 J/cm^2 given as a single 8-msec-duration pulse. Note diminished purpuric response.

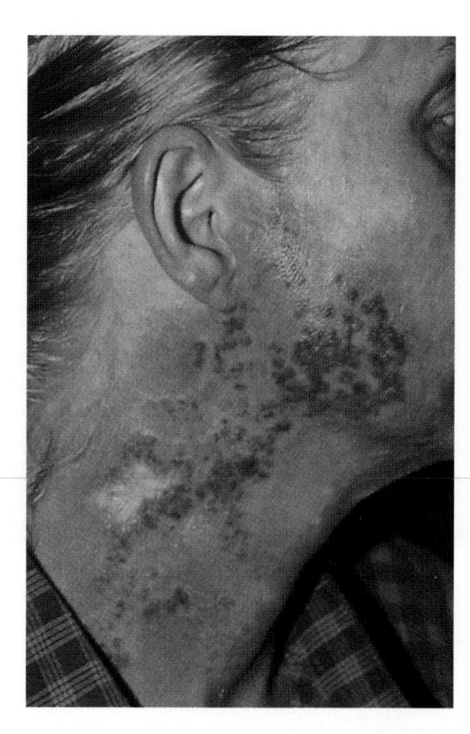

Figure 2-39 PWS on right cheek and lateral neck of 49-year-old woman. Note purpuric and hyperemic response immediately after treatment with FLPDL at 7 J/cm^2. Total of 286 5-mm pulses were given. Patient was given 75 mg of diphenhydramine (Benadryl) 1 hour before the procedure without diminishing hyperemic flare. (White scar in posterior distal PWS was from radiation treatment as a child.)

ment of a neck PWS has appeared in the literature.[173] Although the mechanism for enhancing scarring is speculative and the length of time from cessation of treatment to "safety" is unknown, it would seem prudent to avoid laser treatment within 1 to 2 years of isotretinoin use.

Numerous retrospective studies have detailed adverse sequelae. A study of 133 patients (89 females, 44 males) with PWS who had been treated with the FLPDL over a 2-year period showed good or excellent results in 84% of the PWSs.[46] The average number of treatments increased from 1.7 to 2.3 to 3.5 as the clinical results improved from slight to good to excellent, accordingly. After a treatment session, discoloration and purpura were seen in all patients, crusting in 51.9%, and scaling or peeling in 19.6%. Three patients reported swelling, and two reported blisters. Many patients reported crusting only after their first treatment and not with subsequent treatments. The average duration of these immediate skin changes was reported to be 7 to 14 days. Longterm skin changes with FLPDL therapy included hyperpigmentation in six patients, hypopigmentation in five, and isolated punctate depressions in two. Pigmentation changes in patients who had completed therapy lasted an average of 6 months. Atrophic surface changes noted in two patients involved small areas of excoriation. No hypertrophic scarring was noted. This apparent scarring was transient in nature, and both episodes resolved completely within 12 months. No significant differences in adverse sequelae were apparent between original lesions that were flat or raised.

An additional study of 500 patients treated with the FLPDL found an incidence of atrophic scarring of less than 0.1%. Hyperpigmentation was seen in 1% of patients and transient hypopigmentation in 2.6%.[169] Patients with atrophic scarring were treated in the early stages of the FLPDL development, when problems with the dosage meter were common.

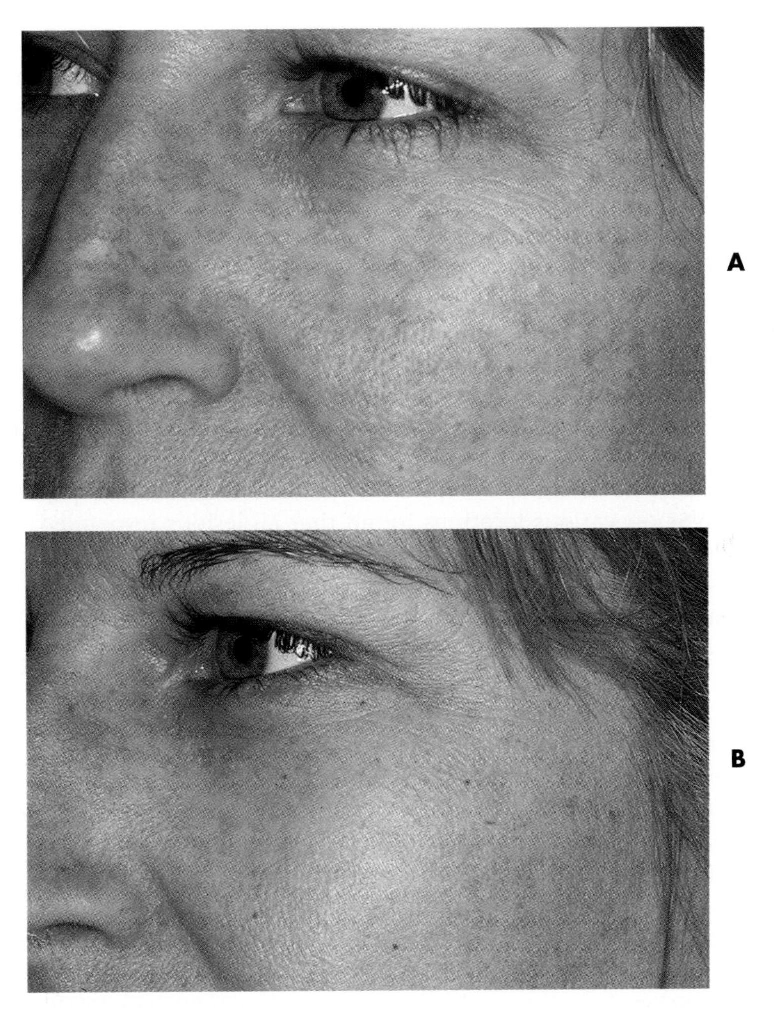

Figure 2-40 **A,** Facial telangiectasia in 32-year-old woman 3 years after one treatment with the FLPDL at 7.0 J/cm² with 5-mm-diameter spot. Note hypopigmented circles and persistent telangiectasia. **B,** Ten months after three treatments with PhotoDerm VL. First treatment was with 570-nm cutoff filter at 37 J/cm² given as a double pulse of 2.4 and 2.4 msec with a delay time of 10 msec. Second and third treatments given 4 weeks apart, 4 weeks later through a 550-nm cutoff filter at 40 J/cm² given as a 2.4- and 4.0-msec double pulse with a 10-msec delay. Note complete resolution of the telangiectasia and hypopigmented circles.

A study of 701 patients who received 3877 full treatments with the FLPDL using a 5- or 7-mm-diameter spot and fluences of 5.5 to 9.5 J/cm² with the Candela and the Cynosure systems reported severe blistering in 1.08%, severe crusting in 0.13%, hypopigmentation in 0.26%, hyperpigmentation in 1.7%, atrophic scarring in 0.7%, and hypertrophic scarring in 0.13% of treatments.[174] Seven patients developed atrophic scarring despite uneventful test area treatments. Thirty percent of patients with scarring had clinical resolution over 6 to 12 months. Hypertrophic scarring also occurred after an uneventful test and four or five uneventful treatments. Hypertrophic scarring showed no resolution in these patients.

Complaints of discomfort from treatment were rated as moderate in 49.1% of patients, which is higher than previously reported.[41] However, pain in adults was not a limiting factor in treatment. Although patients, in retrospect, have rated treatment pain as moderate, treatment was not discontinued because of pain in any patient.

Variable treatment response by lesion location and size

In addition to an obvious decrease in responsiveness to treatment on the extremities compared with the face (see next), PWSs responded differently even within the same anatomic location. The centrofacial regions (medial aspect of the cheek, upper cutaneous lip, nose) respond less favorably than the periorbital, forehead, temple, lateral cheek, neck, and chin areas.[29,166] Evaluation by dermatomal distribution revealed that V_2 lightened on average 74%, whereas combined dermatomes V_1 and V_3 lightened on average 82% when treated with the FLPDL at 585 nm, 5-mm-diameter spot size, and 5.75 to 8.5 J/cm^2 in an average of four treatments. V_2 lesions also require more treatments to reach maximal clearance than V_1 or V_3 lesions. (Figure 2-41). The factors that account for this different therapeutic response are speculative. V_2 skin could be slightly thicker with more adnexal structures and thus more vasculature and nerve endings.

Lesion size may be an independent factor determining lesion response. A study of 74 adult PWSs on various locations found that all lesions responded, with 25% to 90% lightening.[175] However, only 36.5% achieved 50% clearing despite 4 to 19 treatments, depending on the size of the lesion. No lesions had greater than 75% clearance despite 6 to 15 treatments when their size was greater than 60 cm^2, and no lesions had greater than 50% clearance despite a mean of 17 treatments when their size was larger than 100 cm^2 (Figure 2-42).

FLPDL treatment of extremity lesions

The poor response of lesions located on the distal extremities has been seen in our practice and reported by others. In one review, 7 of 10 patients with PWS on the extremities responded only slightly or poorly.[169] This finding might reflect an artifact of fewer treatments because the average number of treatments was 2.6 (Figure 2-43). In contrast, those lesions on the face and neck that responded slightly or poorly had an average of only 1.1 treatments. Twenty-seven patients with lower limb PWS treated with the FLPDL at fluences up to a maximum of 8.5 J/cm^2 also had a poor response.[170] In this population, only one patient had greater than 95% clearance, despite these patients having an average of 9.4 treatments. Overall, 26% of these patients had no response, 22% had a poor response, 33% had less than 50% lightening, 15% had 50% to 75% lightening, and only one had greater than 95% clearance after seven treatments. In addition, 18% of patients developed hyperpigmentation, which lasted for an undisclosed period.

The effect of decreased response to treatment with lesions located in extremities was also noted by Orten et al,[166] who found only 33% lightening despite a mean of approximately six treatments, compared with 80% to 90% lightening of PWS lesions in fewer or similar number of treatments in other locations. Lanigan[176] also reported poor response to treatment in 23 patients with lower limb PWS. Ten patients had no discernible lightening after one treatment at 7.75 J/cm^2. Seventeen patients with a median of seven treatments at a median fluence of 7.25 J/cm^2 showed median lightening of 40%. Of those responding, only three patients had lightening of 70% or greater after six, ten, and five treatments. However, some authors have reported a similar treatment efficacy despite lesion location with a similar average number of treatments.[165]

The reason PWSs on the distal limbs respond slowly is unknown but may be related to gravitational or deoxygenation effects on circulation. Distal vessels have a thicker wall, which may require increased thermal effects for irreversible damage (see p. 137). Because distal areas respond more poorly than more proximal areas, early treatment of extremity lesions, before ambulation, may be beneficial. We have found this to be true in the small number of patients we have treated at an early age with distal limb PWS (Figure 2-44).

A

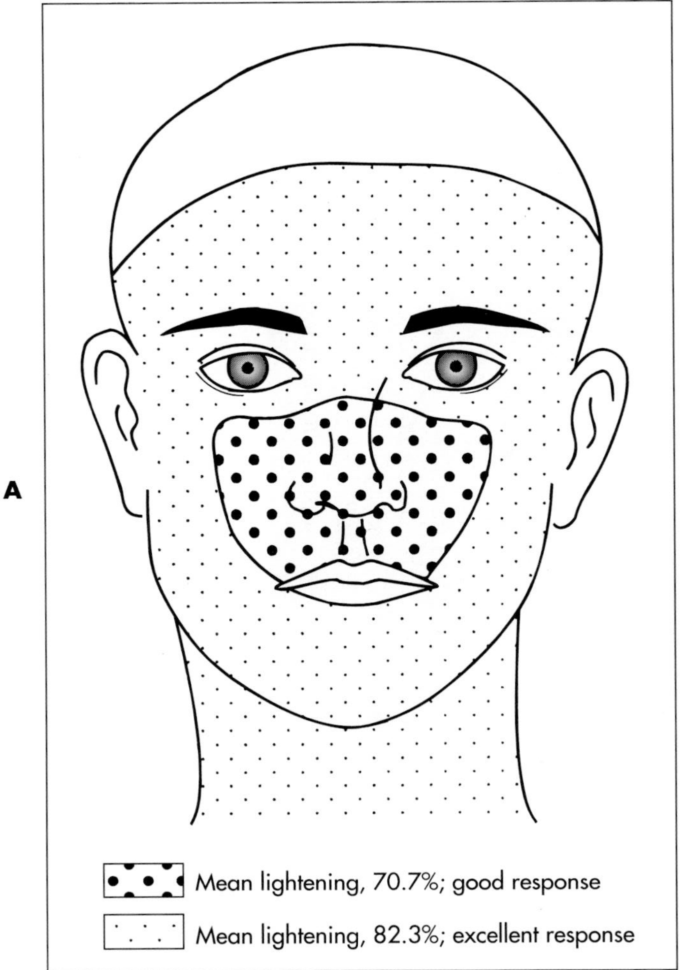

B

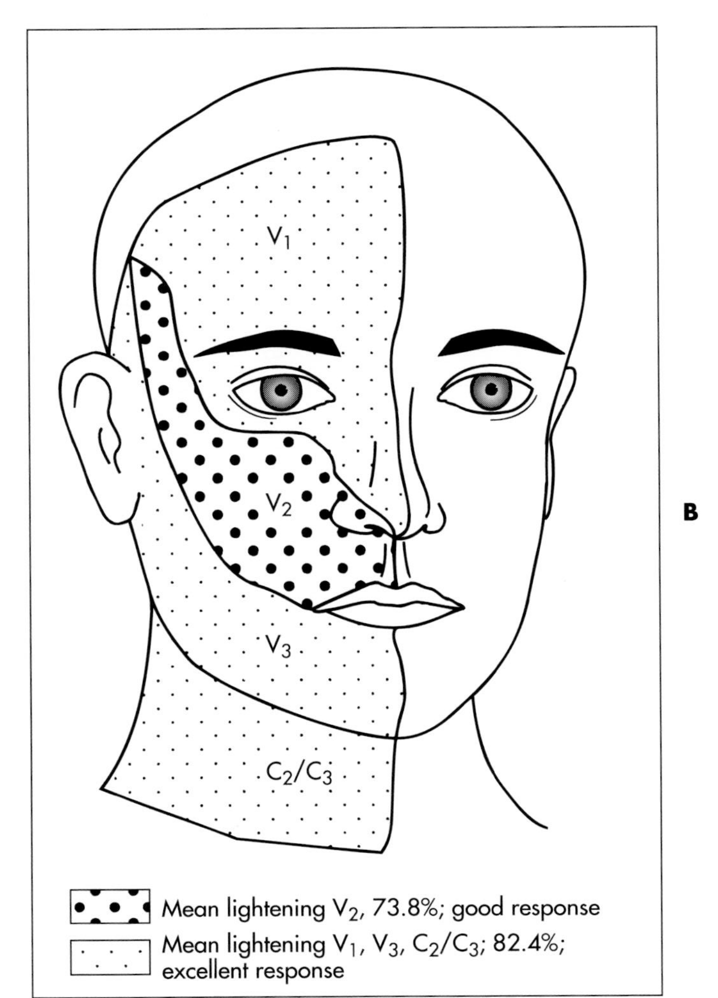

Figure 2-41 **A,** Anatomic subdivision of therapeutic response of PWS to FLPDL treatment. **B,** Dermatomal distribution of therapeutic response of PWS to FLPDL treatment. (From Renfro L, Geronemus RG: *Arch Dermatol* 129:182, 1993.)

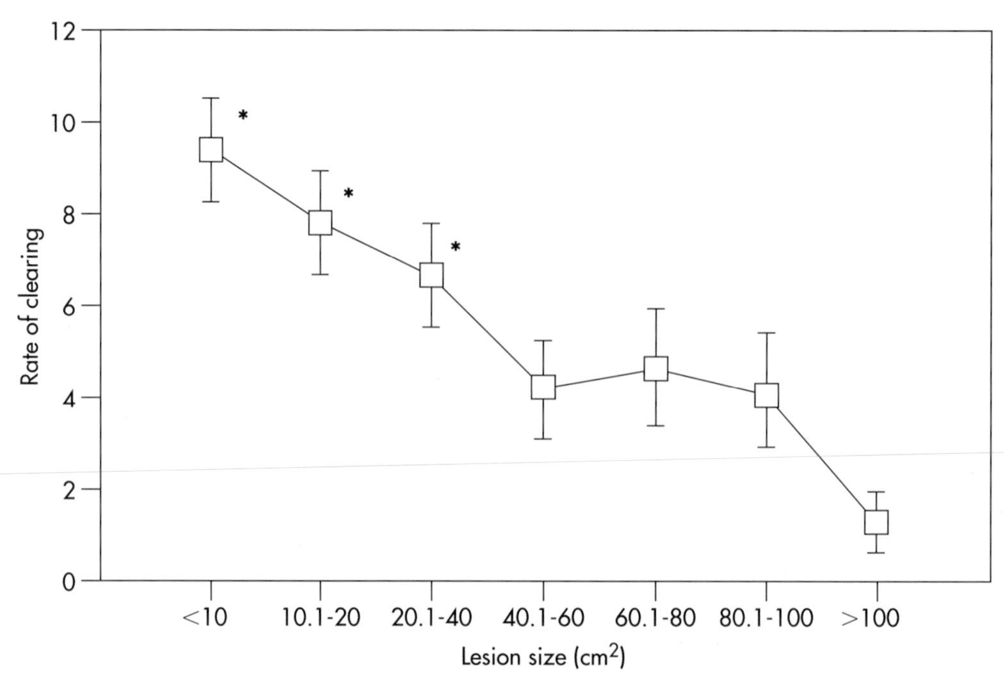

Figure 2-42 Facial PWS lesion size affects rate of clearing after FLPDL treatment in adults. Data are represented as mean ± standard error of mean for each lesion-size category. Asterisk (*) designates significant difference ($p < 0.05$) in rate of clearing versus size category of greater than 100 cm². (From Yohn JJ, Huff JC, Aeling JL et al: *Cutis* 59:267, 1997.)

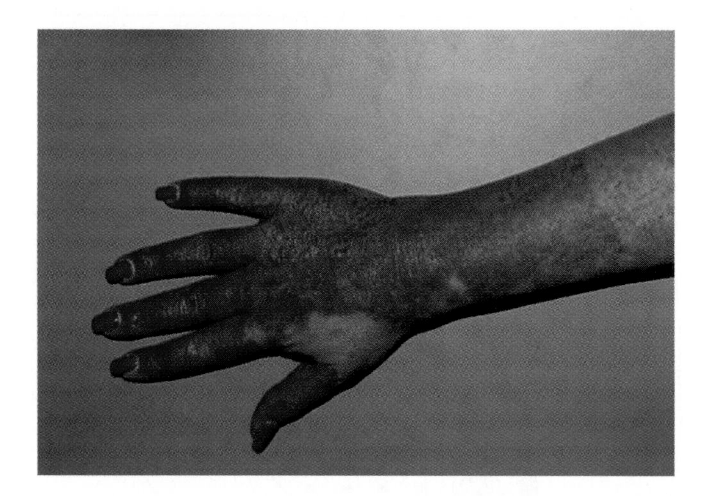

Figure 2-43 PWS on entire right hand, arm, and chest of 38-year-old woman. Photograph was taken 2 years after treatment of hand and arm. Right dorsal hand has been treated three times with the FLPDL at fluences ranging between 7 and 7.5 J/cm². Area from wrist to elbow has been treated once at an energy of 7 J/cm². Area of demarcation from midforearm to lateral aspect of photograph was treated a second time with a fluence of 7.5 J/cm². Note significant improvement in proximal forearm without noticeable improvement (by comparison) of distal forearm, dorsal hand, or fingers.

As previously mentioned, even treating extremity lesions with high-energy fluences has been unsuccessful. Near-complete resolution in only two treatments has been reported when fluences of 9 J/cm² are used. However, this degree of laser energy poses a risk of pigmentary and nonspecific epidermal changes.[163] Therefore epidermal cooling may allow these necessary higher fluences to be used.

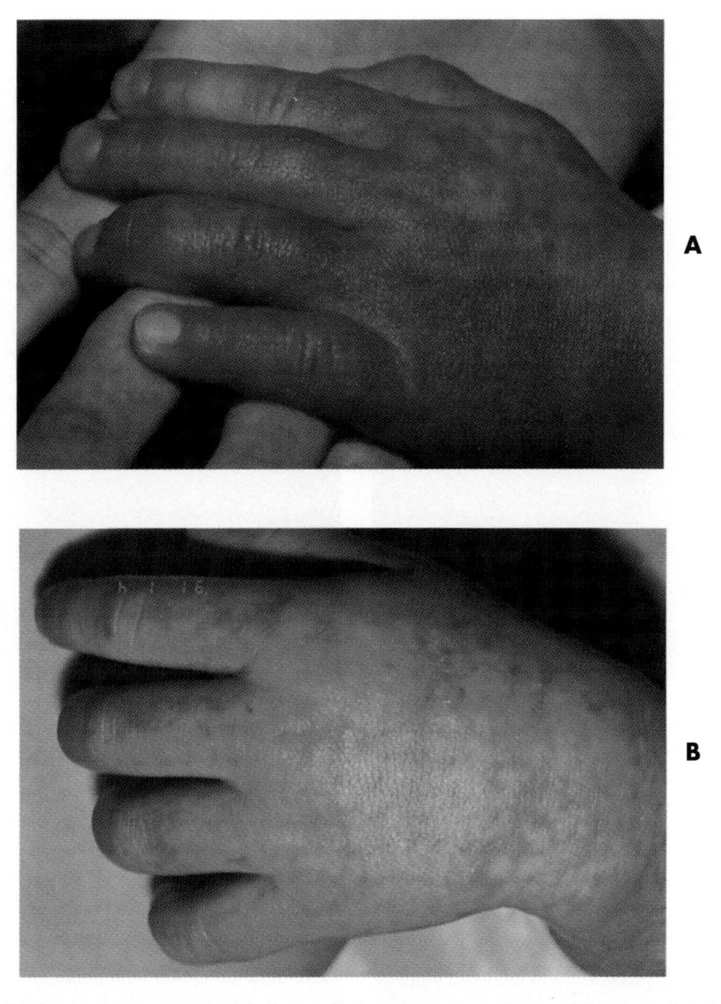

Figure 2-44 Extensive PWS of left hand, forearm, and chest of 18-month-old boy. **A,** Before treatment. **B,** Six months after two treatments to dorsal hand with FLPDL using a fluence of 6.75 J/cm^2. Total of 80 5mm impacts were given during each treatment session. Note significant resolution of PWS.

Treatment protocol

The treatment protocol involves first performing a test of several different energy densities to determine efficacy. Immediately after impact, a dark-purple discoloration occurs. Conversely, if the site does not discolor, too low an energy fluence may have been chosen. If edema, blistering, or blackening of the impact site occurs, too high an energy density may have been chosen. Generally, three or four energy fluences are tested and evaluated at approximately 6 weeks (Figure 2-45). The most effective one is then chosen for treatment. If none of the test sites shows improvement, a second series of test energies is chosen. With experience, the test period may be eliminated and the treatment energy chosen by evaluation of the laser's immediate effects.

Treatment of the entire lesion or a portion of the lesion may be accomplished by covering the treatment area with laser impacts that overlap 10% to 15%. Overlapping can minimize a mottled "egg crate" appearance (Figure 2-46). However, as previously described, the degree of overlapping is determined by the type of FLPDL used, with the Cynosure FLPDL better used without any overlapping, except with a "fuzzy spot." Overlapping may also be achieved with the Candela FLPDL by use of the so-called fuzzy spot.[177] With this treatment modification, the laser handpiece is

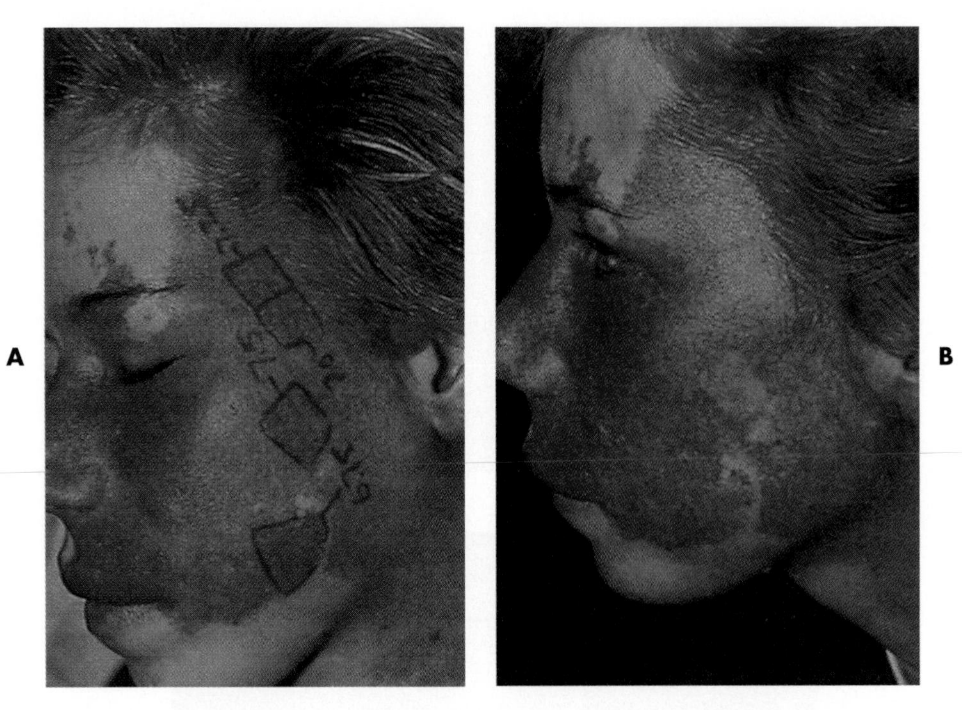

Figure 2-45 **A,** Immediately after application of test doses with FLPDL at laser energies specified. **B,** Four months after test doses. Note significant clearing in all areas, with maximum clearing at fluences of 7.0 and 7.25 J/cm^2. Patch treated at 7.5 J/cm^2 shows light-brown hyperpigmentation. Treatment will therefore proceed at an energy of 7.0 J/cm^2.

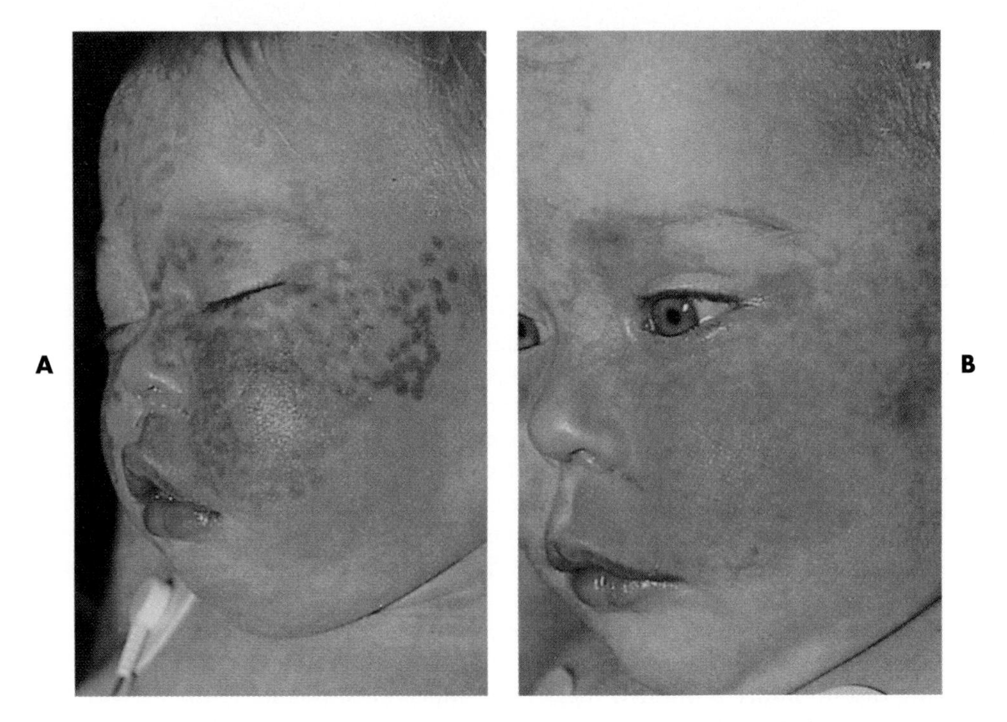

Figure 2-46 Same patient as in Figure 2-34. **A,** Note purpuric response immediately after treatment with FLPDL at 6.25 J/cm^2. **B,** Mottled resolution of PWS 4 months after treatment.

moved away from the skin beyond the laser's focal point, resulting in a larger, defocused impact spot. This has a lower energy density than that indicated for the focused spot and also a more indistinct or "fuzzy" border that blurs the edges of clearing from a single treatment. Re-treatments are generally done at $1\frac{1}{2}$- to 4-month intervals.

The use of overlapping pulses should be undertaken with caution, however, because biopsies of PWSs treated with single impact and consecutive double-impact therapy reveal an additive thermal effect resulting in nonspecific thermal damage to the superficial dermis and epidermis (Figures 2-47 and 2-48) This double-pulsing technique does promote greater resolution of nodular, thicker, and darker lesions but results in loss of specificity.

The reason for multiple treatments is the layered nature of ectatic vessels of a PWS. Modeling studies using the histologically correct layered vessel demonstrate that the more superficial vessels receive most of the delivered energy. The deeper vessels receive less energy and are therefore not thermocoagulated because of mutual shadowing of the superficial vessels[178] (Figure 2-49).

FLPDL, 600 nm. Increased efficacy has been predicted with the advent of the FLPDL with a longer pulse duration of 1.5 msec and longer wavelengths of 590, 595, and 600 nm. These newer parameters may allow treatment of deeper and larger

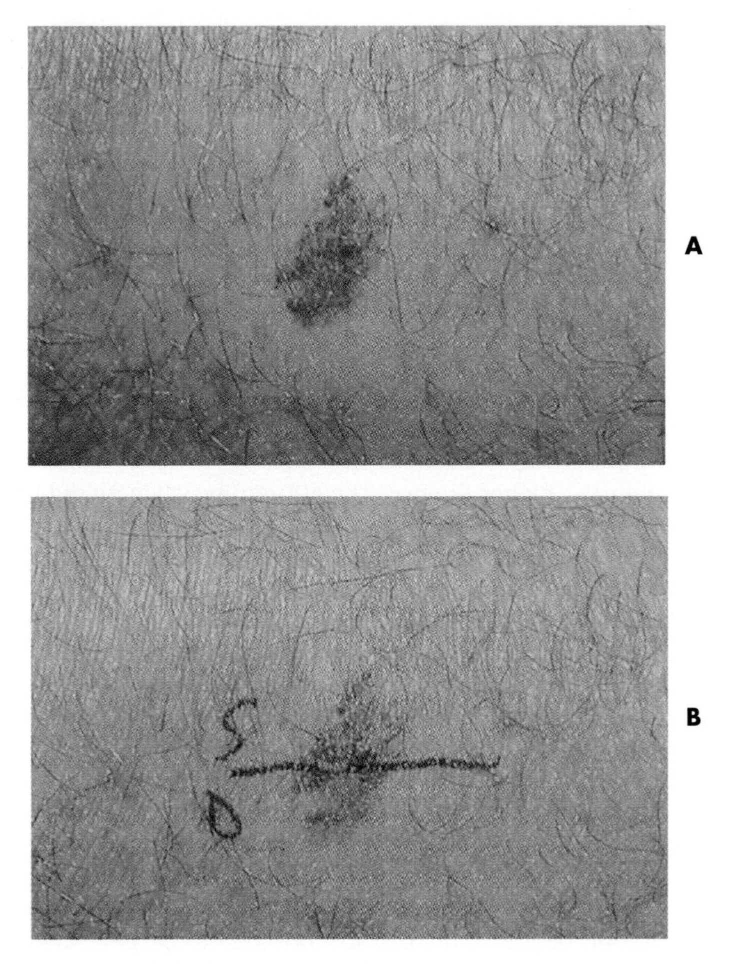

Figure 2-47 Congenital PWS on thigh of 66-year-old man. **A,** Before treatment. **B,** Immediately after treatment with FLPDL at 7 J/cm^2. *S,* Area treated with single pulse; *D,* area treated with double pulse. Double-pulse area has darker pigmentation.

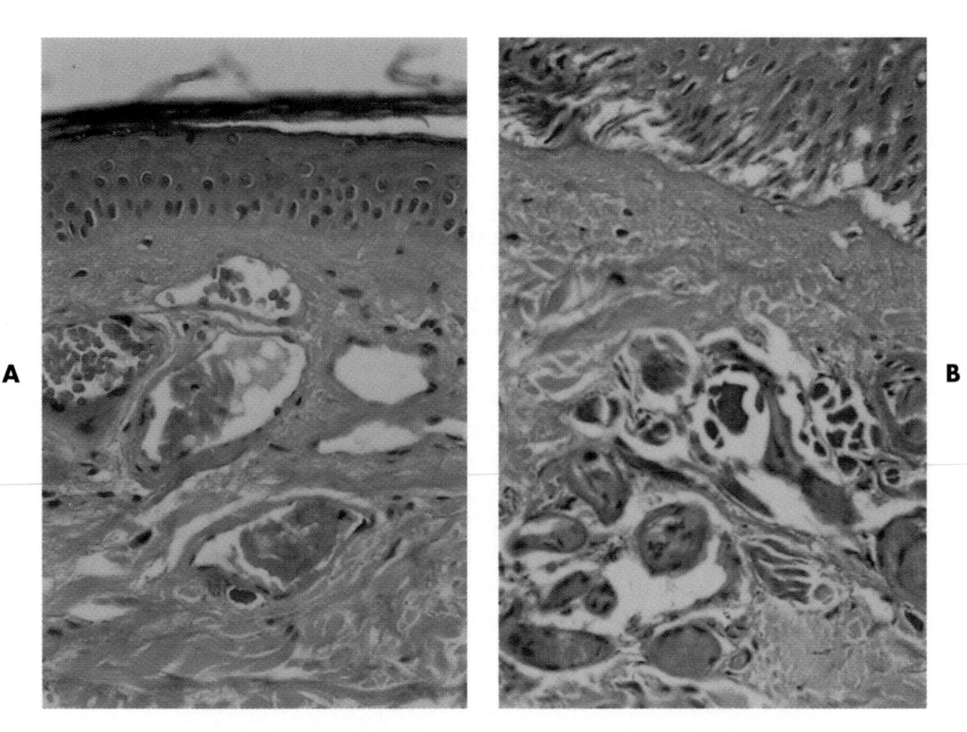

Figure 2-48 **A,** Biopsy specimen immediately after single pulse as described in Figure 2-47, *A*. Note coagulation of superficial dermal ectatic blood vessels without any change in overlying epidermis or perivascular tissue. (Hematoxylin-eosin; ×40.) **B,** Biopsy specimen immediately after double-pulse technique as described in Figure 2-47, *B*. Note nonspecific thermal damage to overlying epidermis and perivascular tissue. Ectatic blood vessels in superficial papillary dermis are thrombosed with evidence of perivascular collagen homogenization. (Hematoxylin-eosin; ×40.)

PWSs, as described later. One report comparing treatment of PWS with 585 versus 600 nm demonstrated that 1.5 to 2 times the fluence was required to achieve similar efficacy with 600 nm than the fluence used by the 585-nm parameter.[179] However, 11 of 22 cases showed at least a 20% increase in lightening with the 600-nm wavelength at a higher fluence. The 600-nm wavelength did not tend to be more effective in darker lesions. Also, no difference was seen in the incidence of temporary adverse sequelae between the two wavelengths. Another preliminary study[180] demonstrated increased clearing with FLPDL at 600 nm, 5-mm-diameter spot size at 13 J/cm^2, compared with FLPDL at 585 nm, 10-mm-diameter spot size at 5 J/cm^2. Therefore, the longer wavelength, even though it is absorbed less efficiently by Hb and HbO_2, may demonstrate increased clearing when a high energy fluence is used. This concept is also used by the PhotoDerm VL (see later).

Other factors in treatment response

In addition to size and location of the PWS (lesions on extremities), other factors may be important in predicting responsiveness to treatment. PWSs that are dark red or purple may be less responsive to laser treatment. The relative difficulty in treating these lesions results from the presence of deeper, larger vessels that are beyond the laser's penetration depth[39,41] or that are too large to be photocoagulated completely within treatment parameters of the FLPDL.[102] (As discussed previously, the thermal relaxation time of target vessels is related to their diameter, with the effective wavelength related to their depth.) However, purple lesions are not completely or always unresponsive to treatment. We found that although purple lesions are graded most often as excellent responders (52%), they also are the leading group of

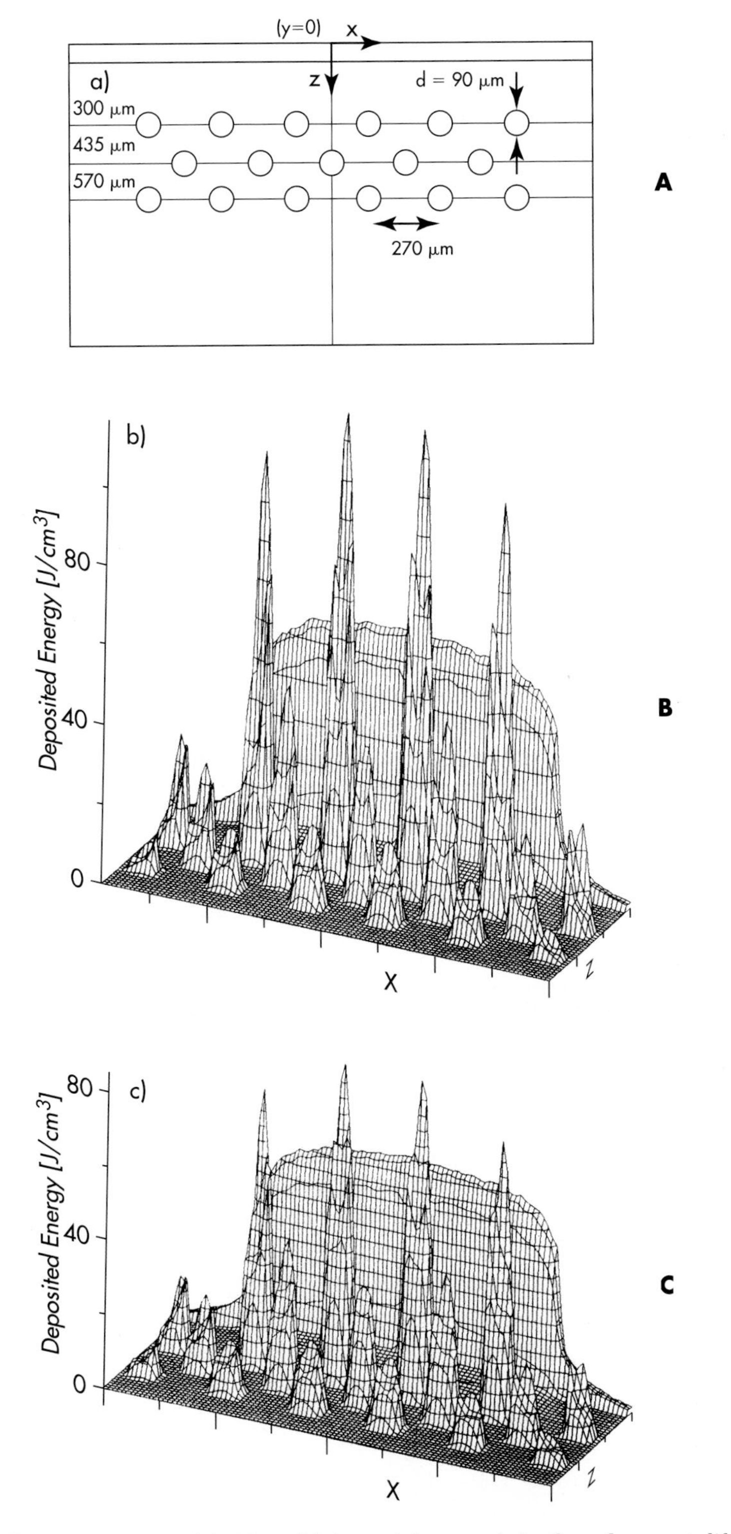

Figure 2-49 **A,** Geometry with 17 multiple straight vessels in three layers at different depths *z* of 300, 435, and 570 μm, and lateral spacing between vessels' centers of 270 μm. Energy deposition in multi–blood vessel geometry for **B,** wavelength 577 nm, and **C,** wavelength 585 nm. Laser beam diameter is 1 mm. Upper vessels receive most of the energy. Deeper vessels receive less energy by decreasing light fluence with depth and also by mutual shadowing of vessels. (From Lucassen GW, Verkruysse W, Keijzer M et al: *Lasers Surg Med* 18:345, 1996.)

poorly responsive lesions (21%).[46] This paradox may occur because two distinct populations of purple lesions exist: macular and nodular. Exophytic nodular lesions respond well, whereas purple and macular lesions respond poorly because of deeper and larger dermal vessels.

Paradoxically, lesions that respond poorly may appear clinically similar to good responders. In these lesions, biopsy demonstrates vessel walls that are thicker despite a vessel diameter that is smaller than 0.056 to 0.102 mm.[181,182] Such lesions are usually on the trunk or extremities. Alternatively, lesions with deeper vessels respond poorly, because the FLPDL at 585 nm and 6 to 8 J/cm² has been found to coagulate the entire vessel wall only to a maximum depth of 0.65 mm (mean 0.37 mm), even in vessels not shielded by more superficial vessels.[183] Superficial PWS vessels up to 0.15 mm in diameter were found histologically to coagulate completely without nonspecific damage to epidermal or perivascular tissues (Table 2-7 and Figure 2-50).

Therefore both vessel size and vessel depth in addition to vascular wall thickness are important determinants in predicting treatment efficacy. Vessel size has an important effect because the entire vessel (not just the superficial portion) must be thermocoagulated. This assumes that for vessel coagulation, heating the center of the vessel is necessary for thermal radiation to the entire vessel wall.

Table 2-7
Treatment of port-wine stains with flashlamp-pumped pulsed dye laser (FLPDL, 6.5 J/cm²): lightening per vessel size and depth

Measurement (μm; mean ± SD)	Poor Lightening (n = 8)	Moderate Lightening (n = 12)	Good Lightening (n = 22)
Diameter	19 ± 7	38 ± 17	38 ± 19
Depth	280 ± 46	315 ± 89	202 ± 56
Wall thickness	5.3 ± 1.8	5.4 ± 2.1	4.5 ± 1.7

From Fiskerstrand EJ, Svaasand LO, Kopstad et al: *J Invest Dermatol* 107:671, 1996.

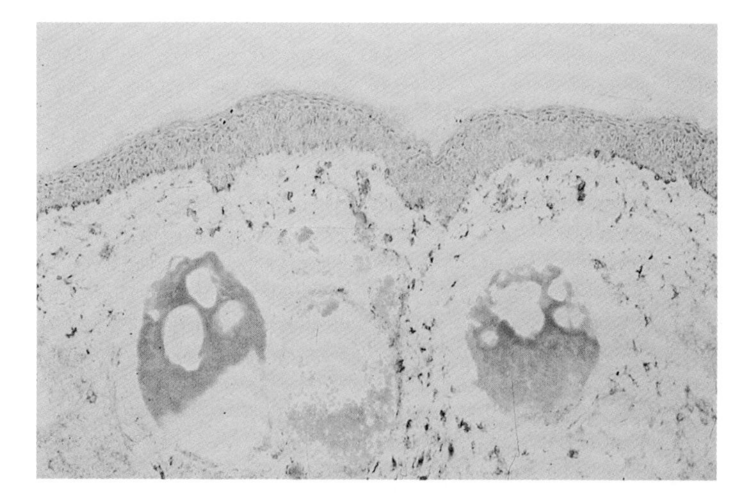

Figure 2-50 Biopsy of PWS on face of 43-year-old female. Lesion is violaceous and thick immediately after treatment with FLPDL at 6.5 J/cm². There is complete coagulation of red blood cells (RBCs) and vessel wall in a 150-μm vessel (*right*) and no damage to the lower third of RBCs and vessel wall in a larger vessel (*arrow*). Note steam bubble formation in upper half of vessels and perivascular dermal coagulation zone (*asterisks*). (Bar = 100 μm.) (From Hohenleutner U, Hilbert M, Wlotzke U et al: *J Invest Dermatol* 104:798, 1995.)

This requires both an adequate wavelength (for depth of penetration) and an adequate pulse duration (thermal relaxation).

Finally, Waner[184] has proposed that autonomic innervation is an important determinant of treatment efficacy. In a study of 118 PWSs in 102 patients, recurrence of the PWS depended on the time lapsed since the completion of treatment. Although only 3% of patients showed evidence of recurrence at 1 year, 20% and 40% showed evidence for recurrence at 1 to 2 and 2 to 3 years after treatment, respectively. Cutaneous venules of the PWS vasculature are innervated by sympathetic postganglionic neurons as well as sensory neurons.[185,186] The apparent underlying cause of a venular malformation is an absolute or relative deficiency of autonomic innervation of the cutaneous vascular plexus. Smaller and Rosen[185] demonstrated a deficit in the number of perivascular nerves in PWS. Kane et al[187] also found a decrease in autonomic innervation in six patients with poorly response PWS despite 5 to 21 treatments with the FLPDL at fluences up to 10 J/cm^2.

Therefore Waner[184] postulates and we concur that even though effective treatment decreases the number of ectatic vessels significantly, the remaining milieu allows for a continuing course of progressive ectasia. Recurrence of completely resolved capillary malformations, however, has not been observed by the authors.

Dark-skinned patients. Patients with darkly pigmented skin are generally less responsive to treatment because of competition from epidermal melanin for the laser energy. This results in preferential absorption of laser energy within melanosome-containing epidermal cells, leading to necrosis and interference with laser light penetration to deeper target vessels. Patients with darker skin generally require more treatment sessions to reach the same degree of clearing.[46] One Fitzpatrick type-V-VI–skinned male with a congenital PWS on the arm treated with the FLPD laser at 7.75 J/cm^2 developed persistent postinflammatory hyperpigmentation with epidermal necrosis. Posttreatment histology showed no damage to the underlying ectatic vessels.[188] As previously mentioned, epidermal cooling may allow limited treatment of PWS in pigmented skin.[114]

Multiple treatments

Improvement and clearance are gradual and usually require 5 to 10 treatments, although some lesions may not fully clear despite more than 20 separate treatments. It is sometimes difficult to determine when a lesion has reached a point of maximum improvement, but treatments should be continued as long as each results in an increment of improvement. We have found the point of diminishing return to occur about the seventh treatment.[47] Finally, areas within a PWS that fail to respond to treatment should be closely examined because we and others have reported the development of basal cell carcinoma within a PWS.[189]

A retrospective photographic analysis was performed on 69 patients who failed to achieve greater than 75% lesional lightening in nine treatment sessions with the FLPDL at typical treatment parameters.[190] Re-treatment at similar parameters with a 5-mm-diameter spot size and fluences of 5.75 to 8.0 J/cm^2 resulted in continued improvement in these patients. An additional 25% to 100% lightening was achieved in these patients treated up to 25 separate times. Extensive surface area involvement and limb lesions were the slowest to respond.

As mentioned previously, the dominant vessel size in childhood PWS is 10 to 50 μm in diameter. The average thermal relaxation time of PWS vessels is estimated at 1.2 msec.[37] As the child grows to adulthood, progressive ectasia results in larger and deeper vessels up to 300 μm in diameter with a thermal relaxation time of approximately 10 msec. It is reasonable to assume that these larger vessels would be more common in the darker, thicker lesions of adults. Although the FLPDL has been shown to be very effective in the treatment of adult PWS,[35,42,44,46] larger vessels in these lesions are not ideally suited for the specific parameters of this laser. Therefore other laser or pulsed light sources or photodynamic therapy may be useful.

Recurrence of port-wine stains

The use of the FLPDL in treating PWS has been widely practiced for more than 10 years. Recently, we and others have begun to evaluate our patients treated in the early years for signs of persistent or recurrent lesions. Although we have not seen a significant number of patients returning to our practice with progressing lesions, other physicians have reported recurrence after completion of treatment. Orten et al[166] have evaluated a small number of patients who were 2, 3, and 4 years posttreatment. They have reported recurrence (darkening of the lesion) in 5 of 24 patients at 2 years, 4 of 10 patients at 3 years, and 2 of 4 patients at 4 years posttreatment. The most obvious patient, an adult female whose PWS was on the midlateral cheek, had near-complete clearance of the PWS only to have almost total recurrence after 42 months. Whether these recurrent lesions would respond more favorably to alternative treatment modalities (e.g., PhotoDerm VL) or respond equally as well to additional treatment is unknown. Recurrence of PWS in a subset of patients may support a "neuronal" theory of PWS evolution.

Although there has yet to be a presentation of significant numbers of patients treated with the PhotoDerm VL who previously received FLPDL treatment, Raulin et al[191] reported complete resolution of a facial PWS in a 35-year-old male that did not respond to a single treatment with the FLPDL at 6.5 J/cm^2. They used a 550-nm cutoff filter with single and double pulses of 25 J/cm^2 3 msec in duration. Treatments were given every 8 weeks until clearance occurred after the fourth treatment.

Treatment with other lasers

Table 2-8 compares PWS response to treatment with various lasers.

Carbon dioxide laser. In our opinion, nodular lesions are best treated with the UltraPulse CO_2 ($UPCO_2$) laser (see Chapter 6) or the PhotoDerm VL high-intensity pulsed light source. With the $UPCO_2$ laser the lesion can be sculpted to reestablish a normal facial contour in addition to thermocoagulating the ectatic blood vessels. The advantages of the $UPCO_2$ laser are its precise hemostasis and avoidance of nonspecific thermal damage (Figure 2-51). After normal contours are obtained, the FLPDL or PhotoDerm VL can be used to lighten the remaining erythema.

Copper vapor laser. The CVL has been advocated for treating large-vessel lesions.[59] The microspot tracing technique using the argon-pumped tunable dye laser has also been reported to be a successful technique.[23,192,193] However, multiple treatments are necessary, and many lesions do not completely resolve[194] (Figure 2-52). The argon laser and CVL have been used with a robotized handpiece, the Hexascan[32,33] (Figure 2-23).

Table 2-8
Port-wine stain response to laser therapy

Laser Type	Macular Lesion	Mildly Hypertrophic Lesion	Very Hypertrophic Lesion
Flashlamp-pumped pulsed dye (FLPD)	Excellent	Very good	Poor
Continuous-wave (CW) dye, argon, krypton, copper vapor/copper bromide, and pulsed train	Fair	Good	Good
CW dye and pulsed train (with scanner)	Very good	Good	Good
Carbon dioxide	Poor	Fair	Good
Nd:YAG/CW	Poor	Poor	Good
PhotoDerm VL	Excellent	Excellent	Excellent

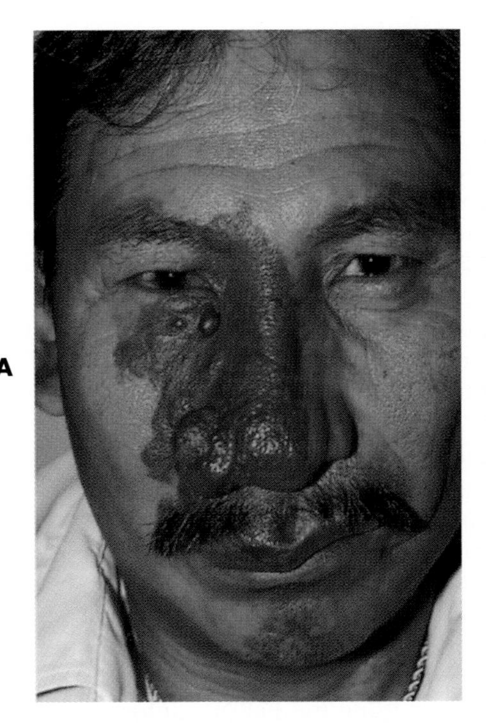

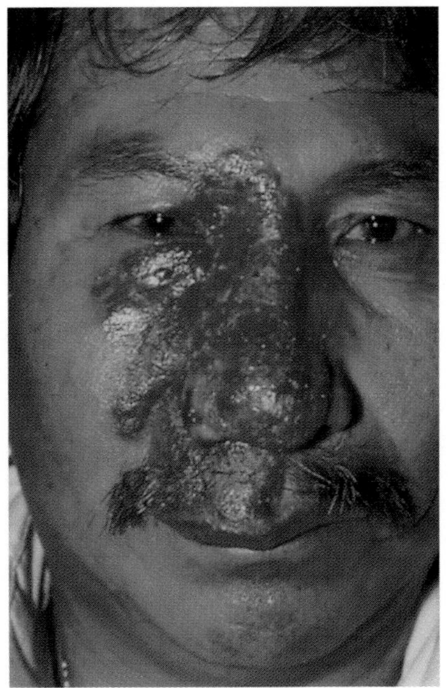

Figure 2-51 **A,** Congenital PWS with large hypertrophic mass on right lateral distal nose and nodules on right inner canthus present in 47-year-old Hispanic man. Over last 20 years, lesion has grown progressively darker in appearance as well as developing nodular hypertrophies. **B,** Three weeks after treatment with Coherent Ultra Pulse CO_2 Laser (Coherent Laser Corp., Palo Alto, Calif) at 250 mJ, pulse width of 794 msec at 20 W, 80 pulses per second, in continuous-wave mode with 2-mm spot.

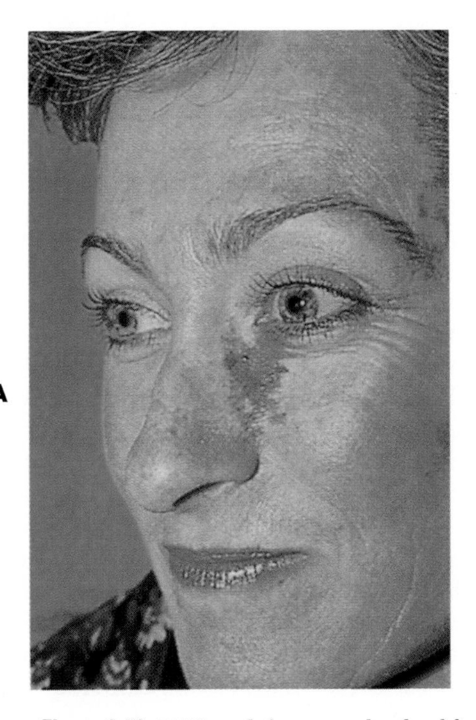

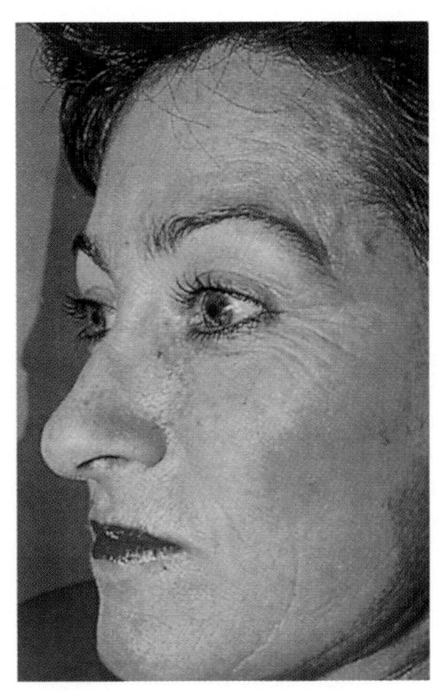

Figure 2-52 PWS on left upper cheek of female patient treated under general anesthesia with copper bromide laser (CBL); actual treatment required about 15 minutes. **A,** Before treatment. **B,** After treatment with exposure time of 7 msec, 2.5 W, and spot size of 0.7 to 1.0 mm (4.5 J/cm^2), with 10 msec (6.5 J/cm^2) for darker areas. (Courtesy Sue McCoy, MD.)

Meticulous tracing of vessels in a PWS using magnification and a 100-μm spot size with a CW dye laser (577 nm) has been shown to be safe and effective in children.[56,159] This technique has been advocated to minimize thermal damage,[23] but others have found that increasing laser beam diameter from 0.2 to 1.0 mm or more causes a typical blood vessel to require 2.5 times more energy fluence to achieve photocoagulation, while the energy absorbed by the epidermis remains the same.[163,195] Thus some degree of scarring and textural change to the skin is to be expected. Unfortunately, this technique is also tedious, time-consuming, difficult to master, and therefore only poorly reproducible.

Dinehart et al[196] recommend treating dark and thicker PWSs with the CVL first before switching to the FLPDL. Interestingly, a study of four patients with PWS treated with the argon laser or dye laser at 577 nm demonstrated no difference in therapeutic outcome between the two CW lasers. This observation was confirmed in a study of 31 adult PWSs treated with the CVL, 532-nm Nd:YAG laser, and argon laser with pulse widths of 30 to 50 msec and 13 J/cm^2 through a Hexascan delivery system.[197] This fact demonstrates the importance of delivering the laser energy within the vessel's thermal relaxation time, as previously described.[198]

McCoy[199] notes that pale-pink lesions respond poorly with the CVL, with best results occurring in dark, nodular lesions or in red lesions with distinct blood vessels. She achieves an average 30% to 50% lightening with the first treatment and proportionately lower percent lightening with subsequent treatments. Once pale-pink skin has been achieved, she also recommends using the FLPDL. Unfortunately, as previously described, adverse sequelae may occur when treating PWSs with the CVL, because the long pulse times allow excessive thermal diffusion and may result in tissue damage beyond the targeted vessels.

An additional report using the CVL with the Hexascan to produce minimal blanching with threshold fluences of 12 to 15 J/cm^2 showed excellent results in 24% of 25 patients and no response in 20%.[200] Eleven of 25 patients did develop slight atrophic scarring or hypopigmentation. Thus the CVL, although successful in treating some patients with PWS, has a high degree of adverse sequelae with little reproducibility between patients.

Potassium titanyl phosphate laser. The 532-nm Starpulse KTP laser (LaserScope) has been used in conjunction with a scanner to treat adults with PWS. Best clearing of the test sites was obtained with 3- or 5-msec pulses at 15 or 20 J/cm^2. Posttreatment purpura developed at all effective treatment sites. No scarring or ulceration occurred. Histology showed that selective vessel closure was achieved without hemorrhage. Perivascular collagen damage was always present at the effective treatment sites. These findings show that a 532-nm laser pulsed in the 1- to 30-msec domain is capable of inducing selective vessel closure.[201]

Nd:YAG long-pulse laser, 532 nm. By extending the pulse duration to within the thermal relaxation time of the vessel treated, purpura is avoided without loss of efficacy (see earlier). This laser has been effective in treating PWSs that have sometimes proved to be recalcitrant to treatment with other laser modalities (Figure 2-53). Formal studies have yet to be published, but our experience in using this modality, both with and without epidermal cooling, has been variable but positive.

PhotoDerm VL. As discussed in other sections in this chapter, the PhotoDerm VL is an effective high-intensity pulsed light source to treat vascular lesions, including PWS. Although most lasers use a pulse duration of less than 1 msec to treat the ectatic vessels in PWS, the thermal relaxation times of PWS vessels probed in vivo were found to respond best between 1 and 10 msec.[202] Purpura threshold and diffusion theory were used to reach the calculations in this study.

Eckhouse and Kreindel[203] have calculated the temperature distributions in the epidermis and target vessels of a PWS with diameters of 60 to 120 μm and depths of 300 to 600 μm treated with a lower cutoff wavelength of 550 nm, fluence of

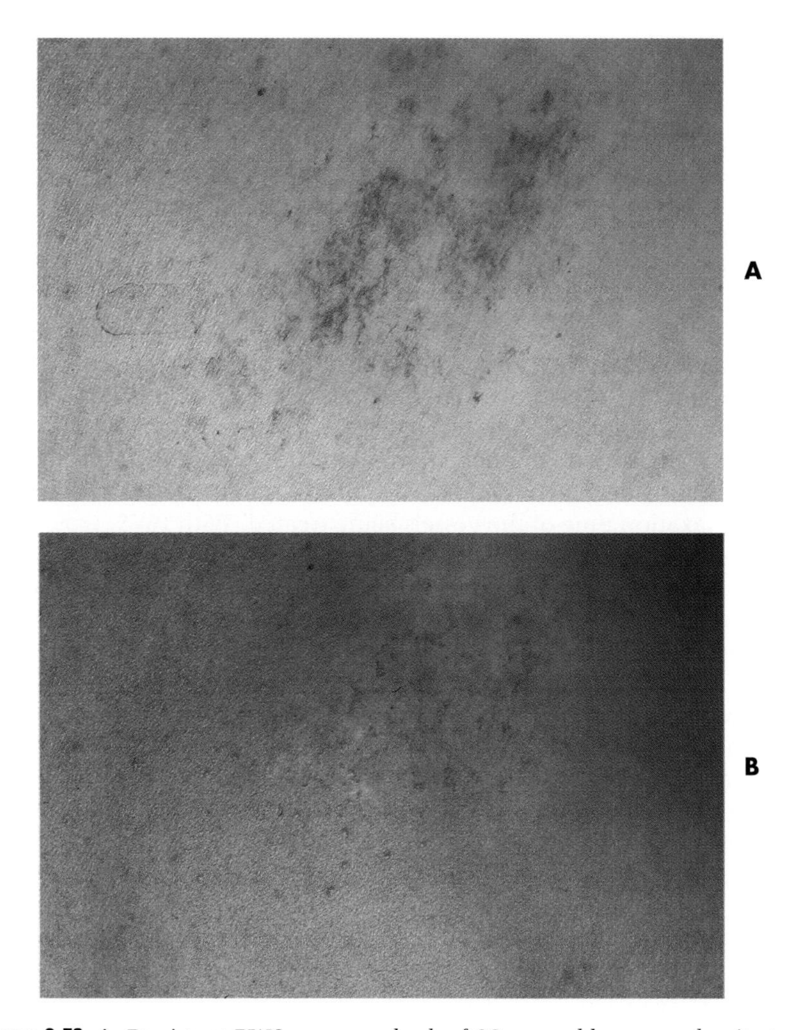

Figure 2-53 **A,** Persistent PWS on upper back of 28-year-old woman despite two treatments with PhotoDerm VL at 42 and 45 J/cm² with a 570-nm and a 550-nm cutoff filter double-pulsed at 2.4 msec and 4.0 msec, respectively, with a 10-msec delay between pulses. **B,** After three treatments at 8-week intervals with Versapulse using epidermal cooling to 4° C at 7.5 J/cm², 7-msec pulse, 4-mm-diameter spot; 9.0 J/cm², 10-msec pulse, 4-mm-diameter spot; and 13 J/cm², 10-msec pulse, 3-mm-diameter spot.

25 J/cm², and pulse duration of 2.5 msec. These parameters produced thermocoagulation of vessels to 80° to 100° C with an epidermal temperature of 60° C.

These calculated parameters compare favorably with our experience. We have treated PWS patients with the PhotoDerm VL with excellent results. The PhotoDerm VL at various fluences, wavelengths, and pulse durations has been found to be effective in treating a variety of PWSs (Figure 2-54). Each treatment session results in a degree of clearance. We usually vary treatment parameters between treatment sessions, with the more superficial parameters with single pulses and short cutoff wavelength filters used first and double and triple pulsing at higher cutoff filter wavelengths used with subsequent treatments. The only immediate response is slight erythema or purpura, which disappears within 48 hours. In particular, dark purpura, seen with FLPDL treatment, does not occur.[204]

The PhotoDerm VL can generate fluences in the range of 3 to 90 J/cm² on the skin in single-, double-, or triple-pulse modes. The pulse duration of each pulse can be varied from 2 to 20 msec and the delays between pulses vary from 10 to 300 msec. The PhotoDerm VL has a spot size of 8 × 35 mm. These parameters allow for treatment of larger and deeper vessels than those treated with the FLPDL.

The PhotoDerm VL is a good alternative to FLPDL treatment, especially in "laser-resistant" PWS. The PhotoDerm VL has the advantage of being capable of treating a large PWS in a short time with a small number of pulses because its very large spot size. Rarely, scarring has occurred when high fluences are used in single pulses. Therefore we advise using double and triple pulses to deliver to required energy fluence. Finally, unlike the 3 to 6 months time between treatments required for complete clearing with the FLPDL, the PhotoDerm VL achieves maximal clearance in 4 to 6 weeks so that additional treatments can be given sooner than with the FLPDL. This allows for more rapid resolution of the entire lesion with a similar number of treatments.[205]

The PhotoDerm VL uses similar operating principles to the FLPDL for the treatment of cutaneous vascular lesions. Selectivity is achieved by combining the optimal spectrum that will have a high interaction with HbO_2, minimal interaction with the skin, and sufficiently deep penetration. The pulse length is chosen so that it is within the thermal relaxation time of the vessels being treated. With PWS, typical pulse durations of 3 to 12 msec are selected. Although these pulse durations are within the thermal relaxation times of the smallest vessels that need to be treated, the pulse duration is long enough to prevent vessel rupture with the generation of purpura, which is typical to FLPDL treatment.

Previously treated port-wine stains

Previous treatments to PWSs with continuous-output lasers invariably result in an alteration of the epidermis and/or dermis because of their nonspecific nature, as previously described. Depigmented hypertrophic scars and subtle changes in dermal structures are often noted. Patients must realize that treatment with the FLPDL may not correct the previous therapy's adverse sequelae. In fact, hypopigmentation from

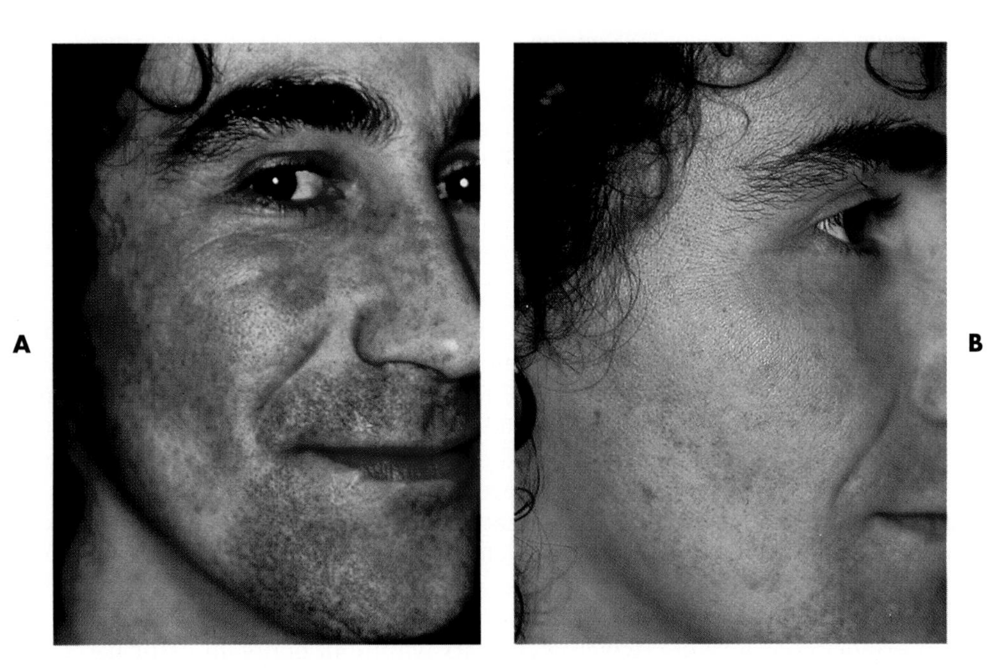

Figure 2-54 **A,** PWS on face of 28-year-old male before treatment. **B,** Three weeks after two treatments with PhotoDerm VL with 550-nm cutoff filter at 25 to 28 J/cm² given in a single short pulse. (From Raulin C, Goldman MP, Weiss MA, Weiss RA: *Dermatol Surg* 23:594, 1997.)

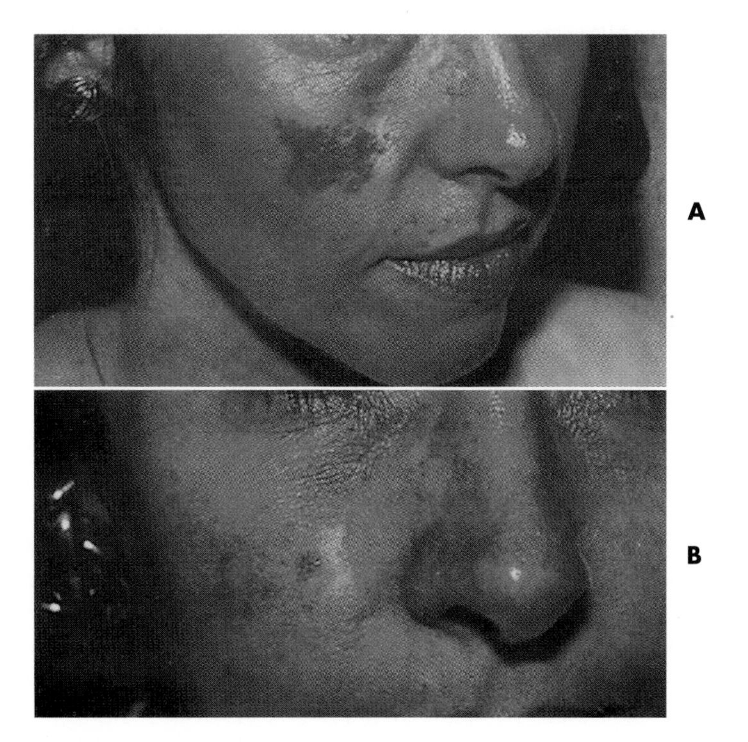

Figure 2-55 **A,** Congenital PWS on right cheek of 38-year-old woman treated 6 years previously with argon laser, resulting in a hypopigmented scar with cutaneous necrosis occurring at therapy. **B,** After four treatments with FLPDL at a fluence of 7.5 J/cm^2.

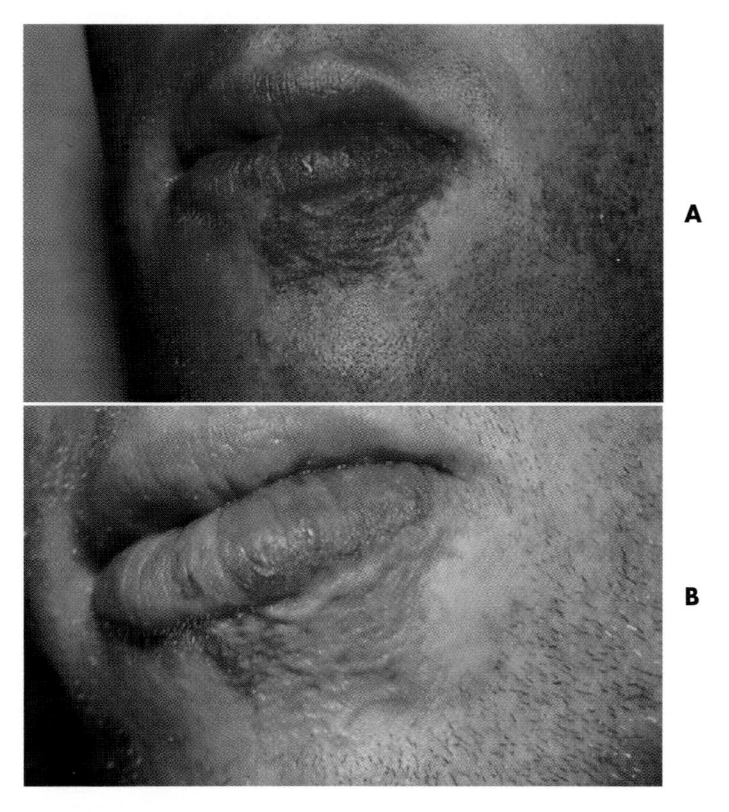

Figure 2-56 **A,** Congenital PWS under lip of 29-year-old male treated 7 years previously with argon laser, resulting in hypertrophic scar with minimal response to laser treatment. **B,** After four treatments with FLPDL. First three treatments were performed at 7.5 J/cm^2 and fourth treatment at 8 J/cm^2. Note near-complete resolution of PWS with persistence of underlying scarring process.

previous treatment may appear more pronounced after the PWS resolves with FLPD laser treatment (Figures 2-55 and 2-56).

When hypertrophic scars or skin textural changes are present, higher laser energies (increases of 0.5 to 1 J/cm^2) may be required to effect PWS resolution. It is hypothesized that higher fluences compensate for light scattering in dermal scar tissue. In addition, Alster et al,[14] using histology, optical profilometry, and clinical assessment, established that FLPD treatment of PWSs previously treated with the argon laser improved the skin texture. Finally, an increased number of laser treatments may be required for complete resolution. Nevertheless, excellent results can be obtained (Figure 2-56).

HEMANGIOMA

The treatment of hemangiomas remains a challenge. Part of the problem in evaluating published reports and in designing rational therapeutic plans resides in the confusion in terminology that still exists.

Hemangiomas are benign vascular tumors composed of proliferative, plump, endothelial cells. They can occur in skin, mucous membranes, and other soft tissues. A hemangioma often begins as a field transformation, frequently in multiple sites simultaneously or over a large area of skin.[206] The tumor may begin in subcutaneous tissue or muscle or may infiltrate the skin densely without elevating it, giving an appearance similar to that of a PWS.[207] However, whether superficial, deep, or mixed, the lesion is thought to have the same histologic and biologic behavior pattern throughout.[206] Hemangiomas typically present with both a superficial component and a deep cutaneous component as well as a subcutaneous proliferation of ectatic vessels.

The term *cavernous* is confusing. At times this term is used to refer to the deep dermal component of a hemangioma. Other times it is used to (mis)label a noninvoluting "cavernous hemangioma," which in reality is a venous malformation with spongy architecture.[207] A venous malformation may be difficult to differentiate clinically from a deep hemangioma. Failure to evacuate blood with compression occurs in hemangiomas, not in venous malformations, and this is a useful maneuver to differentiate the two conditions.

Natural History

Hemangiomas are the most common tumor of infancy; 60% occur on the head and neck, 25% on the trunk, and 15% on the extremities.[208] Eighty percent of hemangiomas are present as a single, well-circumscribed lesion 0.5 to 5.0 cm in diameter, and the remainder occur as multiple cutaneous and visceral lesions.[207] The lesions are generally absent at birth, but a localized area of pallor or macular erythema or telangiectasia may be present. The majority of hemangiomas (70%-90%) appear during the first month of life, and by age 12 months the incidence is reported to be in the 10% to 12% range.[121,209,210]

Hemangiomas present at birth result from in utero growth. They are difficult to diagnose with routine ultrasonic evaluation, even when associated with Kasabach-Merritt syndrome. They tend not to grow after birth and usually regress by 14 months, leaving atrophic, redundant, or scarred skin.[211]

Congenital hemangiomas of eccrine glands have also been reported.[212] These rare lesions usually appear at birth as bluish, slightly elevated tumors. None shows evidence of hyperhidrosis, and all resolve spontaneously. Diagnosis is made on histologic examination of dilated capillary-like vessels located around sweat glands.

The female/male ratio for hemangiomas is estimated to be 3:1.[208,213] Caucasian infants have been reported to have an increased incidence over other racial groups.[189,209,210] The clinical appearance is related to the depth of the proliferating lesion. Superficial lesions are raised and bright red (Figure 2-57). Deeper dermal lesions appear as bluish subcutaneous nodules. The overlying skin may have a fine network of telangiectasia (Figure 2-58). With regression, superficial lesions leave a flaccid, pedunculated, waxy yellow-colored skin (Figure 2-59). Deep lesions usually leave a smooth skin surface with overlying telangiectasia. A mottled grayish mantle spreads towards the periphery of the lesion and is less tense to palpation. Parents note that deep lesions do not swell as much as superficial lesions when the child cries.

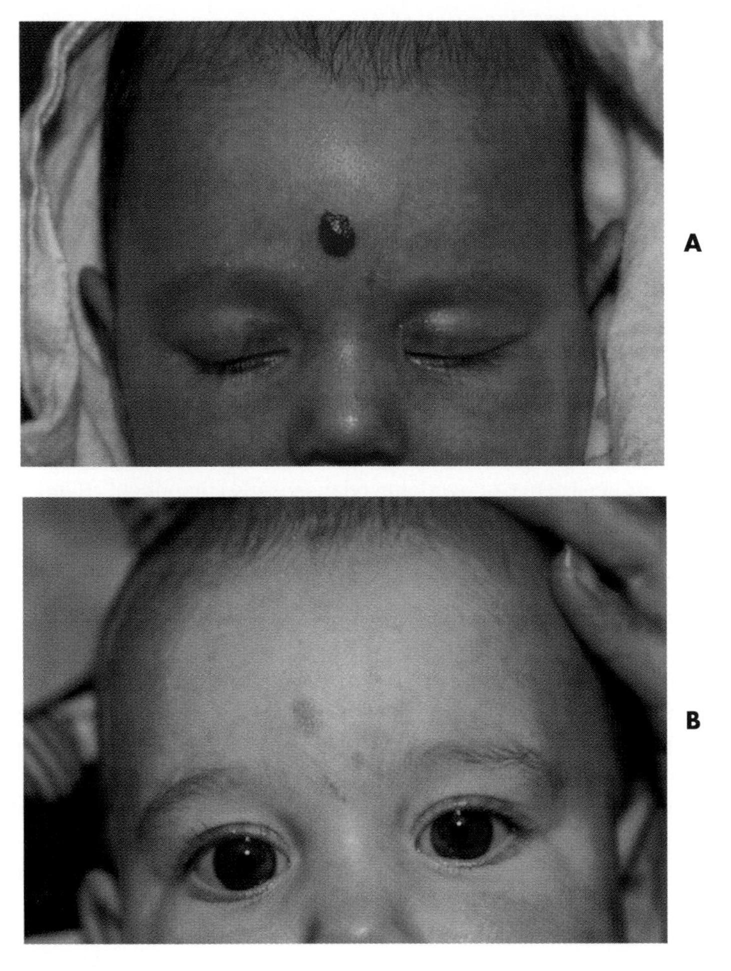

Figure 2-57 Hemangioma on forehead of infant appeared at 2 weeks of age and gradually enlarged. **A,** Appearance at 9 weeks of age. **B,** Clinical appearance 4 months after initial laser treatment and 1 month after fifth treatment with FLPDL at a fluence of 7 J/cm^2. Treatments were given at 3-week intervals. Although some persistence of the lesion is seen clinically as a faint pink macule, parents elected to discontinue treatment. (From Fitzpatrick RE: *Am J Cosmetic Surg* 9:107, 1992.)

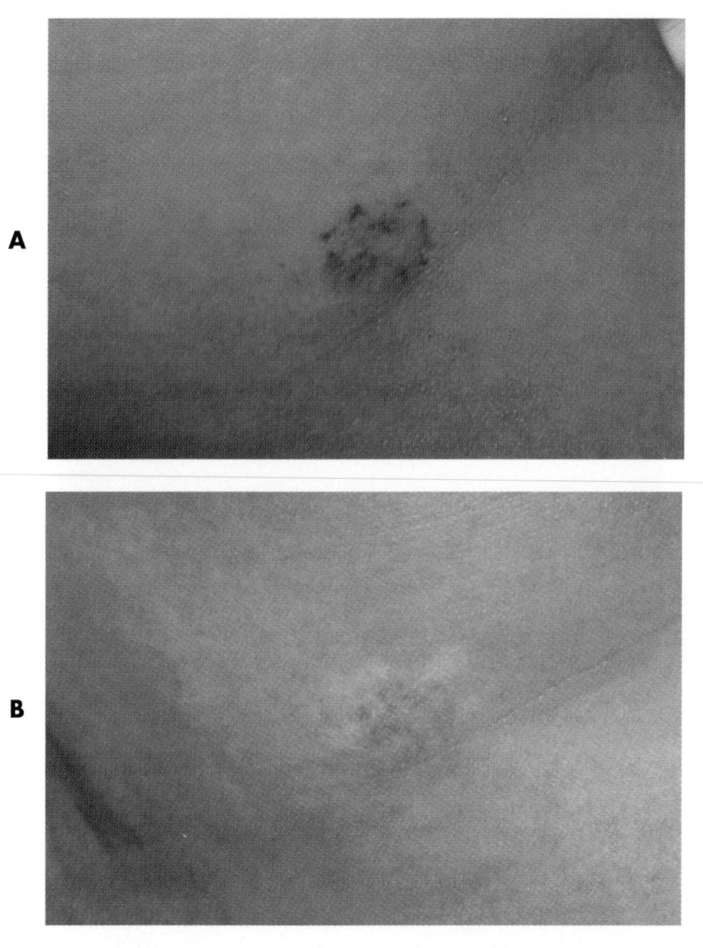

Figure 2-58 **A,** Clinical appearance of deep hemangioma with overlying telangiectasias on lateral trunk of 3-month-old girl. **B,** After five treatments with FLPDL at a fluence of 7 J/cm^2. Note complete resolution of hemangioma with only very faint persistence of overlying telangiectatic component. Hypopigmented area was present before any treatment commenced.

The hallmark of hemangiomas is a *rapid proliferative phase*. Immunohistochemical cellular markers that indicate proliferation include type IV collagenase, vascular endothelial growth factor, basic fibroblast growth factor, and other endothelial markers (CD31 and von Willebrand factor).[214] Growth is particularly rapid during the first 6 months of life but may continue until 12 months of age. Gradual spontaneous involution begins between the sixth and tenth month.[120,121,215] These stages are not distinct, because proliferation continues while involution slowly begins to dominate.[207] The first sign of regression is a change in color from crimson to dull purple. Clinical studies indicate that involution proceeds on the same time schedule for both deep and superficial hemangiomas.[208,213] Lesions located on the nose and lips are thought to involute more slowly.[213]

Adult hemangiomas are composed of mature, capillary-sized vessels approximately 100 μm in diameter, resembling dermal venules with virtually no endothelial growth.[216] Basement membrane thickness ranges from 0.6 to 14 μm because of multiple superimposed layers of basal lamina. At times an ingrowth of dermal collagen fibers is seen in the vessel wall. Pericytic cells are also immersed in the basement membrane, further thickening the vessel wall. Therefore, although response to laser treatment occurs, it may not be as dramatic as in thinner-walled hemangiomas of infancy.

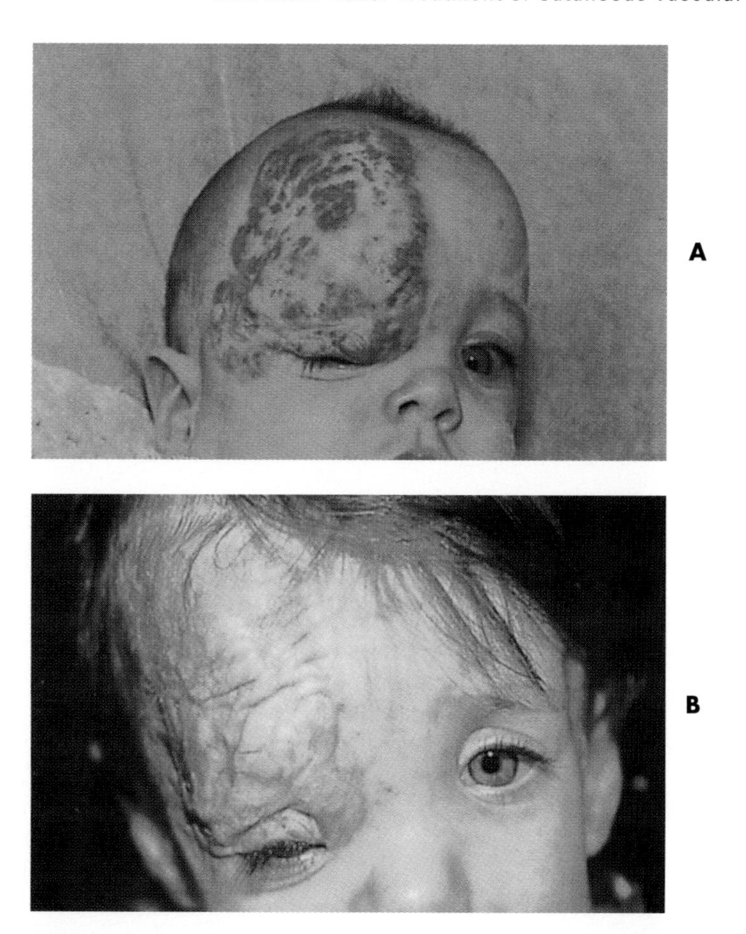

Figure 2-59 Extensive hemangioma on right forehead and upper eyelid of 9-month-old girl. **A,** Clinical appearance before any therapy. **B,** Clinical appearance 7 months after systemic prednisolone therapy per protocol described in this text, plus six separate treatments with FLPDL at a fluence of 7 J/cm^2. CT scan demonstrated no intracranial connection with hemangioma. Severe orbital dystopia will be corrected when her bones are more fully developed at age 6. In addition, periorbital atrophy and loss of subcutaneous tissue in area of hemangioma will be corrected with surgical excision after bony correction has been achieved. (From Fitzpatrick RE: *Am J Cosmetic Surg* 9:107, 1992.)

Studies of the natural history of hemangiomas reveal that complete resolution occurs in 50% of children by age 5 and in 70% by age 7, with continued improvement in the remaining children until ages 10 to 12.[121,122,209,215-217] However, 15% to 25% of lesions do not completely involute, and lesions that do not show significant signs of regression by age 6 to 8 years are not likely to regress completely.[217,218] Rate and extent of resolution are unrelated to lesion size[213] (Figure 2-60).

Complications and Adverse Sequelae

Complications from the proliferative phase include *ulceration* (5% to 11% of patients) and *infection,* which is more common on the lip and genitoanal areas, where abrasion is common[120,219] (Figure 2-61). Bleeding from trauma is an annoying and relatively common problem that usually responds to pressure. At times, superficial ulcerations appearing on buttock, sacral, or lip skin in infants can precede the development of hemangiomas by a few weeks. The reason for this evolution in some infants is unknown.[220]

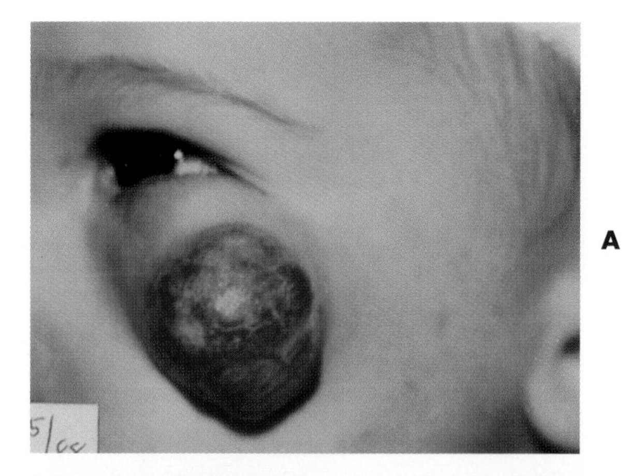

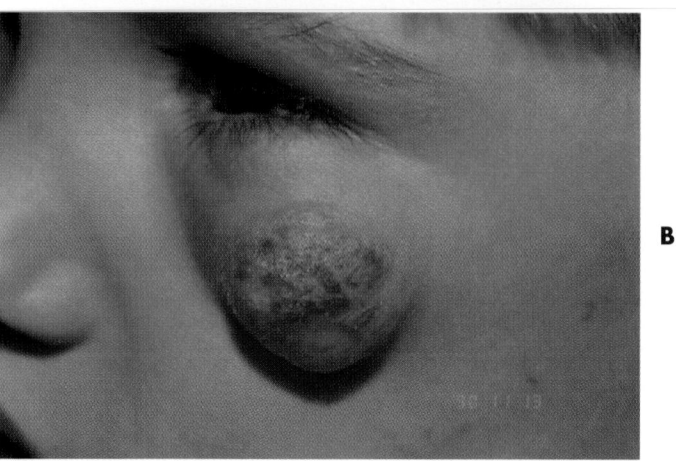

Figure 2-60 **A,** Hemangioma on left cheek of 15-month-old child. Lesion arose at 3 weeks of age and increased in size over first year before beginning a short resolution. Patient was treated with oral prednisolone at 6 weeks of age until 6 months of age without noticeable effect on size of hemangioma.
B, Appearance at 3 years of age. Note redundant skin with some superficial atrophic scarring and persistent superficial telangiectasia.

Skeletal distortion is rare but may occur from a mass effect on underlying bone. Lesions of the nasal tip often distort underlying cartilage (Figure 2-62). Deviation of facial bones or orbital enlargement may occur.[221]

Lesions of the upper eyelid may obstruct the visual axis, causing *deprivation amblyopia* with failure to develop binocular vision.[222] Interruption of vision in infancy for as briefly as 1 to 2 weeks can cause permanent damage, with longer periods of obstruction being more harmful. Upper eyelid lesions may also distort the growing cornea by direct pressure producing refractive errors *(strabismic amblyopia)*.[223] Large hemangiomas of the lower eyelid may result in similar problems, but even the smallest hemangioma within the upper eyelid can cause visual disturbances.[198] Therefore all children with hemangiomas involving either the upper or the lower eyelid should be referred to an ophthalmologist promptly, even if vision appears normal.

Other *functional problems* may occur because of the sheer bulkiness of lesions in critical locations causing obstruction. Lesions of the nose may interfere with breathing. Lesions in the subglottic airway may obstruct the larynx, causing life-threatening asphyxiation.[224] Lesions may obstruct the external auditory canal and

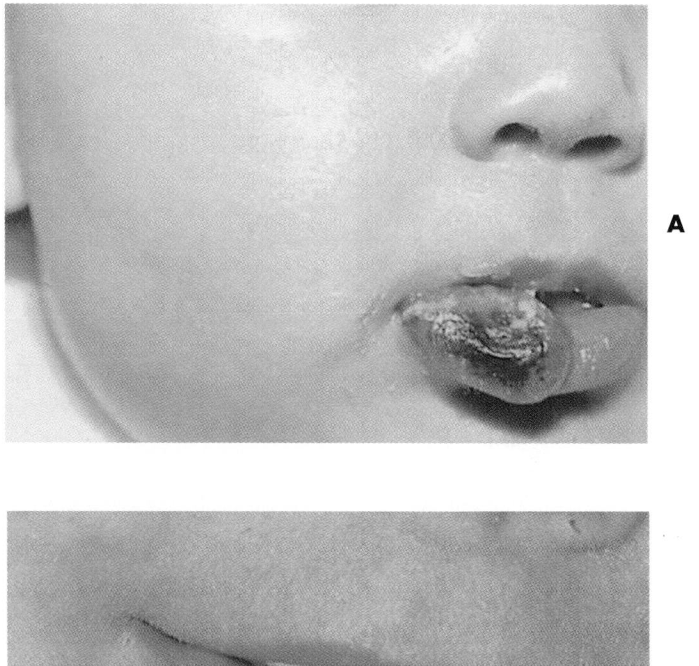

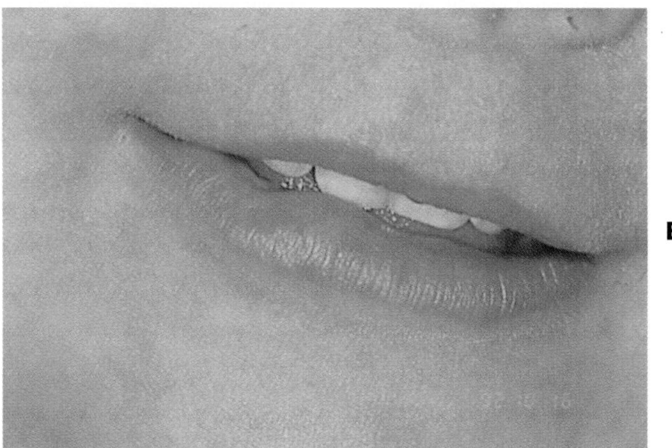

Figure 2-61 **A,** Three-month-old girl with hemangioma on right lower lip that was flat and pink at birth and slowly enlarged during first 2 months before rapid enlargement over last 4 weeks, at which point it interfered with eating and was bleeding. **B,** Clinical response 2 years later and 1 year after last treatment with FLPDL. Total of nine laser treatments were given at 4- to 6-week intervals with a fluence of 7 J/cm^2. Within 2 weeks of first laser treatment, definite improvement with rapid resolution of lesion was seen, as well as near-immediate resolution of pain associated with eating. Slight depression appears in midportion of lower lip underlying previous hemangioma. However, there is no distortion of the vermilion border. (From Fitzpatrick RE: *Am J Cosmetic Surg* 9:107, 1992.)

cause a mild to moderate hearing loss. Lesions in the anogenital area may cause obstruction, pressure, or tenderness when ulcerated and inflamed.

Medical complications include the *Kasabach-Merritt syndrome*[225]: generalized bleeding from profound thrombocytopenia associated with a large hemangioma or extensive hemangiomatosis. Congestive heart failure is a potentially lethal complication in an infant with multiple cutaneous and visceral hemangiomas.[226]

Extensive facial hemangiomas may also be associated with *cardiac and abdominal anomalies.* Associated anomalies can be right-sided aortic arch coarctation, a supraumbilical midabdominal raphe defect, associated laryngeal and duodenal hemangiomas, and posterior brain fossa abnormalities such as Dandy-Walker malformations.[227-231] The constellation of findings consisting of large facial hemangiomas, posterior fossa malformations, arterial anomalies, coarctation of the aorta and cardiac

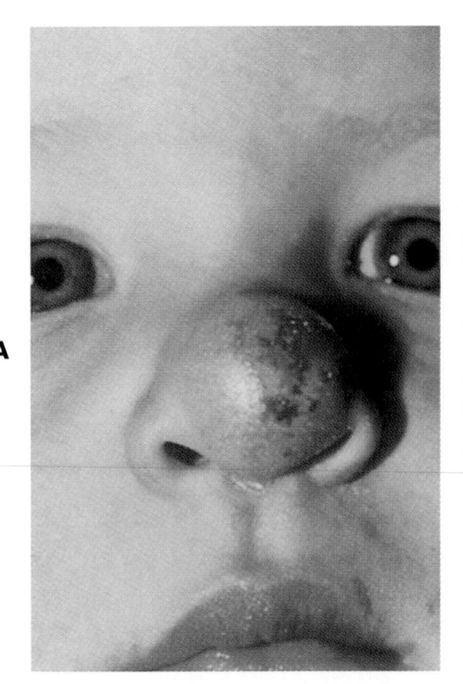

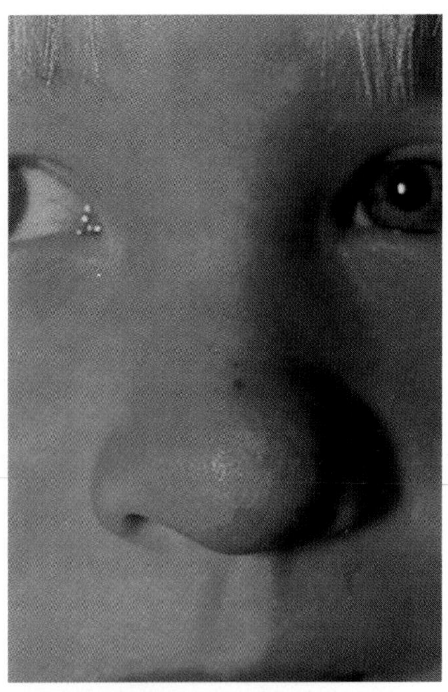

Figure 2-62 **A,** Five-month-old boy with 1.5-cm hemangioma on tip of nose and overlying 4 × 8–mm strawberry-red mark in center of lesion, which is very fluctuant. Hemangioma was present at birth and is continuing to enlarge. **B,** Approximately 3 years later, after four treatments with FLPDL at a fluence beginning initially at 6.75, then 7.5, 8.0, and 8.5 Jcm^2. In addition to laser treatment, patient received intralesional injection of triamcinolone, with a total of 10 mg given over five injections Although nose has assumed normal appearance, it is still slightly boggy and increases in size with hot weather and when patient cries.

defects, and eye abnormalities has been given the acronym *PHACE syndrome*.[231] This syndrome represents a spectrum of malformations of varying degrees of severity caused by a common morphogenetic event or events in utero.[230,232]

The facial hemangiomas seen in the PHACE syndrome are usually plaquelike in quality and cover at least one dermatome; 88% occur in females. Infants who have large facial hemangiomas should be evaluated with head circumference measurements and neurologic studies, including brain imaging with cranial ultrasound and MRI scans. These patients also appear at risk for developing airway abnormalities and should be evaluated closely for cardiac defects as well.

Sacral hemangiomas have also been associated with several anomalies, including imperforate anus, genitourinary abnormalities (absent or hypoplastic kidney, abnormal genitalia), and tethered spinal cord without neurologic dysfunction.[233,234]

In a study of 175 cases of severe superficial hemangiomas, defined as lesions involving large surface areas, symptomatic visceral hemangiomas were present in 11.4% and associated malformations in 6.9%.[235] The authors found that MRI was the best imaging modality to detect the deep growth. Hemangiomas give signals that are different from lymphatic or arteriovenous malformations. It may also indicate the rapidity of blood flow movement. Color-flow duplex ultrasonography was helpful but could not accurately distinguish a hemangioma from an AVM because both may have a high-flow pattern.

As described later, many hemangiomas resolve spontaneously without any form of treatment. However, even when resolution is complete, the skin that remains after involution exhibits mild atrophy, has a wrinkled texture with a few telangiectatic vessels, or is paler than the surrounding skin.[207] Resolution that is considered cosmetically acceptable has been said to occur in 70% to 82% of patients.[219] However, in an analysis of 298 hemangiomas, 80% that had not involuted by age 6 left a significant residual cosmetic deformity.[236] In addition, 38% of those lesions that had completely resolved by age 6 left a significant residual deformity. Scarring after ulceration generally leaves a white, flat area of fibrosis. When the hemangioma has been large, there is often redundant skin and a residual subcutaneous fibrofatty tissue mass.[207] Therefore our opinion, supported by the clinical studies detailed next, is to treat lesions at the first available opportunity.

In addition to medical complications, including persistent scarring, the psychologic consequences are real. A child develops a sense of self-awareness between 18 and 24 months of age. This awareness may be transmitted to psychosocial developmental disorders. Parental guilt, anger, and disappointment as well as overprotectiveness are common. These feelings may affect the dynamics of the entire family.

Traditional Treatment

Treatment of hemangiomas has been oriented toward waiting for natural regression to occur since Lister's article in 1938 outlined a predictable course for these lesions.[217] However, contemporaries of Lister recognized the effectiveness of early treatment before and during the proliferative stage of growth.[237] Therapeutic intervention historically has been reserved for lesions causing recurrent bleeding, ulceration, infection, or serious distortion of facial features and lesions that interfere with normal physiologic functions, such as breathing, hearing, eating, vision, and bladder and bowel function. Despite these therapeutic guidelines, there is tremendous pressure on anguished, concerned parents observing an enlarging hemangioma on their child, particularly when it is a facial lesion of any size. Because of this, there have been many ill-advised attempts at treatment that have resulted in excessive scarring.[238]

Surgical intervention,[239] x-ray therapy,[150,238,240] sclerotherapy,[238, 241] diathermy,[242] CO_2 snow cryotherapy,[243] and electrocautery[244] have all been attempted, resulting in significant scarring. A *basal cell carcinoma* (BCC) presenting 58 years after thorium X applications to a birthmark when the patient was 3 years old has been reported.[245] Thorium X, a rich source of alpha radiation, was frequently used for treating hemangiomas until the 1960s.[246,247] BCC developing after thorium X treatment of hemangiomas has also been reported.[248] *Angiosarcomas* have also occurred after radiation treatment of hemangiomas, with a review of the literature uncovering 11 such cases.[249] The prognosis is poor, with a 10% 5-year survival rate.

Thus these prior methods of treatment, because of unacceptable side effects and lack of efficacy, have been replaced with laser therapy as a destructive and antiproliferative modality and with other antiproliferative medical treatments. As discussed later, some patients require multiple forms of therapy.

When the pathogenesis of these lesions is considered, an antiangiogenic agent that would prevent proliferation and induce involution of the entire lesion is the most logical therapeutic approach.[196] At present, the only treatment of this type is the use of systemic steroids with or without interferon-alpha.

Systemic and Intralesional Corticosteroids

If a hemangioma is steroid responsive (30%-60% of cases),[196,235] the result is often immediate and dramatic.[238] A treatment schedule of 2 to 3 mg/kg/day of *prednisone*, rapidly tapered, when the tumor has reduced in size, is given for a cycle of 4 to 6 weeks, followed by a rest period. Complications have been few.[196] In patients who fail to respond, however, increasing the dose of prednisone to 4 to 5 mg/kg/day may trigger growth of the lesion.[235] Loss of appetite and diminished growth rate have been observed but resolve quickly when steroids are discontinued. However, because the proliferative activity of the tumor continues for 6 to 12 months, the need for prolonged steroid suppression persists, with rebound growth of the hemangioma occurring when treatment is discontinued. This often results in an escalating steroid dosage or abandonment of this regimen because of concern regarding potential steroid side effects.

A second steroid schedule has been used throughout the entire proliferative phase of the hemangioma. *Prednisolone* is given in a dosage of 3 to 5 mg/kg/day for 2 to 4 weeks until control of growth of the hemangioma is achieved. An alternate-day schedule is then instituted by doubling the dose on the "on" day and eliminating the alternate-day dosage gradually over 2 weeks. Prednisolone is then tapered every 2 weeks by 5 mg if the hemangioma does not enlarge.[250] This treatment schedule is maintained for 6 to 10 months. In 43 infants treated, only one infant had transient side effects. However, it is advisable to use the lowest effective dose of steroid for the shortest period until the hemangioma enters the regression phase (Figure 2-63).

A 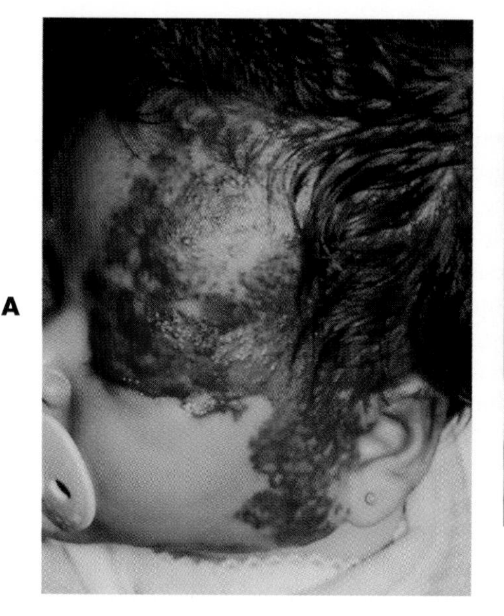

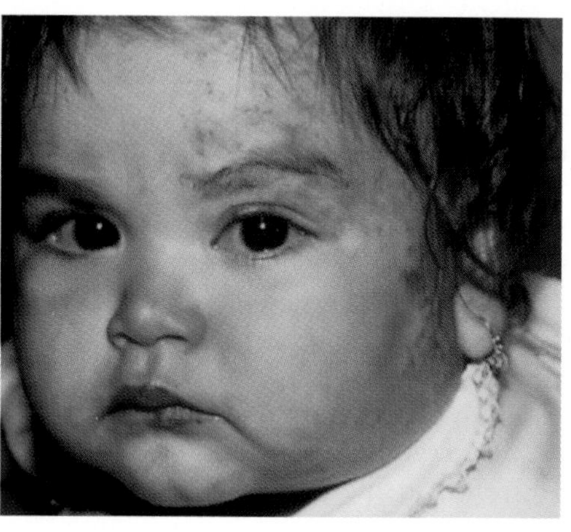 B

Figure 2-63 **A,** Large hemangioma over right side of face of 4-week-old girl. This lesion began as a red macule 5 mm in diameter, first noted over right cheek 2 days after birth. Hemangioma spread rapidly over left forehead, cheek, neck, and eyelid over only 2 to 3 days. Patient was initially treated with FLPDL alone at a fluence of 7.25 J/cm². However, when seen 2 weeks later, although there was definite improvement in laser-treated site, hemangioma was continuing to enlarge rapidly, involving entire orbit and right parotid and neck area. Subcutaneous masses were present, and prednisolone was begun at a dosage of 4.5 mg/kg/day. Laser treatment was continued at a fluence of 7.5 J/cm² at 2-week intervals. Almost immediately after institution of oral prednisolone, hemangioma stopped growing and began a resolution phase. Prednisolone dosage was tapered 2 weeks after institution. When it was discontinued totally on pediatrician's advice 6 weeks later, hemangioma again began to enlarge. We therefore restarted prednisolone therapy, increasing it to a dosage of 5 mg/kg/day to initiate resolution of hemangioma. During this time, lesion was continually treated at 2- to 3-week intervals with Candela FLPDL at fluences ranging from 7.0 to 7.5 J/cm². Interestingly, on alternate-day prednisolone therapy, patient's parents noticed hemangioma increasing in size during the day off therapy, with it regressing in size during the day on prednisolone therapy. Prednisolone therapy was tapered over 2 years before being discontinued. **B,** Patient, now 11 months old, has marked resolution of hemangioma. At this point she is continuing to have prednisolone therapy and has had total of nine treatments with Candela FLPDL, with last treatment 4 months previous to this photograph. (From Fitzpatrick RE:, *Am J Cosmetic Surg* 9:107, 1992.)

Intralesional steroids have been used successfully in the treatment of periorbital hemangiomas.[251,252] Soft tissue atrophy is common but seems to be temporary.[251] Intralesional steroid injection carries a risk of hemorrhage or hematoma in the retrobulbar space, which is a threat to vision.[230] It may cause occlusion of the central retinal artery and damage to the optic nerve.[253] When the hemangioma extends posterior into the orbital cone, systemic steroids should be considered.[238]

A study of 70 children with 74 hemangiomas treated with intralesional corticosteroids showed more than 75% reduction in volume in 58% of patients, 50% to 75% improvement in 22%, 25% to 50% improvement in 12%, and less than 25% improvement in 8%.[254] No patient had regrowth after treatment with a mean follow-up of 14 months. The authors used doses of 10 to 120 mg per injection of triamcinolone and betamethasone acetate (1.5-18 mg/injection) given in a total volume of 0.5 to 6.0 ml depending on the hemangioma's size. Side effects included temporary cushingoid facies and hypopigmentation, each in two patients. No apparent correlation existed between response and lesion location or size or patient gender or age.

Enjolras and Mulliken[255] advise giving 3 to 5 mg/kg/procedure (either intralesional or systemic) of triamcinolone with or without cortisone acetate. They believe that intralesional and systemic corticosteroids have a similar response rate. They advise caution when injecting hemangiomas of the upper eyelid because particles in the steroid suspension can potentially occlude retinal or choroidal microvessels or the central retinal artery.

Interferon

Interferon is the second-line drug for treating severe, large hemangiomas. Interferon-alpha$_{2a}$ (IFN-α_{2a}) is a potent, fairly well-tolerated cytokine that requires liver and hematologic monitoring during therapy. Long-term treatment carries the risk of thyroid dysfunction and neurologic complications. Interferon is known to inhibit angiogenesis, probably through inhibition of vascular smooth muscle cells and capillary endothelial cells.[256]

In a study of 20 patients with vision-threatening hemangiomas resistant to corticosteroids, 18 patients had more than 50% regression after an average of 8 months of treatment.[257]

Combination Therapy

At times, especially when treating large or extensive hemangiomas and conditions such as diffuse neonatal hemangiomatosis, multiple modalities may be required. In these patients, systemic prednisone with or without interferon, embolization of hemangiomas, surgical debulking and excision of the dermal component, and FLPDL treatment to superficial lesions may all be used[258] (Figure 2-64). Although one might believe that the laser is cosmetic, its use in these patients prevents cutaneous hemorrhage and facilitates routine skin care.

Early therapeutic intervention with laser photocoagulation of the vessels of a hemangioma when it is in a thin, flat stage or on initial presentation as localized telangiectasia is advocated to minimize enlargement of the tumor, ulceration, bleeding, and obstruction of vital organs.[48,50] This may be effective theoretically if the laser is capable of reaching all the vessels present. However, the notion that superficial photocoagulation will initiate regression of the entire hemangioma, including adjacent untreated tumor, does not appear to be true. Our experience, along with that of several colleagues, is that the deep portion of hemangiomas beyond the depth of laser penetration continues to proliferate despite involution of the superficial components treated by laser.[47,48,50]

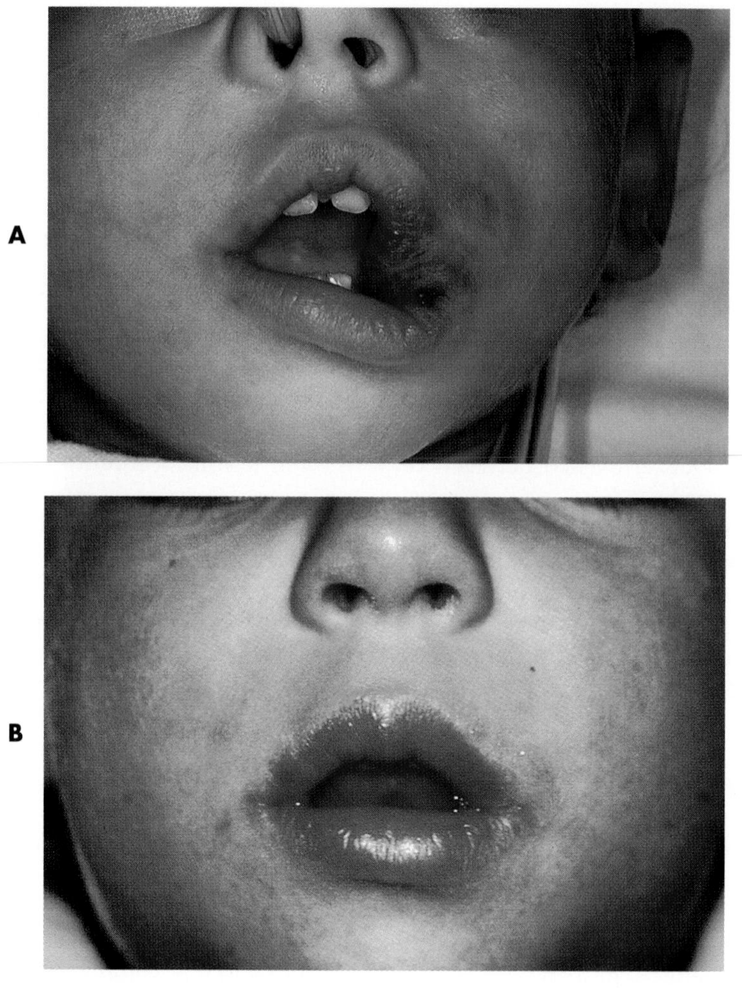

Figure 2-64 **A,** Venous malformation involving lip and mucosa before treatment. **B,** After therapy with Nd:YAG laser delivered as two separate treatments 6 weeks apart. Laser was used with 600-μm filter in noncontact mode and energy fluence of 30 W delivered in 0.2-sec pulses to shrink malformation. This was followed 6 weeks later by surgical resection. This photograph is clinical appearance 6 months after surgery. (Courtesy Milton Waner, MD.)

Laser Treatment

The necessary requirements for any laser or pulsed light source to thermocoagulate effectively the ectatic vessel of a hemangioma are its depth of penetration, energy fluence, and pulse duration. Lasers with short wavelengths (<585 nm) can only deliver sufficient energy required for thermocoagulation to a depth less than 1 mm. Pulse durations necessary range from 0.5 to 10 msec, depending on the size of the ectatic vessels. Energy fluences should be greater than 6 J/cm^2. With these parameters, many different pulsed-light modalities have demonstrated efficacy (Table 2-9).

Argon laser

The argon laser[259-261] and the Nd:YAG laser[68] have both been used effectively to treat hemangiomas. The potential benefit of the argon laser is limited by its depth of penetration into the dermis (<1 mm) and its tendency to cause hypertrophic scarring through nonspecific thermal injury, as reported in children with PWS.[25] However, with PWSs thicker than 1 mm, nonspecific thermal injury may be advantageous

Table 2-9
Response of selected vascular lesions to laser therapy

Laser Type	Strawberry Hemangiomas	Capillary-Cavernous Hemangiomas	Limited Venous Malformations
FLPD	Very good	Fair	Fair
CV/CB, KTP, krypton, 532-nm Nd:YAG	Fair	Fair	Fair
Continuous-wave dye or argon	Good	Fair	Good
Carbon dioxide	Fair	Fair	Fair
Nd:YAG, 1064 nm	Fair	Fair	Good
PhotoDerm VL	Very good	Very good	Very good

FLPD, Flashlamp-pumped pulsed dye; *CV/CB,* copper vapor/copper bromide; *KTP,* potassium titanyl phosphate; *Nd:YAG,* neodymium:yttrium-aluminum-garnet.

with a physician experienced in the laser's use. In addition, one physician noted atrophic, hypopigmented scarring in three of five cases of hemangioma treated with the argon laser.[262]

Nd:YAG laser

The Nd:YAG laser at 1064 nm can penetrate deeply into tissue (2-8 mm) but produces widespread tissue injury because of its nonspecific absorption. This tends to result in scar formation. The Nd:YAG laser has been successful in shrinking large symptomatic lesions through nonspecific thermal injury,[68] but the risk of scarring, which always occurs to some extent,[263] must be weighed against potential benefits.

Some physicians believe the Nd:YAG laser should be limited to treating mucous membrane lesions (e.g., oral mucosa). Treatment technique also makes a difference. Treatment using 3- to 4-mm-diameter spots with 6- to 8-mm untreated lesion between spots has been advocated as a method to decrease scarring while still effectively debulking a lesion.

In 160 patients treated with the Nd:YAG laser at energy fluences of 400 to 1600 J/cm^2 in a continuous manner with pulses of 0.5 sec, 13% had excellent results, 55% had a reduction in hemangioma size by more than 50%, by less than 50% in 35%, and with negligible results in 2%.[264] Ten percent of patients had scarring from superficial necrosis. The incidence of textural or pigmentary changes to the overlying skin was not reported. The authors noted an advantage of surgical resection of bulky tumors after thermocoagulation was obtained with the Nd:YAG laser.

Dr. Berlien in Germany has successfully used the Nd:YAG laser to coagulate tissue, with its fluence being transferred to the bulk of the tumor through a 600-μm bare fiber at 8 to 10 W on a continuous mode until tumor coagulation occurs. The fiber is introduced through an 18-gauge Teflon cannula, and the skin is monitored with a thermal probe and cooled to minimize thermal injury to the epidermis. The fiber is slowly extracted at a rate approximating 0.5 mm/sec, and monthly treatments are given to allow resorption of coagulated tissue. Postoperative edema and some pain occur for about 6 hours.

Use of the sapphire-tip contact probe with the Nd:YAG laser allows excision of vascular lesions with control of bleeding and offers another therapeutic approach in debulking the lesion.[265,266] However, a retrospective analysis of 11 patients treated with this technique demonstrated only three "aesthetically acceptable" results despite four separate treatments.[267] In contrast, Afpelberg[268] has reported total removal without complications or side effects in 16 patients treated in this manner. The difference in treatment results may be related to preoperative preparation of the patient with intralesional corticosteroids or waiting until the lesion is in a stable or regressive stage before proceeding with surgical correction.

Cryogen spray cooling of the epidermis overlying hemangiomas may protect the epidermis and papillary dermis while achieving deep tissue photocoagulation during Nd:YAG laser irradiation.[269] A preliminary study on the highly vascularized chicken comb demonstrated 6.1-mm-deep photocoagulation while preserving epidermal integrity. To be effective, however, surface temperature monitoring must occur simultaneously with laser treatment and cooling to prevent epidermal damage. Therefore this technique may allow treatment of thick hemangiomas with a deep component.

Potassium titanyl phosphate laser

The KTP laser used through an intralesional 0.6-mm-diameter bare fiber has been found to shrink hemangiomas.[270] With this technique the fiber is passed through a 20-gauge needle positioned in the center of the hemangioma. Laser energy is then delivered at 15 J until shrinkage is seen or the overlying skin begins to feel warm to the touch. However, this is inaccurate and potentially dangerous because once the overlying skin is warm, excessive nonspecific damage has probably occurred. In a series of 12 patients 1 month to 3½ years of age, 92% had a greater than 50% reduction in the hemangioma size at 3 months, with 8% maintaining this reduction at 6 months. To achieve these results, 50% required two treatments and 8% three

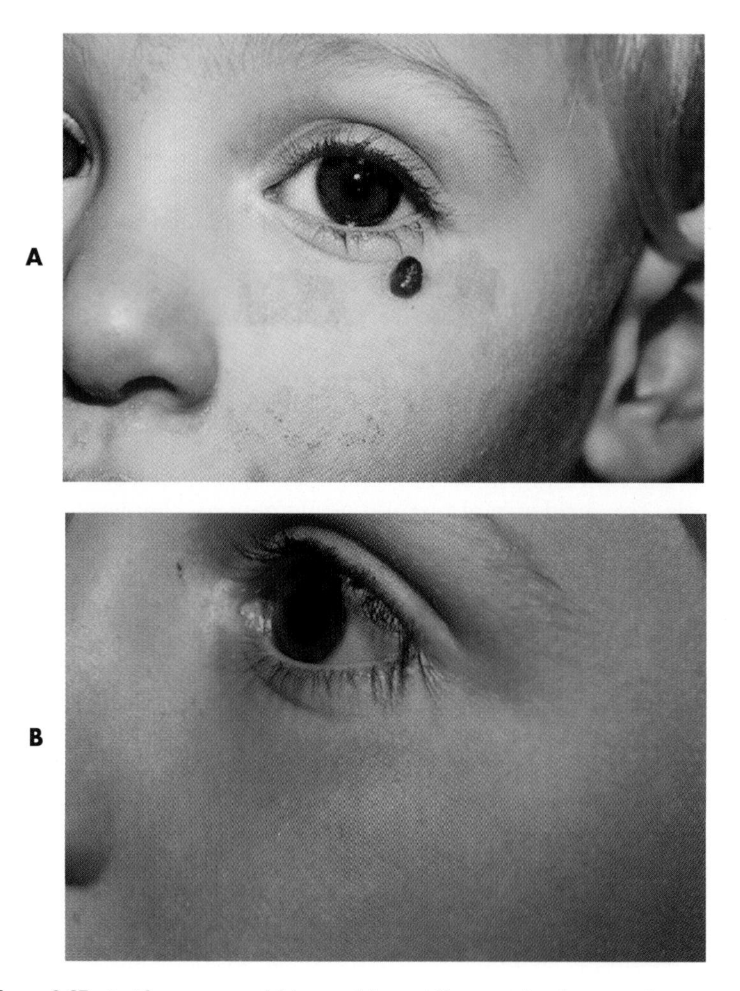

Figure 2-65 **A,** Three-year-old boy with rapidly growing hemangioma over last 5 weeks. Lesion failed to respond to two treatments with FLPDL at 7 J/cm^2. **B,** Four weeks after single treatment using a Coherent superpulsed CO_2 laser (Ambulase). Note excellent resolution of hemangioma with imperceptible scar.

treatments; 33% of hemangiomas ulcerated after therapy. Thus this aggressive form of treatment is best reserved for large, voluminous hemangiomas that have functional significance (e.g., airway obstruction, visual change). We believe that this technique is too poorly controlled to be valuable.

Carbon dioxide laser

The CO_2 laser is also useful as a scalpel to excise and debulk vascular tissue with minimal blood loss. It has been used to excise laryngeal lesions causing airway obstruction,[48,224] oral hemangiomas,[271-273] and facial lesions.[274] Because this treatment modality has also been associated with a higher rate of scarring, it is not recommended for cutaneous lesions and is most efficacious in treating internal and mucosal hemangiomas.[48] However, when used with high-fluence, short-pulse parameters, improved clinical results can be obtained (Figure 2-65). In our practice the $UPCO_2$ laser has been used to resurface scarred hemangiomas and tighten those with redundant and stretched tissue with excellent results (Figure 2-66).

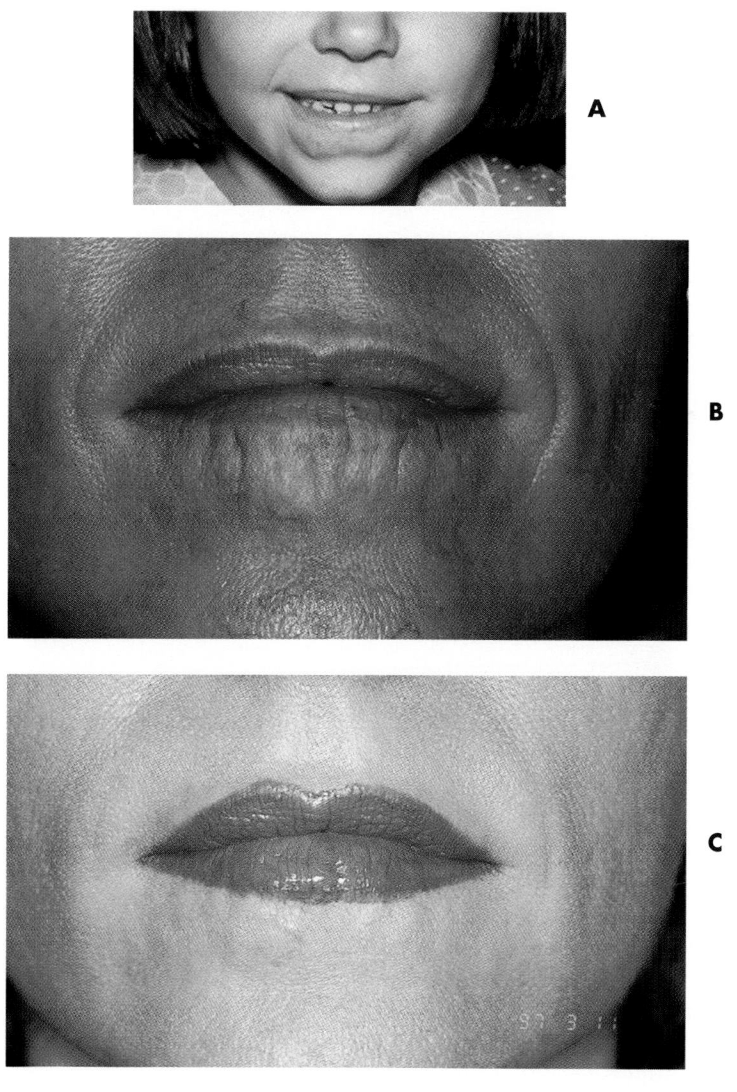

Figure 2-66 **A,** Appearance of hemangioma in 5-year-old girl. **B,** Clinical appearance 30 years later. Note flaccid, wrinkled skin. **C,** Six months after resurfacing with Coherent Ultra Pulse CO_2 Laser. Three passes were given at 500 mJ through 3-mm collimated spot size handpiece.

Flashlamp-pumped pulsed dye laser

The laser with the greatest potential use in the treatment of hemangiomas is the FLPDL. Although initially developed to treat vessels present in PWS, the similar vessel diameter and depth in hemangiomas explains the FLPDL's clinical efficacy. The depth of penetration of 585 nm is 0.6 to 1.2 mm, which limits its efficacy to relatively superficial lesions. Its safety and specificity are the reasons for its appeal. Early studies have demonstrated efficacy in hastening resolution of lesions beyond the proliferative phase,[47,50] as well as slowing or arresting proliferative growth.[47,48,50] The FLPDL is best utilized and most effective in eradicating lesions in a macular stage before proliferation.[48,50]

The FLPDL will not affect hemangioma vasculature below 1.5 mm, because proliferation of deeply situated hemangioma vessels proceeds despite involution of superficial laser-treated areas.[48,50,196]

When the lesion is proliferating, the FLPDL appears to be effective in initiating or hastening involution. Because the depth of penetration is limited, a series of treatments is usually necessary gradually to reach deeper layers of vessels. We recommend a treatment schedule of every 2 to 3 weeks for three to six treatments, using a fluence of 5 to 7 J/cm^2 for most lesions. Lesions with only a superficial component are very responsive to treatment because 90% will completely involute (Figure 2-57). Those with a deep component and a superficial component may require intralesional steroid therapy for the deep component and laser therapy for the superficial component (Figures 2-62 and 2-63). Widespread and deep lesions may require laser therapy and systemic steroids to arrest the growth of the deep component. Treatment at the earliest opportunity is critical in determining success in these cases.

A 1.5-msec 595-nm FLPDL has been introduced by both Candela (Sclerolaser) and Cynosure. Kauvar[99] presented the experience with this longer-pulsed, longer-wavelength FLPDL in the treatment of 10 hemangiomas. Two superficial lesions cleared in two or three treatments, and eight lesions with both a superficial and a deep component cleared in two to four treatments. In the latter group, the superficial component cleared completely, but with only a 10% to 50% reduction in the deep component. Kauvar recommends the following parameters:

- Infants: 7-mm-diameter spot, 7 J/cm^2
- Adults: 7-mm-diameter spot, 8 J/cm^2
- Hypertrophic lesions: 7-mm-diameter spot, 9 J/cm^2

Surgical Treatment

Surgical therapy should be considered for certain lesions. Hemangiomas of the vermilion border, mucous membranes, and nasal tip are very slow to involute and may seriously interfere with a child's self-esteem. In these cases, excision before entering school may be considered.[238] Microsurgical techniques with hemostatic lasers have been successful.[275] The use of tissue expansion further improves excision cosmesis.[276] Facial or neck hemangiomas that have incompletely resolved with sagging skin or excessive fibrofatty residuum may be excised.[277]

Ideally a team approach should be used in treating extensive hemangiomas. Multiple specialties, including but not limited to vascular surgeons, radiologists, dermatologists, plastic surgeons, and pediatricians, may combine their expertise to optimize patient care. Apfelberg et al[265,278] have reported the use of the Nd:YAG laser with sapphire tip in conjunction with intralesional steroids and also in a team approach using superselective embolization before resection.

Clinical Studies

Of 50 patients (mean age 13 months) treated with the FLPDL an average of 3.8 times, 53% had significant improvement in color without an appreciable reduction in lesion bulk.[279] Four of seven patients with flat lesions completely cleared after two treatments, with the remaining three patients achieving satisfactory results requiring no further treatment. Eight flat, ulcerated hemangiomas healed completely with FLPDL treatment after one to three treatments. Ten patients with slightly raised lesions required a mean of 5.2 treatments to achieve clearance in four and a good degree of flattening and improvement in the remaining six patients. Red raised lesions with a significant subcutaneous component showed elimination of the red coloration and any ulcerations without change in lesion bulk.

Morelli and Weston[280] reported their 2-year experience in treating 55 lesions. Five patients with hemangiomas less than 3 cm^3 treated once or twice with the FLPDL in the proliferative phase had a good response with arrest of lesion growth. An additional five patients with large lesions greater than 20 cm^3 had an excellent response and resolution of lesions in those who continued treatment. Twenty patients with superficial and deep lesions had resolution of the superficial component only. Purely nodular older lesions resisted treatment. Ulcerated painful hemangiomas, when treated, heal and become painless, providing the best indication for treatment. Morelli et al[281] reported a total of 37 infants with ulcerated hemangiomas treated with the FLPDL between 2 and 40 weeks of age. All ulcerations healed with one to three treatments at 2- to 4-week intervals at fluences of 6.0 to 6.5 J/cm^2. Almost 70% healed within 2 weeks after a single laser treatment.

Garden et al[282] have reported that the best results occur when the hemangioma is elevated 3 mm or less and advise treatment in the first weeks of life. They studied 33 hemangiomas in 24 patients 2 weeks to 7 months of age in whom a 93.9% lightening occurred in the superficial lesions in 4.1 treatment sessions. Seven lesions 4 mm or more in thickness lightened 83.7% in seven treatment sessions. They found that compressing the hemangioma with a glass slide to bring the deeper vascular component closer to the surface did not increase efficacy.

A report on treating 68 infants with 100 hemangiomas within 12 weeks of their development further confirms FLPDL efficacy.[283] Seventy-three lesions required a single treatment and 27 up to five treatments; 23% of lesions showed complete remission, 55% showed partial remission, and 14% stopped growing. Only 8% of lesions continued to grow despite treatment. This efficacy occurred with virtually no serious adverse sequelae.

Proliferative hemangiomas causing functional impairment in seven patients 8 to 24 weeks of age showed significant reduction in size, normalization of color, and resolution of superficial ulceration.[284] Lesions were treated at fluences of 7.0 to 9.25 J/cm^2 at 4- to 8-week intervals (two to six times) until the hemangioma completely regressed or stopped regressing further. As reported in the previous studies, all patients with ulceration responded to treatment. Four of seven patients had complete resolution of the hemangioma. No adverse events or complications were noted.

Our experience is similar to that of most reports.[285] The following is a summary of our experience with a total of 34 infants and children. We used the FLPDL at fluences of 6.25 to 8.0 J/cm^2 at 2- to 3-week intervals with spots overlapping 10% to 15% to produce an endpoint of homogenous darkening of the entire lesion until one of the following circumstances: resolution occurred, the treatment was judged to be ineffective, or the parents discontinued treatment for unrelated reasons. Treatment was offered to all parents of children with hemangiomas after explanation of the natural resolution history of the lesions and the potential benefits and risks of laser therapy and steroid therapy. Some patients had medical reasons for treatment (visual obstruction, interference with feeding or breathing, or lesional bleeding), but treatment was also offered to patients with lesions that caused concern because of proliferative activity, tissue distortion, or cosmetic disfigurement.

Seventeen hemangiomas had only a superficial component, with 13 of these less than 1 cm in diameter, averaging 7 mm. The lesions appeared as a red macule initially, at an average age of 15 days. The lesions typically began to proliferate, causing parental concern. The average age at first treatment was 5.5 months. The most common reason for the delay in treatment was difficulty in finding an appropriate treatment center. The average patient received 3.6 treatments over 3.3 months. The average fluence used was 6.8 J/cm². Nine patients (53%) cleared completely. Those lesions not clearing had an average improvement of 67% (Table 2-10).

Seventeen infants had hemangiomas classified as mixed, with both a superficial and a deep component. All these lesions were large, some encompassing the entire side of the face. Eight lesions were treated relatively early, during the proliferative phase, and nine lesions were treated later, during the involution-dominant phase (Table 2-11).

Those hemangiomas treated early had appeared at an earlier age (average age 6 days). Treatment was initiated at an average age of 4.5 months and continued for an average 7.4 months, during which time 4.5 treatments were administered, using

Table 2-10
Superficial capillary hemangiomas: FLPDL treatment

No. of Lesions	Diameter <1 cm	Average Age Lesion Appeared	Average Age First Treatment	Average No. of Treatments	Average Time of Treatment	Average Treatment Fluence	Complete Clearing	Average Improvement if Not Clear
17	13	15 days	5.5 mo	3.6	3.35 mo	6.8 J/cm²	9 (53%)	67%

Table 2-11
Mixed superficial/deep capillary hemangioma: early FLPDL treatment

No. of Lesions	Diameter >1 cm	Average Age Lesion Appeared	Average Age First Treatment	Average No. of Treatments	Average Time of Treatment	Average Treatment Fluence	Adjunctive Steroid Therapy	Average Improvement	
								Superficial	Deep
8	8	6 days	4.5 mo	4.5	7.4 mo	6.8 J/cm^2	4 (50%)	96%	73%

Table 2-12
Mixed superficial/deep capillary hemangioma: late FLPDL treatment

No. of Lesions	Diameter >1 cm	Average Age Lesion Appeared	Average Age First Treatment	Average No. of Treatments	Average Time of Treatment	Average Treatment Fluence	Adjunctive Steroid Therapy	Average Improvement	
								Superficial	Deep
9	8	40 days	41 mo	3.5	7.2 mo	6.9 J/cm^2	2 (22%)	62%	32%

an average fluence of 6.8 J/cm^2. Four patients (50%) received adjunctive therapy with steroids during this period, two receiving systemic prednisolone and two receiving intralesional steroids. Interestingly, in these four patients, treatment with steroids abruptly halted the proliferation of the deep component and resulted in shrinking this deep portion, but it had no visible effect on the superficial component. Likewise, the FLPDL treatment abruptly halted proliferation and resulted in clearance of the superficial component without apparent effect on the deep component, which continued to proliferate unless steroids were used. Treatment resulted in near-complete (96%) clearing of the superficial component in all patients and an average improvement of 73% in the deep component (Table 2-11).

Lesions treated later in their course appeared at an average age of 40 days but were not treated until an average age of 41 months. These nine lesions received an average of 3.5 treatments, using an average fluence of 7.2 J/cm^2 and a treatment interval averaging 9 weeks. Two patients received intralesional steroids in an attempt to shrink the persistent deep component of the lesion. These nine patients achieved a much more modest degree of improvement than the other eight patients treated early, with the superficial component improving an average 62% and the deep component only 32% (Table 2-12).

Most authors report cessation of the proliferative phase as a consequence of treatment with the FLPDL.[48,49,282] Controversy has surrounded the question of whether early treatment can prevent the proliferative phase and especially whether it may have an effect on the deep component that the FLPDL cannot reach.[33] Indeed, the case reported by Glassberg et al[48] showed deep proliferation despite cutaneous involution during FLPDL therapy. Mulliken[238] reported his experience of the same phenomenon. This was our experience as well: four patients with superficial and deep components showed response of only the superficial component to treatment with the FLPD laser, while the deep component continued to proliferate. Interestingly, the opposite was true as well; only the deep component was responsive to steroid therapy, the superficial component being unaffected. Glassberg et al[48] also have mentioned this point.

The cases reported by Glassberg et al,[48] Sherwood and Tan,[49] and us well illustrate that the FLPDL can rapidly and dramatically halt the proliferative superficial component. In two of these three series, the hemangiomas were very extensive and were responsive throughout the superficial component.

High-intensity Pulsed-light Treatment

In addition to monochromatic light, noncoherent light has also been found to be effective in treating hemangiomas when used within an adequate wavelength range and with proper fluence and pulse duration. We have used the PhotoDerm VL with a cutoff filter at 550, 570, or 590 nm to treat multiple hemangiomas with excellent results (Figure 2-67). We have used this light source to treat evolving as well as long-established tumors. One 66-year-old patient developed a hemangioma after trauma 15 years before treatment. One treatment with a 570-nm cutoff filter at 80 J/cm^2 given as a double pulse of 9 and 13 msec separated by a 50-msec delay resulted in 100% resolution. The lesion immediately became purpuric, then crusted before completely involuting (Figure 2-68).

Foster and Gold[286] reported 90% involution of a 7.5 × 4–cm ulcerated cavernous hemangioma on the abdomen of an 11-week-old black infant. They used a 550-nm cutoff filter at a fluence of 38 J/cm^2 in a triple-pulse mode (T_1 3 msec, T_2 2 msec, T_3 1.7 msec) with a 10-msec delay between pulses. Two additional treatments at 2-week intervals with a 570-nm cutoff filter at fluences of 30 and 38 J/cm^2 using a triple pulse (T_1 4 msec, T_2 3 msec, T_3 2 msec) with a 20-msec delay between pulses resulted in maximal resolution with minimal hypopigmentation.

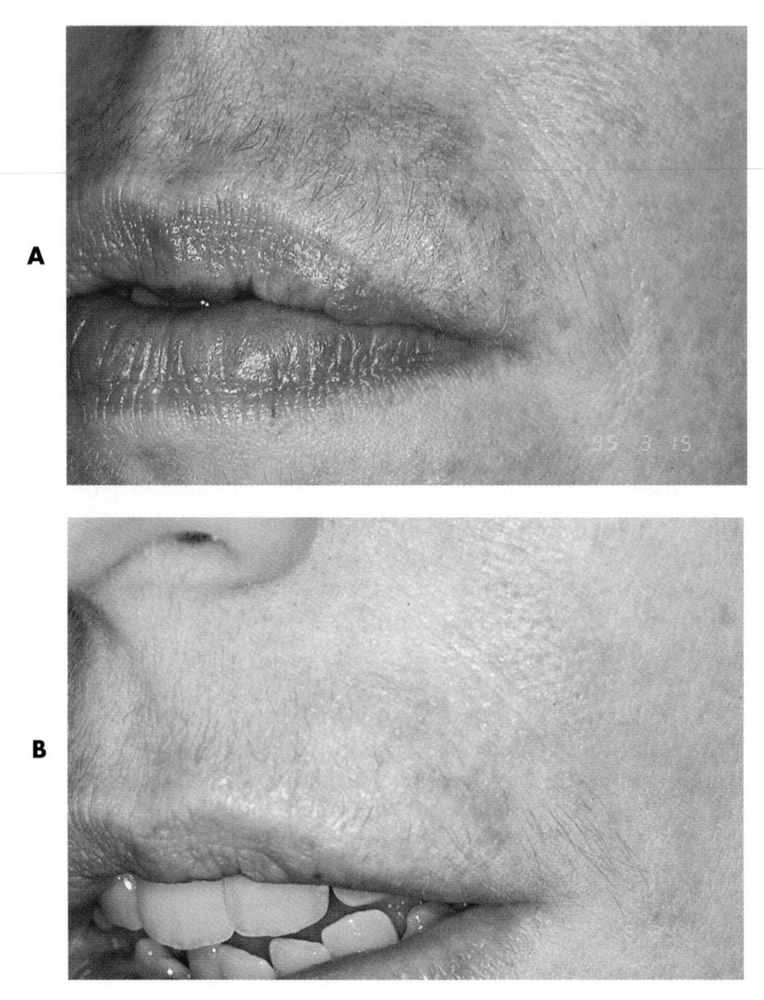

Figure 2-67 **A,** Persistent hemangioma/venous malformation despite four treatments with argon laser (0.5-sec pulses at 2 W) and one treatment with the FLPDL (8 J/cm^2 with 5-mm-diameter spot size). **B,** After three treatments with Photoderm VL with 590-nm cutoff filter, double pulse of 4.2 and 7.7 msec with 300-msec delay between pulses at 65, 71, and 69 J/cm^2, respectively.

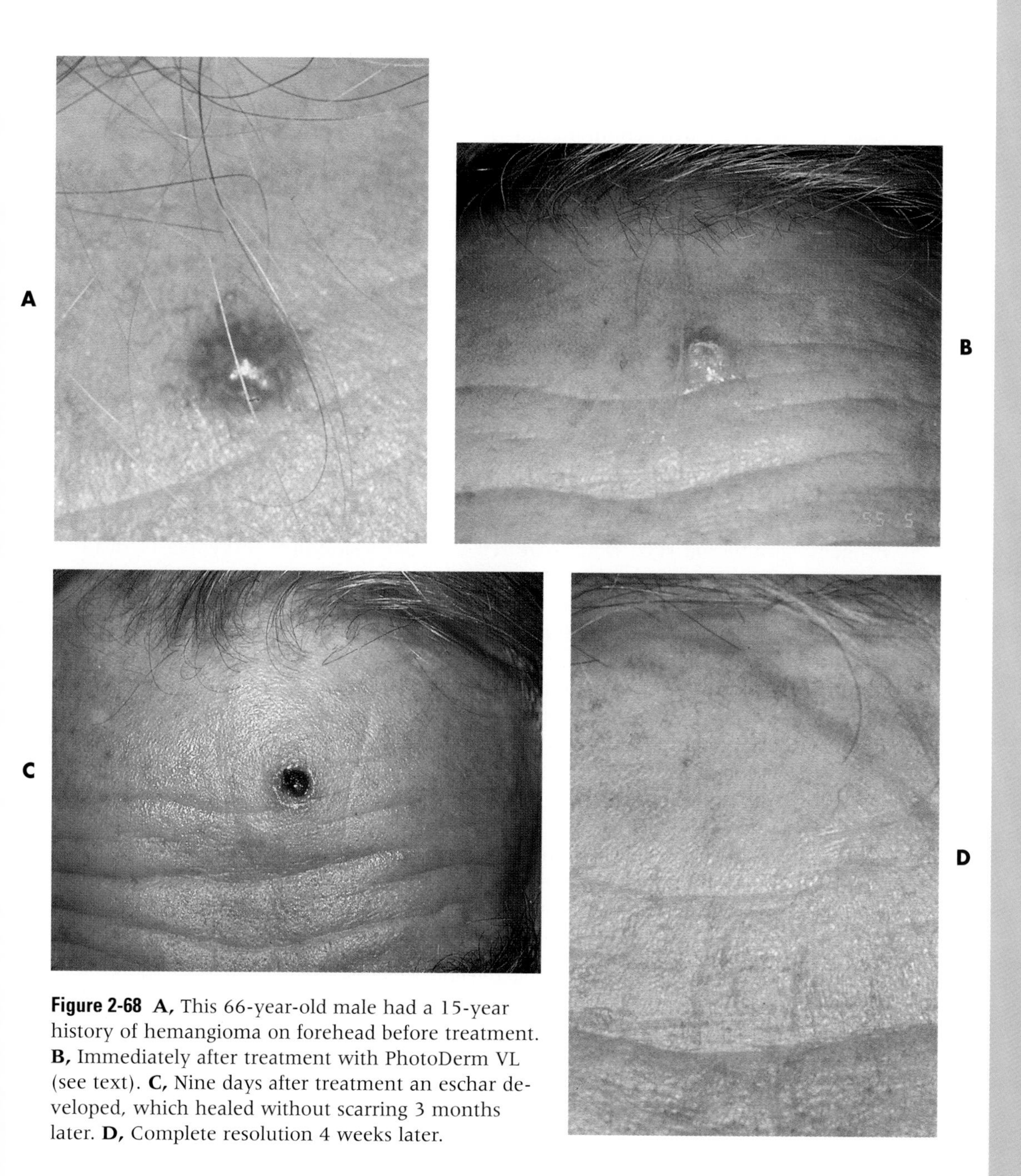

Figure 2-68 **A,** This 66-year-old male had a 15-year history of hemangioma on forehead before treatment. **B,** Immediately after treatment with PhotoDerm VL (see text). **C,** Nine days after treatment an eschar developed, which healed without scarring 3 months later. **D,** Complete resolution 4 weeks later.

Summary Recommendations

Mulliken[206] correctly calls for a biologic approach to the treatment of hemangiomas of infancy. He points out that the only antiangiogenic agents currently available are corticosteroids and that they may afford dramatic benefit without significant risks as one might expect. When this therapeutic approach is considered in light of the recent information available regarding laser responsiveness of the superficial component, we conclude that the FLPDL should be used at the earliest sign of a capillary hemangioma and certainly as soon as active proliferation begins. In conjunction with this treatment, intralesional or systemic steroids should be given to halt the proliferation of the deep component when that portion proceeds despite laser therapy. The risks of therapy have been demonstrated to be minimal.

Extensive hemangiomas that have not responded to other treatments have reduced with PhotoDerm VL treatment.[287]

The recommendations of the American Academy of Dermatology's Guidelines of Care Committee for treatment of hemangiomas are summarized as follows[288]:

1. Prevent or reverse life-threatening or function-threatening complications.
2. Prevent permanent disfigurement left by residual skin changes.
3. Minimize psychosocial stress.
4. Avoid scarring procedures.
5. Prevent or treat ulcerative lesions to minimize scarring, infection, and pain.

PYOGENIC GRANULOMA

Pyogenic granuloma (PG) is an acquired vascular lesion, a true neoplasm distinct from granulation tissue, usually solitary, 0.5 to 2.0 cm in diameter, bright red, and pedunculated.[289-291] The surface is soft, bleeding easily with trauma. It may become ulcerated and develop a granulomatous surface with a brown or black crust. Lesions usually appear suddenly and may enlarge rapidly. There is no history of preceding trauma or infection in most patients (75%),[292] although this typically is assumed.[293] These lesions also frequently occur as a superimposed growth on the surface of a PWS.[222] Repeated episodes of bleeding and unresponsiveness to electrocautery have been reported in up to 50% of patients.[292] This may be secondary to the extension of vascular proliferation deep into the dermis, often with a unique lobular arrangement of capillaries.[294]

The argon laser,[295] as well as the CO_2 laser,[296] has been shown to be effective in treating PGs. The PG is photocoagulated until the entire lesion blanches and turns a dusty gray color. Treatments are repeated at 3- to 4-week intervals as needed.

PG lesions have been unpredictably responsive to the FLPDL.[155] They have been shown to respond,[116,293,297,298] but in most cases lesions are too thick for the laser to penetrate throughout the lesion in one treatment. Tan and Kurban[297] use a glass slide to compress the superficial ectatic vessels and use the laser through the glass to treat the deeper component of this lesion. This maneuver presumably allows treatment of deep vessels, after which the slide is removed and the treatment is repeated to coagulate more superficially located vessels. When effective by itself, the FLPDL must be used with multiple, 100% overlapping pulses to turn the lesion deep purple. As previously demonstrated, this technique produces nonselective photothermolysis and is therefore no different than CW argon, copper vapor, or 577-nm dye lasers.

A study of 18 patients with PG treated with the FLPDL demonstrated both symptomatic and clinical clearing in 16 patients with excellent cosmetic results.[299] Seven of the lesions had been previously treated with electrosurgery or excision. The authors flattened the lesions with a glass slide and used fluences of 6.5 to 9.0 J/cm^2 in an overlapping manner to cover the lesion completely. Treatments were repeated up

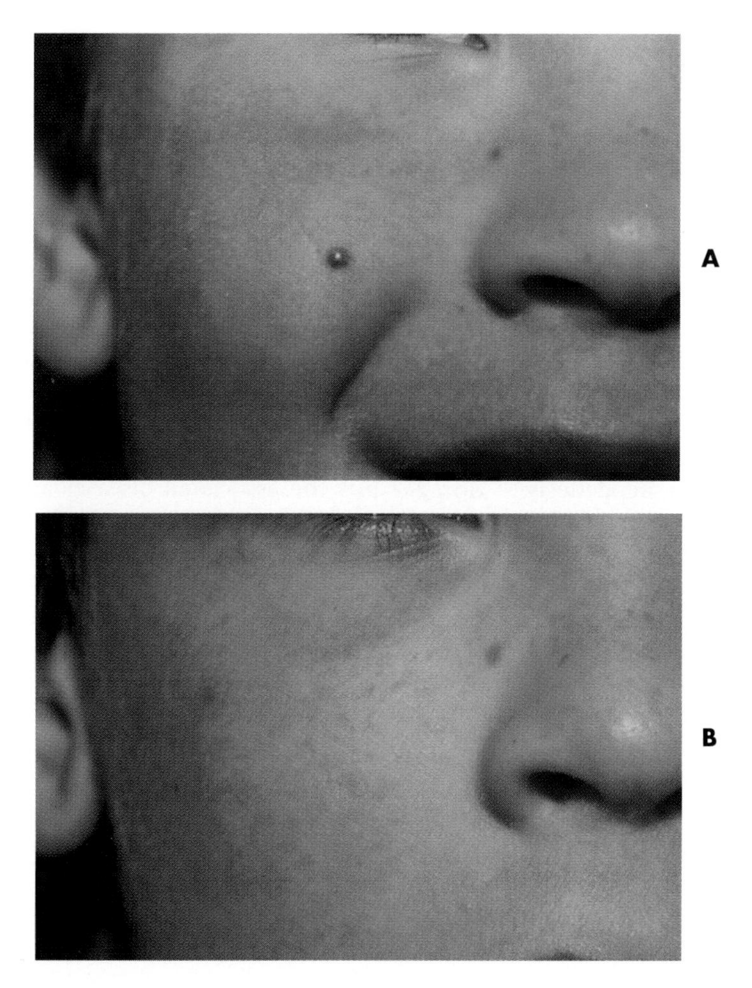

Figure 2-69 **A,** Clinical appearance of rapidly growing pyogenic granuloma on right cheek of 4-year-old boy. **B,** After shave excision followed by two treatments with FLPDL at 7.5 J/cm^2, 8 weeks after final treatment. Note slight atrophic depression.

to four times to achieve success. Treatment outcomes were excellent, but two postoperative photos showed textural changes that resembled a scar, although this was not noted by the authors.

We have not been able to achieve uniform success in treating PG lesions with or without the diascopy maneuver with the FLPDL. In addition, multiple treatments are impractical because of the ease with which lesions are traumatized between sessions. We therefore recommend shave excision of the lesion's papular component if a histologic specimen is necessary or CO_2 vaporization of the lesion followed by FLPDL therapy to the remaining flat macular lesion if necessary (Figure 2-69).

TELANGIECTASIA

The term *telangiectasia* refers to superficial cutaneous vessels visible to the human eye.[300] These vessels measure 0.1 to 1.0 mm in diameter and represent a dilated venule, capillary, or arteriole. Telangiectasia that are arteriolar in origin are small in diameter, bright red in color, and do not protrude above the skin surface. Those that arise from venules are wider, blue in color, and often protrude above the skin surface. Telangiectasia arising at the capillary loop are often initially fine, red lesions but become larger and purple or blue with time because of venous backflow from increasing hydrostatic pressure.[301]

Telangiectasia have been subdivided into four classifications based on clinical appearance: (1) simple or linear, (2) arborizing, (3) spider, and (4) papular[302] (Figure 2-70). *Red linear and arborizing telangiectasia* are very common on the face, especially the nose, midcheeks, and chin. These lesions are also seen relatively frequently on the legs. *Blue linear and arborizing telangiectasia* are most often seen on the legs but also may be present on the face. *Spider telangiectasia* are described in the next section. *Papular telangiectasia* are frequently part of genetic syndromes, such as Osler-Weber-Rendu disease, and also are seen in collagen vascular diseases.

All forms of telangiectasia are thought to occur through the release or activation of vasoactive substances under the influence of a variety of factors, such as anoxia, estrogen, corticosteroids (topical or systemic), various chemicals, multiple types of bacterial or viral infection, and multiple physical factors, with resultant capillary or venular neogenesis.[301] Box 2-2 lists the associated diseases and causes of telangiectasia.

Telangiectasia of the face are most often seen in patients with fair complexion (Fitzpatrick types I and II skin). These lesions are especially common on the nasal alae, nose, and midcheeks and are probably caused by persistent arteriolar vasodilatation resulting from vessel wall weakness. The vessels dilate further when damage to the surrounding connective and elastic tissue occurs from factors such as chronic sun exposure or use of topical steroids. These lesions have a definite familial or genetic component. Rosacea may be an accompanying condition.

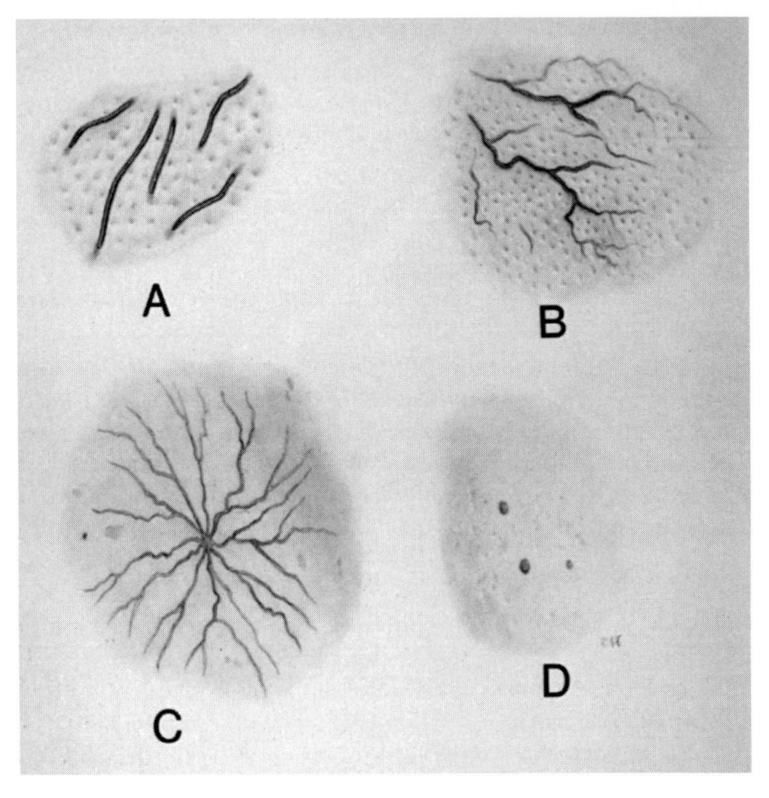

Figure 2-70 Four types of telangiectasia: **A,** simple; **B,** arborized; **C,** spider; and **D,** papular. (From Goldman MP, Bennett RG: *J Am Acad Dermatol* 17:167, 1987.)

Spider Telangiectasia

Spider telangiectasia represent telangiectasia with a central feeding arteriole. They typically appear in preschool and school-age children. The peak incidence appears to be between ages 7 and 10,[303] and as many as 40% of girls and 32% of boys less than 15 years old have at least one lesion.[304,305] The incidence in healthy adults is about 15%.[306] The difference between these stated incidences implies that 50% to 75% of childhood lesions regress. However, this is not easily observable because most lesions seem to persist without change and become a source of cosmetic concern when present on the face.

Treatment in the past included electrocautery and the argon laser. Both modalities have the disadvantages of being painful and prone to causing punctate scarring. In addition, recurrence is common if treatment is done lightly to avoid scarring. The FLPDL has proved to be a very effective treatment for these benign lesions.[307,308]

Geronemus[307] reported 100% success without any adverse sequelae in 12 children treated with the FLPDL for facial spider telangiectasia.

Box 2-2 Causes of cutaneous telangiectasia

Genetic
Vascular nevi
- Nevus flammeus
- Nevus araneus

Congenital neuroangiopathies
- Ataxia telangiectasia
- Sturge-Weber syndrome
- Maffucci syndrome
- Klippel-Trenaunay-Weber syndrome

Congenital poikiloderma (Rothmund-Thomson syndrome)
Bloom syndrome
Cockayne syndrome
Hereditary hemorrhagic telangiectasia (Osler-Weber-Rendu disease)
Essential progressive telangiectasia
Generalized essential telangiectasia
- Familial (autosomal dominant)
- Acquired (hormonal or infectious stimulation)

Unilateral nevoid telangiectatic syndrome
Diffuse neonatal hemangiomatosis
Hereditary benign telangiectasia

Acquired disease with secondary cutaneous component: Collagen vascular diseases
Lupus erythematosus (especially periungual)
Dermatomyositis
Progressive systemic sclerosis (especially periungual, and with the *c*alcinosis, *R*aynaud, *e*sophageal dysmotility, *s*clerodactyly, and *t*elangiectasia [CREST] syndrome)
Cryoglobulinemia

Other
- Telangiectasia macularis eruptiva perstans (mastocytosis)
- Carcinoma telangiectasia (metastatic tumors)

Component of a primary cutaneous disease
Rosacea
Varicose veins
Basal cell carcinoma
Merkel cell tumor
Necrobiosis lipoidica diabeticorum
Poikiloderma vasculare atrophicans
Capillaritis (purpura annularis telangiectodes)
Xeroderma pigmentosum
Pseudoxanthoma elasticum
Degos disease
Superficial epithelium with sebaceous differentiation

Hormonal
Pregnancy
Corticoid induced
- Cushing syndrome/disease
- Iatrogenic (from systemic, topical, or intralesional use)
- Estrogen therapy (usually with high dose)

Physical damage
Actinic dermatitis
Radiodermatitis
Postsurgical, especially in suture lines under tension and after rhinoplasty
Physical trauma

Modified from Goldman MP, Bennett RG: *J Am Acad Dermatol* 17:167, 1987.

We retrospectively evaluated the response to treatment with the FLPDL in 23 children with 55 spider telangiectasia.[308] Lesions were treated at energy fluences of 6.5 to 7.5 J/cm^2 (mean 6.9 J/cm^2). One or two pulses were given to the central punctum of the "spider," with additional pulses with a 10% overlap given to the radiating "arms" of the lesion if the lesion was greater than 5 mm in diameter. Local anesthesia was not used. Seventy percent of lesions resolved completely with one treatment. Twelve lesions required a second treatment for complete resolution. The remaining five lesions not treated a second time had an average clearance of 78% (Table 2-13 and Figure 2-71). The three patients with five lesions who did not have

Table 2-13
Childhood spider telangiectasia: FLPDL treatment

No. of Lesions	No. of Patients	Average Age	Age Range	Average No. of Treatments	Average Treatment Fluence	Average Improvement	Total Clearing	Average Improvement if Not Clear
55	23	6.7 yr	1-14 yr	1.2*	6.9 J/cm^2	90%	90 %	78%

*22% of lesions were treated a second time.

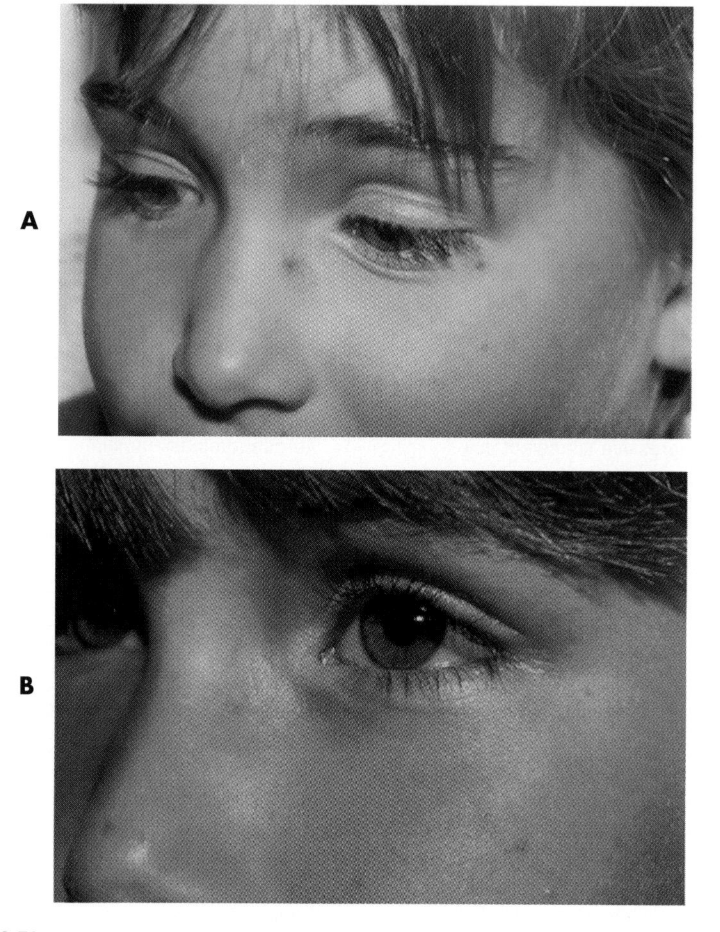

Figure 2-71 **A,** Two spider telangiectasia on left inner canthal area and outer canthal area of 10-year-old girl for 6 months. **B,** Four weeks after single treatment with FLPDL at 7 J/cm^2. Note complete resolution of telangiectasia without any evidence of cutaneous changes. (From Fitzpatrick RE: *Am J Cosmetic Surg* 9:107 1992.)

a second treatment were either satisfied with the degree of resolution from their first treatment or were unavailable for further treatment.

Spider telangiectasia respond equally as well in adults, with 93% of patients having total resolution with one treatment between 6.5 and 7.0 J/cm^{2}[116] (Figure 2-72).

With the FLPDL, lesions become purpuric immediately after laser treatment. Purpura resolves within 7 to 10 days. We have not seen permanent pigmentary changes or scarring. Although adverse effects from treating spider telangiectasia are extremely rare, one case of granuloma telangiectaticum (pyogenic granuloma) after argon laser therapy has been reported.[309] This complication occurred 3 months after the central vessel was treated at 5 W, 50 msec, with a 0.5-mm-diameter spot size. The authors speculated that laser trauma, in addition to the lack of complete destruction of the spider telangiectasia endothelium, led to a focal capillary proliferation. This effect has also been reported with laser treatment of PWS, with development of "hemangiomas" within the treated areas.

The PhotoDerm VL has also been useful in treating these lesions, because its quartz light guide (even the small light guide 12 × 8–mm treatment interface) is larger than most lesions. Because one needs only to treat the lesion, we use a hole punch or scissors to cut out an open area in a sheet of white paper to match the lesion's diameter. A simple sheet of white paper, cardboard, or self-sticking label is sufficient to block out the light delivered through the quartz light guide. Fluences of

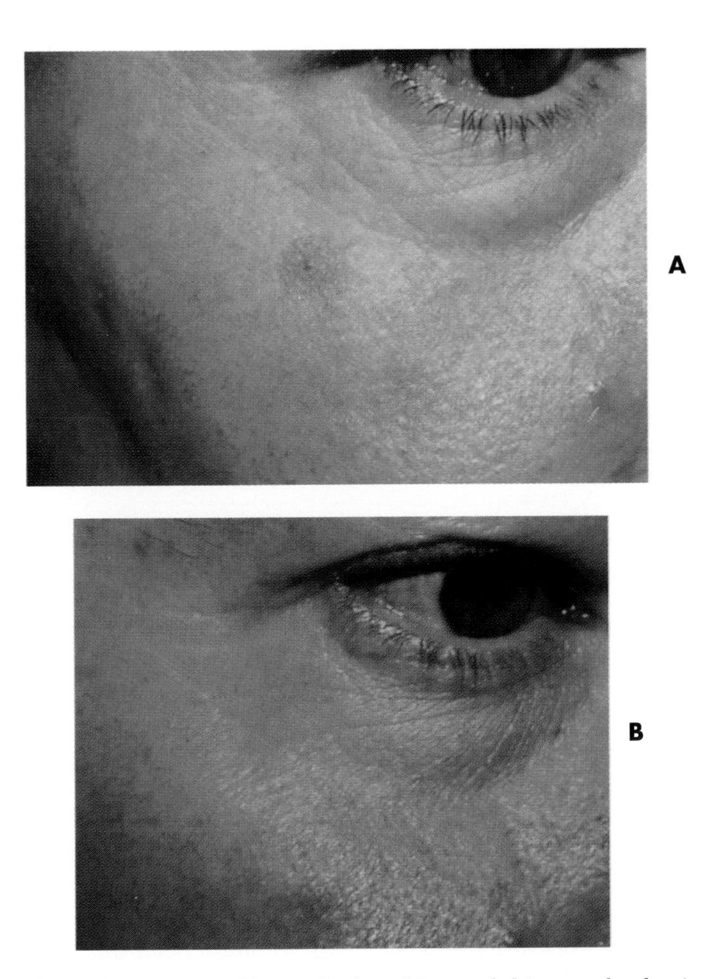

Figure 2-72 **A,** This 44-year-old man had an 18-month history of enlarging spider telangiectasia on right cheek. **B,** Six months after single treatment with FLPDL at 7 J/cm^{2}. Total of six 5-mm pulses were given, with complete resolution of telangiectasia.

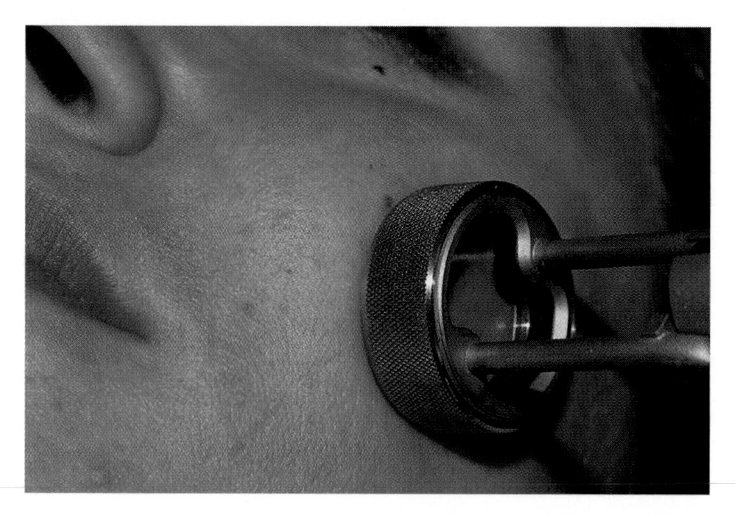

Figure 2-73 Cooling head is attached to handpiece of Versapulse 532-nm laser and placed on skin over target vascular lesion. Laser energy is then given through this cooling device.

35 to 40 J/cm² delivered in a double pulse of 2.4 and 4.0 msec with a 10-msec delay through a 550-nm cutoff filter usually gives near-100% efficacy with almost no pain. Even small children and male adults tolerate the treatment without complaint. Lesions are rarely purpuric and usually without adverse sequelae, making this modality a treatment of choice.

An additional nearly painless treatment modality is the long-pulse 532-nm laser (Versapulse). Parameters found to be efficacious in treating this lesion are a 3- to 4-mm-diameter spot with an energy fluence of 12 to 14 J/cm² delivered in a 10-msec pulse. The treatment is almost painless because the laser beam is delivered through a double-chambered clear quartz crystal cooled in its center to 4° C with water (Figure 2-73). The quartz cooling device is placed over the lesion on the skin surface, and the laser fluence is delivered 1 to 3 times until the lesion blanches. This laser has an efficacy of almost 100% for this treatment in our practice.

Poikiloderma of Civatte

Poikiloderma of Civatte is a variant of telangiectasia involving the neck and upper chest and occurring from accumulated ultraviolet exposure and associated photosensitization of various chemicals, most notably fragrances.[310] Poikiloderma consists of a combination of telangiectasia, irregular pigmentation, and atrophic changes of the skin. Histologic changes on biopsy confirm this clinical combination. These changes are best treated by addressing the telangiectatic and pigmentary components simultaneously.

In the past, poikiloderma treatment focused on the telangiectatic component and solely on various laser modalities. Fair efficacy was reported, but treatments were lengthy because of the large surface areas involved and multiple sessions required. The argon laser is only partially successful and frequently results in areas of hypopigmentation with a low incidence of scarring. The FLPDL, as reported by Tan and Kuran,[297] Wheeland and Applebaum,[311] and us, has good efficacy at fluences of 6 to 7 J/cm² with a 5-mm-diameter spot size. Our recommended fluence at a 7-mm diameter is 5 to 6 J/cm². Problems with the FLPDL include extensive purpura, multiple treatments because of large surface area, and mottled response with circular imprints (Figure 2-74). In addition, by mainly targeting the vascular component, these treatments often do little to change the hyperpigmentation.

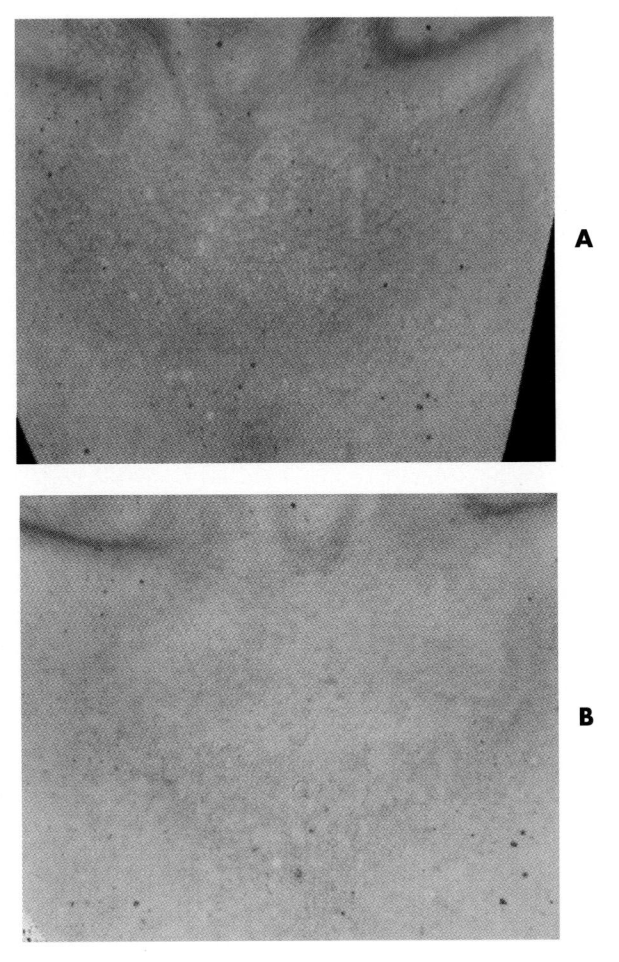

Figure 2-74 **A,** Extensive poikilodermic changes from sun damage on central chest of 36-year-old woman. **B,** After three treatments with FLPDL at a fluence of 7 J/cm² during each treatment session. Between 200 and 300 5-mm impact pulses were given at each session. Note excellent clearing of poikilodermic changes. Somewhat mottled pigmentation remains between laser impact sites and on peripheral aspect of poikiloderma.

Our results using an intense pulsed light source (PhotoDerm VL) have been very favorable. With this pulsed light system, the target is both vascular and epidermal and dermal melanin. Multiple wavelengths are used, usually with a 515-nm filter first. This filter is used with a single pulse of 3 msec at a fluence of 22 to 25 J/cm². These treatment parameters are effective in removing epidermal melanin and very superficial telangiectasia. A second or third treatment spaced at least 4 weeks apart is usually necessary and typically uses a 550-nm cutoff filter with a double pulse of 2.4 and 4 msec with a 10-msec delay. This is helpful in treating slightly larger or deeper telangiectasia. A total fluence from 35 to 42 J/cm² is usually necessary to achieve an optimal clinical result. With these parameters, few or no side effects have been noted in our patients (Figures 2-75 and 2-76).

Approximately 75% improvement occurs after one treatment. Side effects include transitory erythema from 24 to 72 hours. Purpura occurs only 10% of the time and only with some pulses in variable locations. This purpura is different from that seen with the FLPDL in that it is intravascular and resolution occurs within 3 to 5 days. A slight stinging pain during treatment is easily tolerated for up to 60 pulses per session. No anesthesia is required, and the entire neck and chest area can be treated during one treatment session.

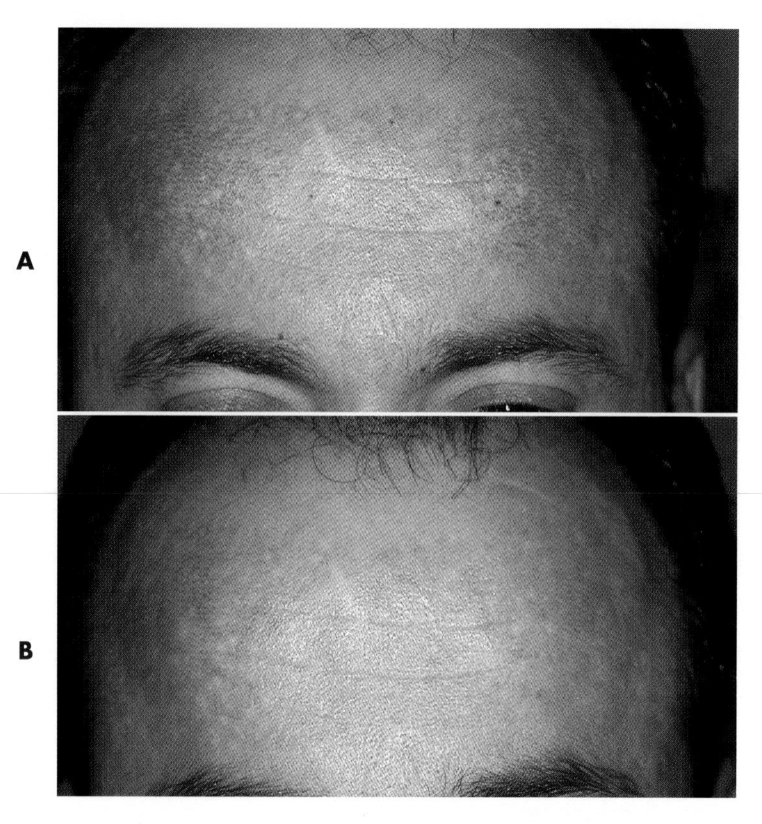

Figure 2-75 **A,** Poikiloderma of Civatte in 44-year-old male before treatment. **B,** One month after second treatment with PhotoDerm VL using 550-nm cutoff filter at 40 J/cm² given as a double pulse of 2.4 and 4.0 msec separated by 10-msec delay.

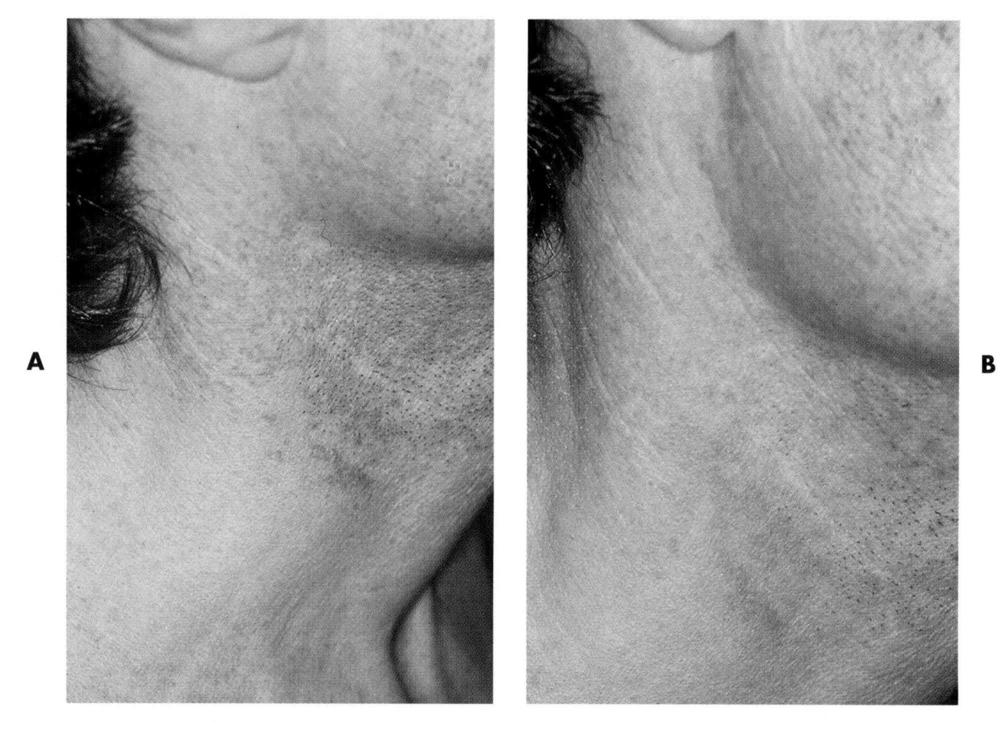

Figure 2-76 **A,** Poikiloderma of Civatte in 52-year-old male before treatment. **B,** Six months after third treatment with PhotoDerm VL using 550-nm cutoff filter at 37 to 40.5 and 43.5 J/cm² given over three treatments as a double pulse of 2.4 and 2.4 msec with 10-msec delay between pulses.

Facial Telangiectasia Treatment

Patients with facial telangiectasia of various types seek treatment primarily because of cosmetic concerns. Therefore it is important that the procedure be relatively risk free without unsightly scarring. A short discussion of traditional treatment methods for this common condition follows.

Electrosurgery

Electrodesiccation is typically used to treat facial telangiectasia. The vessel must be cauterized or electrocoagulated every 2 to 3 mm with very-low-amperage current (1-2 amps).[312,313] *Electrodesiccation* is a process in which heat is generated from resistance of tissues to the passage of a highly damped current from a single electrode. Dehydration occurs in the tissue immediately adjacent to the needle point, and as cellular fluids are evaporated, tissue destruction results.[306] Some degree of superficial necrosis always occurs. Multiple treatments are typically necessary for successful treatment. Punctate white or pigmented scars may occur as well as keloids.[313] Electrosurgery is not usually effective and has a higher risk of scarring for arborizing lesions or mats of telangiectasia. Electrodesiccation is best reserved for the smallest of telangiectasia.

Sclerotherapy

Sclerotherapy refers to the injection of a foreign substance into the lumen of a vessel to cause endothelial and mural damage with resulting thrombosis, vessel wall necrosis, and subsequent fibrosis. When performed on telangiectasia, the procedure is referred to as *microsclerotherapy*.[314] Successful microinjection of telangiectasia was first described in 1934.[315] Best results are obtained on superficial vessels of the legs or vessels greater than 0.4 mm in diameter. The reader is referred to Goldman and Bennett's article[301] for details of therapy.

Facial telangiectasia are less responsive to microsclerotherapy than leg telangiectasia and are more prone to complications common to sclerotherapy.[301,306,316,317] Because many facial telangiectasia, especially those that are bright red and less than 0.2 mm in diameter, are arteriolar in origin, injecting a sclerosing solution into these vessels may produce necrosis of the overlying skin. When a sclerosing solution is injected into a high-flow arterial system, complete endothelial and mural destruction does not occur. Superficial and patchy endothelial necrotic cells along with necrotic red and white blood cells combine to form microemboli and sludge, which lodge in vessels downstream.[318] This manifests as *punctate cutaneous necrosis*. In addition, arterial vasospasm may also occur, producing ischemia at the point of injection.[319]

When a detergent-type sclerosing solution (polidocanol, sodium tetradecyl sulfate, morrhuate sodium, or ethanolamine oleate) is injected into a slow-flow venular system (which is represented by a blue-green facial venule greater than 0.4 mm in diameter), its destructive action may occur far from the site of injection. The sclerosing effect within veins may continue for up to 6 cm from the point of injection.[318] Therefore, when performing sclerotherapy on facial venules, one should use an osmotic sclerosing solution, such as hypertonic saline or hypertonic saline/dextrose solutions. With the osmotic agent, endothelial and mural fibrosis occurs in a localized area. This limits the fear of sclerosing deeper and more distal venular drainage patterns, such as the retroorbital venous plexus. Unfortunately, osmotic solutions can be painful to inject and have the risk of ulceration and hyperpigmentation with extravasation. Therefore sclerotherapy should be used only on selected facial veins greater than 0.4 mm in diameter, with osmotic solutions, and with minimal volumes injected in each site.

Laser treatment

Table 2-14 compares response of facial telangiectasia to various lasers.

Carbon dioxide laser. The CO_2 laser has been used for treatment of facial telangiectasia.[4] Because tissue destruction is nonselective with this laser, occurring by vaporization of water within cells, the skin surface and dermis overlying the telangiectasia are destroyed as well as the vessel. Because of this nonselective action, the CO_2 laser has no advantage over electrosurgery in the treatment of telangiectasia.

Argon laser. The argon laser has often been used for treatment of facial telangiectasia. Treatment parameters have varied, with laser powers of 0.8 to 2.9 W; exposure times of 50 msec, 0.2 sec, and 0.3 sec; and continuous output with spot sizes of 0.1 and 1 mm. Although the success rate has been reported to be good to excellent in 65% to 99% of patients treated,[2,320] pitted and depressed scars, hypopigmentation, hyperpigmentation, and recurrence of veins have been noted.[3,321] One area of particular concern is the nasal alae and nasolabial creases, where depressed scarring is relatively common, although resolution gradually occurs over time.[3]

Adverse healing may occur with the argon laser because of nonspecific thermal damage to perivascular tissue and the overlying epidermis. This is caused by competition for absorption of laser fluence from epidermal melanin and extensive radial diffusion and dissipation of heat from the target blood vessels.[36] Both these factors result in relatively nonspecific thermal destruction. To minimize these effects, a small beam size (100 μm) has been advocated to trace vessels precisely,[23,56,159] and a low power or pulsing with a 50-msec shutter has been recommended.[13,21,23] As mentioned previously, these parameters must be monitored closely, because the successful treatment of vascular lesions with the argon laser requires experience and artful expertise. As described previously, the use of a very small beam (100 μm) greatly increases the scattering of laser photons within the dermis and limits treatment to the most superficial of dermal vessels. With these parameters, many physicians find the argon laser effective in treating facial telangiectasia, with only minimal risk of adverse healing. This application is its most successful use.

To limit heat diffusion with the argon laser, robotized scanning laser handpieces have been used (see earlier section on treatment of PWS in adults). The use of this device has been reported to be successful in the treatment of facial and leg telangi-

Table 2-14
Response of telangiectasia to laser therapy

Laser Type	Spider (Face, Trunk)	Small Diameter (Face, Trunk)	Large Diameter (Face, Trunk)	Small Diameter: <0.2 mm (Legs)	Large Diameter: 1-3 mm (Legs)
FLPD	Excellent	Excellent	Fair	Very good	Poor
CV/CB, KTP, Krypton, 532-nm Nd:YAG	Good	Good	Fair	Poor	Poor
Continuous-wave dye or argon (with scanner)	Excellent	Good	Fair	Fair	Poor
Nd:YAG, 1064 nm	Poor	Poor	Poor	Poor	Poor
PhotoDerm VL	Excellent	Excellent	Excellent	Excellent	Good

See Table 2-9 for abbreviations.

ectasia when the telangiectasia occur in densely interlacing mats.[32] This technique is effective and greatly reduces the risk of adverse response, but it is not well suited for individual or widespread isolated telangiectasia.

Argon-pumped tunable dye laser. The argon-pumped tunable dye laser (ATDL) is a CW laser, although mechanically shuttered pulses as short as 20 msec are achievable. Beam size may be varied from 50 μm to 6.0 mm. Yellow light (577-595 nm) is usually chosen for treatment of vascular lesions. The tracing technique using a 100-μm beam with this laser has been used extensively and advocated by Scheibner and Wheeland[23] as a technique that produces good to excellent results with minimal risk in a variety of cutaneous vascular lesions,[56,159] including facial telangiectasia.[322] The proper endpoint of treatment is disappearance of the vessel, not blanching, blistering, or charring of the overlying skin. Because the tracing hand motion cannot be accurately quantified, treatment parameters are difficult to teach except by direct monitoring. In addition, this technique is more tedious and time-consuming than the FLPDL, even when one becomes a skilled operator. Multiple treatments are usually required, with hypopigmentation rarely occurring.[323] The laser also may be used with a robotized scanning device if large areas of matted telangiectasia are to be treated.[32,33] However, multiple treatments are required, including spot vessel tracing to eliminate the hexagonal appearance.

A prospective, side-by-side comparison of the ATDL with the FLPDL in 14 patients found better efficacy with the FLPDL.[324] The ATDL used was a modified ophthalmic laser at 585 nm, focused to a 0.1-mm circular spot with a power of 0.7 to 0.8 W at a pulse duration of 0.1 sec (Coherent Medical). Treatment times were about three times longer for the ATDL than the FLPDL. The FLPDL was more painful than the ATDL. Swelling and erythema was similar between the two lasers, but hyperpigmentation was greater with the ATDL. Excellent clearance occurred with the FLPDL in 78% of patients compared with 28% with the ATDL.

Copper vapor/copper bromide laser. The CVL or CBL operates at two specific wavelengths, 578 nm (yellow) and 511 nm (green), and delivers a "quasi-continuous wave" composed of pulsed laser light energy in 20-nsec pulses at a frequency of 15,000 pulses per second. This train of pulses interacts with tissue in the same manner as a continuous beam because of the accumulation of heat with the large number of pulses delivered. Because of resulting thermal diffusion, it may be necessary to gate the pulse electronically with 20- to 50-msec secondary pulses or to use a scanning device.

The ability to pulse the CVL between 20 and 50 msec allows this laser to work within the thermal relaxation time of many telangiectasia (Figure 2-77). When the laser is used with these refinements, it is somewhat safer and more effective than the argon laser for treatment of facial telangiectasia and has the advantage of leaving only very minor superficial crusts overlying treated vessels, in contrast to the very visible, dark purpuric impact spots of the FLPDL.[325] A comparison of the CVL with the FLPDL in 10 adults with facial telangiectasia resistant to electrosurgical therapy demonstrated no difference in efficacy or adverse sequelae.[58] However, Dinehart et al[196] report a 10% incidence of transient hyperpigmentation. Whether this represents melanin or hemosiderin is unknown.

Of 33 patients with facial telangiectasia treated with the CVL, 69% had good to excellent results and 19% had poor results.[200] Treatment occurred with a 1-mm-diameter spot size at pulse durations of 50 to 200 msec at energy densities from 8 to 32 J/cm^2 or continuous until vessel blanching occurred. Best results were seen on the cheeks,with poor results on the nose or nasolabial folds. Atrophic scarring was reported on nasal lesions (7 of 33 patients), and edema lasting 1 to 3 days occurred on the cheeks and lower eyelids.

Thibault[326] reported the results of a patient questionnaire of 180 patients treated with the CVL with or without sclerotherapy for facial telangiectasia. He used a CVL (VisErase 3w, Visiray Pty Ltd., Hornsby, NSW, Australia) with a 200-μm fiber

A

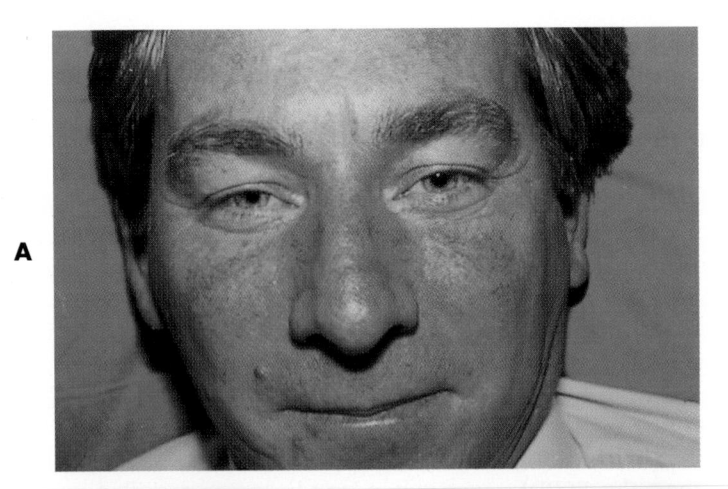

B

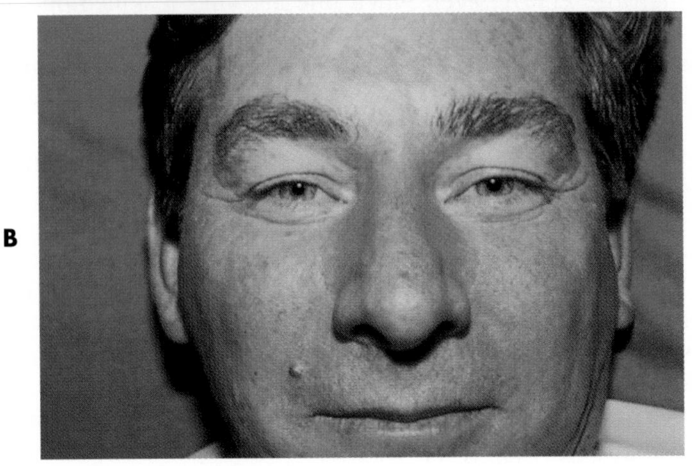

Figure 2-77 This man with telangiectasias was treated for about 20 minutes on two occasions with a copper bromide laser. **A,** Before treatment. **B,** After treatment. First treatment was at 2.2 W and 0.7 mm spot size, with 20-msec pulses (11.4 J/cm^2) for smaller vessels and 30-msec pulses (17.1 J/cm^2) for larger vessels. Second treatment 2 months later was at 2 W with 20-msec pulses for all remaining vessels (10.4 J/cm^2). (Courtesy Sue McCoy, MD.)

delivering a spot size of 150 to 400 μm. A clinical endpoint of vessel blanching was used, which required a power of 600 to 700 mW impinging on the vessel for less than 1 sec delivered continuously. Patients developed blistering 24 to 48 hours after treatment, with crusting lasting 7 to 17 days. Edema usually lasted 3 days. Almost half of patients treated with the CVL alone developed hypopigmentation. Good results were seen in 47% of vessels treated with the CVL alone, and these patients were satisfied with treatment, versus 86% of patients who had combination treatment with CVL and sclerotherapy being satisfied with treatment.

Waner et al[327] compared the CVL with the FLPDL in 12 patients with facial telangiectasia. Treatment times and patient satisfaction were equivalent. Postoperative swelling and prolonged healing occurred with the FLPDL. The CVL used was the Vasculase (Metalaser), with a spot size of 150 μm at a power of 0.35 to 0.55 W chopped at 0.2-sec intervals. Waner concludes that both lasers have equal efficacy, with most patients preferring the CVL.

McCoy[328] has reported her results in treating 570 patients with facial telangiectasia. Similar results were reported in another study of 23 patients evaluated in a blinded manner.[329] In both studies, greater than 75% clearance was achieved in 70% of patients, 50% to 75% clearance in 17%, and less than 50% clearance in

13%. Vessels on the cheeks cleared much better than nasal telangiectasia, which only had an excellent response in 26% of patients. Vessels less than 100 μm or greater than 300 μm did not respond as well as vessels 100 to 300 μm in diameter. McCoy used the CBL at 578 nm only (Norseld CuB D-10, Adelaide, South Australia) in a train of 30-nsec pulses at 16 kHz. The average power through the 600-μm fiber was 2 W. The fiber was used in a slightly defocused mode to produce a 0.9-mm-diameter spot. Although the chopped pulse duration varied from 7 to 60 msec, the treatment endpoint was vessel spasm without epidermal blanching. About 45% of patients required one treatment, and 35% of patients required two treatments. The remaining 20% of patients received three to five treatments. Treatment sessions ranged from 5 to 60 minutes, with the average treatment requiring 16.7 minutes. Moderate erythema occurred in most patients and lasted 2 to 3 hours. Swelling and crusting were rare. There were no reports of scarring or hyperpigmentation.

McCoy[328] postulates that the reduced effectiveness in treating vessels less than 100 μm results from the thermal relaxation time being much less than the delivered pulse durations. The reduced effectiveness in vessels greater than 300 μm results from absorption of laser fluence in the superficial portion of the vessel with "protection" to the deeper endothelium. McCoy recommends using sclerotherapy for vessels greater than 300 μm in diameter.

When used with the modulating influence of a secondary shuttered pulse or scanning device, the risk of adverse response is further minimized without significant change in clinical effectiveness. In a comparison of 144 patients treated with the point-by-point technique and 105 patients treated by the Hexascan, French investigators determined that the incidence of hypertrophic scarring was less than 1% in the Hexascan group versus 7% in the point-by-point group. Treatment time was also reduced to 20% of the point-by-point time. Patients treated by Hexascan also experienced less pain, and local anesthesia was rarely required.[81] The balance between these two results (vessel obliteration and adverse healing) must be weighed and the treatment technique altered to be consistent with the goals of treatment.

StarPulse (532-nm KTP laser). The Starpulse KTP laser (LaserScope) operates at 532 nm and emits a train of 1-msec Q-switched pulses at 25 kHz. What distinguishes this system from other frequency-doubled Nd:YAG lasers is that the arc lamp is modulated and can provide pulse durations ranging from 1 to 50 msec. This produces very-high-energy pulses that can be projected onto the skin in spots ranging in diameter from 0.25 to 4.0 mm while still maintaining fluences within the 5 to 10 J/cm^2 therapeutic range. The combination of high-energy pulses and ability to adjust pulse duration to match the thermal relaxation time of blood vessels allows modulated KTP lasers to remove vascular lesions with less purpura than the FLPDL (Figures 2-78 and 2-79).

A comparison study of the KTP laser (Starpulse) with the FLPDL found less swelling, pain, bruising, and redness with the KTP laser.[330] The Starpulse was used with a 2-mm-diameter spot size, 17 J/cm^2, 10 msec. The FLPDL was used with a 3-mm-diameter spot size at 6.8 J. No significant difference in efficacy was found between the two lasers.

Q-switched Nd:YAG laser, 532 nm. Even without consideration for the thermal relaxation time of vascular lesions, the 532-nm laser has been shown to be effective in clearing facial telangiectasia. Ten patients treated with the Nd:YAG laser at 532 nm in the Q-switched mode with 5-nsec pulses at 1 to 2 and 3 to 4 J/cm^2 demonstrated clearance.[331] Excellent results occurred in 30% of patients treated at 1 to 2 J/cm^2 versus 70% of patients having excellent results when treated at 3 to 4 J/cm^2. However, at 3 to 4 J/cm^2, purpura occurred in all patients, with hyperpigmentation developing in 20% at 30 days and 10% at 60 days. The effectiveness and pigmentation were probably caused by the explosive effects to the absorption of the laser energy in a very short time (5 nsec) with rupture of

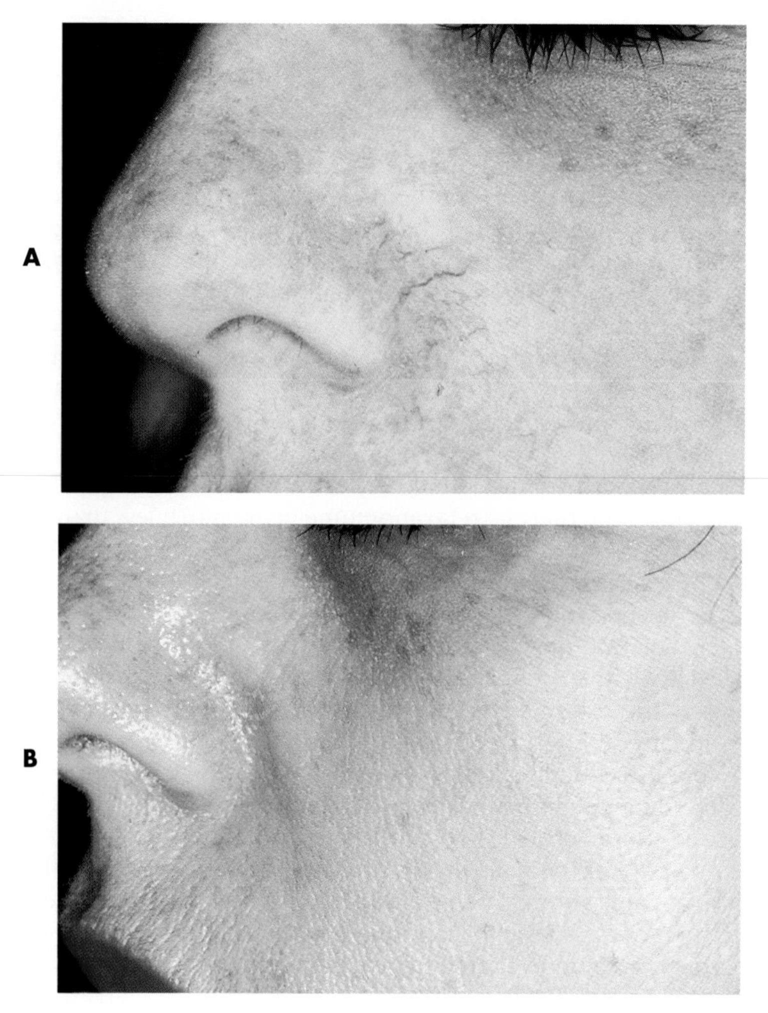

Figure 2-78 **A,** Perinasal telangiectasia before treatment. **B,** Two weeks after treatment with Orion potassium titanyl phosphorus (KTP) at 5 W, tracing vessels once with 250-μm spot Dermastat with 10-msec exposure duration, 5 pulses per second (pps). (Courtesy Burton E Silver, MD.)

the vessel and release of hemosiderin. Larger comparative studies are needed to determine the relative efficacy and safety of this laser.

Long-pulse Nd:YAG laser, 532 nm. By extending the pulse duration to within the thermal relaxation time of the vessel treated, purpura is avoided without loss of efficacy (see earlier discussion) (Figure 2-80). This laser has been effective in treating facial telangiectasia that have sometimes proved to be recalcitrant to treatment with other laser modalities[322] (Figure 2-81). Our experience in using this modality both with and without epidermal cooling has been variable but positive.

Krypton laser. The krypton laser is a gas-medium laser that produces wavelengths of 520, 530, and 568 nm. It is a CW laser that can be shuttered to a pulse duration of 50 msec. The HGW K1 krypton laser (HGM, Inc.) produces a maximum 1.5 W of light at 520 and 530 nm and 1 W at 568 nm. When using a 1-mm-diameter spot size, all three wavelengths combined produce an energy fluence of 16 J/cm^2, which is more than sufficient for coagulating telangiectasia.

Thibault[333] reported that 64% of his patients surveyed had large to total reduction of their facial lesions, with 84% reporting good to very good response. Unfortunately, 11% of patients reported atrophic scarring, and 38% claimed a change in their skin texture (Figures 2-82 and 2-83).

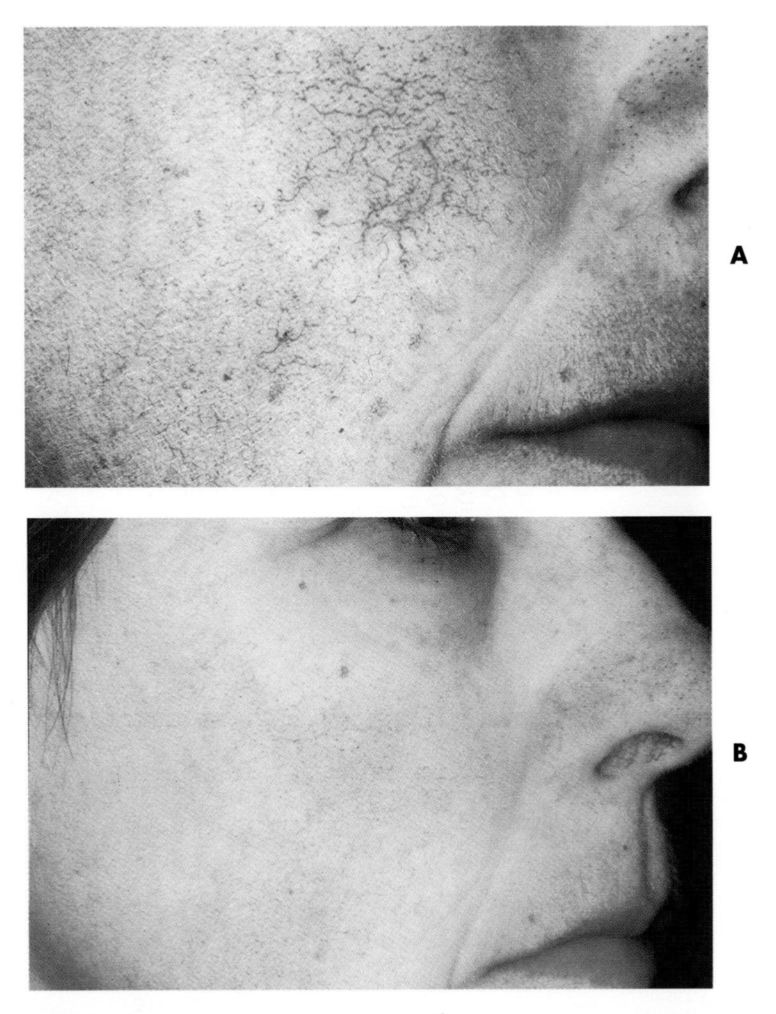

Figure 2-79 **A,** Facial telangiectasia before treatment. **B,** Three months after treatment with Orion KTP at 40 W, 4-mm Dermastat with 20-msec exposure duration, 1 pps. (Courtesy Burton E Silver, MD.)

Sadick[334] confirmed Thibault's findings in 40 patients with nasal telangiectasia using different parameters (longer pulse durations at lower fluences with a larger spot size; specifically, 0.6 J/cm², 0.2-sec pulses at 568 nm with a 6-mm-diameter spot size). He found crusting in 40% of patients, resulting in 15% of patients having epidermal textural changes, including tracking scars and persistent exaggerated erythema. Only 35% of his patients achieved 75% improvement. The similar results reported by Sadick and Thibault most likely relate to their use of the clinical endpoint of lesion blanching, which can be achieved through treatment of the telangiectasia in multiple pulses.

Flashlamp-pumped pulsed dye laser. The FLPDL operates at 585 nm with a 450-msec pulse. A newer version of this laser operates with a 1.5-msec pulse at wavelengths of 595 and 600 nm. To date, no published studies have reported its effectiveness in treating facial telangiectasia, with reports of its efficacy in treating leg telangiectasia variable. The clinical treatment technique involves delivering a train of pulses overlapping 10% to 20%, tracing the vessels to be treated with a 2-, 3-, or 5-mm delivery spot, and treating an area of interlacing telangiectasia with overlapping spots to cover the involved area. Delivery energies range from 5 to 8 J/cm² and are adjusted according to lesion response and location. Disruption of blood flow occurs with resultant purpura but without excessive swelling or crusting. Patients with type I Celtic skin may be treated with fluences of 5 to 6 J/cm² without loss of

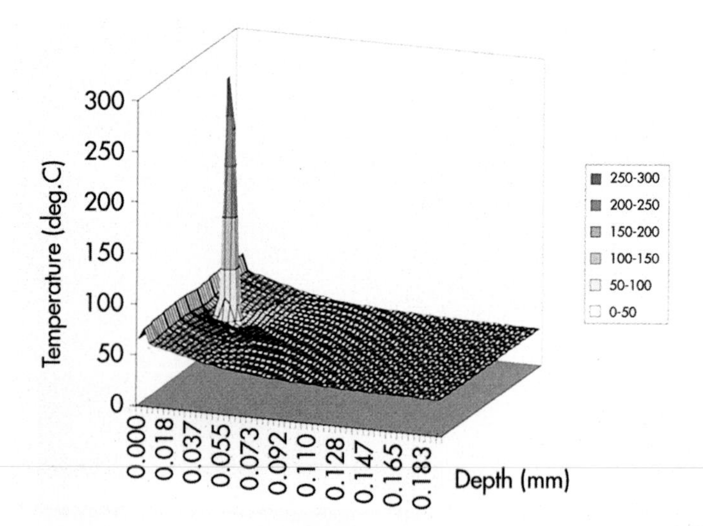

Figure 2-80 Temperature distribution achieved in treating 0.1-mm-diameter, 0.2-mm deep vessel with 532-nm laser with 2-msec pulse duration, 5-mm-diameter spot size, 15 J/cm² with epidermal cooling to 4° C. (Courtesy ESC Medical, Inc.)

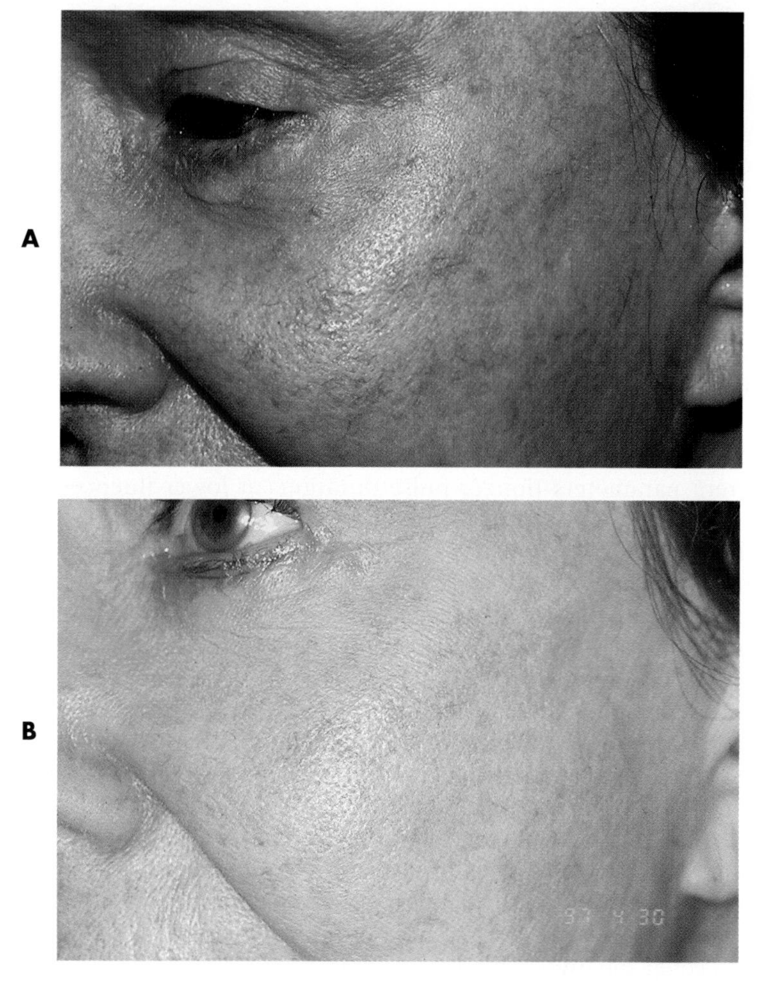

Figure 2-81 **A,** Facial telangiectasia on cheek of 60-year-old woman before treatment. **B,** Two months after single treatment with Versapulse, 532 nm at 10-msec pulse duration, 3-mm-diameter spot size, 10 J/cm² with epidermal cooling to 4° C.

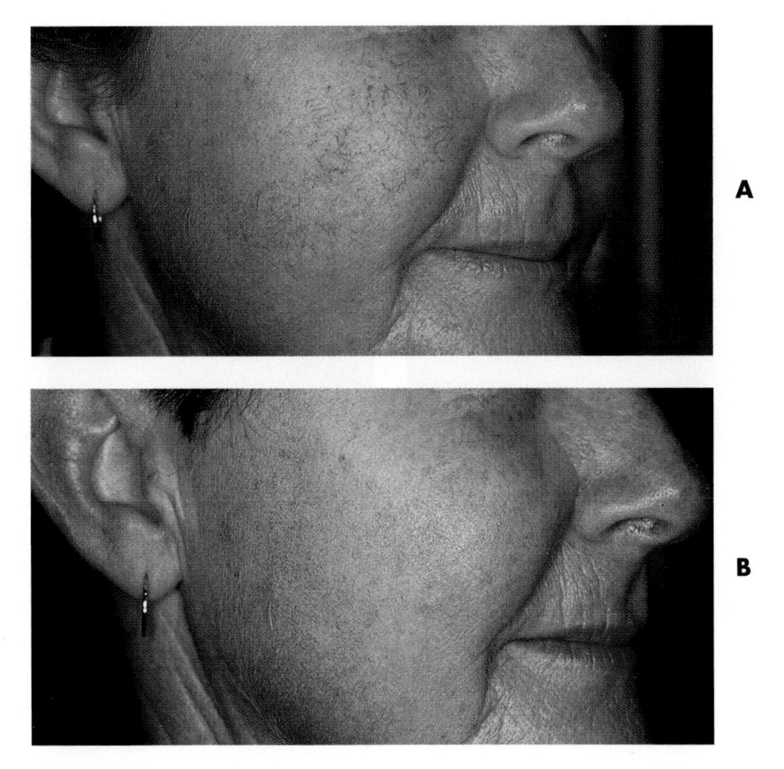

Figure 2-82 **A,** Facial telangiectasia before treatment. **B,** Three years after treatment with HGM krypton laser, 1-mm-diameter spot, 16 J/cm^2, 1 W, at 568 nm and 1.5 W at 532 nm plus sclerotherapy with sodium tetradecyl sulfate 0.2%. (Courtesy Paul Thibault, MD, Newcastle, Australia.)

efficacy. Treatments of telangiectasia are generally done without the use of test spots, although these may be used if the patient or physician is unsure and wants to observe response in a small area. If test spots are used, the entire length of the vessel must be treated to eliminate the vessel (Figure 2-84).

A 2-mm spot size is available. Geronemus and Greiken[335] reported clearing in 70% of 35 patients with linear telangiectasia, with no cases of scarring, skin texture change, or hypopigmentation. Reduced purpura was the major advantage. However, high fluences of 8.5 to 9.5 J/cm^2 were needed to produce vessel clearing.

Sadick[334] reported that a long-pulse, 1.5-msec, 595-nm version of the FLPDL (Sclerolaser, Candela) resulted in less purpura than the original FLPDL. In a series of 40 patients, 90% achieved greater than 75% improvement with one treatment. He used a fluence of 14 J/cm^2 with a 2 × 7-mm elliptic spot size. Ten percent of his patients developed crusting without significant textural changes.

PhotoDerm VL. This high-energy pulsed light source described previously is very effective in treating facial telangiectasia. Advantages are the almost complete lack of purpura and adverse sequelae. Energy fluences of 25 to 45 J/cm^2 are required for vessel ablation given either as a single 2.5- to 5-msec pulse or over two pulses of 2.4 to 6.0 msec each with a of 10-msec delay between pulses. A 550- or 570-nm cutoff filter works best. Lesions usually clear in one treatment in 90% of patients.[336]

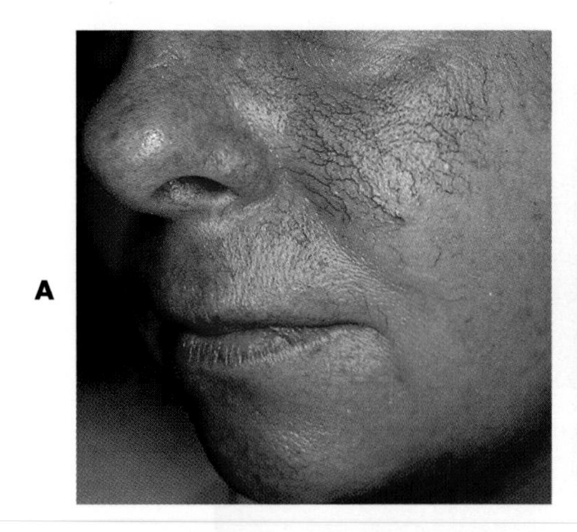

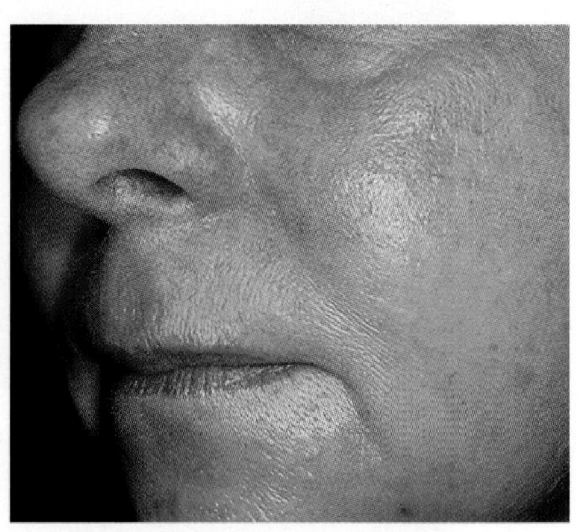

Figure 2-83 Facial telangiectasia treated with HGM krypton laser alone at same parameters as in Fig. 2-82 without sclerotherapy treatment. **A,** Before treatment. **B,** Ten months after treatment. (Courtesy Paul Thibault, MD, Newcastle, Australia.)

Lesions are treated with one or two pulses until initial vessel spasm or slight purpura occurs (Figures 2-85 and 2-86). The only side effects are slight purpura, which lasts 2 to 4 days, or epidermal desquamation when treatment is performed on tanned or type III or IV skin. Epidermal desquamation can be avoided by changing the filter to a longer wavelength or increasing the delay time between double or triple pulses.

Telangiectasia: Clinical Variants

Generalized essential telangiectasia

This telangiectasia generally occurs on the legs but may also involve other cutaneous surfaces. Various treatments have been proposed, with variable efficacy.[301] Tan and Kurban[297] reported successful treatment with the FLPDL at fluences of 6 J/cm^2. We also treated four patients with the FLPDL at fluences ranging from 6.0 to 7.5 J/cm^2. Two patients responded with total resolution, but two patients had almost no improvement in their appearance (Figure 2-87). Therefore we believe that intrinsic factors in these patients may preclude predictable results. We recommend performing a patch test for such patients. PhotoDerm VL treatment has also been found to be effective.[337]

Linear facial telangiectasia

These telangiectasia often carry an unjustified social stigma implying alcoholism. Thus patients are understandably distressed by this otherwise benign condition. Treatment of large vessels on the nasal ala or nasal alar groove is difficult and often leads to noticeable scarring when conventional methods are used. We have found the FLPDL to be a powerful and effective tool in the treatment of these lesions, virtually without the risk of scarring or other permanent skin changes.

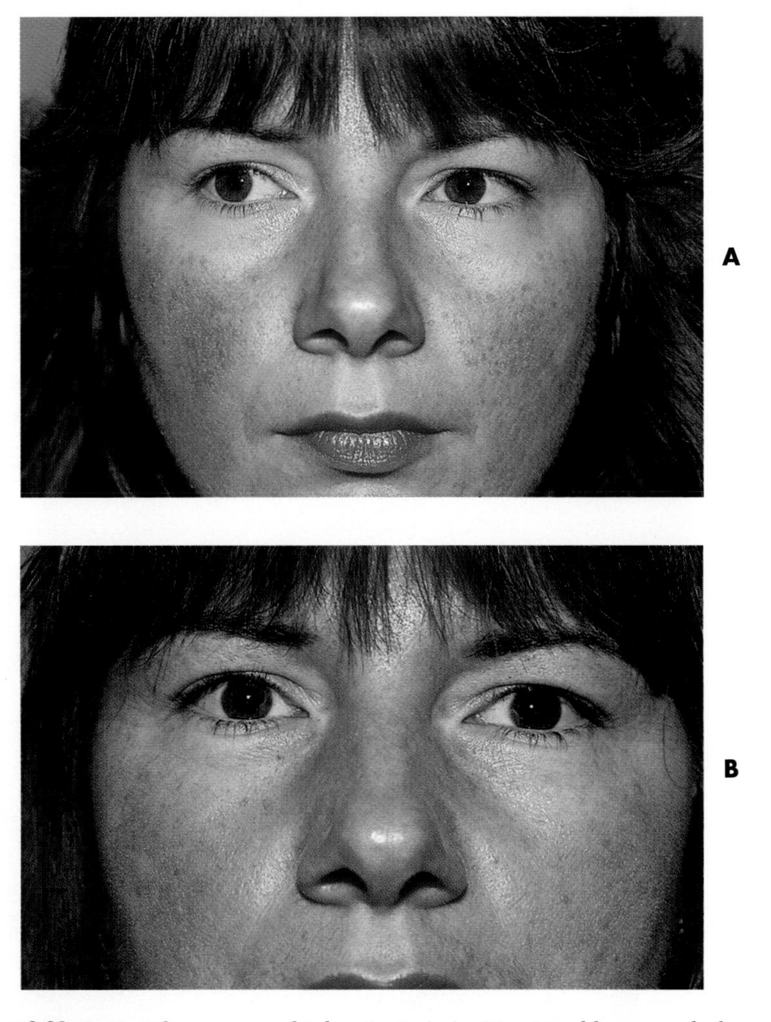

Figure 2-84 **A,** Facial rosacea and telangiectasia in 32-year-old woman before treatment. **B,** Three years after single treatment with FLPDL at 7 J/cm^2 delivered through 5-mm-diameter spot.

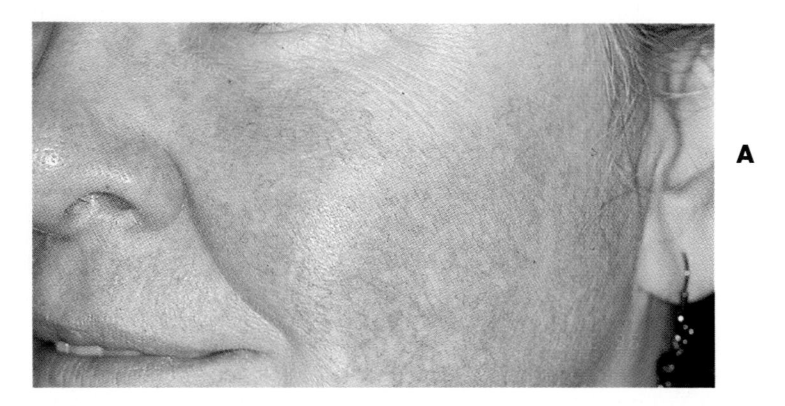

Figure 2-85 **A,** Extensive facial telangiectasia on 55-year-old woman after automobile airbag impacted her face.

Continued

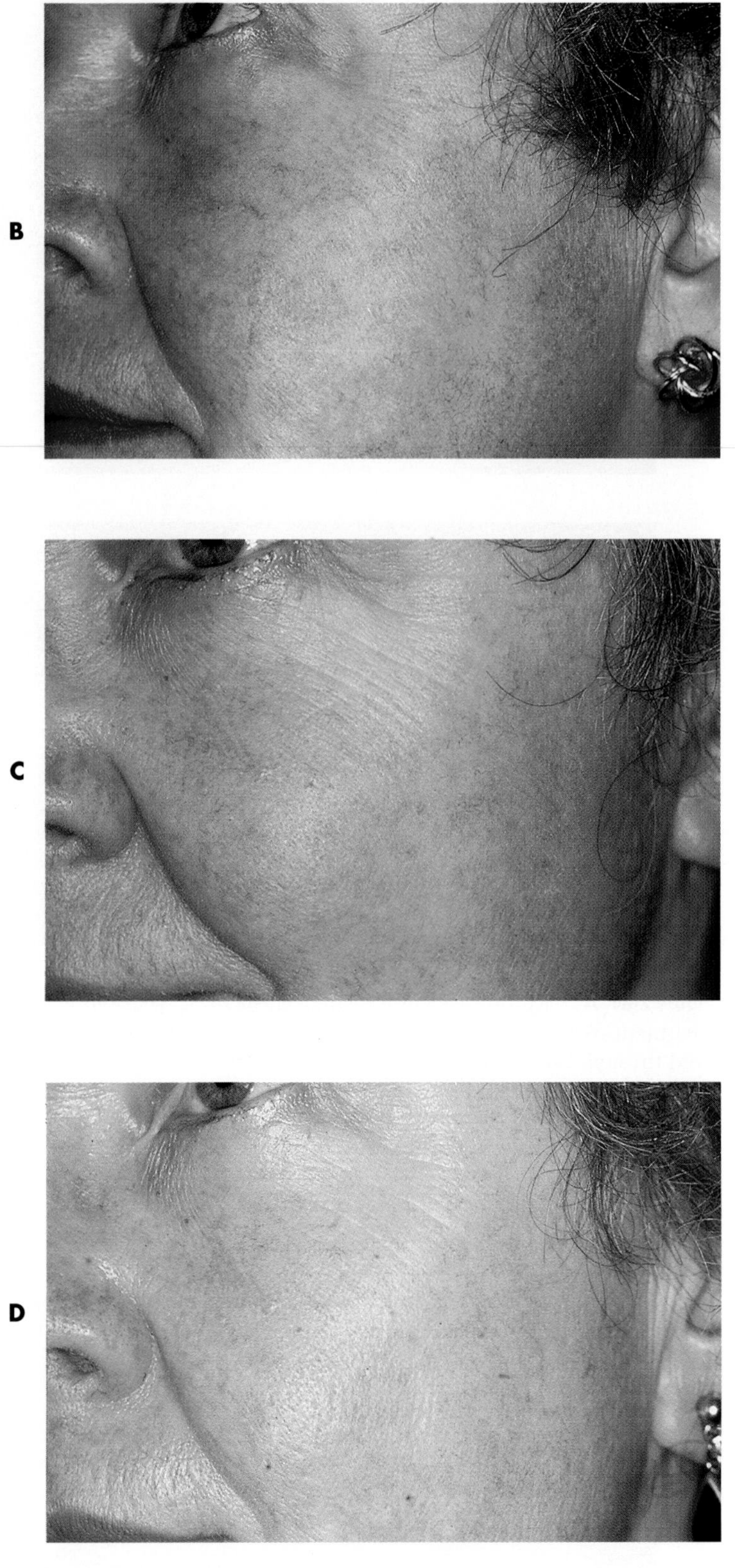

Figure 2-85, cont'd **B,** Eight weeks after treatment with PhotoDerm VL, 550-nm cutoff filter, 40 J/cm², double pulse of 2.4 and 4.0 msec with 10-msec delay. Note 50% improvement. **C,** Four weeks after second PhotoDerm VL treatment with 570-nm cutoff filter, 44 J/cm² delivered in two pulses of 2.4 and 4.0 msec with 10-msec delay. **D,** Complete resolution 8 weeks after third and fourth treatments, with parameters similar to those in **C.**

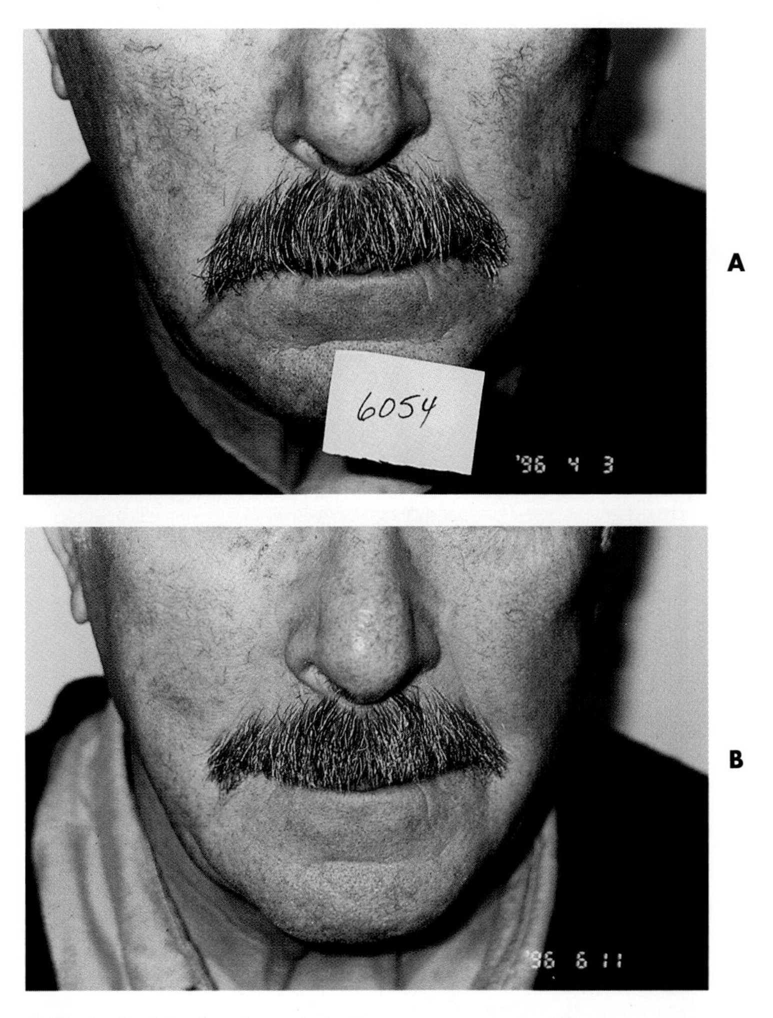

Figure 2-86 **A,** Facial telangiectasia before treatment. **B,** After two treatments with PhotoDerm VL with 570- or 550-nm cutoff filters, 37 J/cm² given as double pulse of 3 and 4 msec with 10-msec delay between pulses. (Courtesy Beverly Kemsley, MD, Calgary, Canada.)

One study reports a 77% response rate to FLPDL treatment of adult facial linear telangiectasia.[116] Although vessel diameter was not measured, larger blue vessels were less responsive than smaller red vessels. The poorer response to treatment of these larger vessels may result from (1) the thermal relaxation time in larger-diameter telangiectasia being longer than the pulse duration of the laser and (2) the deoxygenated Hb absorbing at a lower wavelength of the laser (545 nm.)

Our published series shows 97.5% of 182 patients achieving good to excellent results (14% good, 83.5% excellent), indicating resolution of more than 50% of the treated lesions in one or two treatments[338] (Figures 2-88 and 2-89). In 152 of these patients, more than 75% of their telangiectasia was removed (Table 2-15). Scarring did not occur in any patient, and skin texture remained unchanged. As expected, all patients experienced a transient bluish purple discoloration at the treatment site that resolved spontaneously in 10 to 14 days. This discoloration was well tolerated by our patient population, who were informed in advance of its occurrence. They could therefore modify their social and business schedules accordingly. Typically, makeup foundation was used to camouflage the purpura approximately 5 days after treatment. A small number of patients experienced other transient skin changes at the

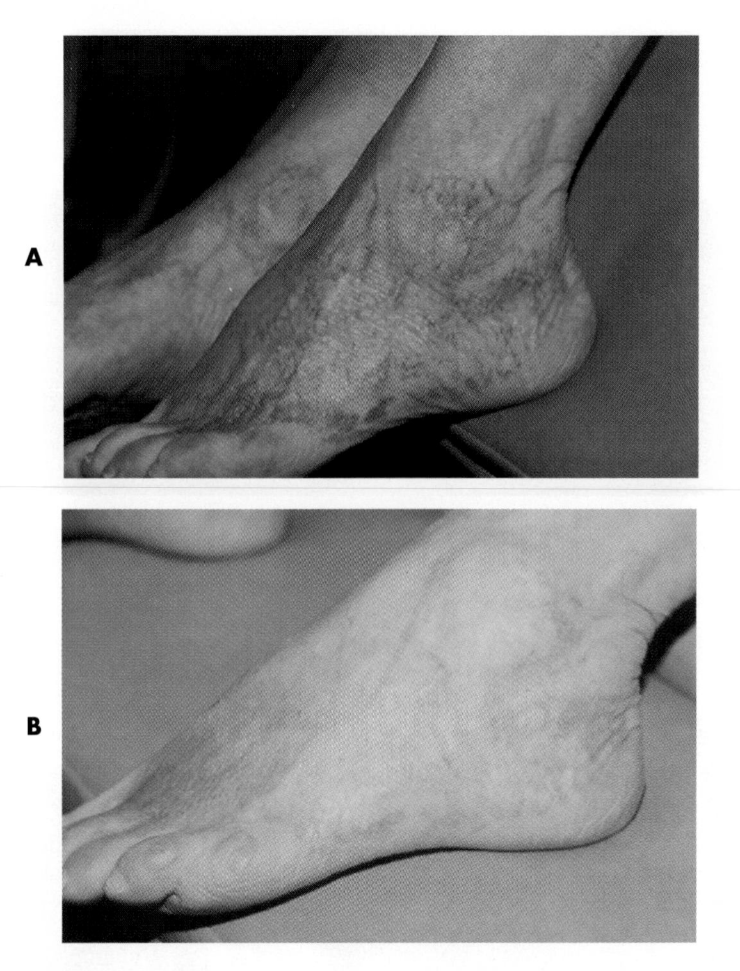

Figure 2-87 Extensive vascular ectasia on both feet of 54-year-old woman. **A,** Before treatment. **B,** Six months after initial treatment and 3 months after second treatment with FLPDL at 7.25 J/cm^2 using 84 and 115 pulses, respectively. (From Goldman MP: *Sclerotherapy: treatment of varicose and telangiectatic leg veins,* ed 2, St Louis, 1995, Mosby.)

treatment site (Table 2-16). Even though no anesthesia was used, patients experienced only mild to moderate discomfort in 93% of the cases.

Most patients (62%) underwent only one treatment, although further improvement and a better response was seen in patients with more than one treatment (Table 2-17). Skin type did not have a measurable influence on response to treatment. The largest percentage of patients had an excellent response with fluences above 7 J/cm^2 (93% versus 78%). There was a noticeable trend toward increasing effectiveness with increasing fluence.[338]

Our experience is that vessels larger than 0.2 mm in diameter require multiple treatments. Vessels larger than 0.4 mm in diameter are poorly responsive to FLPDL treatment and may best be treated with sclerotherapy or in combination with one of the continuous-output or longer-pulsed (1-10-msec) lasers previously described. The PhotoDerm VL is also effective for these vessels. Although treatment is tolerated well by patients without anesthesia, it may be prudent to offer topical anesthetic creams (see Chapter 10).

An additional consideration in limiting temporary purpura may be to treat linear facial telangiectasia with a low-fluence FLPDL (3 J/cm^2). Garden and Bakus[339] treated 10 patients with low-fluence FLPDL and a 10-mm-diameter spot size, which resulted

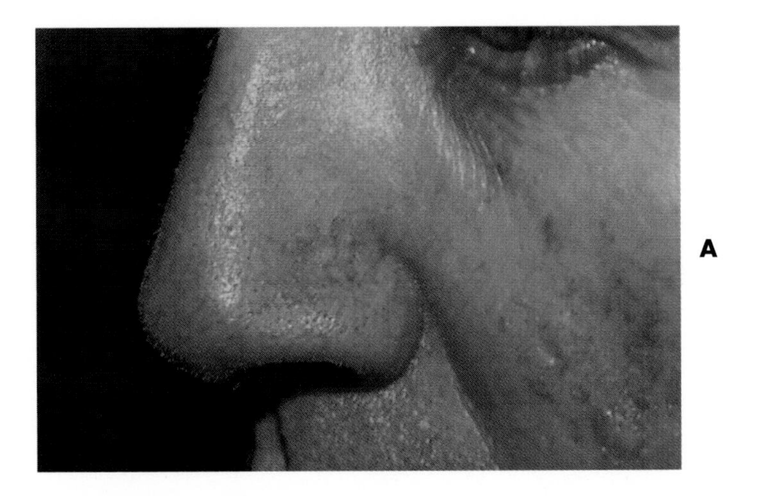

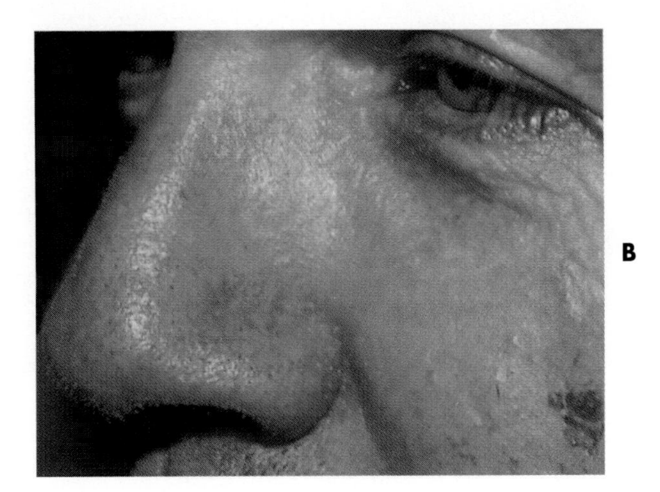

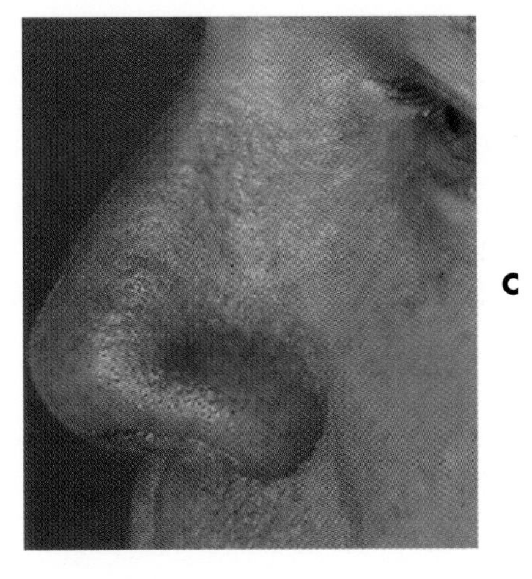

Figure 2-88 **A,** Bright-red linear telangiectasia 0.1 mm in diameter over nasal alar crease in 46-year-old man. **B,** Three months after FLPDL treatment at 7 J/cm². Note complete resolution of nasal alar telangiectasia. **C,** One year after laser treatment. Note persistent resolution of nasal telangiectasia.

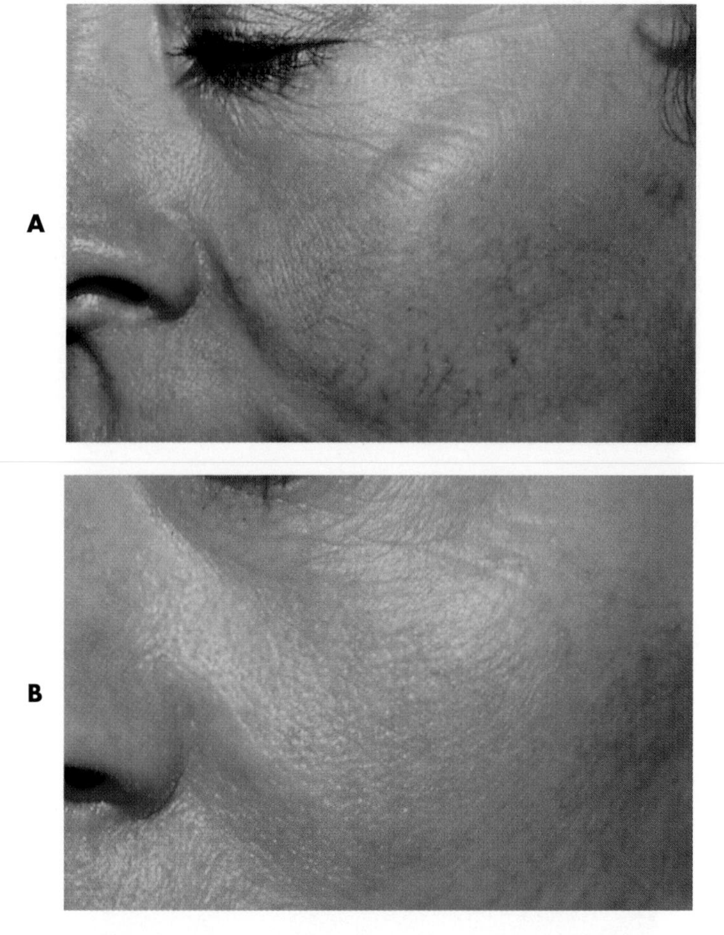

Figure 2-89 **A,** Extensive telangiectasia bilaterally on cheeks of 56-year-old woman. **B,** Six months after one treatment with FLPDL at 7.25 J/cm^2. Total of 40 5-mm impact pulses were given to entire left cheek.

Table 2-15
Linear facial telangiectasia: response to FLPDL treatment in 182 patients

Clinical Response (%)	No. (%) of Patients
None to poor (0-25)	2 (1)
Slight (26-50)	3 (1.6)
Good (51-75)	25 (14)
Excellent (76-100)	152 (83.5)

in temporary erythema without purpura. They graded the response rate after one treatment at 41 ± 5%. Small-diameter vessels responded best. Thus select linear facial telangiectasia may respond to FLPDL treatment without adverse sequelae.

Rosacea

Rosacea is essentially a cutaneous vascular disorder. It is best thought of not as a disease but as a typology of a cluster of patients with a characteristic combination of cutaneous stigmata consisting of telangiectasia, papules, pustules, and rhinophyma.[340] Telangiectasia represents the later phase of vascularization and probably results from a reduction in mechanical integrity of the upper dermal

Table 2-16
Linear facial telangiectasia: skin changes after FLPDL treatment in 182 patients

Skin Change	No. (%) of Patients
Bluish purple discoloration	182 (100)
Scaling	22 (12)
Crusting	8 (4)
Blistering	1 (0.5)
Increased pigmentation (up to 7 mo)	3 (1.6)
Decreased pigmentation (up to 12 mo)	3 (1.6)
Scarring	0 (0.1)

Table 2-17
Linear facial telangiectasia: response according to number of FLPDL treatment(s)

Average No. of Treatments	Treatment Response
1	None
1	Slight
1.2	Good
1.5	Excellent

connective tissue, allowing a passive dilatation of capillaries. Inflammation and associated angiogenesis may contribute to the telangiectasia.

Rosacea-associated telangiectasia and erythema respond well to treatment with the FLPDL. We have reported good to excellent results in 24 of 27 patients (89%).[338,341] In addition to the cosmetic improvement resulting from elimination of the vascular component of this disorder, FLPDL treatment also appears to alter the pathophysiology of this condition because a decrease in papule and pustule activity occurs in up to 59% of patients (Figure 2-90). After FLPDL treatment, patients who responded to treatment with elimination of the vascular component required less or no topical or systemic antibiotic therapy to maintain disease resolution.[341] Anecdotal reports from Tan and Kurban[297] confirm our more formal evaluations.

In assessing the overall success and potential risk of each laser used in the treatment of facial telangiectasia with rosacea, we believe that the FLPDL provides effective and relatively risk-free results. However, purpura resulting after treatment is an inconvenience that must be recognized in advance in scheduling treatment.

Both the CVL and the 577-nm ATDL offer reasonable alternatives to the FLPDL with the potential advantage of causing less visible crusting over treated vessels instead of purpura. However, some perivascular thermal damage with both lasers can cause scarring and hypopigmentation. These CW are also generally more time-consuming to operate. These three lasers are all superior to the argon laser, which, although successful with expert technique, must be used with discretion. The CO_2 laser has no advantage over electrosurgery and in our opinion should not be used for treating facial telangiectasia.

A study of 47 patients treated with the KTP 532-nm laser with variable-sized handpieces depending on the type of telangiectasia showed good results.[342] Matted telangiectasia were treated with a 4-mm-diameter spot and 20-msec pulse width at an average energy of 0.7 W. Vessels 0.1 to 0.3 mm in diameter were treated with a 0.25-mm-diameter spot size and 20-msec pulse width at an average energy of 0.12 W. Vessels greater than 0.3 mm in diameter were treated with a 1-mm-diameter spot

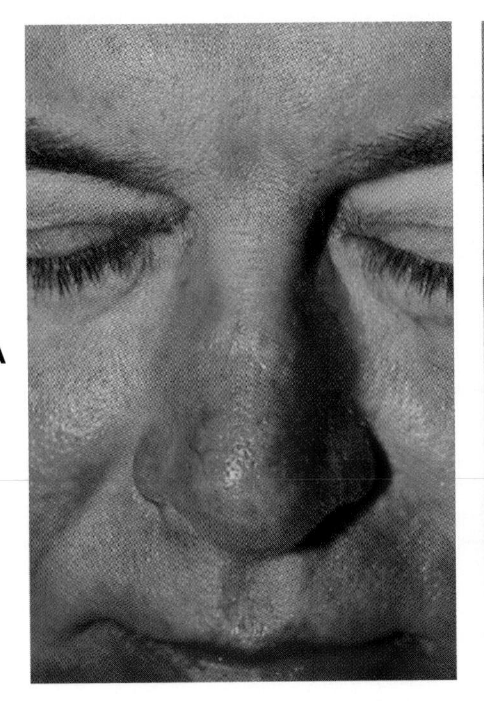

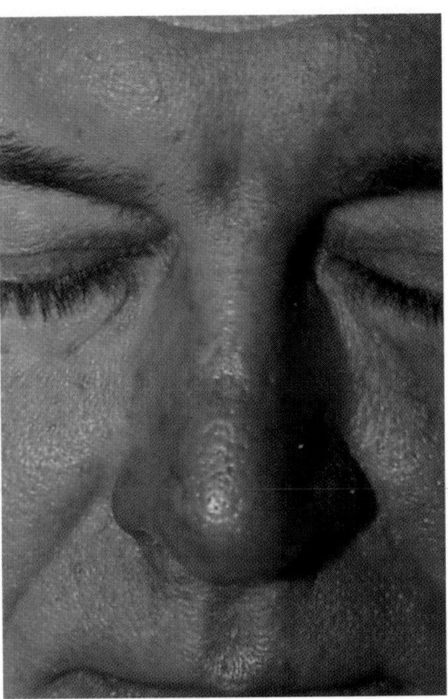

Figure 2-90 **A,** Acne rosacea and extensively telangiectatic nose in 54-year-old man. **B,** One year after two treatments with FLPDL at a fluence of 7.25 J/cm². First treatment used 106 and second 65 5-mm pulses.

and 10-msec pulse width at an average energy of 0.2 W. Vessels were treated by tracing them with the laser until they disappeared. This required one to several tracings. Of the 47 patients, 38% had more than 70% resolution of their telangiectasia, and 32% required a second treatment to achieve the same result. The only adverse effect consisted of linear crusting along the path of the telangiectasia.

The PhotoDerm VL has also been found to be effective in treating rosacea. As described previously, this light source has the advantage of relatively quick vessel elimination without significant purpura or crusting (Figures 2-91 and 2-92).

Telangiectasia macularis eruptiva perstans

Telangiectasia macularis eruptiva perstans (TMEP) is a form of mastocytosis characterized by truncal telangiectasia. A 10-year-old girl with extensive truncal TMEP treated with the FLPDL had complete clearance of lesions, but with recurrence of 70% of lesions 14 months postoperatively.[343] The best results for TMEP were achieved at a fluence of 7 J/cm², with complete fading occurring at 2 months with a single treatment. To limit the development of urticarial lesions after treatment from excessive histamine release, the patient was pretreated with the H_1 blocker diphenhydramine, 25 mg four times a day, and the H_2 blocker ranitidine, 75 mg twice a day, preoperatively and postoperatively. Doxepin, 10 mg three times a day 1 day preoperatively and 7 days postoperatively, also prevented urticarial reactions.

Scar Telangiectasia and Hypertrophic Scar

Scar telangiectasia are those vessels that cause a scar to be persistently red. They may represent ectatic dermal vessels, which give the scar a pink hue or may be superimposed over a scar as linear or arborizing arteriolar telangiectasia. When present as overlying telangiectasia, scars are more visible than they would otherwise be.

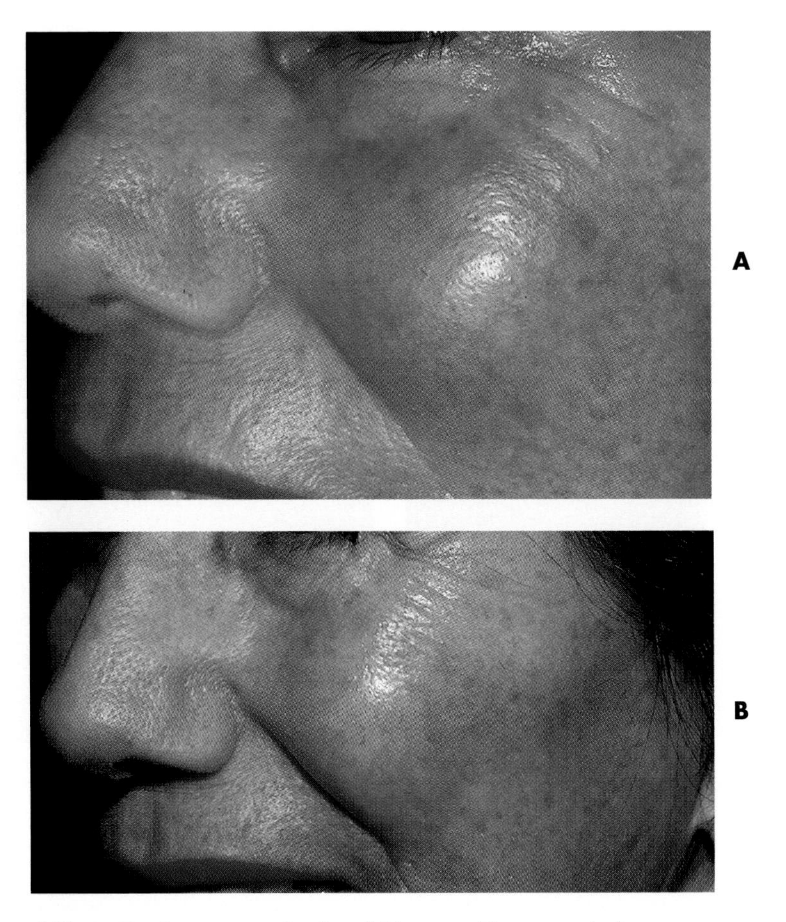

Figure 2-91 **A,** Erythematous cheeks of 66-year-old woman before treatment. **B,** After three treatments with PhotoDerm VL using 570-nm cutoff filter and 12-msec pulse at 52 J/cm^2; followed 4 weeks later by 590-nm cutoff filter and 12-msec pulse at 55 J/cm^2; then followed 4 weeks later by 550-nm cutoff filter at 44 J/cm^2 given as double pulse of 4.2 and 7.7 msec with 20-msec delay.

Neovascularization occurs in response to various angiogenic stimuli. Capillary endothelial cells release plasminogen activators and collagenases in response to angiogenic factors. Early scars are hyperemic from angiogenesis. As the scar matures, angiogenesis decreases with fading of the red color. Unfortunately, a scar may remain red for a long time, possibly from persistence of angiogenic stimuli or a retarded regression of the capillaries, as in hypertrophic scars and keloids.

We have found that scar telangiectasia respond as facial telangiectasia do. A series of treatments may be necessary. Each of the appropriate vascular lasers may be used with the same precautions as in treatment of facial telangiectasia. Some evidence indicates that elimination of these vessels also may reduce the swelling and bulkiness of the scar and normalize the surface texture.[344]

Various lasers have been shown to have an effect on collagen metabolism. The Nd:YAG laser has been shown to have a photobiologic effect on collagen metabolism.[345-347] Collagen production was selectively inhibited, whereas fibroblast deoxyribonucleic acid (DNA) replication and cell viability were spared. The Nd:YAG laser appears to address most appropriately the described pathobiology of keloid scars.

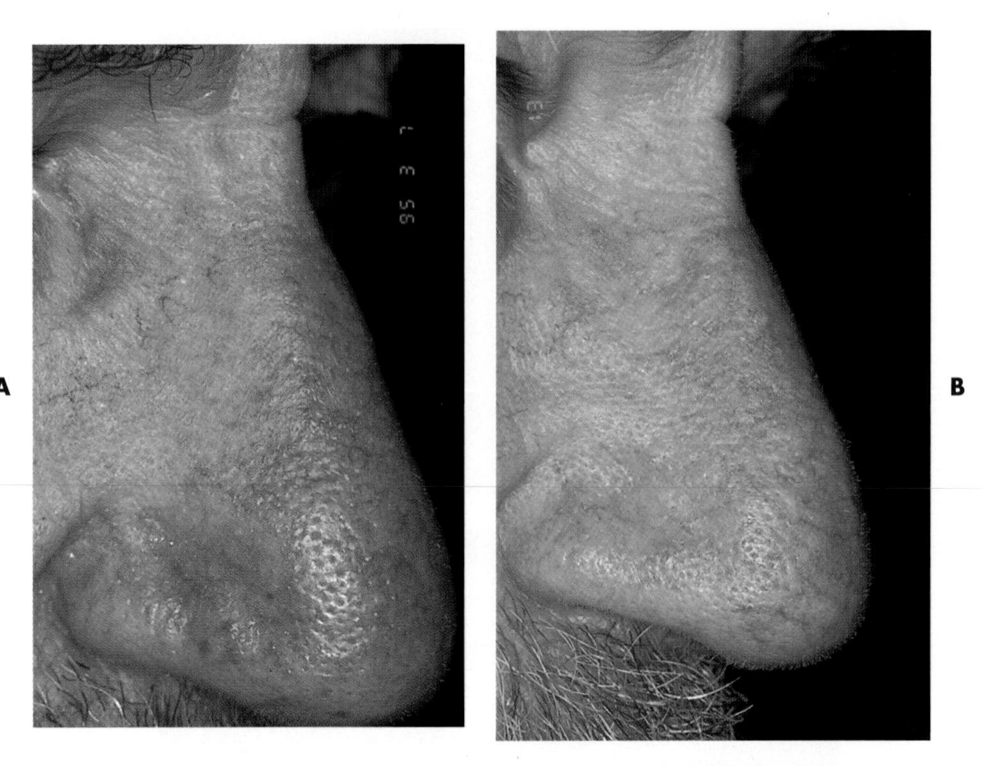

Figure 2-92 **A,** Diffusely red telangiectatic nose of 68-year-old male. **B,** After two treatments with PhotoDerm VL using 550-nm cutoff filter at 40 J/cm^2 given as single pulse of 8 msec at 4-week intervals.

Successful treatment of hypertrophic and keloid scars with the argon laser has been reported.[348,349] The blue-green argon laser light is highly absorbed by the HbO_2 of blood, leading to coagulation of the capillary plexus. An area of localized anoxia causes lymphatic plugging and vasculature disruption at the site of laser impact. Excessive amounts of lactic acid are produced by glycolysis. Granulocytes are extremely sensitive to low pH and are lysed, releasing their enzymes, including collagenase.[350] The increase in tissue levels of collagenase is thus a direct result of the laser, but it can also be an indirect effect by decreasing alpha$_2$-macroglobulin, a collagenase inhibitor. Through increasing collagenase, directly or indirectly, lysis of collagen increases, thereby altering the balance between collagen synthesis and collagen lysis, as seen in a keloid scar. In theory the FLPDL can have the same effect on collagen metabolism by selectively targeting the increased microcirculation in hypertrophic scars (Figure 2-93).

In addition to decreasing scar erythema, elimination of scar telangiectatic vessels may promote resolution of scar hypertrophy. Data suggest that patients with hypertrophic scars have increased microcirculatory perfusion.[351,352] Type V collagen has been found to be increased in hypertrophic scars that have numerous capillaries.[353] Therefore laser-induced destruction of cicatricial capillaries may decrease endothelial stimulation of type V collagen deposition with subsequent flattening of hypertrophic scars. Capillary endothelium may also play a direct role in stimulating collagen synthesis. An association between vascularity of granulation tissue and type V collagen has been demonstrated.[354] High levels of collagen and transforming growth factor beta$_1$ (TGF-β_1) messenger ribonucleic acid (mRNA) in fibroblasts and endothelial cells are found near blood vessels of hypertrophic scars and keloids.[355,356] Thus destruction of the microvasculature may eliminate the source of these factors to effect scar resolution. Finally, hypoxia induced by laser destruction of capillaries may alter the rate of collagen metabolism so that catabolism becomes dominant.[357]

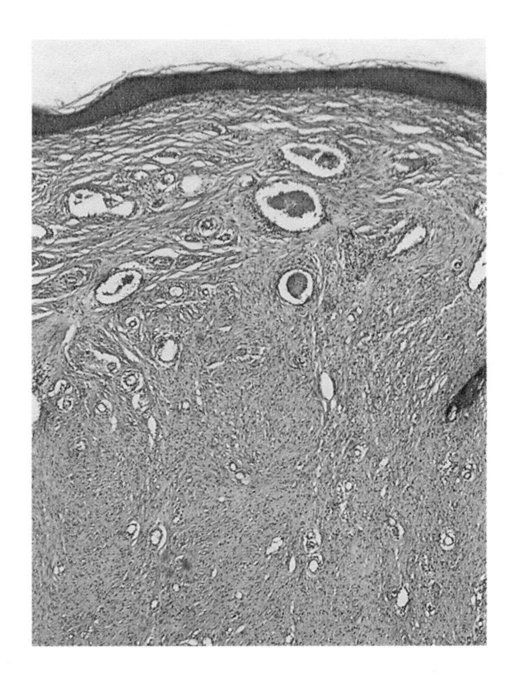

Figure 2-93 Biopsy of erythematous hypertrophic scar immediately after treatment with FLPDL at 7.0 J/cm^2. Note thrombosis of all vessels into deep papillary dermis and no apparent effect on overlying epidermis or perivascular tissue. (Hematoxylin-eosin; ×100.) (From Goldman MP, Fitzpatrick RE: *Dermatol Surg* 21:685, 1995.)

Alster and Williams[358] have suggested that an increase in local mast cell population after laser irradiation indirectly affects collagen turnover through histamine release because normal and keloid fibroblast growth is stimulated by histamine.[359] Conversely, degranulation of mast cells with release of histamine, interleukins, heparin, and tumor necrosis factor (TNF) may all increase the production of collagenase, which acts to decrease scar collagen hypertrophy. In addition to direct effects on dermal fibroblast and vessels, there may be other, as yet unknown mechanisms in scar resolution.

Clinical studies

Erythematous hypertrophic scars on the cheek, temple, neck, nose, thigh, and chest of 10 patients 15 to 20 months after argon laser treatment of their PWSs were evaluated histologically and with a computerized analysis of skin surface impressions *(optical profilometry)*.[14] These scars showed a decrease in skin surface markings and a variable degree of hypertrophy. They were treated with the FLPDL at a pulse duration of 360 μsec and a fluence of 6 to 7 J/cm^2 every 7 to 8 weeks for a total of five treatments. Posttreatment analysis demonstrated improvement with flattening of the hypertrophic portions of the scars and reappearance of skin surface markings in the atrophic areas. Normalization of dilated vascular channels within the scars also occurred.

Based on the clinical efficacy described previously (and also seen by us when treating PWSs in patients previously scarred with other laser modalities), we treated 15 patients with erythematous hypertrophic surgical scars with the FLPDL at 585 nm, a pulse duration of 450 μsec, with fluences of 7.0 to 7.5 J/cm^2.[344] An average 1.7 treatments resulted in an average 78% improvement in erythema and thickness, and 46% of patients had a 100% improvement after one to three treatments (Figure 2-94). These patients had received previous treatments without success, including plastic surgery (Z-plasty), radiotherapy, intralesional corticosteroid injection (alone or in combination with 5-fluorouracil), excision with the CO_2 laser, and treatment with the argon laser. Although the number of patients sustaining scars through different mechanisms was small, superficially induced scars, such as abrasions, thermal scars, or chemical peeling burns, appeared to respond better than excisional scars. Facial scars tended to respond better with a single treatment than scars on the extremities or buttocks. Multiple treatment sessions seemed to continue to

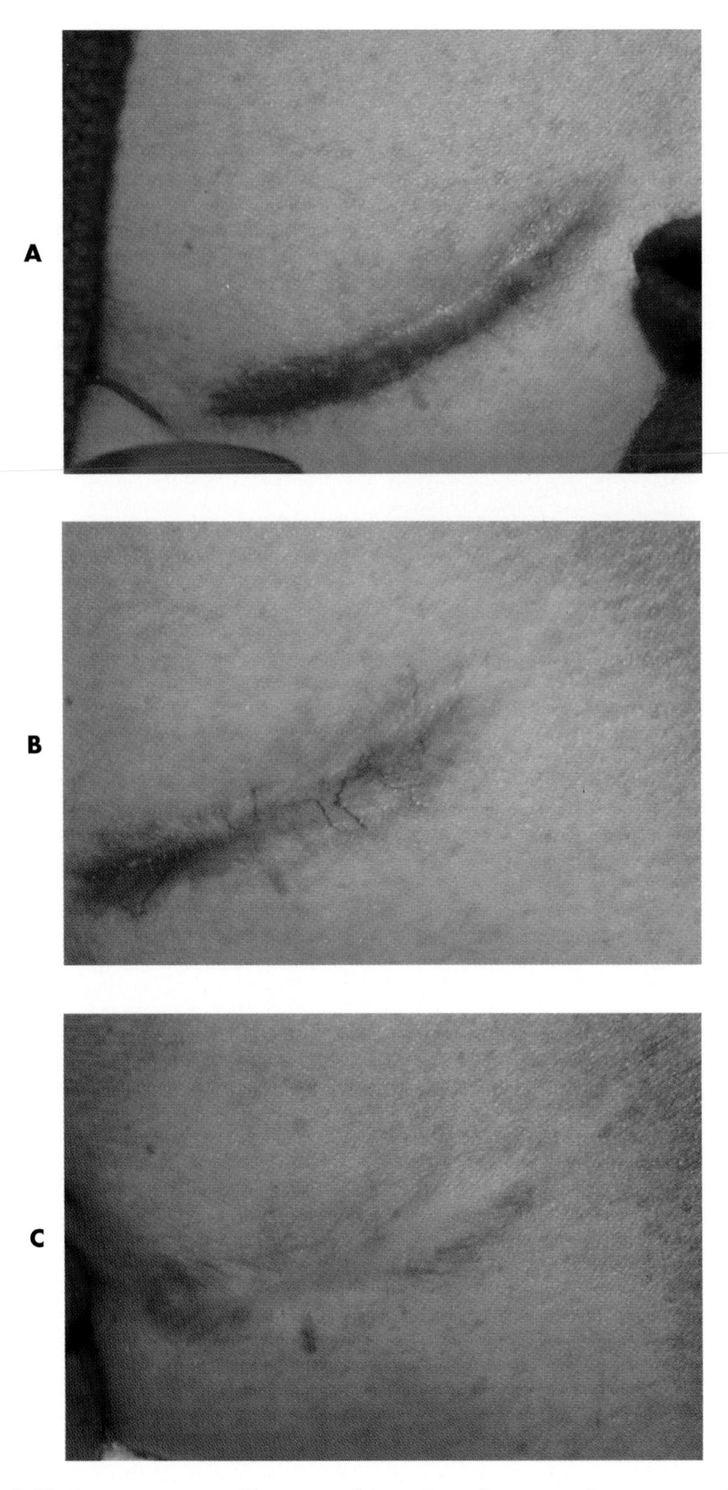

Figure 2-94 **A,** Appearance of hypertrophic and erythematous burn scar on lateral aspect of breast of 56-year-old woman 2 months after burn injury. **B,** Appearance of scar, now flattened and telangiectatic, after five intralesional injections of triamcinolone (40 mg/ml solution mixed 1:1 with 5% 5-fluorouracil). Total of 0.2 to 0.3 ml of solution was injected in each treatment session at monthly intervals. Photograph taken immediately before laser treatment. **C,** After one treatment with FLPDL at 7 J/cm². Note total resolution of erythematous component of scar, which is now almost totally flat, 1 year after treatment.

improve the response. This preliminary report has been substantiated by additional patients treated in our practice and further reports in the literature (Figure 2-95).

Alster[360] examined 14 patients with erythematous and hypertrophic scars 2 to 10 years old resulting from surgical excisions treated with the FLPDL. One or two treatments were given over 8 weeks at a fluence of 6.5 to 6.75 J/cm². Optical profilometry showed a near normalization of skin surface markings. Clinical improvement was graded subjectively at 57% with one treatment and 83% with two treatments.

We expanded our original study to examine long-term results with maximal treatment in 48 patients with erythematous and hypertrophic scars.[361] Of scars appearing on the face for less than 1 year, 73% totally resolved in an average 2.3 treatments; 20% of scars on the face longer than 1 year had a total resolution in 4.4 treatments, with an average improvement of 88%. Scars on nonfacial areas for less than 1 year had a 25% incidence of total resolution over an average of 2.5 treatments, with an average improvement of 81%. Scars in nonfacial distributions older than 1 year had a 12% total resolution, with an average 62% improvement over 2.2 treatments (Table 2-18). Patients were treated at fluences ranging from 6.0 to 7.5 J/cm² delivered through a 5- or 7-mm-diameter handpiece at 4-week intervals. Eleven of 48 patients also received intralesional triamcinolone

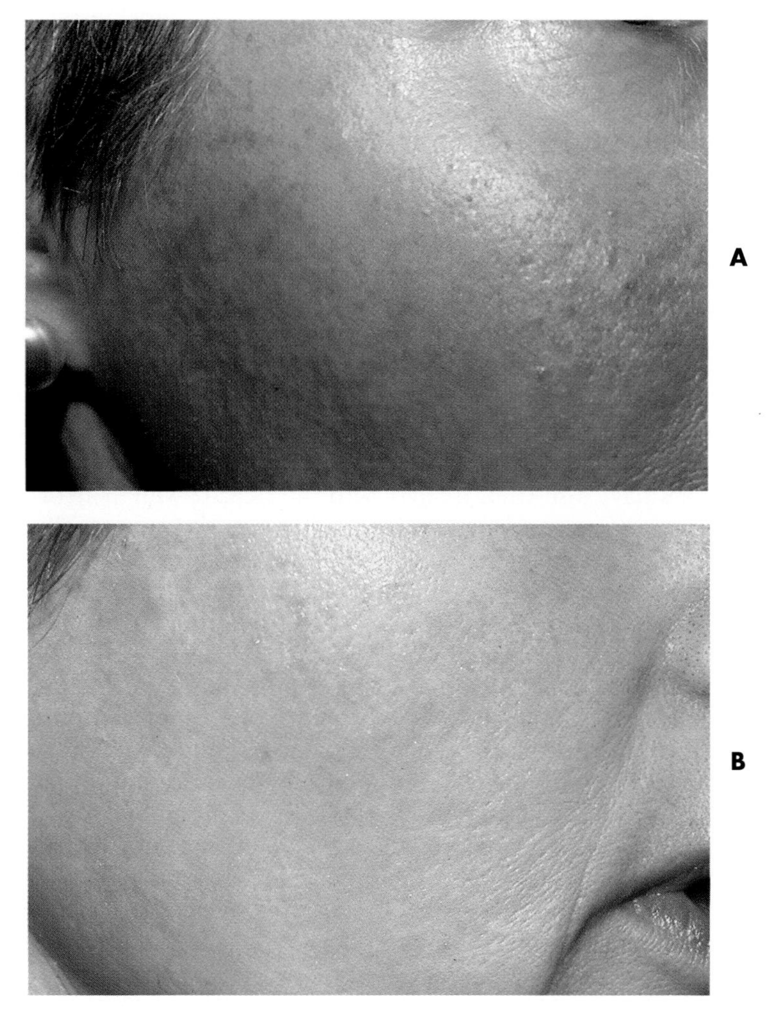

Figure 2-95 **A,** Erythematous textural changes occurred after "Obaji chemical peel" 2 years previously. **B,** Four months after single treatment with FLPDL at 6 J/cm², and 7-mm-diameter spot size.

Table 2-18
Erythematous/hypertrophic scars: Age, location, and response to FLPDL treatment in 48 patients

Scar Location	No. of Patients	No. with Adjunctive Therapy*	Average Improvement (%)	Treatments	Total Resolution (%)
Face (<1 yr)	14	5	95	2.3	75 (5/5)
Face (>1 yr)	5	0	88	4.4	20
Off Face (<1 yr)	12	2	81	2.5	25 (1/2)
Off Face (>1 yr)	17	4	62	2.2	12 (1/1)

From Goldman MP, Fitzpatrick RE: *Dermatol Surg* 21:685, 1995.
*Intralesional triamcinolone (5-10 mg/ml).

(5-10 mg/ml) at the time of laser treatment. No patient had adverse sequelae. Biopsy immediately after treatment showed thrombosis of all vessels into the deep papillary dermis.

In contrast to excellent results reported for hypertrophic scars, however, keloid scars have been less responsive to treatment. As shown previously with hypertrophic scars, 10 of 14 patients with keloids reported improvement from itching or pain after FLPDL treatment at fluences from 6.5 to 8.5 J/cm^2.[362] Three of eight white patients noted greater than 50% flattening of the keloid. Hypopigmentation developed in all six black patients, with no change in the keloid's appearance.

Alster and Williams[358] treated 16 patients with hypertrophic and keloid sternotomy scars with the FLPDL, as previously described. A mean fluence of 7.0 J/cm^2 was used with two treatments 6 to 8 weeks apart. All patients had clinical improvement. All patients (except one) who complained of pruritus of their scars before treatment noted total cessation of itching in the treated area. Significant improvement occurred in erythema, thickness, surface texture, and scar pliability.

Acne scars have also been noted to improve with FLPDL treatment.[363] Twenty-two patients were treated once or twice with the FLPDL at an average fluence of 6.5 J/cm^2. Average scar duration was 10.5 years (range 1 to 30 years). Average clinical improvement was 67.5% with one treatment and 72.5% with two treatments.

Old burn scars have also been treated with the FLPDL. Nine patients with burn scars for 1 to 34 years were treated with the FLPDL at fluences ranging from 5 to 10 J/cm^2 (5- and 7-mm diameter spot size).[364] Three patients with constricting burn scars of the hand present for 1, 6, and 30 years had greater than 75% improvement with two to four treatments. Improvement in scar texture and pliability was "dramatic and long lasting."

At this time the FLPDL at 585 nm, 0.45-msec pulse duration, and 6 to 7 J/cm^2 is the recommended laser for treating hypertrophic scars. However, other laser and pulsed–light source treatments are being evaluated to enhance efficacy. An in vitro study of implanted hypertrophic scar tissue in athymic mice found that a 585-nm wavelength inhibited implant growth by 70% at 6 J/cm^2 and 92% at 10 J/cm^2.[365] Significant inhibition of implant growth (72%) occurred when the wavelength was increased to 590 nm, and 65% inhibition occurred at 595 nm. However, minimal inhibition of growth occurred with a 600-nm wavelength. Because increased depth of penetration occurs at 595 nm versus 585 nm, the authors recommend the 590-mm wavelength.

The PhotoDerm VL at 550-nm and 570-nm cutoff filters with a double pulse of 2.4 and 4.0 msec separated by 10 to 20 msec at 30 to 40 J/cm^2 has also been found to decrease the erythema and normalize the epidermal changes of a hypertrophic scar. Although a formal study has yet to be reported in the literature, case reports show remarkable efficacy (Figure 2-96).

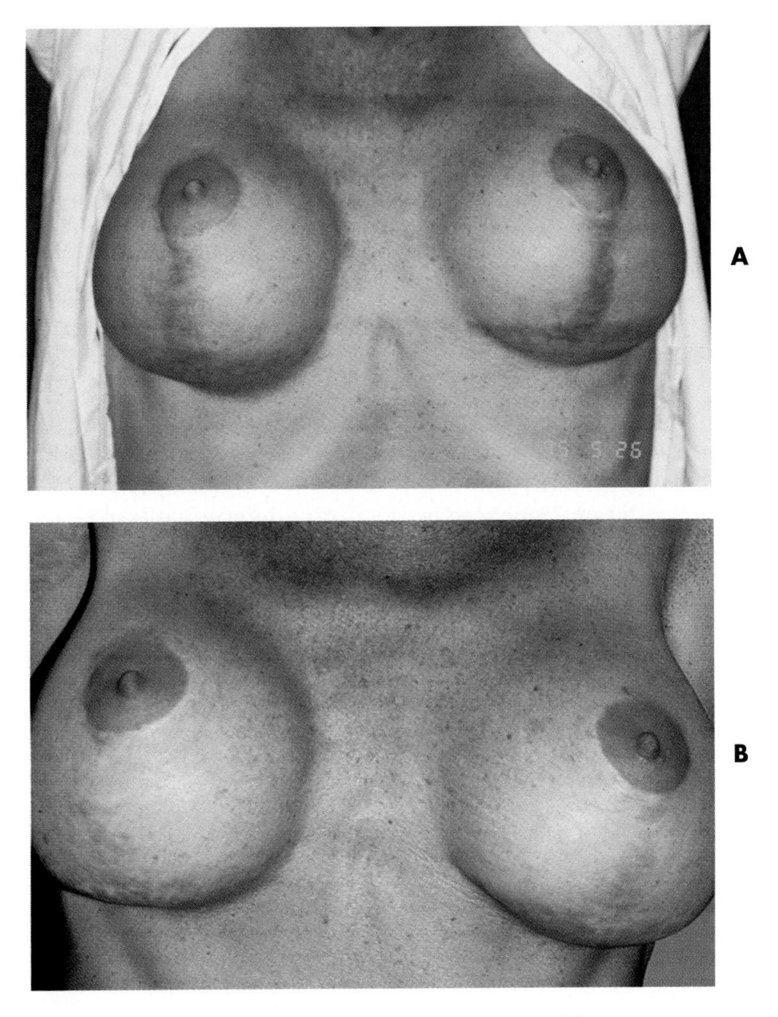

Figure 2-96 **A,** Persistent erythematous scars in 45-year-old woman 2 years after breast reduction and implantation. **B,** Two months after final treatment. Treatments 1 to 3 were with FLPDL at 6 J/cm^2, 7-mm-diameter spot. When no further improvement was noted, treatments 4 to 7 were performed using PhotoDerm VL using either 550-nm or 570-nm cutoff filter at 26 J/cm^2 as single 3-msec pulse.

Striae Distensae (Atrophicae)

Striae, or stretch marks, represent dermal scars with overlying epidermal erythematous atrophic changes.[366,367] They occur at sites of skin expansion caused by weight gain or gain in muscle mass. They may also occur in overlying areas after excessive use of topical steroids. Thus both mechanical and hormonal changes lead to their development.

Striae initially appear erythematous before becoming reddish purple in color. With time they become paler than surrounding skin. Despite their red color, histologic changes in early lesions consist mostly of thin, densely packed collagen bundles oriented in a parallel array horizontal to the epidermis within the papillary dermis. Over time the abnormal collagen penetrates into the deeper dermis. Elastin fibers are randomly arranged and appear thinner, more tangled, and curlier than normal elastic fibers.[368]

Because striae are dermal scars, the same rationale presented previously for the treatment of hypertrophic scars may explain the reported efficacy of treatment with the FLPDL. One study used the FLPDL with a 7- or 10-mm-diameter spot size and fluences of 2.0, 2.5, 3.0, and 4.0 J/cm² to treat striae.[369] Of 39 striae treated, those sections treated with a fluence of 3.0 J/cm² through a 10-mm spot appeared to return toward the appearance of normal skin. Maximal clinical improvement was not seen until 6 months after treatment. Up to 50% improvement was noted on subjective evaluation. Objective analysis was provided with optical profilometry, which noted significant improvement as well, although the authors noted difficulty in interpretation because of multiple technical factors.

Histologic examination of two specimens showed they regained normal-appearing elastin content when examined with hematoxylin-eosin and elastin stains. The increase in elastin content of treated lesions toward normal levels was reported to be remarkable.

Fifty patients with striae were treated with the 585-nm FLPDL with a 10-mm-diameter spot size at a fluence of 3 to 4 J/cm².[370] Ten patients showed no response to treatment, but the majority showed 50% to 75% improvement. Location, age of striae, and etiology did not appear to be significant determinants in response. Small-diameter striae responded better than larger striae. The mechanisms of the variabilities in response remain to be elucidated.

Leg Telangiectasia

Unsightly or symptomatic venulectases and telangiectasia on the legs occur in 29% to 41% of women and 6% to 15% of men in the United States.[371] These smaller vessels are most often directly or indirectly connected to larger reticular or varicose "feeding" veins. A family history of varicose or telangiectatic leg veins ranges from 43%[372] to 90%.[373] Approximately one third of patients first note the development of these veins during pregnancy. Between 20% and 30% of patients developed these veins before pregnancy, with 18% of women noting the onset while ingesting progestational agents. Therefore the development of "spider leg veins" is probably a partially sex-linked, autosomal dominant condition with incomplete penetrance and variable expressivity.

Even though up to 53% of patients have associated symptoms with these veins, the most common reason patients seek treatment is cosmetic.[374] Therefore any treatment that is effective should be relatively free of adverse sequelae. Unfortunately, all forms of treatment to date have some side effects.[301] The most common method for treating leg telangiectasia is sclerotherapy. Up to 30% of patients treated with sclerotherapy will develop postsclerosis pigmentation[375] or telangiectatic matting.[373] Postsclerosis hyperpigmentation is caused by the extravasation of erythrocytes through vessels damaged or destroyed by sclerotherapy.[375] This is more likely to occur if sclerosing agents of excessive strength are used but may occur even with optimum treatment.[375,376] Telangiectatic matting is also thought to be related to the use of excessively strong sclerosing agents with the development of "excessive" perivascular inflammation or "excessive" thrombus formation.[301,320] This adverse reaction usually resolves within 6 months but, if persistent, is usually recalcitrant to further sclerotherapy treatment.

Various lasers have been used in an effort to enhance clinical efficacy and minimize the adverse sequelae of sclerotherapy. Unfortunately, most have also been associated with many more adverse responses than those associated with sclerotherapy. This is related to both the nonspecificity of the laser used and the lack of treatment of the "feeding" venous system.

Varicose veins most likely lead to the development of telangiectasia either through associated venous hypertension with resulting angiogenesis or vascular dilatation[301] and/or through an associated increased distensibility of the telangiectatic vein wall. Although telangiectasia associated with varicose veins may appear at first as erythematous streaks, over time they turn blue. Often they are directly associated with underlying varicose veins so that the distinction between telangiectasia and varicose veins becomes blurred.[377-380] Multiple studies using Doppler and duplex ultrasonography have demonstrated that telangiectasia are associated with underlying reticular veins.[377,381-383] These veins were separate from any truncal varicosities that might have been present. Fifty percent of patients with blue reticular veins demonstrate reflux from incompetent perforating calf veins. In this scenario, treatment of the feeding varicosity results in treatment of the distal telangiectasia. A direct connection from telangiectasia to the deep venous system was also found in 2 of 15 radiographed patients.[384] Finally, when no apparent connection exists between deep collecting or reticular vessels, the telangiectasia may arise from a terminal arteriole or arteriovenous anastomosis.[378] Red telangiectasia have an oxygen saturation of 76%, whereas blue telangiectasia have an oxygen concentration of 69%.[383] Thus each type of telangiectasia may have a slightly different optimal absorption despite its relative size and depth.

Leg telangiectasia may be associated with underlying venous disease even when no obvious reticular or varicose veins are present. Duplex imaging and venous Doppler ultrasonography revealed that 23% of patients without clinically apparent varicose veins demonstrated incompetence of the superficial venous system.[385] In addition, 1.2% had incompetence of a perforator vein. Nineteen patients with one clinically abnormal leg and one clinically normal leg were also evaluated. Interestingly, 37% of clinically normal legs demonstrated incompetence of the superficial system. The abnormal legs in this group had a 74% incidence of incompetence of the superficial system, with 21% having saphenofemoral incompetence. This study demonstrates the need for a clinical or noninvasive diagnostic workup in patients with telangiectatic leg veins and reinforces the view that "spider leg veins" arise from underlying varicose veins via venous hypertension.

A proposed mechanism for the development of leg telangiectasia associated with underlying venous disease is that preexisting vascular anastomotic channels open in response to venous stasis.[386,387] The resulting capillary hypertension leads to opening and dilatation of normally closed vessels. Alternatively, relative anoxia as a result of reversed venous flow may lead to angiogenesis.[386]

The hormonal influence in the development of telangiectasia is well known. Perhaps the most common physiologic condition that leads to the development of telangiectasia is *pregnancy*. Almost 70% of women develop telangiectasia during pregnancy, the majority of which disappear between 3 and 6 weeks postpartum.[388] Pregnant women often develop telangiectasia on the legs within a few weeks of conception, even before the uterus has enlarged to compress venous return to the pelvis. In addition, pregnant women and those taking oral contraceptives have an increase in the distensibility of vein walls.[389] This increase in distensibility has also been noted to fluctuate with the normal menstrual cycle.[390] Thus some hormonal influence is involved in the development of varicose veins and their associated telangiectasia in women. Finally, an apparent association exists between excess estrogen states and development of telangiectatic matting after sclerotherapy of "spider leg veins." Twenty-nine percent of women who developed "new" telangiectasia were taking systemic estrogens compared with 19% of patients taking hormones who did not develop telangiectatic matting.[391]

Histology

The venules in the upper and middle dermis usually run in a horizontal orientation. The diameter of the postcapillary venule ranges from 12 to 35 μm.[392] Collecting venules range from 40 to 60 μm in the upper and middle dermis and enlarge to 100 to 400 μm in diameter in the deeper tissues.[393] One-way valves are found at the subcutis- (dermis-)adipose junction on the venous side of the circulation.[394] Valves are usually found in the area of anastomosis of small to large venules and also within larger venules not associated with branching points. The free edges of the valves are always directed from the smaller to larger vessel so that blood flows toward the deeper venous system.

Histologic examination of simple telangiectasia demonstrates dilated blood channels in a normal dermal stroma with a single endothelial cell lining, limited muscularis, and adventitia.[379,395] Most leg telangiectasia measure 26 to 225 μm in diameter. Electron microscopic examination of "sunburst" varicosities of the leg has demonstrated that these vessels are widened cutaneous veins.[379] They are found 175 to 382 μm below the stratum granulosum. The thickened vessel walls are composed of endothelial cells covered with collagen and muscle fibers. Elastic fibers are also present. Electron microscopy reveals an intercellular collagenous dysplasia, lattice collagen, and some matrix vesicles. These findings suggest that telangiectatic leg veins, as with varicose veins, have an alteration of collagen metabolism of their walls. Therefore, like varicose veins, these veins are dysplastic. Alternatively, arteriovenous anastomoses may be involved in the pathogenesis of telangiectasia and were demonstrated in 1 of 26 biopsy specimens of leg telangiectasia.[378]

Unlike leg telangiectasia, the ectatic vessels of a PWS are arranged in a loose fashion throughout the superficial and deep dermis. They are more superficial (0.46-mm depth) and much smaller than leg telangiectasia, usually measuring 10 to 40 μm in diameter. This may explain the lack of efficacy reported by many physicians who treat leg telangiectasia with the same laser parameters as PWSs.

Sclerotherapy

Treatment of varicose veins by first closing off the high-pressure reflux points with either surgical ligation or sclerotherapy then using sclerotherapy for remaining abnormal vessels forms the basis for rational therapy.[376] Because, in the vast majority of cases, "spider veins" are in direct connection to underlying varicose veins either directly or through tributaries, as with varicose veins, treatment should first be directed to "plugging" the leaking high-pressure outflow at its point of origin. An appropriate analogy is to think of spider veins as the fingers and the feeding varicose vein as the arm. Treatment should first be directed to the feeding "arm" and only if necessary directed to the spider "fingers." This systematic approach has a number of advantages. Spider veins often disappear without their direct treatment. The larger feeding vein is both easier to cannulate and less likely to rupture with injection of the sclerosant, thus minimizing the extent of extravasated RBCs and sclerosant. Theoretically, this method should minimize treatment complications.

A complete discussion of sclerotherapy treatment is beyond the scope of this chapter. The reader is referred to a recent textbook on the subject.[396] However, the essential point is that all leg telangiectasia that can be cannulated with a 30-gauge needle should be treated before considering laser surgery. Treatment should proceed from the largest to the smallest vessel. Only those vessels that do not respond to sclerotherapy or those vessels that are too small to be injected should be considered for laser treatment. By adhering to these principles, physicians can provide cost-effective, efficient, and logical care to their patients.

Laser treatment

Carbon dioxide laser. The CO_2 laser has been used for the obliteration of venules and telangiectatic vessels.[306,397-399] The rationale for using the CO_2 laser in the treatment of telangiectasia is to produce precise vaporization without significant damage to tissue structures adjacent to the penetrating laser beam. However, the skin surface, as well as the dermis overlying the blood vessel, is destroyed. CO_2 laser penetration of vessels has also been reported to cause occasional brisk bleeding from the vessel, which required pressure bandages for 48 hours.[398] Pain during treatment is moderate to severe but of short duration. All reported studies demonstrate unsatisfactory cosmetic results. Treated areas show multiple hypopigmented punctate scars with either minimal resolution of the treated vessel or neovascularization adjacent to the treatment site (Figure 2-97). Because of this nonselective action, the CO_2 laser has no advantage over the electrodesiccation needle and has not been successfully used in treating leg telangiectasia.

Nd:YAG laser. The Nd:YAG laser, 1064 nm, has also been used to treat leg telangiectasia.[397] The average depth of penetration in human skin is 0.75 mm, and reduction to 10% of the incident power occurs at a depth of 3.7 mm.[32] Thus this laser should be well suited to treat blood vessels within the middermis. However, the wavelength is absorbed by water and to a certain degree by melanin and Hb. Therefore, as with the CO_2 laser, tissue damage is relatively nonspecific. Apfelberg et al[397] treated leg telangiectasia with the Nd:YAG laser equipped with a 1.5-mm sapphire contact probe. Treatment complications included linear hypopigmentation and depressions overlying the skin of the treated vessel. Re-treatment was needed at 6-week intervals. In addition, the cost is high because the disposable sapphire tips are expensive. In summary, as with the CO_2 laser, this modality produces unsatisfactory cosmetic results and has yet to be found useful in treating leg telangiectasia.

Argon laser. Argon laser treatment of telangiectasia or superficial varicosities of the lower extremities may result in purple or depressed scars. In a report of 38 patients treated by Apfelberg et al,[400] 49% had either poor or no results from treatment, and only 16% had excellent or good results. In addition, almost half the patients had hemosiderin bruising. In another series, Dixon et al[24] noted significant improvement in only 49% of patients. They speculated that after initial improvement, incomplete thrombosis, recanalization, or new vein formation produced reappearance of the vessels after 6 to 12 months.

In an effort to enhance therapeutic success with leg vein sclerotherapy, the argon laser has been used to interrupt the telangiectasia every 2 to 3 cm before injection of a sclerosing agent.[401] In 11 of 16 patients who completed treatment, two developed punctate depigmented scars and three developed hyperpigmentation.

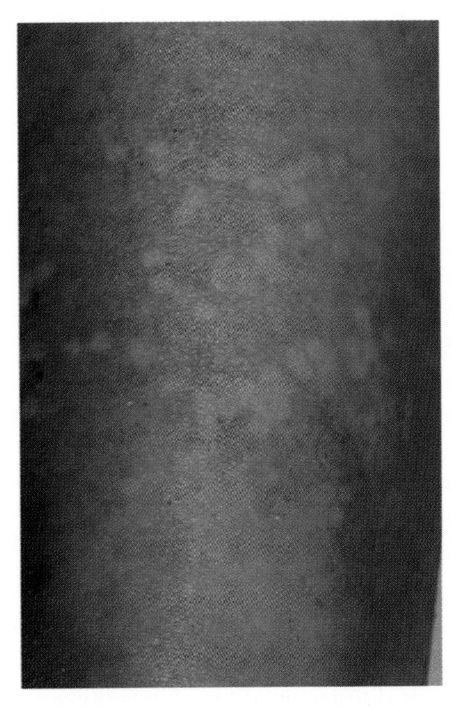

Figure 2-97 Hypopigmented scars with skin textural changes 5 years after treatment of leg telangiectasia with CO_2 laser. (From Goldman MP: *Sclerotherapy: treatment of varicose and telangiectatic leg veins,* ed 2, St Louis, 1995, Mosby.)

However, 93.7% of patients were reported to have "satisfactory" results. Cooling the skin simultaneously with argon or tunable dye (577 nm, 585 nm) laser treatment has been demonstrated to produce improvement in 67% of leg telangiectasia 1 mm in diameter.[110] This may be secondary to temperature-related vasomotor changes in blood flow.[402] Overall, argon laser therapy appears to be not only relatively ineffective in treating leg telangiectasia, but also associated with an unacceptably high risk of adverse sequelae.

Potassium titanyl potassium laser, 532 nm. Modulated KTP lasers have been reported to be effective at removing leg telangiectasia using pulses between 1 and 50 msec in duration. The most effective results have been achieved by tracing vessels with a 1-mm projected spot. Typically the laser is moved between adjacent 1-mm spots, which still allows vessels to be traced at 5 to 10 mm/sec. Immediately after laser exposure, the epidermis is blanched. Lengthening the pulse duration to match the vessel's diameter optimizes treatment (see Table 2-1).

A long-pulse 532-nm laser (Versapulse) has been reported to be somewhat effective in treating leg veins less than 1 mm in diameter that are not directly connected to a feeding reticular vein.[403] When used with a 4° C chilled tip, a fluence of 12 to 15 J/cm² is delivered in a 3-mm-diameter spot size as a train of pulses to trace the vessel until spasm or thrombosis occurs. Some overlying epidermal scabbing is noted, with hypopigmentation possible in dark-skinned patients (Figure 2-98). Individual physicians report considerable variation in results, with most finding this laser ineffective for treating leg veins (Figure 2-99). Thus, the long-pulse laser is best used for vessels recalcitrant to other laser and sclerotherapy treatment.

Flashlamp-pumped pulsed dye laser, 585 nm. As previously described, the FLPDL is highly efficacious in treating cutaneous vascular lesions. The depth of vascular damage is estimated to be 1.5 mm at 585 nm. Therefore the FLPDL can penetrate to reach the typical depth of leg telangiectasia.[97] However, telangiectasia over the lower extremities have not responded as well, with less lightening and more posttherapy hyperpigmentation.[404] This may be caused by the larger diameter of leg telangiectasia compared with dermal vessels in PWS or the failure to recognize the importance of high-pressure vascular flow from feeding reticular and varicose veins.

Polla et al[404] treated 35 superficial leg telangiectasia with the FLPDL. The exact laser parameters were not given, except that vessels were treated an average of

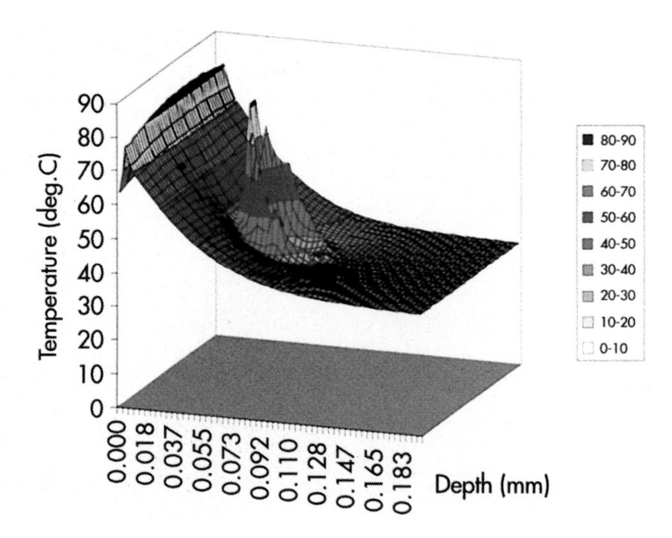

Figure 2-98 Temperature distribution achieved in treating 0.5-mm-diameter, 0.5-mm-deep vessel with 532-nm laser using 10-msec pulse duration at 20 J/cm², 5-mm-diameter spot size, and epidermal cooling to 4° C. (Courtesy ESC Medical, Inc.)

2.1 times with a maximum of four separate treatments. These vessels were described as being red-purple and raised or blue and flat. No mention was made regarding the association of reticular or varicose veins or vessel diameter. Fifteen percent of treated vessels had greater than 75% clearing, with 73% of treated areas showing little response to treatment. The only lesions that responded at all were red-pink tiny telangiectasia. Almost 50% of the treated patients developed persistent hypopigmentation or hyperpigmentation.

As illustrated by this study, it is difficult to compare the clinical and experimental results of laser treatment of leg telangiectasia with those of PWSs. The former typically do not report the diameter, location, or type of vessel treated. In addition, no mention is made of feeding reticular veins or of postlaser compression. Therefore we systematically examined the clinical effects of various powers of the FLPDL in specific leg telangiectasia. We chose red telangiectasia less than 0.2 mm in diameter and vessels arising as a function of telangiectatic matting for examination, because these vessels are the most difficult to treat with standard sclerotherapy techniques.

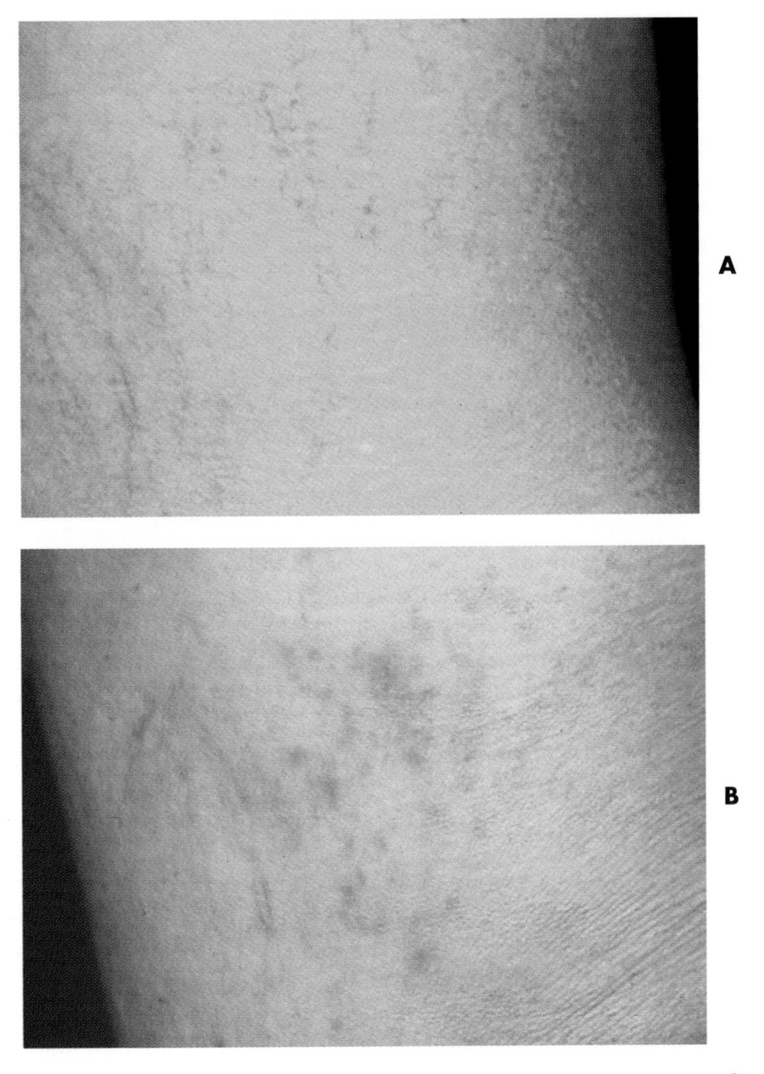

Figure 2-99 **A,** Leg telangiectasia on medial thigh before treatment. **B,** Twelve weeks after treatment. Telangiectasia treated with 595-nm 1.5-msec FLPDL shows hyperpigmentation. Medially located telangiectasia treated with KTP laser shows minimal improvement. (Courtesy Tina Alster, MD, and Tina West, MD.)

The FLPDL produces vascular injury in a histologic pattern that is different than that produced by sclerotherapy. In our studies of the rabbit ear vein, approximately 50% of vessels treated with an effective concentration of sclerosant demonstrated extravasated RBCs. With FLPDL treatment, extravasated RBCs were apparent in only 30% of vessels treated. Thus the FLPDL may produce less posttherapy pigmentation because of a decreased incidence of extravasated RBCs.

The etiology of telangiectatic matting is unknown but has been thought to be related to either angiogenesis[405] or dilatation of existing subclinical blood vessels by promoting collateral flow through arteriovenous anastomoses.[406] One or both of these mechanisms may occur. Obstruction of outflow from a vessel (the endpoint of successful sclerotherapy) is one of the most important factors contributing to angiogenesis.[407] In addition, endothelial damage leads to the release of histamine and other mast cell factors which promotes both dilatation of existing blood vessels and angiogenesis.[408,409] Thus sclerotherapy, by its very mechanism of action, provides the means for new blood vessel formation to occur. Indeed, it is remarkable that one does not see a higher incidence of postsclerosis telangiectatic matting with sclerotherapy treatment.

Telangiectatic matting has not been reported to be a side effect of argon, FLPD, or dye laser treatment of any vascular disorders, possibly because of the production of intravascular fibrin that occurs during laser treatment.[410-412] This is believed to occur through thermal alteration of fibrin complexes or proteolytic cleavage of fibrinogen. Fibrin deposition has been demonstrated to promote angiogenesis.[408] Interestingly, sclerotherapy-induced vascular injury has not been associated with the appearance of fibrin strands. Therefore either factors other than those associated with the absence of fibrin deposition or the intravascular consumption of fibrin-promoting factors must limit angiogenesis in laser treatment of cutaneous vascular disease.

Another possible mechanism for the absence in telangiectatic matting in laser-treated blood vessels may be a decrease in perivascular inflammation. Rabbit ear vein treatment with the FLPDL results in a relative decrease in perivascular inflammation compared with vessels treated with sclerotherapy alone.[412] Multiple factors associated with inflammation have been demonstrated to promote both dilatation of existing blood vessels and angiogenesis.[409]

Goldman and Fitzpatrick[413] examined these theoretic advantages and methods for treating leg telangiectasia with the FLPDL or combined FLPDL and sclerotherapy. Thirty female patients with an average age of 38 years (range 20-67) were treated for treatment of telangiectatic leg veins. Telangiectasia measured less than 0.2 mm in diameter and were red. Thirteen of 101 telangiectatic patches were noted to have an associated reticular feeding vein 2 to 3 mm in diameter, which was not treated. Seven patients with 25 patches of telangiectatic matting after previous sclerotherapy were also treated.

FLPDL 5-mm-diameter spots were overlapped slightly, with every effort made to treat the entire vessel. After treatment a chemical ice pack (Kwik Kold, American Pharmaseal Co., Valencia, Calif) was applied to the treated area until the laser-induced sensation of heat resolved (5-15 minutes). Thirty-nine telangiectatic patches, chosen randomly, were treated with laser energies between 7 and 8 J/cm^2 and compressed with a rubber "E" compression pad (Vascular Products Ltd., Bristol, England) fixed in place with Microfoam 100-mm tape (3M Medical-Surgical Division, St. Paul, Minn). A 30- to 40-mm-Hg graduated compression stocking was then continuously worn over this dressing for approximately 72 hours.[413]

As hypothesized, telangiectatic matting and persistent pigmentation did not occur with FLPDL treatment of leg telangiectasia. FLPDL-induced hyperpigmentation completely resolved within 4 months. There were no episodes of cutaneous ulceration, thrombophlebitis, or other complications. However, hypopigmentation was noted in some patients with tanned skin treated for telangiectatic matting (Figure 2-100). The laser impact sites usually remain hypopigmented for years and may be permanent. Brown hyperpigmentation typically occurs but resolves within 6 months.[413]

With FLPDL treatment, the most effective fluence appears to be between 7 and 8 J/cm². At these laser parameters, approximately 67% of telangiectatic patches completely faded within 4 months[413] (Figure 2-101).

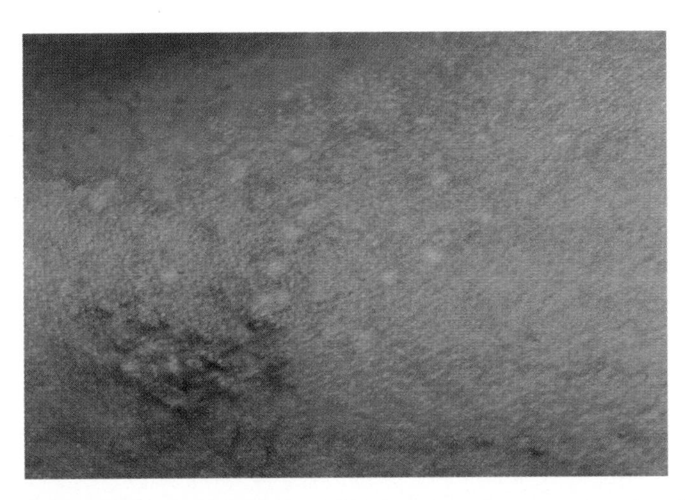

Figure 2-100 Temporary hypopigmentation that lasted for 6 months developed in this 32-year-old woman with type III tanned skin. Anterior thigh was treated with FLPDL at 7.5 J/cm². (From Goldman MP: *Sclerotherapy treatment of varicose and telangiectatic leg veins,* ed 2, St Louis, 1995, Mosby.)

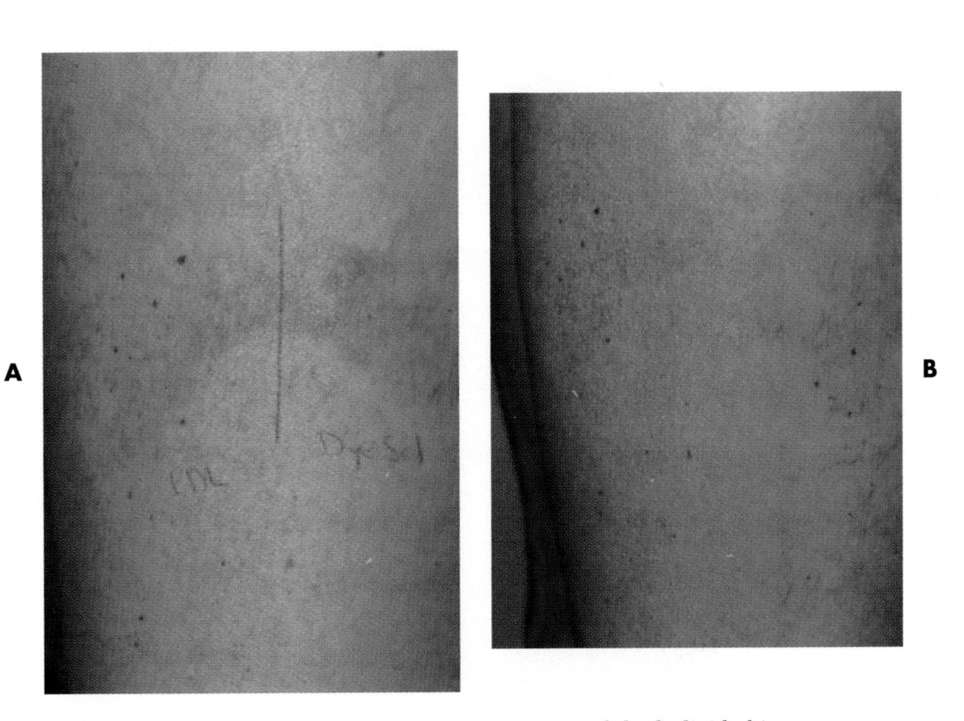

Figure 2-101 **A,** Telangiectatic flare on lateral aspect of thigh divided into two treatment sites. Anterior aspect was treated with FLPDL at 6 J/cm² and 50 5-mm pulses immediately before sclerotherapy with 2 ml of polidocanol 0.25%. Posterior aspect was treated with FLPDL at 7 J/cm² and 5-mm pulses. **B,** Three months after treatment. Note complete resolution in both treatment sites. (From Goldman MP: *Sclerotherapy: treatment of varicose and telangiectatic leg veins,* ed 2, St Louis, 1995, Mosby.)

The response to FLPDL treatment does not appear to differ between linear leg telangiectasia and telangiectatic matting vessels. In these seven patients with 25 sites treated, 72% of the treated sites completely faded at laser fluences of 6.5 to 7.5 J/cm^2 (Figure 2-102). Telangiectatic matting vessels did not respond to treatment in only one patient with four areas of matting. Less than 100% resolution occurred in 16% of treated areas.

The reason for the greater efficacy of treatment in our report[413] compared with others[404,414] may result from the rigid criteria by which patients were selected for treatment. Our patients who responded well to treatment had red telangiectasia less than 0.2 mm in diameter without associated feeding reticular veins.

Many physicians have found that vessel location may affect treatment outcome, with vessels on the medial thigh being the most difficult to eradicate completely. However, with the FLPDL, vessel location appears to be unrelated to treatment outcome if telangiectatic patches with untreated feeding reticular veins are excluded. In addition, there appeared to be no obvious difference in treatment efficacy between telangiectatic patches treated with or without compression.

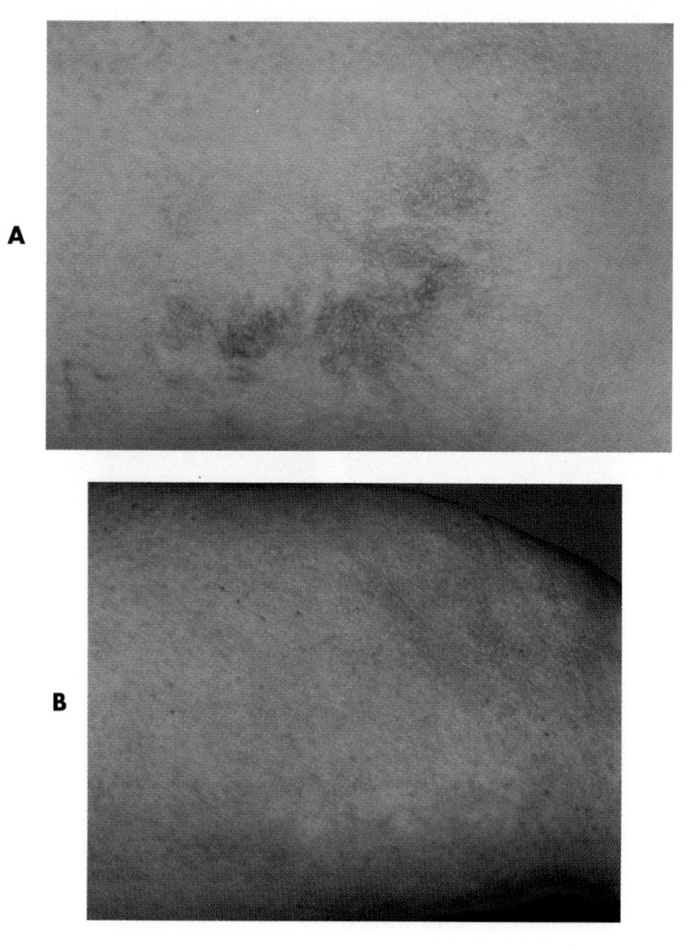

Figure 2-102 **A,** Telangiectatic matting 9 months after sclerotherapy treatment of leg telangiectasia on medial aspect of thigh immediately before treatment. **B,** One year after treatment of entire area with FLPDL at 7.25 J/cm^2 and 46 5-mm pulses. Note complete resolution of telangiectatic mat without pigmentary or textural change. (From Goldman MP: *Sclerotherapy: treatment of varicose and telangiectatic leg veins,* ed 2, St Louis, 1995, Mosby.)

Evaluation of combined FLPDL and sclerotherapy treatment

Twenty-seven patients had either bilaterally symmetric telangiectatic patches or a large "sunburst" telangiectatic flare that could be divided into two separate treatment sites. Patients were treated at one site with the FLPDL alone or with laser fluences 1 to 2 J/cm^2 less than those used with the FLPDL alone immediately before injection of the telangiectasia with polidocanol (POL), 0.25%, 0.5%, or 0.75%, with a volume of 0.1 to 0.25 ml per injection site.[412]

Forty-four percent of combination-treated areas completely resolved. Little difference in efficacy and adverse sequelae was seen with POL concentrations of 0.25% to 0.75%. There did appear to be an increased efficacy of treatment with laser energies of 7.5 to 7.75 J/cm^2. As with the FLPDL alone, treatment site did not appear to affect outcome significantly except for an increased incidence of complications in the ankle and knee areas.

The most significant difference between the FLPDL alone and combination treatment was the incidence of complications. With combination treatment, posttreatment ulceration and telangiectatic matting occurred in 11% of treated areas compared with no adverse sequelae with FLPDL alone. Six of 23 nonulcerated treatment sites developed persistent pigmentation beyond 1 year. Two of 27 sites developed telangiectatic matting, which lasted longer than 1 year. Four of 27 treatment sites developed superficial ulceration. In these ulcerated patients, laser fluences were 6.5 J/cm^2 or greater and POL concentration was 0.5% or greater.

The FLPDL is an effective modality for treating red leg telangiectasia 0.2 mm or less in diameter. FLPDL treatment is efficacious for both essential telangiectasia and vessels of telangiectatic matting. This form of treatment alone has a remarkably low incidence of adverse sequelae. The optimal clinically useful laser fluence is 7 to 8 J/cm^2. Treatment is most efficacious if all vessels larger than 0.2 mm in diameter, especially varicose and reticular feeding veins, are treated first with sclerotherapy. Results are not affected by vessel location. Posttreatment compression of this type of vessel appears unnecessary. Combination treatment appears to offer no advantage to sclerotherapy alone and to have a significant degree of complications when treatment is limited to red telangiectasia less than 0.2 mm in diameter.

Preliminary evidence suggests that combination treatment may be more efficacious than either FLPDL or sclerotherapy alone in the rabbit ear vein model.[412] In this model the FLPDL alone was only effective in establishing a histologic and clinical resolution of the vessel with an energy of 10 J/cm^2. In combination with immediate injection of the sclerosant, a significant degree of clinical and histologic resolution of the vessel occurred with all tested laser fluences (8-10 J/cm^2). Pilot studies using a combination of sclerotherapy with POL 0.25% and laser fluences of 6 and 7 J/cm^2 demonstrated no endothelial damage in vessels treated with POL alone at 8 days. Combination-treated vessels receiving 6 and 7 J/cm^2 did demonstrate endothelial vacuolization. Thus FLPDL fluences less than 5 J/cm^2 may be successfully combined with sclerotherapy in human leg veins to provide effective therapy. In addition, a relative decrease in the extent of extravasated RBCs and perivascular inflammation was noted with both FLPDL-only treatment and combination treatment.

Long-pulse FLPDL

In an effort to thermocoagulate larger-diameter blood vessels, the pulse duration of the FLPDL has been lengthened to 1.5 msec and the wavelength increased to 600 nm (Figure 2-99). One study using a 595-nm FLPDL at 1.5 msec found greater than 50% clearance of leg veins at a fluence of 15 J/cm^2 and approximately 65% clearance at 18 J/cm^2.[415] In this limited study of 18 patients, vessels ranging in diameter from 0.6 to 1 mm were treated with an elliptic spot size of 2 × 7 mm through a transparent hydrogel-based wound dressing. No adverse sequelae were noted at the 5-month follow-up visit.

Lee and Lask[416] treated 25 women with leg telangiectasia less than 1 mm in diameter with the Candela Sclerolaser. Each patient had four areas treated: two at a wavelength of 595 nm with fluences of 15 and 20 J/cm^2 and two at a 600-nm wavelength at 15 and 20 J/cm^2, respectively. A maximum of three treatments were performed at 6-week intervals. All patients showed improvement, with the 595-nm wavelength at 20 J/cm^2 providing the best results. Treatment response was variable and unpredictable, with some patients having complete resolution and some only slight improvement. Three patients had superficial scabbing, which resolved without apparent scarring. Most patients experienced purpura and hyperpigmentation, which resolved after several weeks. Reasons for the variable efficacy were not reported.

High-intensity pulsed light: PhotoDerm VL

In an effort to maximize efficacy in treating leg veins, a high-intensity pulsed light source was developed (PhotoDerm VL, ESC Medical, Inc., Newton, Mass). Because leg venules are substantially larger and have thicker walls than the ectatic vessels in PWSs and hemangiomas, thermal heat diffusion from absorbed RBCs must require longer times to damage the vein wall effectively. This has been estimated to be 1 to 10 msec or more (Table 2-1). In addition, leg veins are not composed primarily of oxygenated Hb as are PWSs and hemangiomas. Leg veins are filled with predominantly deoxygenated Hb, thus their blue color. Therefore a more selective wavelength would be approximately 545 nm. Finally, because leg veins are located deeper in the dermis than telangiectasia, a longer wavelength or protection of the epidermis and superficial dermis from thermal damage is necessary for ideal treatment.

Optical properties of blood are mainly determined by the absorption and scattering coefficients of its various HbO_2 components. Figure 2-6 shows the HbO_2 absorption and scattering coefficient depth of penetration into blood.[417] The main feature to note in the curve is the strong absorption at wavelengths below 600 nm with less absorption at longer wavelengths. However, a vessel 1 mm in diameter absorbs more than 67% of light even at wavelengths longer than 600 nm. This absorption is even more significant for blood vessels 2 mm in diameter. Therefore, using a light source above 600 nm would result in deeper penetration of thermal energy without negating absorption by HbO_2. This is because the absorption coefficient in blood is higher than that of surrounding tissue for wavelengths between 600 and 1000 nm.

Theoretically, a phototherapy device that produces a noncoherent light as a continuous spectrum longer than 550 nm should have several advantages over a single-wavelength laser system. First, both oxygenated and deoxygenated Hb will absorb at these wavelengths. Second, blood vessels located deeper in the dermis will be affected. Third, thermal absorption by the exposed blood vessels should occur with less overlying epidermal absorption because the longer wavelengths will penetrate deeper and be absorbed less by the epidermis.

Using these theoretic considerations, a pulsed light source radiating in the 515- to 1000-nm range was used at varying energy fluences (5-90 J/cm^2) and various pulse durations (2-25 msec) to treat the dorsal marginal rabbit ear vein ranging in size from 0.4 to 0.8 mm in diameter. The rabbit ear vein was then analyzed as pre-

Figure 2-103 **A,** Clinical appearance of 0.6-mm-diameter vessel on distal calf before treatment. **B,** Immediately after treatment with PhotoDerm VL with 590-nm cutoff filter, 41 J/cm^2 given as double pulse of 6.5 and 15 msec with a 10-msec delay time. **C,** Five weeks after treatment showing partial resolution. **D,** Ten weeks after treatment with complete resolution. (From Goldman MP: Laser and noncoherent pulsed light treatment of leg telangiectasia and venules. In Goldman MP, Bergan JJ, editors: *Ambulatory treatment of venous disease: an illustrative guide,* St Louis, 1995, Mosby.)

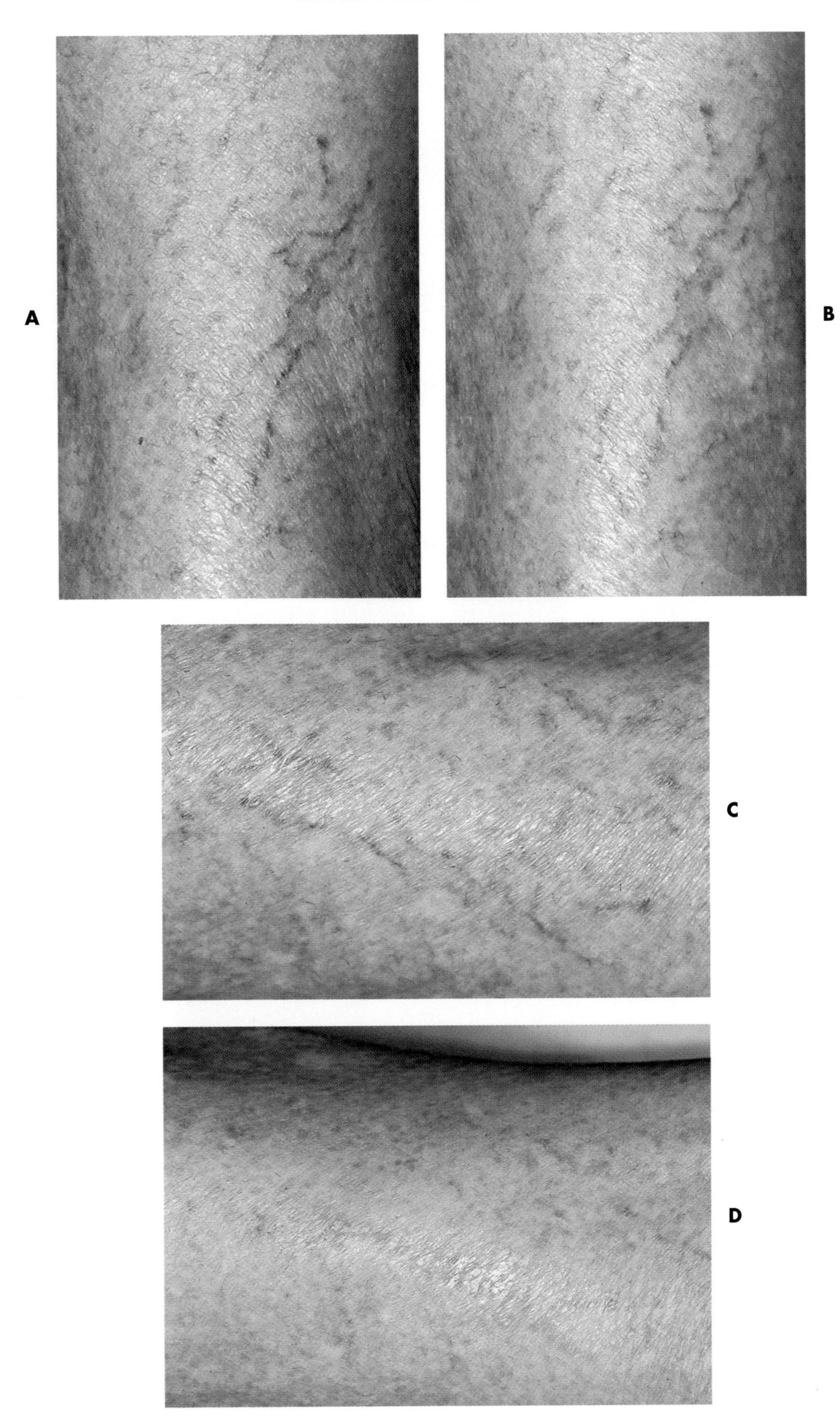
A
B
C
D

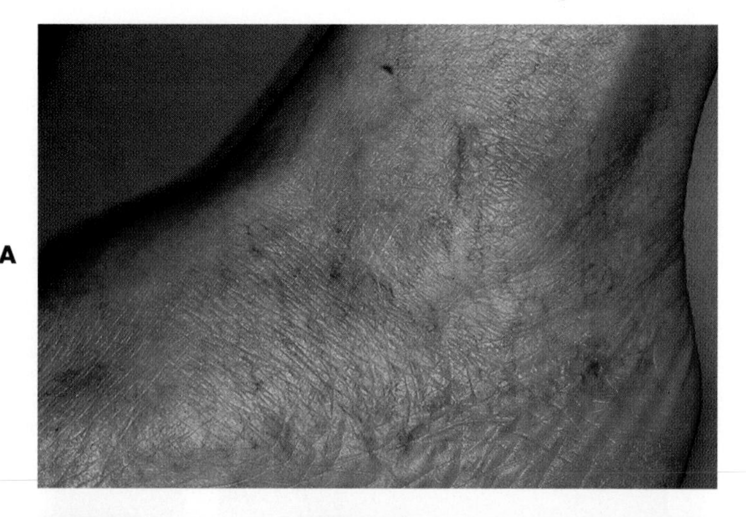

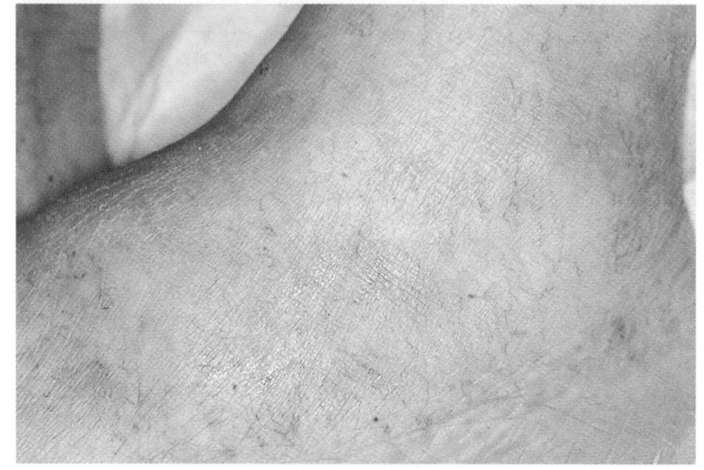

Figure 2-104 **A,** Ankle telangiectasia before treatment. **B,** Six weeks after single treatment with PhotoDerm VL at 40 J/cm² given as double pulse of 2.4 and 4.0 msec with 10-msec delay.

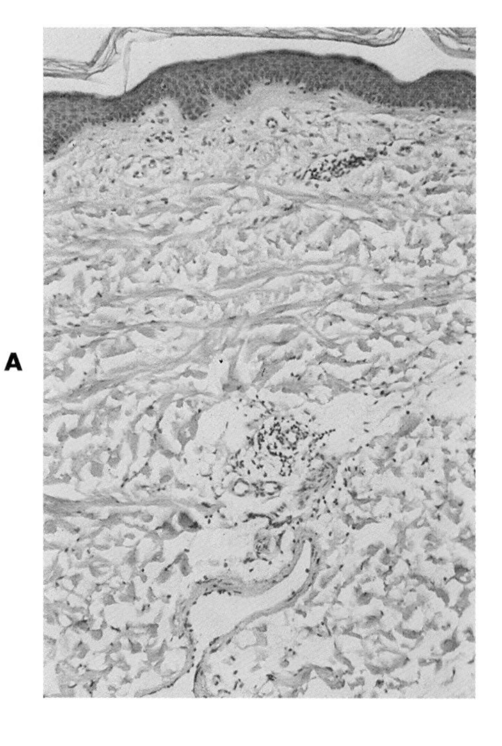

Figure 2-105 **A,** Appearance of venule 1 mm in diameter 48 hours after treatment with PhotoDerm VL at 26 J/cm², delivered in double pulse of 6 and 15 msec with 50-msec delay. Note size and depth of vessel, which appears collapsed from biopsy and processing artifacts but devoid of blood. (Hematoxylin-eosin; original magnification ×50.)

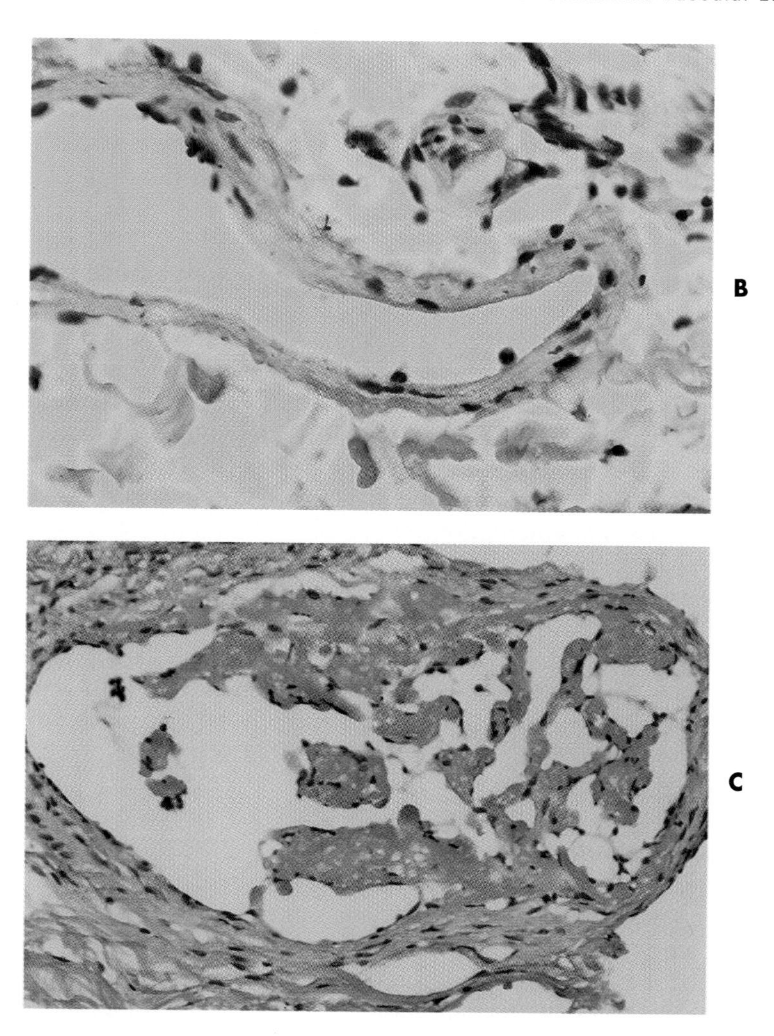

Figure 2-105, cont'd **B,** Same vessel as in **A.** Note intravascular margination of mast cells and lymphocytes with partial destruction of endothelium and vessel wall. (Original magnification ×200.) **C,** Different, 2-mm-diameter vessel 3 weeks after treatment with PhotoDerm VL. Note reorganizing thrombosis. (Original magnification ×50.) (**A** and **B,** from Goldman MP: *Sclerotherapy: treatment of varicose and telangiectatic leg veins,* ed 2, St Louis, 1995, Mosby; **C,** from Goldman MP: Laser and noncoherent pulsed light treatment of leg telangiectasia and venules. In Goldman MP, Bergan JJ, editors: *Ambulatory treatment of venous disease: an illustrative guide,* St Louis, 1995, Mosby.)

viously described.[412] Variable degrees of intravascular coagulation occurred with all tested parameters. A pulse duration of 5 msec at 15 J/cm^2 produced the most specific vascular damage, with evidence of partial vessel fibrosis at 28 days. All longer pulse durations produced nonspecific dermal coagulation. Therefore this experimental treatment modality demonstrated potential for treating human venectasia 0.4 to 2.0 mm in diameter.

Clinical trials using various parameters with the PhotoDerm VL, including multiple pulses of variable duration, demonstrated efficacy ranging from more than 90% total clearance in vessels less than 0.2 mm in diameter, 80% in vessels 0.2 to 05 mm, and 80% in vessels 0.5 to 1 mm in diameter.[418,419] The incidence of adverse sequelae was minimal, with hypopigmentation occurring in 1% to 3% of patients and resolving in 4 to 6 months. Tanned or darkly pigmented patients with Fitzpatrick photoskin type III were likely to develop hypopigmentation and hyperpigmentation in addition to blistering and superficial erosions. These all cleared over a few months. The treatment parameters found to be most successful ranged from a single pulse of 22 J/cm^2 delivered in 3 msec for vessels less than 0.2 mm or a double pulse of 40 J/cm^2 given in 2.4 and 4.0 msec with a 10-msec delay. Vessels 0.2 to 0.5 mm in diameter were treated with the same double-pulse parameters or with a 2.4-msec pulse at 35 J/cm^2 with a 20-msec delay time. Vessels larger than 0.5 mm were treated with a triple pulse of 3.5, 3.1, and 2.6 msec with pulse delays of 20 msec at a fluence of 50 J/cm^2 or with a triple pulse of 3, 4, and 6 msec with a pulse delay of 30 msec at a fluence of 55 to 60 J/cm^2. The choice of a cutoff filter was based on skin color, with a 550-nm filter for light-skinned patients and a 570-nm or 590-nm filter for darker-skinned patients (Figures 2-103 to 2-105).

Weiss and Weiss[420] have reported increased efficacy by increasing the pulse durations to a maximum of 10 msec in two consecutive pulses separated by a 20-msec delay with a 570-nm cutoff filter and fluences of 70 J/cm^2. They have achieved response rates of 74% in two treatments with an 8% incidence of temporary hypopigmentation or hyperigmentation.

Mercury vapor system

Although no studies have been published as yet, a mercury vapor flashlamp system is also being promoted for treating leg telangiectasia. This system, OptoDerm (OptoMed, Inc., Austin, Texas), uses a mercury vapor lamp with wavelength peaks at 436, 546, and 577 nm. The pulse duration is 5 to 50 msec with pulse intervals of 2 secs. An energy fluence up to 50 J/cm^2 delivered as a 5-mm, 5 × 20-mm, or 8 × 13-mm spot size can be used.

Treatment considerations

Because sclerotherapy treatment is relatively cost-effective compared with laser or PhotoDerm VL treatment, when is it appropriate to use this advanced therapy? Obviously, patients who are needle phobic will tolerate the use of this technology even though the pain from both forms of treatment are comparable. In addition, patients who are prone to telangiectatic matting are also appropriate candidates. Vessels below the ankle are particularly appropriate to treat with light because sclerotherapy has a relatively high incidence of ulceration in this area resulting from the higher distribution of arteriovenous anastomoses. Finally, patients who have vessels that are resistant to sclerotherapy are excellent candidates. Efficacy of 75% clearance with two or three treatments occurred in sclerotherapy resistant vessels as well.[421] In this study, a novel treatment regimen using a triple pulse of 50 J/cm^2 in 2-, 3-, and 4-msec pulses with 50-msec pulse delays and a 590-nm cutoff filter was followed a minute later with a single 5-msec pulse of 35 J/cm^2 with a 550-nm cutoff filter. This regimen was hypothesized to treat both deep and superficial components of the vascular network.

In a similar "vein," Weiss and Weiss[422] have reported enhanced efficacy by combining sclerotherapy using hypertonic saline and dextrose with the PhotoDerm VL. This compares favorably with the combined sclerotherapy and FLPDL treatment described previously.

We believe that optimal efficacy in treating common leg telangiectasia will use a combination of sclerotherapy followed by PhotoDerm VL or other laser surgery with a rationale similar to that described earlier for FLPDL and sclerotherapy. This belief is shared by others who have performed comparative studies with other laser systems.[423] Sclerotherapy will treat the feeding venous system, with the PhotoDerm VL or other laser effectively sealing superficial vessels to prevent extravasation with resulting pigmentation, recanalization, and telangiectatic matting. If other nonspecific vascular lasers are used without first treating feeding reticular veins, posttreatment pigmentation can occur and last 6 to 12 months (Figure 2-106).

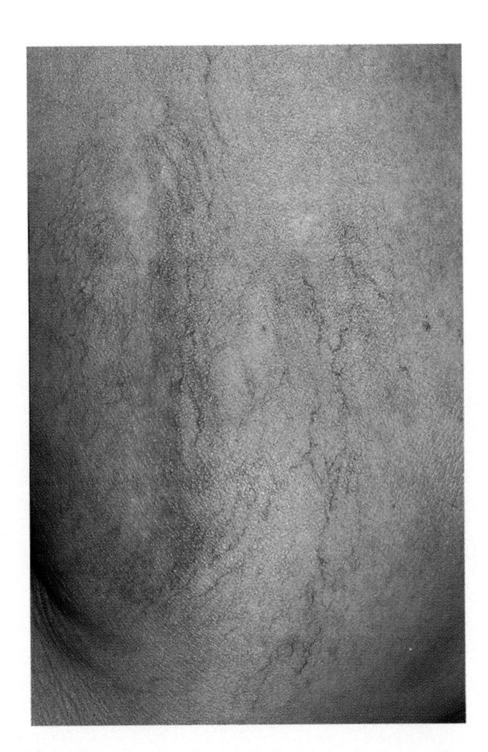

Figure 2-106 Hyperpigmentation and ineffective treatment from 532-nm KTP laser on distal lateral thigh telangiectasia.

VENOUS LAKE

Venous lakes are dilated "lakelike" venules in the upper dermis typically seen on the lips or ears of elderly patients. These lesions are dark-blue to purple, soft, raised nodules, usually 2 to 10 mm in diameter.[424] Patients generally request treatment because of concern over possible medical consequences and recurrent bleeding with trauma or for cosmetic improvement.

Treatment of venous lakes of the lips and ears has been effective with the argon laser, requiring from one to four treatment sessions.[399,425] Use of laser spot size less than 1 mm in diameter may promote excessive bleeding.[426] Lesions less than 5 mm in diameter almost always heal without scarring, whereas those larger than 5 mm healed with scarring in 21% of patients treated in one study.[427] Treatment of venous lakes with electrocautery has been unsatisfactory.[428] The FLPDL has been reported to be successful in treating venous lake lesions [297,338] (Figure 2-107). When using the FLPDL, selective photothermolysis is not the goal. Multiple pulses over the same area with or without diascopy are usually required for efficacy. This has resulted in epidermal and perivascular thermal damage as previously described. A tunable dye laser at 577 nm used with diascopy in a continuous wave at 1 W also gives excellent cosmetic results.[429]

The PhotoDerm VL has also been found to be effective in resolving venous lakes in one or two treatments. Treatment parameters are similar to those used for treating hemangiomas (Figure 2-108).

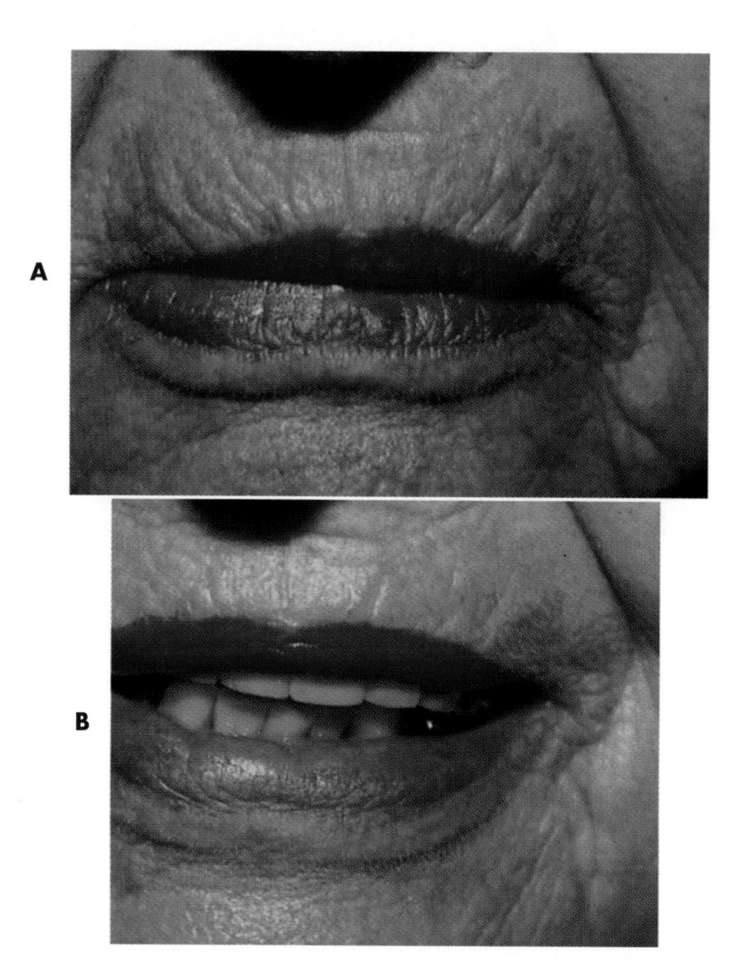

Figure 2-107 **A,** Progressively enlarging venous lake on lower lip of 78-year-old woman for 2 years. **B,** Three months after single treatment with FLPDL at 7.5 J/cm² with total of four 5-mm impacts.

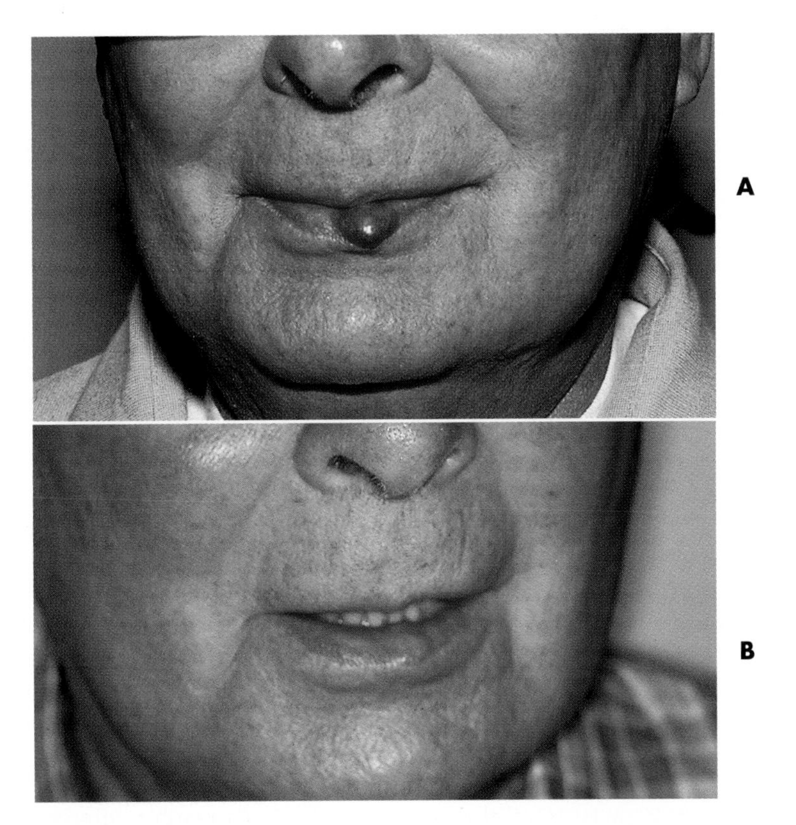

Figure 2-108 **A,** Venous lake present for more than 20 years on lower lip. **B,** Four weeks after second treatment with PhotoDerm VL at 590-nm cutoff filter, 38 J/cm^2 given as double pulse of 3 and 2 msec with 10-msec delay.

VERRUCA VULGARIS

Verrucae represent benign tumors of epidermal cells induced by the human papillomavirus (HPV). They occur in about 10% of adults and children.[430] Verrucae develop from epidermal hyperproliferation in response to viral genome incorporation into epidermal cellular DNA. To maintain a proliferative growth, neovascularization is stimulated. This is reflected histologically in prominent, dilated blood vessels in dermal papillae.[431] Theoretically, vaporization and coagulation of the new capillaries should halt viral replication and promote verrucae resolution. To produce vascular coagulation, the CVL has been reported to treat genital warts effectively.[432]

Nemeth and Reyes[432] postulated that using epidermal melanin as the "surrogate" target produces epidermal-dermal separation with removal of the wart. In a population of resistant warts, only 12 of 137 patients failed to respond to treatment with a CVL. However, one third of patients developed recurrent lesions at the 6-month follow-up.

In an effort to coagulate deeper vessels, using a laser with a longer wavelength should be effective. Therefore we have used the FLPDL to treat common verrucae. Lesions are treated at a fluence of 7.0 to 7.5 J/cm^2 with single pulses to flat warts and double pulses to hypertrophic verrucae. Paring down the warts is recommended but not to the point of bleeding, which would cause the laser light to be absorbed by surface blood. Lesions appear gray to purpuric, immediately becoming black after 24 hours. Patients are retreated every 1 to 2 weeks until resolution. We combined a limited series of patients with those of Webster et al[433] at Jefferson Medical College and found that flat warts were most responsive to treatment, with 71% resolving completely in an average of 2.4 treatments. Palmar and plantar warts had a 65% total resolution response in 2.3 treatments, and periungual warts only cleared completely in 33% of patients despite an average of 3.3 treatments.

Some warts cleared after one treatment, and some required several treatments. There was no significant difference in the number of treatments or fluence used. Very few warts failed to show some response to treatment, with smaller warts responding more quickly than larger warts. None of our patients developed postprocedural debility.

Tan et al[434] treated 39 patients with verrucae recalcitrant to multiple treatment modalities with the FLPDL after paring the warts at fluences ranging from 6.25 to 7.5 J/cm^2. As with our patients, excellent resolution occurred, warts totally clearing in 72% of patients after an average of 1.68 treatments. The more rapid response was most likely related to enhanced efficacy by allowing deeper vascular coagulation through paring the surface of the verrucae. Only one of the patients had a recurrence in the 5- to 6-month follow-up period. The authors examined 15 patients histologically and found marked agglutination of RBCs accompanied by vessel wall necrosis. Necrotic keratinocytes surrounded these vessels.

Kauvar et al[435] have reported the highest efficacy with FLPDL treatment: 93% overall efficacy in treating 142 patients with 703 verrucae that had been recalcitrant to previous treatment with various modalities, including liquid nitrogen and CO_2 laser vaporization. Warts were pared and hemostasis obtained with aluminum chloride 3 weeks before treatment. When warts cleared, they did so in an average of 2.5 treatments (range 2-5). In addition to an enhanced therapeutic response from therapy, 60% of patients reported adverse effects that were minimal enough to prevent a change in their daily activities, and 70% thought FLPDL treatment was less painful than liquid nitrogen cryosurgery. Interestingly, the study found no difference in efficacy among 7, 8, 9, or 10 J/cm^2 fluences, as well as no apparent difference between 2 to 5 pulses or 6 to 10 pulses. The authors concluded that each wart should receive 2 to 3 pulses at a fluence of 6 to 7 J/cm^2 at three-week intervals.

An additional study of 156 warts in 32 individuals treated with the FLPDL at 8 J/cm^2 showed resolution of 68% of recalcitrant warts and 47% of never-treated warts with an average of 1.78 treatments.[436] Recalcitrant warts had a higher clearance rate because they were usually treated up to three times, whereas never-treated were usually only treated once or twice. These patients generally preferred FLPDL treatment to cryosurgery, with only 2 of 32 patients having residual pain lasting 1.5 days to 1.5 weeks.

Increasing the fluence of the FLPDL to 8.1 to 8.4 J/cm^2 has increased clearance. Of 97 verrucae treated at this higher fluence, 70% had 100% clearance.[437]

Unfortunately, some studies do not report the same degree of significant efficacy with FLPDL therapy.[438] A study of 27 patients with 79 recalcitrant palmoplantar, digital, periungual, and body lesion warts found that 36% of the patients had complete resolution of their warts and 59% partially responded. Of the total number of warts treated, only 21% completely resolved.[439] Of those warts that cleared, 40% recurred within 4 months with a mean follow-up of 7 months. Exact treatment parameters and techniques were not noted in this abstract, but this study from a major laser center casts doubt on the absolute efficacy of FLPDL treatment.

Reasons for the difference in therapeutic response is unknown. Because of a wart's tendency toward spontaneous resolution, however, a blinded controlled study of FLPDL versus sham laser is necessary. Nevertheless, the efficacy of this treatment, in addition to its ease and lack of scarring, is encouraging. In addition to the proposed mechanism of vascular coagulation for wart destruction, direct thermal effects from treatment may be significant.

Nonlaser-induced hyperthermia has been demonstrated to result in regression of warts in a high percentage of patients.[440] The mechanism of action for heat may be related to direct epidermal protein coagulation or coagulation of nutritive blood vessels or to the subsequent inflammatory response to thermal injury. Other lasers have been used to produce local hyperthermia, and the term *laserthermia* has been used specifically with Nd:YAG laser therapy.[441,442] As with FLPDL treatment, Nd:YAG laserthermia has advantages over CO_2 laser treatment because the skin remains intact and bleeding usually does not occur. Thirty-one patients with recalcitrant warts (previous unsuccessful cryosurgery, keratolytic treatment, antimitotic therapy, and excision alone or in combination) were treated with the Nd:YAG at 10 W with 8-mm-diameter spot size and irradiation time of 20 sec. These parameters resulted in heating of wart tissue to 40° C for 30 sec. Patients were treated up to three times at 3-week intervals. At 9-month follow-up, 77% of patients cleared completely without scarring or recurrence.[443] Local anesthesia was not necessary because patients felt only a slight burning sensation during and after treatment.

Another system that incorporates both vascular specificity and thermal effects is the PhotoDerm VL. As previously described, this system produces deep vascular coagulation and thermal effects. We have achieved limited success with this modality, but a formal study has not yet been completed.

KAPOSI SARCOMA

Kaposi sarcoma (KS) is a vascular neoplasm appearing as pink to deep-purple macules, nodules, or plaques most often on the lower extremities. Four distinct types have been described. Type I affects elderly men of Jewish or Mediterranean ancestry.[444,445] Type II affects young homosexual men who have acquired immunodeficiency syndrome (AIDS).[446,447] A third variant affects black African natives.[448,449] The fourth type affects immunosuppressed individuals.[450]

The clinical course varies from slowly growing neoplasms confined to the skin in type I patients to extremely aggressive neoplasms that spread to internal organs in type II. The most effective therapies include radiotherapy,[451] intralesional chemotherapy (especially with vincristine and vinblastine),[452,453] interferon,[454] surgical excision,[455] and various forms of laser vaporization.

Nonspecific laser vaporization of KS has been shown to be useful, especially for exophytic or nodular lesions.[456] We have found the ultrapulse CO_2 laser to be especially effective for these lesions. The argon laser has also been reported to be an effective form of palliative therapy, with improvement in both cosmetic and functional status of the patient.[457] In addition, the Nd:YAG laser has been demonstrated to produce excellent results in type I KS lesions.[458]

The FLPDL has also been reported to decrease the size and lighten the color of KS lesions.[459,460] However, because of the limited penetration of photocoagulative effects, total resolution occurs in only 44% of lesions, with recurrent lesions appearing in all patients histologically and clinically within 12 weeks. Therefore the benefits of FLPDL treatment in KS are cosmetic improvements without adverse sequelae, with limited risk of human immunodeficiency virus (HIV) exposure.

SCLERODERMA

Scleroderma is an immunologic disease of enhanced dermal fibrosis that is associated with cutaneous telangiectasia, particularly with the CREST variant (*c*alcinosis, *R*aynaud disease, *e*sophageal dysmotility, *s*clerodactyly, *t*elangiectasia). Patients often have numerous and cosmetically disfiguring matlike telangiectasia on the face, neck, and upper trunk. The FLPDL has been successful in resolving the telangiectatic component.[461,462] Resolution has occurred with fluences of 5 to 7 J/cm^2 within one to four treatment sessions. No clinical evidence of scarring or adverse sequelae has been noted, and the disease has not progressed. Telangiectasia have not recurred during follow-up periods of up to 2 years.

We have seen similar efficacy in our practice without any adverse sequelae. Interestingly, although the FLPDL has been shown to improve hypertrophic scars, no change in dermal and cutaneous fibrosis has been seen in sclerodermoid lesions despite elimination of the hypervascularity.

LUPUS ERYTHEMATOSUS

Telangiectasia and erythema are usual components of lupus erythematosus (LE). As in treatment of other connective diseases, the FLPDL has been found to improve or resolve the telangiectatic component of LE.[463-465] Three to six treatments were required to clear more than 75% of lesions in four patients with a fluence of 7.75 J/cm^2.[463] The FLPDL has been shown to have superior results to the argon laser in LE. Treatment of LE with the argon laser, although effective, caused some scarring and hyperpigmentation.[465,466]

LUPUS PERNIO

Lupus pernio (LP) is a cutaneous manifestation of sarcoidosis that occurs most often on the central face and ears. Lesions appear as violaceous papules or nodules that thicken and coalesce into plaques. Longstanding lesions may be complicated by granulomatous inflammatory destruction of nasal bone and cartilage.

Histologic examination shows dermal noncaseating granulomatous inflammation without a predominant vascular proliferation. However, lesions have a blanchable erythematous component implying a dilated vasculature.

Standard treatments include long-term systemic corticosteroids, methotrexate or dapsone, all of which produce a variable response with associated adverse sequelae.[467] Dermabrasion and skin grafting, although reportedly successful, carry the risk of scarring and pigmentary changes.[468] The FLPDL has been reported to produce a temporary resolution of the erythematous and papular components, lasting approximately 6 months in one patient.[469] The lesion required fluences of up to 8 J/cm^2 for clinical efficacy, and the long-term outcome was not reported. Although we have no experience in treating LP with any laser, efficacy likely occurs in a manner similar to treatment of acne rosacea.

PSORIASIS VULGARIS

Psoriasis vulgaris is a hyperproliferative disease of the epidermis that occurs in the setting of immunologic alterations. To support the hyperproliferative response, an increased dermal vasculature is represented by elongated and twisted capillary loops and an increased microvascular mass in lesional skin. Vascular changes occur as early disease events, suggesting that psoriasis is an angiogenesis-dependent disease.[470-472] Therefore destruction of the increased dermal vasculature may eliminate the necessary substrate for epidermal growth, resolving established lesions in addition to slowing disease progression. In addition, specialized endothelia in psoriatic dermis are capable of mediating specific lymphocyte-endothelial interactions and possibly regulating the traffic of lymphocyte subsets in psoriatic lesions.[473,474] This rationale led to the use of the FLPDL for psoriasis with significant success.[475-477]

A fluence of 7.5 J/cm^2 increased to 8.5 J/cm^2 and delivered through a 5- or 7-mm-diameter spot (if lesions were unresponsive) showed 50% clearance and 100% improvement in patients who completed one to four treatment sessions.[476] Clinical clearing and improvement persisted at least 13 months in some subjects. Clinical improvement correlated with histologic resolution of dermal hypervascularity.

Ros et al[477] found significant clinical benefit in using the FLPDL at similar treatment parameters, but they increased laser penetration by applying a layer of mineral water to the treated area before laser irradiation. In their 10 patients, several treatments tended to have a better effect than a single treatment. The only adverse effect reported was the development of black crusts after treatment, with one patient developing atrophic scarring with healing. Thus the FLPDL may be a reasonable therapeutic modality to treat patients with limited localized disease.

POROKERATOSIS

Porokeratosis is a disorder of epidermal keratinization with several clinical variants: classic Mibelli, palmoplantar, linear, and disseminated superficial actinic porokeratosis (DSAP). The etiology is probably a combination of immunologic causes and a maturation disorder of epidermal cells and dermal fibroblasts. Although these lesions do not demonstrate an increased vascularity, laser vascular coagulation may influence vascular permeability and lead to a decrease in inflammation.

Alster and Nanni[478] have reported the successful treatment of a patient with linear, hyperpigmented, erythematous lesions with the FLPDL. After a total of six treatments with fluences ranging from 6.5 to 6.75 J/cm^2 with a 5- to 7-mm-diameter spot size, all lesions were clinically resolved. No evidence of recurrence was noted at 11 months' follow-up.

FOCAL DERMAL HYPOPLASIA

Focal dermal hypoplasia (Goltz syndrome) is a congenital defect characterized by linear areas of skin thinning with herniation of subcutaneous adipose tissue associated with a variety of mesodermal and ectodermal tissue. An X-linked dominant inheritance, which is lethal in hemizygous males, is presumed because of the predominance of this syndrome in women (88%).[479-481] Cutaneous lesions are noted at birth as erythematous, atrophic linear lesions with telangiectasia. Over time, lesions may become elevated and roughened, associated with itching and burning. The FLPDL has successfully treated the cutaneous lesions in one patient.[482] In this case, both the symptoms and the erythematous, elevated appearance of the lesions were diminished without adverse sequelae (Figure 2-109).

A

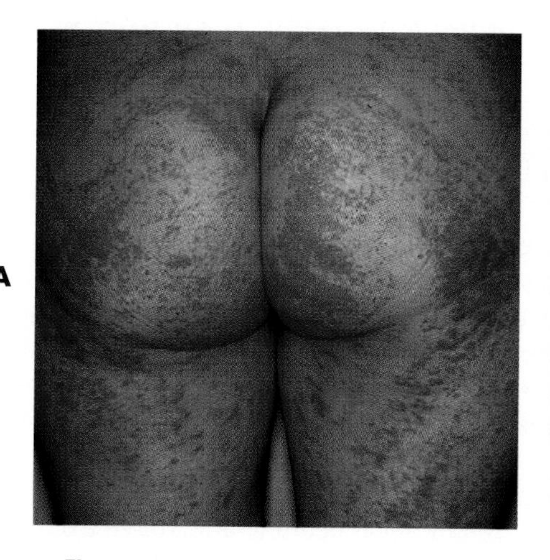

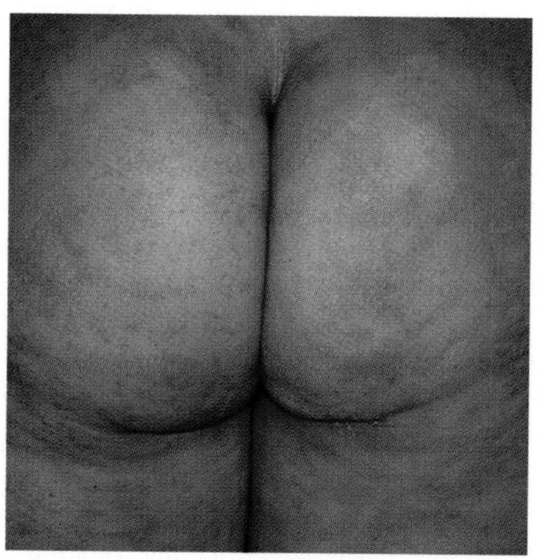

B

Figure 2-109 **A,** Widespread erythematous atrophic patches of Goltz syndrome on extremities. **B,** Extremely flattened lesions with diminished erythema 2 months after therapy with FLPDL at 6.75 J/cm^2. (From Alster TS, Wilson F: *Arch Dermatol* 131:143, 1995.)

ANGIOKERATOMA

Angiokeratomas are dark-red to black papules with ectasia and various degrees of hyperkeratosis. The five types of angiokeratomas[483] are *angiokeratoma circumscriptum* (solitary unilateral plaque), *angiokeratoma of Fordyce* (genital localization), *angiokeratoma of Mibelli* (acral localization), *solitary angiokeratomas*, and *generalized angiokeratomas*, which occur in systemic diseases (e.g., Fabry disease, fucosidosis, sialodosis). Because lesions histologically are composed of an ectasia of vessels in the papillary dermis, treatment with a vascular laser should be efficacious. Two patients with angiokeratomas of Fordyce have been successfully treated with the argon laser without scarring.[484] With the patient under local anesthesia, the argon laser was used at 0.5 to 0.9 W of power with a 1-mm spot size and 0.2-sec exposure times to coagulate the lesions.

INFLAMMATORY LINEAR VERRUCOUS EPIDERMAL NEVUS

Inflammatory linear verrucous epidermal nevus (ILVEN) is a benign epidermal hyperplasia of unknown cause characterized by erythematous papules and plaques most often located on the extremities with pruritus.[485] A 5-year-old girl treated with the FLPDL showed a significant improvement in skin lesions with elimination of pruritus after two treatments.[486] The ILVEN was treated at 6.5 to 6.75 J/cm^2 at 6-week intervals. The author speculated that the pruritus was eliminated because of an alteration of the neural response from elimination of perineural blood vessels and mast cell degranulation of perivascular mast cells.

ANGIOFIBROMA

Angiofibromas are solitary fibrous papules and appear on the face of adults as smooth, firm, dome-shaped, slightly erythematous to skin-colored papules. Histologically, they contain a variable number of stellate fibroblasts in the papillary dermis with ectatic blood vessels.[487] These lesions have been reported to resolve with both argon laser and FLPDL treatment. The ATDL was used at 577 nm with a 4.5 J/cm^2 fluence delivered over a 100-μm area with 298 pulses at 0.05 to 0.1 sec.[488] With the FLPDL a single pulse of 7.0 J/cm^2 was used twice over 3 weeks to obtain complete resolution in four patients.[489] We have had similar experience, with excellent results obtained after a single treatment using the FLPDL at 8.0 J/cm^2 with a 3-mm-diameter spot size.

ADENOMA SEBACEUM (Pringle disease)

Adenomata sebaceum represent facial angiofibromata seen in the neurocutaneous disease *tuberous sclerosis*[490] (Bourneville disease, epoloia), a benign hamartomatous disease of skin, brain, heart, and kidney. Transmitted in an autosomal-dominant pattern with variable expression, nearly two thirds of cases are caused by new mutations. Adenomata sebaceum usually develop after age 5. These lesions are small, erythematous papules located on the cheeks, chin, nasolabial folds, nose, and sometimes central forehead.

These lesions have been treated in the past with many destructive modalities, including cryosurgery, curettage, dermabrasion, chemical peeling, and shave excision in addition to nonspecific argon and CO_2 lasers.[491-496] The CVL proved to be a safe and effective treatment without adverse sequelae in nine patients.[496] In this report the CVL was used at 578 nm and 0.4 to 0.9 mW with a 150- to 267-μm-diameter spot size and a mechanically gated beam of 200 msec on, 100 msec off. Lesions were treated until the vascular component disappeared, as noted by gray coloration. Crusting developed and lasted for 2 to 3 days, with re-treatments performed as necessary in 6 weeks.

An additional study of nine patients treated at 0.4 to 0.6 mW with the 578-nm and at 0.4 to 0.9 mW with the 511-nm component of the CVL showed good to excellent results without any scarring or pigmentary changes.[496] The spot size was usually 150 to 267 μm, and the beam was mechanically gated to be on 200 msec and off 100 msec. Thin, superficial crusting occurred in all patients and resolved in 2 to 3 days. Complete fading of the erythema required 1 to 2 weeks.

The FLPDL has also been used to treat angiofibromata in patients with adenoma sebaceum.[497] Seven patients were treated with mean energies of 6.7 J/cm^2 (range 6.0-7.5 J/cm^2) in a mean number of 5.7 (range 2-10) separate treatment sessions. Treatment efficacy was much less than that reported with the CVL. With the FLPDL, only 1 of 7 patients had an excellent response, with one very good result and three good results. No scarring or pigmentary changes were seen in any patient. Therefore a less specific destructive laser is required to produce optimal results.

ANGIOLYMPHOID HYPERPLASIA WITH EOSINOPHILIA

ALHE is a vascular proliferative disorder that usually affects the head and neck region of young women.[498] Therapy is usually of limited success even with destructive modalities, including surgical excision, cryosurgery, electrodesiccation, argon laser, and CO_2 laser.[499-501] The FLPDL has been reported to treat this lesion effectively with minimal sequelae.[502]

A 30-year-old woman with multiple, discrete, erythematous to violaceous nodules on the preauricular cheek, ear, and scalp was treated with the FLPDL at fluences of 5 to 7.5 J/cm^2, given through a 7- or 10-mm-diameter spot. Seven treatments at monthly intervals resulted in marked improvement without scarring or postinflammatory pigmentation. One-year follow-up showed no recurrence.

TUFTED ANGIOMA AND ANGIOBLASTOMA

Tufted angioma and angioblastoma are benign childhood lesions involving the trunk or neck. Lesions have their onset in early childhood, with 14% occurring at birth and 49% before 1 year of age. They progressively enlarge and may grow to significant size.[503] Typically, lesions occur on the neck, trunk, and back and may be mistaken for PWS or early hemangioma. They usually appear as dull-red to red-brown or red-blue patches or plaques and are frequently tender. Lesions represent a collection of blood vessels described as round to ovoid cellular tufts of capillaries, either superficial or deep dermal or both. Treatment of these lesions has shown variable results, with one report of satisfactory clearance with the FLPDL[504] and one report demonstrating a lack of efficacy with FLPDL treatment.[505] The lack of efficacy of laser treatment likely results from the deep nature of the vascular abnormality.

XANTHELASMA PALPEBRARUM

Xanthelasmas can erupt from early childhood through late adulthood. They appear as singular or coalescing papules on the upper and lower eyelids. Various non-specific destructive treatments are used to remove these cosmetically disfiguring lesions. The CO_2 or erbium:YAG lasers can vaporize lesions entirely but produce punctate erosions that can heal with atrophic, hypopigmented scars. The argon laser has been used with good clinical results.[506] The FLPDL has also been used with good results at a fluence of 7 J/cm^2. However, five treatment sessions were necessary for complete resolution of the lesion.[507] The mechanism of action of this vascular-specific laser is presumed to be destruction of capillaries in the lesion, which have an abnormal permeability to deposit lipids.

RHYTIDS (WRINKLES)

At times, when treating vascular lesions, other effects are noted in addition to improvement of the lesion. As detailed previously, treatment of PWS previously treated with the argon laser with resultant scarring led to the observation that the FLPDL can significantly improve hypertrophic scarring. This improvement was hypothesized to be secondary to both vascular effects and direct effects on dermal collagen. This observation and hypothesis led to treating striae with the FLPDL, which also showed improvement through presumed effects on dermal collagen. In a similar manner, many laser surgeons, including us, and many patients have noticed an improvement in skin texture and even smoothing of rhytids after treating facial telangiectasia and PWS with the FLPDL and PhotoDerm VL. We treated a small number of patients with neck rhytids with the FLPDL 5 years ago and noted softening of wrinkling in some patients but not others. Our study was abandoned when we developed laser resurfacing with the CO_2 laser (see Chapter 7).

Kilmer and Chotzen[508] initiated a pilot study to examine this effect and noted that five of five patients who had the left lateral periorbital region treated with the FLPDL at 5 to 10 J/cm^2 with a 5- to 7-mm-diameter spot size had improvement in their mild degree of wrinkling. Two of five patients had greater than 50% improvement and three more than 75% improvement at 6 and 12 weeks' follow-up.

The mechanism for wrinkle improvement is speculative but may be secondary to the thermal effects on dermal collagen that cause its contraction.

REFERENCES

1. Solomon H et al: Histopathology of the laser treatment of port-wine lesions, *J Invest Dermatol* 50:141, 1968
2. Apfelberg DB, Maser MR, Lash H: Argon laser management of cutaneous vascular deformities: a preliminary report, *West J Med* 124:99, 1976.
3. Dolsky RL: Argon laser skin surgery, *Surg Clin North Am* 64:861, 1984.
4. Kaplan I, Peled I: The carbon dioxide laser in the treatment of superficial telangiectases, *Br J Plast Surg* 28:214, 1975.
5. Levine H, Bailin P: Carbon dioxide laser treatment of cutaneous hemangiomas and tattoos, *Arch Otolaryngol* 108:236, 1982.
6. Bailin PL: Treatment of port-wine stains with the CO_2 laser: early results. In Arndt KA, Noe JM, Rosen S, editors: *Cutaneous laser therapy: principles and methods,* Chickester, NY, 1983, Wiley & Sons.
7. Cosman B: Experience in the argon laser therapy of port-wine stains, *Plast Reconstr Surg* 65:119, 1980.
8. Apfelberg DB, Maser MR, Lash H: Extended clinical use of the argon laser for cutaneous lesions, *Arch Dermatol* 115:719, 1979.
9. Hobby LW: Treatment of port-wine stains and other cutaneous lesions, *Contemp Surg* 18:21, 1981.
10. Noe JM et al: Port-wine stains and the response to argon laser therapy: successful treatment and the predictive role of color, age, and biopsy, *Plast Reconstr Surg* 65:130, 1980.
11. Apfelberg DB et al: Progress report on extended clinical use of the argon laser for cutaneous lesions, *Lasers Surg Med* 1:71, 1980.

12. Apfelberg DB, Maser MR, Lash H: Argon laser treatment of cutaneous vascular abnormalities: progress report, *Ann Plast Surg* 1:14, 1981.
13. Cosman B: Role of retreatment in minimal-power argon laser therapy for port-wine stains, *Lasers Surg Med* 2:43, 1982.
14. Alster TS, Kurban AK, Grove GL et al: Alteration of argon laser–induced scars by the pulsed dye laser, *Lasers Surg Med* 13:368, 1993.
15. van Gemert MJC, Hulsbergen-Henning JP: A model approach to laser coagulation of dermal vascular lesions, *Arch Dermatol Res* 270:429, 1981.
16. A new ray of hope for port-wine stains, *Lancet* 1:480, 1981 (editorial).
17. Apfelberg DB et al: Analysis of complications of argon laser treatment for port-wine hemangiomas with reference to striped technique, *Lasers Surg Med* 2:357, 1983.
18. Gilchrest BA, Rosen S, Noe JM: Chilling port-wine stains improves the response to argon laser therapy, *Plast Reconstr Surg* 69:278, 1982.
19. Barsky SH et al: The nature and evolution of port-wine stains: a computer-assisted study, *J Invest Dermatol* 74:154, 1980.
20. Finley JL et al: Healing of port-wine stains after argon laser therapy, *Arch Dermatol* 117:486, 1981.
21. Fitzpatrick RE, Feinberg JA: Low dose argon laser therapy of port-wine stains, *ICALEO '83 Proc* 6:47, 1984.
22. Ohmori S, Huang CK, Takada H: Experiences upon the utilization of argon laser for treatment of port-wine stains, *Transactions of Seventh International Congress, Plastic and Reconstructive Surgery,* Rio de Janeiro, 1979.
23. Scheibner A, Wheeland RG: Argon-pumped tunable dye laser therapy for facial port-wine stain hemangiomas in adults: a new technique using small spot size and minimal power, *J Dermatol Surg Oncol* 15:277, 1989.
24. Dixon JA, Rotering RH, Huethner SE: Patient's evaluation of argon laser therapy of port-wine stain, decorative tattoos, and essential telangiectasia, *Lasers Surg Med* 4:181, 1984.
25. Dixon J, Huether S, Rotering R: Hypertrophic scarring in argon laser treatment of port-wine stains, *Plast Reconstr Surg* 73:771, 1984.
26. Carruth JAS, van Gemert MJC, Shakespeare PG: The argon laser in the treatment of port-wine stain birthmark. In Tan OT, editor: *Management and treatment of benign cutaneous vascular lesions,* Philadelphia, 1992, Lea & Febiger.
27. Tan OT, Mortemedi M, Welch AJ et al: Spot size effects on guinea pig skin following pulsed irradiation, *J Invest Dertamol* 90:877, 1988.
28. Mortemedi M, Welch AJ, Tan OT et al: Non-linear changes in optical behavior of tissue during laser irradiation, *Laser Surg Med* 7:72, 1987.
29. Renfro L, Geronemus RG: Anatomical differences of port-wine stains in response to treatment with the pulse dye laser, *Arch Dermatol* 129:182, 1993.
30. Hulsbergen-Henning JP: Personal communication, Veldhoven, The Netherlands. Cited in Carruth JAS, van Gemert MJC, Shakespeare PG: The argon laser in the treatment of port-wine stain birthmark. In Tan OT, editor: *Management and treatment of benign cutaneous vascular lesions,* Philadelphia, 1992, Lea & Febiger.
31. Pickering JW, Walker EP, Butler PH et al: Copper vapor laser treatment of port-wine stains and other vascular malformations, *Br J Plast Surg* 43:273, 1990.
32. Rotteleur G et al: Robotized scanning laser handpiece for the treatment of port-wine stains and other angiodysplasias, *Lasers Surg Med* 8:283, 1988.
33. McDaniel DH, Mordon S: Hexascan: a new robotized scanning laser handpiece, *Cutis* 45:300, 1990.
34. Brooks SG, Ashley S, Fisher J et al: Exogenous chromophores for the argon and Nd:YAG lasers: a potential application to laser-tissue interactions, *Lasers Surg Med* 12:294, 1992.
35. Glassberg E et al: The flashlamp-pumped 577 nm pulsed tunable dye laser: clinical efficacy and in vitro studies, *J Dermatol Surg Oncol* 14:1200, 1988.
36. Greenwald J et al: Comparative histological studies of the tunable dye (at 577 nm) laser and argon laser: the specific vascular effects of the dye laser, *J Invest Dermatol* 77:305, 1981.
37. Anderson RR, Parrish JA: Microvasculature can be selectively damaged using dye lasers: a basic theory and experimental evidence in human skin, *Lasers Surg Med* 1:263, 1981.
38. Anderson RR, Parrish JA: Selective photothermolysis: precise microsurgery by selective absorption of pulsed radiation, *Science* 220:524, 1983.

39. Tan OT, Sherwood K, Gilchrest BA: Treatment of children with port-wine stains using the flashlamp-pulsed tunable dye laser, *N Engl J Med* 320:416, 1989.
40. Garden JM, Tan OT, Parrish JA: The pulsed dye laser: its use at 577 nm wavelength, *J Dermatol Surg Oncol* 13:134, 1987.
41. Garden JM, Polla LL, Tan OT: The treatment of port-wine stains by the pulsed dye laser. analysis of pulse duration and long-term therapy, *Arch Dermatol* 124:889, 1988.
42. Garden JM et al: The pulsed dye laser for the treatment of port-wine stains, *J Dermatol Surg Oncol* 12:757, 1986.
43. Rios WR: Flashlamp-excited dye laser: treatment of vascular cutaneous lesions, *Facial Plast Surg* 6:167, 1989.
44. Morelli JG, Tan OT, Garden J: Tunable dye laser (577 nm) treatment of port-wine stains, *Lasers Surg Med* 6:94, 1986.
45. Reyes BA, Geronemus R: Treatment of port-wine stains during childhood with the flashlamp-pumped pulsed dye laser, *J Am Acad Dermatol* 23:1142, 1990.
46. Fitzpatrick RE et al: Flashlamp-pumped dye laser for port-wine stains, *Lasers Surg Med,* 1993.
47. Goldman MP, Fitzpatrick RE, Ruiz-Esparza J: Treatment of port-wine stains (capillary malformation) with the flashlamp-pumped pulsed dye laser, *J Pediatr* 122:71, 1993.
48. Glassberg E et al: Capillary hemangiomas: case study of a novel laser treatment and a review of therapeutic options, *J Dermatol Surg Oncol* 15:1214, 1989.
49. Sherwood KA, Tan OT: Treatment of a capillary hemangioma with the flashlamp-pumped dye laser, *J Am Acad Dermatol* 22:136, 1990.
50. Ashinoff R, Geronemus RG: Capillary hemangiomas and treatment with the flashlamp-pumped pulsed dye laser, *Arch Dermatol* 127:202, 1991.
51. Dinehart SM, Flock S, Waner M: Beam profile of the flashlamp-pumped pulsed dye laser: support for overlap of exposure spots, *Lasers Surg Med* 15:277, 1980.
52. Jackson BA, Arndt KA, Dover JS: Are all 585 nm pulsed dye lasers equivalent? *J Am Acad Dermatol* 34:1000, 1996.
53. Verkruysse W, Lucassen GW, Oosterdi JK et al: Spectral and temporal effects of two commercial flashlamp-pumped dye lasers for port-wine stain treatment, *Lasers Surg Med Suppl* 7:54, 1995.
54. McMeekin TO, Goodwin DP: A comparison of spot size: 7 mm versus 5 mm of pulsed dye laser treatment of benign cutaneous vascular lesions, *Lasers Surg Med Suppl* 7:55, 1995.
55. Lanigan SW, Cartwright P, Cotterill JA: Continuous wave dye laser therapy of port-wine stains, *Br J Dermatol* 121:345, 1989.
56. Scheibner A, Wheeland RG: Use of the argon-pumped tunable dye laser for port-wine stains in children, *J Dermatol Surg Oncol* 17:735, 1991.
57. Dover JS, Geronemus R, Stern RS et al: Dye laser treatment of port-wine stains: comparison of the continuous-wave dye laser with a robotized scanning device and the pulsed dye laser, *J Am Acad Dermatol* 32:237, 1995.
58. Dinehart SM, Waner M: Comparison of the copper vapor and flashlamp-pulsed dye laser in the treatment of facial telangiectasia, *J Am Acad Dermatol* 24:116, 1991.
59. Waner M, Dinehart S: Lasers in facial plastic and reconstructive surgery. In Davis RK, Shapstray S, editors: *Lasers in otolaryngology/head and neck surgery,* Philadelphia, 1989, Saunders.
60. Murdock L, Waner M, Griffin E: The treatment of vascular and pigmented malformations with a copper vapor laser. Presented at the International Conference on Photodynamic Therapy and Medical Laser Applications, London, 1988.
61. Tan OT, Stafford TJ, Murray S et al: Histologic comparison of the pulsed dye laser and copper vapor laser effects on pig skin, *Lasers Surg Med* 10:551, 1990.
62. Jonell R, Larko O: Clinical effect of the copper vapor laser compared to previously used argon laser on cutaneous vascular lesions, *Acta Derm Venerol (Stockh)* 74:210, 1994.
63. Sheehan-Dare RA, Cotterill JA: Copper vapor laser treatment of port-wine stains: clinical evaluation and comparison with conventional argon laser therapy, *Br J Dermatol* 128:546, 1993.
64. Sheehan-Dare RA, Cotterill JA: Copper vapor laser (578 nm) and flashlamp-pumped pulsed dye laser (585 nm) treatment of port-wine stains: result of a comparative study using test sites, *Br J Dermatol* 130:478, 1994.
65. Chung J-H, Koh W-S, Youn J-I: Histological responses of port-wine stains in brown skin after 578 nm copper vapor laser treatment, *Lasers Surg Med* 18:358, 1996.

66. Haedersdal M, Wulf HC: Pigmentation-dependent side effects to copper vapor laser and argon laser treatment, *Lasers Surg Med* 16:351, 1995.
67. Haedersdal M, Wulf HC: Risk assessment of side effects from copper vapor and argon laser treatment: the importance of skin pigmentation, *Lasers Surg Med* 20:84, 1997.
68. Shapshay SM, David LM, Zeitels S: Neodymium-YAG laser photocoagulation of hemangiomas of the head and neck, *Laryngoscope* 97:323, 1987.
69. Landthaler M, Haina D, Brunner R: Neodymium-YAG laser therapy for vascular lesions, *J Am Acad Dermatol* 14:107, 1986.
70. Dixon JA, Gilbertson JJ: Argon and neodymium YAG laser therapy of dark nodular port-wine stains in older patients, *Lasers Surg Med* 6:5, 1986.
71. Apfelberg DB, Smith T, Lash H et al: Preliminary report on use of the neodymium-YAG laser in plastic surgery, *Lasers Surg Med* 7:189, 1987.
72. Adams SJ, Swain CP, Mills TN et al: The effect of wavelength, power and treatment pattern on the outcome of laser treatment of port-wine stains, *Br J Dermatol* 117:487, 1987.
73. Apfelberg DB, Bailin P, Rosenberg H: Preliminary investigation of KTP/532 laser light in the treatment of hemangiomas and tattoos, *Lasers Surg Med* 6:38, 1986.
74. Keller GS: Use of the KTP laser in cosmetic surgery, *Am J Cosmetic Surg* 9:177, 1992.
75. Routteleur G, Mordon S, Brunetaud JM: Argon 488-415, Nd:YAG 532, and CW dye 585 lasers for port-wine stain treatment using the Hexascan, *Lasers Surg Med Suppl* 3:68, 1991.
76. Tong AKF, Tan OT, Boll J et al: Ultrastructure: effects of melanin pigment on target specificity using a pulsed dye laser (577 nm), *J Invest Dermatol* 88:747, 1987.
77. Tan OT, Kerschmann R, Parrish JA: The effect of epidermal pigmentation on selective vascular effects of pulse dye laser, *Lasers Surg Med* 4:365, 1986.
78. Margolis RJ, Dover JS, Polla LL et al: Visible action spectrum for melanin-specific selective photothermolysis, *Laser Surg Med* 9:389, 1989.
79. Alhara H, Tanino R, Osada M et al: Attempt to obtain greater depth of vascular injury using dye-enhanced laser technique: a new approach, *Lasers Surg Med* 18:260, 1996.
80. Apfelberg DB et al: Dot or pointillistic method for improvement in results of hypertrophic scarring in the argon laser treatment of port-wine hemangiomas, *Lasers Surg Med* 6:552, 1987.
81. Mordon SR et al: Comparison study of the "point-by-point technique" and the "scanning technique" for laser treatment of port-wine stain, *Lasers Surg Med* 9:398, 1989.
82. Chambers IR, Clark D, Bainbridge C: Automation of laser treatment of port-wine stains, *Phys Med Biol* 7:1025, 1990.
83. Branner GJ: Laser scanners in dermatologic surgery, *Am J Cosmetic Surg* 9:197, 1992.
84. Apfelberg DB et al: Histology of port-wine stains following argon laser treatment, *Br J Plast Surg* 32:232, 1979.
85. Neumann RA, Knobler RM, Leonhartsberger H et al: Histochemical evaluation of the coagulation depth after argon laser impact on a port-wine stain, *Lasers Surg Med* 11:606, 1991.
86. Maser MR, Apfelbert DB, Lash H: Argon laser treatment of cutaneous vascular lesions, *West J Med* 133:57, 1980.
87. Fitzpatrick RE, Feinberg JA: Comparative histology of low-dose argon laser therapy versus high-dose argon laser therapy of port-wine stains, *Lasers Surg Med Suppl* 1:45, 1984.
88. Finley JC et al: Argon laser–port-wine stain interaction, *Arch Dermatol* 120:613, 1984.
89. van Gemert MJC, Welch AJ, Amin AP: Is there an optimal treatment for port-wine stains? *Lasers Med Surg* 6:76, 1986.
90. Neumann RA et al: Enzyme histochemical analysis of cell viability after argon laser–induced coagulation necrosis of the skin, *J Am Acad Dermatol* 25:991, 1991.
91. Goldman L et al: Treatment of port-wine marks by an argon laser, *J Dermatol Surg Oncol* 2:385, 1976.
92. Goldman MP et al: Sclerosing agents in the treatment of telangiectasia: comparison of the clinical and histologic effects of intravascular polidocanol, sodium tetradecyl sulfate, hypertonic saline in the dorsal rabbit ear vein model, *Arch Dermatol* 123:1196, 1987.
93. Hanschell HM: Treatment of varicose veins, *Br Med J* 2:630, 1947.
94. Goldman MP: A comparison of sclerosing agents: clinical and histologic effects of intravascular sodium morrhuate, ethanolamine oleate, hypertonic saline (11.7%) and Sclerodex in the dorsal rabbit ear vein, *J Dermatol Surg Oncol* 17:354, 1991.

95. Martin DE, Goldman MP: A comparison of sclerosing agents: clinical and histologic effects of intravascular sodium tetradecyl sulfate and chromated glycerine in the dorsal rabbit ear vein, *J Dermatol Surg Oncol* 16:18, 1990.
96. Pickering JW, Butler PH, Ring BJ et al: Computed temperature distributions around ectatic capillaries exposed to yellow (578 nm) laser light, *Phys Med Biol* 34:1247, 1989.
97. Garden JM, Tan OT, Kerschmann R et al: Effect of dye laser pulse duration on selective cutaneous vascular injury, *J Invest Dermatol* 87:653, 1986.
98. Garden JM et al: Pulse dye laser treatment of port-wine stain, 450 μsec vs 750 μsec pulse. Presented at the 15th Annual Meeting of the American Society for Laser Medicine and Surgery, San Diego, April 1995.
99. Kauvar A: Long-pulse and high energy pulsed dye laser treatment of port-wine stains and hemangiomas. Presented at 24th Annual meeting of the American Society of Dermatologic Surgery, Boston, May 1997.
100. Tan OT, Murray S, Kurban A: Action spectrum of vascular specific injury using pulsed irradiation, *J Invest Dermatol* 92:868, 1989.
101. van Gemert MCJ et al: Can physical modeling lead to an optimal laser treatment strategy for port-wine stains? In Wolbarsht ML, editor: *Laser applications in medicine and biology*, vol 5, New York, 1991, Plenum.
102. Pickering TW, van Gemert MJC: 585 nm for the laser treatment of port-wine stains: a possible mechanism, *Lasers Surg Med* 11:616, 1991 (letter).
103. Niechajev IA, Clodius L: Histology of port-wine stains, *Eur J Plast Surg* 13:79, 1990.
104. Tan OT, Morrison P, Kurban AK: 585 nm for the treatment of port-wine stains, *Plast Reconstr Surg* 86:1112, 1990.
105. van Gemert MJC, Pickering JW, Welch AJ: Modeling laser treatment of port-wine stains. In Tan OT, editor: *Management and treatment of benign cutaneous vascular lesions*, Philadelphia, 1992, Lea & Febiger.
106. Garden JM, Bakus AD: Effective wavelength on port-wine stain therapy. Presented at 14th Annual Meeting of the American Society for Laser Medicine and Surgery, Toronto, April 1994.
107. Tan OT, Whitaker D, Garden J et al: Pulsed dye laser (577 nm) treatment of port-wine stains: ultrastructural evidence of neovascularization and mast cell degranulation in healed lesions, *J Invest Dermatol* 90:395, 1988.
108. Gilchrist BA, Rosen S, Noe JM: Chilling port-wine stains improves the response to argon laser therapy, *Plast Reconstr Surg*, 69:278, 1982.
109. Dreno B, Patrice T, Litoux P et al: The benefit of chilling in argon laser treatment of port-wine stains, *Plast Resconstr Surg* 75:42, 1985.
110. Chess C, Chess Q: Cool laser optics treatment of large telangiectasia of the lower extremities, *J Dermatol Surg Oncol* 19:74, 1993.
111. Nelson JS, Milner TE, Anvari B et al: Dynamic epidermal cooling during pulsed laser treatment of port-wine stain, *Arch Dermatol* 131:695, 1995.
112. Adrian RM: Pulse dye laser treatment of port-wine stain: cooling facilitated high fluence. Presented at the 15th Annual Meeting of the American Society for Laser Medicine and Surgery, San Diego, April 1995.
113. Nelson JS, Milner TE, Anvari B: Dynamic epidermal cooking in conjunction with laser-induced photothermolysis of port-wine stain blood vessels, *Lasers Surg Med* 19;224, 1996.
114. Waldorf HA, Alster TS, McMillian K et al: Effects of dynamic cooling on 585-nm pulsed dye laser treatment of port-wine stain birthmarks, *Dermatol Surg* 23:657, 1997.
115. Archauer BM, Vander Kam VM, Padilla III JF: Clinical experience with the tunable pulsed-dye laser (585 nm) in the treatment of capillary vascular malformations, *Plast Reconstr Surg* 92:1233, 1993.
116. Gonzalez E, Gange RW, Momtaz K: Treatment of telangiectases and other benign vascular lesions with the 577 nm pulsed dye laser, *J Am Acad Dermatol* 27:220, 1992.
117. Swinehart JM: Hypertrophic scarring resulting from flashlamp-pumped pulsed dye laser surgery, *J Am Acad Dermatol* 25:845, 1991.
118. Nunez M, Perez B, Boixeda P et al: Transient cutaneous pustulosis as a complication of flashlamp pulsed dye laser treatment, *J Dermatol Treat* 6:249, 1995.
119. Mulliken JB: Classification of vascular birthmarks. In Mulliken JB, Young Ag, editors: *Vascular birthmarks, hemangiomas and malformations*, Philadelphia, 1988, Saunders.

120. Margileth AM, Museles M: Cavernous hemangiomas in children: diagnosis and conservative management, *JAMA* 194:523, 1965.
121. Jacobs AH, Walton RG: The incidence of birthmarks in the neonate, *Pediatrics* 58:218, 1976.
122. Pratt AG: Birthmarks in infants, *Arch Dermatol* 67:302, 1953.
123. Warner M: Personal communication, 1996.
124. Metzker A, Shamir R: Butterfly-shaped mark: a variant form of nevus flammeus simplex, *Pediatrics* 85:1069, 1990.
125. Motley RJ, Lanigan SW, Katugampola GA: Videomicroscopy predicts outcome in treatment of port-wine stains, *Arch Dermatol* 133:921, 1997.
126. Mulliken JB: Capillary (port-wine) and other telangiectatic stains. In Mulliken JB, Young AE, editors: *Vascular birthmarks, hemangiomas, and malformations,* Philadelphia, 1988, Saunders.
127. Susan JO et al: The "tomato catsup" fundus in Sturge-Weber syndrome, *Arch Ophthalmol* 92:69, 1974.
128. Bebin EM, Gomez MR: Prognosis in Sturge-Weber disease: comparison of unihemispheric and bihemispheric involvement, *J Child Neurol* 3:181, 1988.
129. Paller AS: The Sturge-Weber syndrome, *Pediatr Dermatol* 4:300, 1987.
130. Iwach AG et al: Analysis of surgical and medical management of glaucoma in Sturge-Weber syndrome, *Ophthalmology* 97:904, 1990.
131. Uram M, Zubillaga C: The cutaneous manifestations of Sturge-Weber syndrome, *J Clin Neurol Ophthalmol* 2:245, 1982.
132. Tallman B, Tan OT, Morelli JG et al: Location of port-wine stains and the likelihood of ophthalmic and/or central nervous system complications, *Pediatrics* 87:323, 1991.
133. Roach ES: Congenital cutaneovascular syndromes. In Vinkin PV, Bruyn GW, Klawans HL, editors: *Handbook of clinical neurology: vascular diseases,* vol 2, Amsterdam, 1989, Elsevier.
134. Stern R: Syndromes associated with port-wine stains. In Arndt K, Noe J, editors: *Cutaneous laser therapy: principles and methods,* New York, 1983, Wiley & Sons.
135. Jessen RT, Thompson S, Smith EB: Cobb syndrome, *Arch Dermatol* 113:1587, 1977.
136. Tay Y-K, Morelli J, Weston WL: Inflammatory nuchal-occipital port-wine stains, *J Am Acad Dermatol* 35:811, 1996.
137. Geronemus RG, Ashinoff R: The medical necessity of evaluation and treatment of port-wine stains, *J Dermatol Surg Oncol* 17:76, 1991.
138. Wilson BB, Brewer PC, Cooper PH: Spontaneous improvement of port-wine stain, *Cutis* 55:93, 1995.
139. Holloway KB, Ramos-Caro FA, Brownlee RE Jr et al: Giant proliferative hemangiomas arising in a port-wine stain, *J Am Acad Dermatol* 31:675, 1994.
140. Wagner KD, Wagner RF: The necessity for treatment of childhood port-wine stains, *Cutis* 45:317, 1990.
141. Malm M, Calberg M: Port-wine stain: a surgical and psychological problem, *Ann Plast Surg* 20:512, 1988.
142. Lanigan SW, Cotterill JA: Psychological disabilities amongst patients with port-wine stains, *Br J Dermatol* 121:209, 1989.
143. Dieterich CA, Cohen BA, Liggett J: Behavioral adjustment and self-concept of young children with hemangiomas, *Pediatr Dermatol* 9:241, 1992.
144. Ashinoff R, Geronemus RG: Flashlamp-pumped pulsed dye laser for port-wine stains in infancy: earlier versus later treatment, *J Am Acad Dermatol* 24:467, 1991.
145. Tan E, Vinciullo C: Pulsed dye laser treatment of port-wine stains, *Dermatol Surg* 22:119, 1996.
146. Masclarelli PC: Living with a port-wine birthmark. In Tan OT, editor: *Management and treatment of benign cutaneous vascular lesions,* Philadelphia, 1992, Lea & Febiger.
147. McClean K, Hanke CW: The medical necessity for treatment of port-wine stains, *Dermatol Surg* 23:663, 1997.
148. Clodius I: Excision and grafting of extensive facial haemangiomas, *Br J Plast Surg* 30:185, 1977.
149. Clodius I: Surgery for the extensive facial port-wine stain? *Aesthetic Plast Surg* 9:61, 1985.
150. Wilson GM, Kilpatrick R, Eckert H: Thyroid neoplasms following irradiation, *Br Med J* 2:929, 1958.

151. Hidano A, Ogihara Y: Cryotherapy with solid carbon dioxide in the treatment of nevus flammeus, *J Dermatol Surg Oncol* 3:213, 1977.
152. Conway H, Montroy RE: Permanent camouflage of capillary hemangiomas of the face by interdermal injection of insoluble pigments (tattooing): indications for surgery, *NY State J Med* 65:876, 1965.
153. Thomson HG, Wright A: Surgical tattooing of the port-wine stain: operative technique, results and critique, *Plast Reconstr Surg* 48:113, 1971.
154. Cosman B: Clinical experience in the laser therapy of port-wine stains, *Lasers Surg Med* 1:133, 1980.
155. Buecker JW, Ratz JL, Richfield DF: Histology of port-wine stains treated with carbon dioxide laser, *J Am Acad Dermatol* 10:1014, 1984.
156. Ratz JL, Bailin PL, Levine HL: CO_2 laser treatment for port-wine stains: a preliminary report, *J Dermatol Surg Oncol* 8:1039, 1982.
157. Lanigan SW, Cotterill JA: The treatment of port-wine stains with the carbon dioxide laser, *Br J Dermatol* 123:229, 1990.
158. Walker EP, Butler PH, Pickering JW: Histology of port-wine stains after copper vapor laser treatment, *Br J Dermatol* 121:217, 1989.
159. Scheibner A, Applebaum J, Wheeland RG: Treatment of port-wine hemangiomas in children, *Lasers Surg Med (Suppl)* 1:42, 1989.
160. Hobby LW: Argon laser treatment of superficial vascular lesions in children, *Lasers Surg Med* 6:16, 1986.
161. Brauner GJ, Schliftman A: Laser surgery for children, *J Dermatol Surg Oncol* 13:178, 1987.
162. Brauner G, Schliftman A, Cosman B: Evaluation of argon laser surgery in children under 13 years of age, *Plast Reconstr Surg* 87:37, 1991.
163. Morelli JG, Weston WL: Pulsed dye laser treatment of port-wine stains in children. In Tan OT, editor: *Management and treatment of benign cutaneous vascular lesions,* Philadelphia, 1992, Lea & Febiger.
164. Morelli JG, Weston WL, Huff JV et al: Initial lesion size as a predictive factor in determining the response of port-wine stains in children treated with the pulsed dye laser, *Arch Pediatr Adolesc Med* 149:1142, 1995.
165. Alster TS, Wilson F: Treatment of port-wine stains with the flashlamp-pumped dye laser: extended clinical experience in children and adults, *Ann Plast Surg* 32:474, 1994
166. Orten SS, Waner M, Flock s et al: Port-wine stains: an assessment of 5 years of treatment, *Arch Otolaryngol Head Neck Surg* 122;1174, 1996.
167. Eppley BL, Sadove M: Systemic effects of photothermolysis of large port-wine stains in infants and children, *Plast Reconstr Surg* 93:1150, 1994.
168. Pao D: Personal communication, 1994.
169. Levine VJ, Geronemus RG: Adverse effects associated with the 577- and 585-nm pulsed dye laser in the treatment of cutaneous vascular lesions: a study of 500 patients, *J Am Acad Dermatol* 32:613, 1995.
170. Lanigan SW: Port-wine stains on the lower limb: response to pulsed dye laser therapy, *Clin Exp Dermatol* 21:88, 1996.
171. Zachariea H: Delayed wound healing and keloid formation following argon laser treatment or dermabrasion during isotretinoin treatment, *Br J Dermatol* 118:703, 1988.
172. Rubenstein R, Roenigk HH, Stegman S et al: Atypical keloids after dermabrasion of patients taking tretinoin, *J Am Acad Dermatol* 15:280, 1986.
173. Bernestein LJ, Geronemus RG: Keloid formation with the 585-nm pulsed dye laser during isotretinoin treatment, *Arch Dermatol* 133:111, 1997.
174. Seukeran DC, Collins P, Sheehan-Dare RA: Adverse reactions following pulsed tunable dye laser treatment of port-wine stains in 701 patients, *Br J Dermatol* 136:725, 1997.
175. Yohn JJ, Huff JC, Aeling JL et al: Lesion size is a factor for determining the rate of port-wine stain clearing following pulsed dye laser treatment in adults, *Cutis* 59:267, 1997.
176. Lanigan SW: Poor response of port wine stains on lower limb to pulsed tunable dye laser therapy, *Lasers Surg Med Suppl* 7:58, 1995.
177. Taylor MB: Flashlamp laser treatment of port-wine stain hemangiomas and other vascular lesions using a defocused "fuzzy spot," *Lasers Surg Med Suppl* 3:68, 1991.

178. Lucassen GW, Verkruysse W, Keijzer M et al: Light distributions in port-wine stain model containing multiple cylindrical and curved blood vessels, *Lasers Surg Med* 18:345, 1996.
179. Wieglebb Edtstrom D, Ros A-M: The treatment of port-wine stains with the pulsed dye laser at 600nm, *Br J Dermatol;* 136:360, 1997.
180. Kauvar ANB: Long-pulse high energy pulsed dye laser treatment of port-wine stains and hemangiomas, *Lasers Surg Med Suppl* 9:36,1997.
181. Fiskerstrand EJ, Dalaker M, Norvang LT: Laser treatment of port-wine stains: a study comparing therapeutic outcome with morphologic characteristics of the lesions, *Acta Derm Venerol (Stockh)* 75:92, 1995.
182. Fiskerstrand EJ, Svaasand LO, Kopstad G et al: Photothermally induced vessel-wall necrosis after pulsed dye laser treatment: lack of response in portwine stains with small sized or deply located vessels, *J Invest Dermatol* 107:671, 1996.
183. Hohenleutner U, Hilbert M, Wlotzke U et al: Epidermal damage and limited coagulation depth with the flashlamp-pumped pulsed dye laser: a histochemical study, *J Invest Dermatol* 104:798, 1995.
184. Waner M: Recurrence of port-wine stains after treatment, *Arch Dermatol,* 1997 (submitted).
185. Smaller RB, Rosen S: Port-wine stains: a disease of altered neural modulation of blood vessels, *Arch Dermatol* 122:177, 1986.
186. Rydh M, Malm M, Jernbeck J et al: Ectatic blood vessels in port-wine stains lack innervation: possible role in pathogenesis, *Plast Reconstr Surg* 87:419, 1991.
187. Kane KS, Smoller BR, Fitzpatrick RE et al: Pulsed dye laser–resistant port-wine stains, *Arch Dermatol* 132:839, 1996.
188. Ashinoff R, Geronemus RG: Treatment of a port-wine stain in a black patient with the pulsed dye laser, *J Dermatol Surg Oncol* 18:147, 1992.
189. Lo JS, Sgouros GN, Laohs FE et al: Basal cell carcinoma within a nevus flammeus: report of a case, *Int J Dermatol* 30:723, 1991.
190. Kauvar AN, Geronemus RG: Repetitive pulse dye laser treatments improve persistent port-wine stains, *Dermatol Surg* 21:515, 1995.
191. Raulin C, Hellwig S, Schonermark MP: Treatment of a non-responding port-wine stain with a new pulsed light source (Photoderm VL), *Lasers Surg Med* 21:203, 1997.
192. Nelson JS: Case 7.13: port-wine stain hemangioma. In Apfelberg DB, editor: *Atlas of cutaneous laser surgery,* New York, 1992, Raven.
193. McDaniel DH: Case 7.15: portwine stain hemangioma. In Apfelberg DB, editor: *Atlas of cutaneous laser surgery,* New York, 1992, Raven.
194. McDaniel DH: Case 7.12: port-wine stain hemangioma of the right face. In Apfelberg DB, editor: *Atlas of cutaneous laser surgery,* New York, 1992, Raven.
195. Keijzer M, Pickering JW, van Gemert MJC: Laser beam diameter for port-wine stain treatment, *Lasers Surg Med* 11:601, 1991.
196. Dinehart S, Waner M, Flock S: The copper vapor laser for treatment of cutaneous vascular and pigmented lesions, *J Dermatol Surg Oncol* 19:370, 1993.
197. Sheehan-Dare RA, Cotterill JA: Are copper vapour and frequency doubled Nd:YAG lasers superior to the argon laser for port-wine stains at pulse widths of 30-50 milliseconds? *Lasers Surg Med* 18:46, 1996.
198. Malm M: *Port-wine stain: laser treatment and evaluation of results,* Stockholm, 1987, Kongl Carolinska Medico Chirargiska Institutet.
199. McCoy: Personal communication, 1992.
200. Neumann RA, Leonhartsberger H, Bohler-Sommereger K et al: Results and tissue healing after copper-vapour laser (at 578 nm) treatment of port-wine stains and facial telangiectasias, *Br J Dermatol* 128:306, 1993.
201. Dierickx CC, Farinelli WA, Flotte T et al: Effect of long-pulsed 532 nm ND-YAG laser on port-wine stains (PWS), *Lasers Surg Med Suppl* 8:188, 1996.
202. Dierickx CC, Casparian JM, Venugopalan V et al: Themal relaxation of port-wine stain vessels robed in vivo: the need for 1-10 millisecond laser pulse treatment, *J Invest Dermatol* 105:709, 1995.
203. Eckhouse S, Kreindel: Personal communication, 1996.
204. Goldman MP: Treatment of benign vascular lesions with the Photoderm VL high-intensity pulsed light source, *Adv Dermatol* 13:503, 1998.

205. Ranlin C, Goldman MP, Weiss MA, Weiss RA: Treatment of adult port-wine stains using intense pulsed light therapy (PhotoDerm VL): brief initial clinical report, *Dermatol Surg* 23:594, 1997.
206. Mulliken JB: A plea for a biologic approach to hemangiomas of infancy, *Arch Dermatol* 127:243, 1991 (editorial).
207. Mulliken JB: Diagnosis and natural history of hemangiomas. In Mulliken JB, Young AE, editors: *Vascular birthmarks, hemangiomas and malformations,* Philadelphia, 1988, Saunders.
208. Finn MC, Glowacki J, Mulliken JB: Congenital vascular lesions: clinical application of a new classification, *J Pediatr Surg* 18:894, 1983.
209. Jacobs AH: Strawberry hemangiomas: the natural history of the untreated lesion, *Calif Med* 86:8, 1957.
210. Holmdahl K: Cutaneous hemangiomas in premature and mature infants, *Acta Paediatr* 44:370, 1955.
211. Boon LM, Enjolras O, Mulliken JB: Congenital hemangioma: evidence of accelerated involution, *J Pediatr* 128:329, 1996.
212. Rositto A, Ranalletta M, Drut R: Congenital hemangioma of eccrine sweat glands, *Pediatr Dermatol* 10:341, 1993.
213. Bowers RE, Graham EA, Tomlinson KM: The natural history of the strawberry nevus, *Arch Dermatol* 82:667, 1960.
214. Takahashi K, Mulliken JB, Kozakewich HPW et al: Cellular markers that distinguish the phases of hemangioma during infancy and childhood, *J Clin Invest* 93:2357, 1994.
215. Bivings L: Spontaneous regression of angiomas in children: twenty-two years' observation covering 236 cases, *J Pediatr* 45:643, 1954.
216. Tuder RM, Young R, Karasek M et al: Adult cutaneous hemangiomas are composed of new replicating endothelial cells, *J Invest Dermatol* 89:594, 1987.
217. Lister WA: The natural history of strawberry naevi, *Lancet* 1:1429, 1938.
218. Baker ER, Manders E, Whitney CW: Growth of cavernous hemangioma with puberty, *Clin Pediatr* 24:596, 1985.
219. Moroz B: The course of haemangiomas in children. In Ryan TJ, Cherry GW, editors: *Vascular birthmarks: pathogenesis and management,* New York, 1987, Oxford University Press.
220. Liang MG, Frieden IJ: Perineal and lip ulcerations as the presenting manifestation of hemangioma of infancy, *Pediatrics* 99:256, 1997.
221. Williams HB: Facial bone changes with vascular tumors in children, *Plast Reconstr Surg* 63:309, 1979.
222. Thomson G et al: Stigmar G. hemangiomas of the eyelid: visual complications and prophylactic concepts, *Plast Reconstr Surg* 63:641, 1979.
223. Robb RM: Refractive errors associated with hemangiomas of the eyelids and orbit in infancy, *Am J Ophthalmol* 83:52, 1977.
224. Healy GB et al: Treatment of subglottic hemangioma with the carbon dioxide laser, *Laryngoscope* 90:809, 1980.
225. Kasabach HH, Merritt KK: Capillary hemangioma with extensive purpura, *Am J Dis Child* 59:1063, 1940.
226. McLean RH et al: Multinodular hemangiomatosis of the liver in infancy, *Pediatrics* 49:563, 1972.
227. Patel SD, Cohen BA, Kan JS et al: Extensive facial hemangiomas associated with cardiac and abdominal abnormalities, *J Am Acad Dermatol* 36:636, 1997.
228. Igarashi M, Uchida H, Kaji T: Supraumbilical midabdominal raphe and facial cavernous hemangiomas, *Clin Genet* 27:196, 1985.
229. Schneeweiss A, Blieden LC, Shem-Tov A et al: Coarctation of the aorta and congenital hemangioma of the face and neck and aneurysm or dilatation of a subclavian or innominate artery, *Chest* 82:186, 1982.
230. Reese V, Frieden IJ, Paller AS et al: Association of facial hemangiomas with Dandy-Walker and other posterior fossa malformations, *J Pediatr* 122:379, 1993.
231. Frieden IJ, Reese V, Cohen D: PHACE syndrome, *Arch Dermatol* 132:307, 1996.
232. Gorlin RJ, Kantaputra P, Aughton DJ et al: Marked female predilection in some syndromes associated with facial hemangiomas, *Am J Med Genet* 52:130, 1994.
233. Goldberg NS, Hebert AA, Esterly NB: Sacral hemangiomas and multiple congenital abnormalities, *Arch Dermatol* 122:684, 1986.

234. Albright AL, Gartner JC, Wiener ES: Lumbar cutaneous hemangiomas as indicators of tethered spinal cords, *Pediatrics* 83:977, 1989.
235. Enjolras O, Gelbert F: Superficial hemangiomas: associations and management, *Pediatr Dermatol* 14:173, 1997.
236. Finn MC, Glowacki J, Mulliken JP: Congenital vascular lesions: clinical applications of a new classification, *J Pediatr Surg* 18:894, 1983.
237. Modlin JJ: Capillary hemangiomas of the skin, *Surgery* 38:169, 1955.
238. Mulliken JB: Treatment of hemangiomas. In Mulliken JB, Young AE, editors: *Vascular birthmarks, hemangiomas and malformations,* Philadelphia, 1988, Saunders.
239. Cherry GW: A review of the role of surgery in the treatment of hemangiomas and port-wine stains. In Ryan TJ, Cherry GW, editors: *Vascular birthmarks: pathogenesis and management,* New York, 1987, Oxford University Press.
240. Bek V, Zahn K: Cataract as a late sequela of contract roentgen therapy of angiomas in children, *Acta Radiol* 54:443, 1960.
241. Tan OT, Gilchrest BA: Laser therapy for selected cutaneous vascular lesions in the pediatric population: a review, *Pediatrics* 82:652, 1988.
242. MacCollum DW: Treatment of hemangiomas, *Am J Surg* 29:32, 1935.
243. Brain RT, Calvan CD: Vascular naevi and their treatment, *Br J Dermatol* 64:147, 1952.
244. Matthews DN: Hemangiomata, *Plast Reconstr Surg* 41:528, 1968.
245. Scerri L, Navaratnam A: Basal cell carcinoma presenting as a delayed complication of thorium X used for treating a congenital hemangioma, *J Am Acad Dermatol* 31:796, 1994.
246. Lomholt S: Alpha and beta ray therapy in dermatology, *Br J Dermatol* 48:567, 1936.
247. Bowers RE: Treatment of haemangiomatous naevi with thorium X, *Br Med J* 1:121, 1951.
248. Courtermarche AD: Thorium X induced BCC: a case report, *Br J Plast Surg* 14:254, 1961.
249. Caldwell JB, Ryan MT, Benson PM et al: Cutaneous angiosarcoma arising in the radiation site of a congenital hemangioma, *J Am Acad Dermatol* 33:865, 1995.
250. Sybert V: Personal communication, 1992.
251. Kushner BJ: The treatment of periorbital infantile hemangiomas with intralesional corticosteroid, *Plast Reconstr Surg* 76:517, 1985.
252. Nelson LB, Melick JE, Harley RD: Intralesional corticosteroid injections for infantile hemangiomas of the eyelid, *Pediatrics* 74:241, 1984.
253. Ellis PO: Occlusion of the central retinal artery after retrobulbar corticosteroid injection, *Am J Ophthalmol* 85:352, 1983.
254. Chowdri NA, Darzi MA, Fazili Z et al: Intralesional corticosteroid therapy for childhood cutaneous hemangiomas, *Ann Plast Surg* 33:46, 1994.
255. Enjolras O, Mulliken JB: The current management of vascular birthmarks, *Pediatr Dermatol* 10:311, 1993.
256. Brousty-Brye D, Zelter BR: Inhibition of cell motility by interferon, *Science* 208:516, 1980.
257. Ezekowitz RA, Mulliken JB, Folkman J: Interferon alpha-2a therapy for life-threatening hemangiomas of infancy, *N Engl J Med* 326:1456, 1992.
258. Stratte EG, Tope WD, Johnson CL et al: Multimodal management of diffuse neonatal hemangiomatosis, *J Am Acad Dermatol* 34:337, 1996.
259. Apfelberg DB, Greene RA, Maser MR: Results of argon laser exposure of capillary hemangiomas of infancy: preliminary report, *Plast Reconstr Surg* 67:188, 1981.
260. Hobby LW: Further evaluation of the potential of the argon laser in the treatment of strawberry hemangiomas, *Plast Reconstr Surg* 71:481, 1983.
261. Achauer BM, VanderKam VM: Argon laser treatment of strawberry hemangioma in infancy, *West J Med* 143:628, 1985.
262. Cases 5.6, 5.7, 5.9, 5.10, 5.11. In Apfelberg DB, editor: *Atlas of cutaneous laser surgery,* New York, 1992, Raven.
263. Cases 6.9, 6.10, 6.19, 6.20. In Apfelberg DB, editor: *Atlas of cutaneous laser surgery,* New York, 1992, Raven.
264. Preeyanont P, Nimsakul N: The Nd:YAG laser treatment of hemangioma, *J Clin Laser Med Surg* 12:225, 1994.
265. Apfelberg DB, Maser MR, Lash H: YAG laser resection of complicated hemangiomas of the hand and upper extremity, *J Hand Surg* 15A:765, 1990.
266. Apfelberg DB, Maser MR, Lash H: High- and low-tech solutions for massive cavernous hemangioma of the face: lasers and leeches to the rescue, *Ann Plast Surg* 23:341, 1989.

267. Thompson HG, Lonigan M: The Cyrano nose: a clinical review of hemangiomas of the nasal tip, *Plast Reconstr Surg* 63:155, 1979.
268. Afpelberg DB: Argon and YAG laser photocoagulation and excision of hemangiomas and vascular malformations of the nose, *West J Med* 163:122, 1995.
269. Hoffman WL, Anvari B, Said S et al: Cryogen spray cooling during Nd:YAG laser treatment of hemangiomas, *Dermatol Surg* 23:635,1997.
270. Achauer BM, Vanderkam VM, Celikoz B: Intralesional bare fiber laser treatment of hemangioma, *Lasers Surg Med Suppl* 9:41, 1997.
271. Kaplan I, Sharon U: Current laser surgery, *Ann NY Acad Sci* 267:247, 1976.
272. Labandter H, Kaplan I: Experience with a continuous laser in the treatment of suitable cutaneous conditions: preliminary report, *J Dermatol Surg Oncol* 3:527, 1977.
273. Apfelberg DB, Maser MR, Lash H et al: Benefits of carbon dioxide laser in oral hemangioma excision, *Plast Reconstr Surg* 75:46, 1985.
274. Apfelberg DB, Maser MR, Lash H: Review and usage of argon and carbon dioxide lasers for pediatric hemangiomas, *Ann Plast Surg* 12:353, 1984.
275. Fujino T: Microsurgical technique in resection of haemangioma in infants, *Ann Plast Surg* 13:190, 1985.
276. Argenta L: Controlled tissue expansion in reconstructive surgery, *Br Plast Surg* 37:520, 1984.
277. Grabb WC et al: Facial hamartomas in children: neurofibroma, lymphangioma and haemangioma, *Plast Reconstr Surg* 66:509, 1980.
278. Apfelberg DB, Lane B, Marx MP: Combined (team) approach to hemangioma management: arteriography with superselective embolization plus YAG laser/sapphire-tip resection, *Plast Reconstr Surg* 88:71, 1991.
279. Scheepers JH, Quaba AA: Does the pulsed tunable dye laser have a role in the management of infantile hemangiomas? Observations based on 3 years' experience. *Plast Reconstr Surg* 95:305, 1995.
280. Morelli JG, Weston WL: Pulsed dye laser treatment of hemangiomas. In Tan OT, editor: *Management and treatment of benign cutaneous vascular lesions,* Philadelphia, 1992, Lea & Febiger.
281. Morelli JG, Tan OT, Yohn JJ: Treatment of ulcerated hemangiomas in infancy, *Arch Pediatr Adolesc Med* 148:1104, 1994.
282. Garden JM, Babus AD, Paller AS: Treatment of cutaneous hemangiomas by the flashlamp-pumped pulsed dye laser: prospective analysis, *J Pediatr* 120:555, 1992.
283. Maier H, Neumann R: Treatment of strawberry marks with flashlamp-pumped pulsed dye laser in infancy, *Lancet* 347:131, 1996.
284. Barlow RJ, Walker NPJ, Markey AC: Treatment of proliferative haemangiomas with the 585 nm pulsed dye laser, *Br J Dermatol* 134:700, 1996.
285. West T, Fitzpatrick RE, Goldman MP, Alster T: Treatment of capillary hemangiomas with the Candela flashlamp-pumped pulsed dye laser and corticosteroids, *Dermatol Surg,* 1998.
286. Foster TD, Gold MH: The successful use of the PhotoDerm VL in the treatment of a cavernous hemangioma in a dark-skinned infant, *Minim Invas Nurs* 10:102, 1996.
287. Raulin C, Raulin SJ, Hellwig S, Schonermark MP: Treatment of benign venous malformation with an intense pulsed light source (Photoderm VL), *Eur J Dermatol* 7:279, 1997.
288. Frieden IJ, Eichenfield LF, Esterly NB et al: Guidelines of care for hemangiomas of infancy, J *Am Acad Dermatol* 37:631,1997.
289. Pasyl KA: Classification and histopathological features of haemangiomas and other vascular malformations. In Ryan TJ, Cherry GW, editors: *Vascular birthmarks: pathogenesis and management,* New York, 1987, Oxford University Press.
290. Bucci FA, Wiener BD: The pyogenic granuloma, *Ariz Med* WLI:794, 1984.
291. Cooper PH, Mills SE: Subcutaneous granuloma pyogenicum: lobular capillary hemangioma, *Arch Dermatol* 118:30, 1982.
292. Patrice SJ, Wiss K, Mulliken JB: Pyogenic granuloma (lobular capillary hemangioma): a clinicopathologic study of 178 cases, *Pediatr Dermatol* 8:267, 1991.
293. Goldberg DJ, Sciales CW: Pyogenic granuloma in children, *J Dermatol Surg Oncol* 17:960, 1991.
294. Mills SE, Cooper PH, Fechner RE: Lobular capillary hemangioma: the underlying lesion of pyogenic granuloma, a study of 73 cases from the oral and nasal mucous membranes, *Am J Surg Pathol* 4:471, 1980.

295. Arndt KA: Argon laser therapy of small cutaneous vascular lesions, *Arch Dermatol* 118:220, 1982.
296. Blickenstaff RD et al: Recurrent pyogenic granuloma with satellitosis, *J Am Acad Dermatol* 21:1241, 1989.
297. Tan OT, Kurban AK: Noncongenital benign cutaneous vascular lesions: pulse dye laser treatment. In Tan OT, editor: *Management and treatment of benign cutaneous vascular lesions,* Philadelphia, 1992, Lea & Febiger.
298. Glass AT, Milgram S: Flashlamp-pumped dye laser treatment for pyogenic granuloma, *Cutis* 49:351, 1992.
299. Gonzalez S, Vibhagool C, Falo LD Jr et al: Treatment of pyogenic granuolmas with the 585nm pulsed dye laser, *J Am Acad Dermatol* 35:428, 1996.
300. Merlen JF: Red telangiectasias, blue telangiectasias, *Soc Franc Phlebol* 22:167, 1970.
301. Goldman MP, Bennett RG: Treatment of telangiectasia: a review, *J Am Acad Dermatol* 17:167, 1987.
302. Redisch W, Pelzer RH: Localized vascular dilatations of the human skin: capillary microscopy and related studies, *Am Heart J* 37:106, 1949.
303. Alderson MR: Spider naevi: their incidence in healthy school children, *Arch Dis Child* 38:286, 1963.
304. Wenzl JE, Burgert EO: The spider nevus in infancy and childhood, *Pediatrics* 33:227, 1964.
305. Oster J, Nielsen A: Nuchal naevi and intrascapular telangiectases, *Acta Paediatr Scand* 59:416, 1970.
306. Bean WB: *Vascular spiders and related lesions of the skin,* Springfield, Ill, 1958, Thomas.
307. Geronemus RG: Treatment of spider telangiectases in children using the flashlamp pumped pulsed dye laser, *Pediatr Dermatol* 8:61, 1991.
308. Goldman MP, Fitzpatrick RE, Ruiz-Esparza J: Treatment of spider telangiectasia in children, *Contemp Pediatr* 10:16, 1993.
309. de Rooij MJM, Neumann HAM: Granuloma telangiectaticum after argon laser therapy of a spider nevus, *Dermatol Surg* 20:354, 1995.
310. Civatte A: Poikilodermie reticulae pigmentaire du visage et du col, *Ann Derm Syph* 6:605, 1923.
311. Wheeland RG, Applebaum J: Flashlamp-pumped pulsed dye laser therapy for poikiloderma of Civatte, *J Dermatol Surg Oncol* 16:12, 1990.
312. Kirsch N: Telangiectasia and electrolysis, *J Dermatol Surg Oncol* 10:9, 1984 (letter).
313. Recoules-Arche J: Electrocoagulation, *Phlebologie* 33:885, 1966.
314. Green AR, Morgan BDG: Sclerotherapy for venous flare, *Br J Plast Surg* 38:241, 1985
315. Biegelseisen HI: Telangiectasia associated with varicose veins: treatment by a microinjection technique, *JAMA* 102:2092, 1934.
316. MacGowen WAL et al: The local effects of intra-arterial injections of sodium tetradecyl sulfate (STD) 3%: an experimental study, *Br J Surg* 59:101, 1972.
317. Fegan WG, Pegum JM: Accidental intra-arterial injection during sclerotherapy of varicose veins, *Br J Surg* 61:124, 1974
318. Staubesand JI, Seydewitz V: Ultrastructural changes following paravascular and intraarterial injection of sclerosing agents: an experimental contribution to the problem of iatrogenic damage, *Phlebologie* 20:1, 1991.
319. Goldman MP: Complications and adverse sequelae of sclerotherapy. In Goldman MP, editor: *Sclerotherapy treatment of varicose and telangiectatic leg veins,* St Louis, 1991, Mosby.
320. Achauer BM, VanderKam VM: Argon laser treatment of the face and neck: 5 years' experience, *Lasers Surg Med* 7:495:1987.
321. Lyons GD, Owens RE, Moriney DF: Argon laser destruction of cutaneous telangiectatic lesions, *Laryngoscope* 91:1322, 1981.
322. Orenstein A, Nelson JS: Treatment of facial vascular lesions with a 100 μm spot 577 nm pulsed continuous wave dye laser, *Ann Plast Surg* 23:310, 1989.
323. Cases 7.6, 7.7, 7.22, 7.30. In Apfelberg DB, editor: *Atlas of cutaneous laser surgery,* New York, 1992, Raven.
324. Broska P, Martinho E, Goodman MM: Comparison of the argon tunable dye laser with the flashlamp pulsed dye laser in treatment of facial telangiectasia, *J Dermatol Surg Oncol* 20:749, 1994.
325. Waner M, Dinehart S: Lasers in facial plastic and reconstructive surgery. In Davis RK, Shapstray S, editors: *Lasers in otolaryngology/head and neck surgery,* Philadelphia, 1989, Saunders.

326. Thibault PK: Copper vapor laser and microsclerotherapy of facial telangiectases, *J Dermatol Surg Oncol* 20:48, 1994.
327. Waner M, Dinehart SM, Wilson MB et al: A comparison of copper vapor and flashlamp pumped dye lasers in the treatment of facial telangiectasia, *J Dermatol Surg Oncol* 19:992, 1993.
328. McCoy SE: Copper bromide laser treatment of facial telangiectasia: results of patients treated over five years, *Lasers Surg Med* 21:329, 1997.
329. McCoy S, Hanna M, Anderson P et al: An evaluation of the copper-bromide laser for treating telangiectasia, *Dermatol Surg* 22:551, 1996.
330. Hevia O: New laser treatment for facial telangiectasias: a randomized study, *Cosmetic Dermatol* 10:53, 1997.
331. Goldberg DJ, Marcus J: The use of the frequency-doubled Q-switched Nd:YAG laser in the treatment of small cutaneous vascular lesions, *Dermatol Surg* 22:841, 1996.
332. Adrian RM, Tanghetti EA: Long pulse 532-nm laser treatment of facial telangiectasia, *Dermatol Surg* 24:71, 1998.
333. Thibault PK: A patient's questionnaire evaluation of krypton laser treatment of facial telangiectasia, *Dermatol Surg* 23:37, 1997.
334. Sadick N: A comparison study of a continuous wave laser (Krypton HGM) vs. long-pulse tunable dye laser (Sclerolaser—Candela) in the treatment of nasal actinic telangiectasia. Presented at 24th Annual Meeting of the American Society for Dermatologic Surgery, Boston, May 1997.
335. Geronemus RG, Greiken: In Candela Corporation brochure, 1992.
336. Weiss RA, Weiss MA, Goldman MP: Photothermal sclerosis of facial telangiectasia using the PhotoDerm VL, *Dermatol Surg,* 1998.
337. Raulin C, Weiss RA, Schohermark MP: Treatment of essential telangiectasias with an intense pulsal light source (PhotoDerm VL), *Dermatol Surg* 23:941, 1997.
338. Fitzpatrick RE et al: Treatment of facial telangiectasia with the flash pump dye laser, *Lasers Surg Med Suppl* 3:70, 1991.
339. Garden JM, Bakus AD: Low energy pulsed dye laser treatment of facial blood vessels, *Lasers Surg Med Suppl* 9:38, 1997.
340. Wilkin JK: Rosacea: pathophysiology and treatment, *Arch Dermatol* 130:359, 1994.
341. Lowe NJ et al: Flashlamp pumped dye laser for rosacea-associated telangiectasia and erythema, *J Dermatol Surg Oncol* 17:522, 1991.
342. Silver BE, Livshots YL: Preliminary experience with the KTP/532 nm laser in the treatment of facial telangiectasia, *Cosmetic Dermatol* 9:61, 1996.
343. Ellis DL: Treatment of telangiectasia macularis eruptiva perstans with the 585-nm flashlamp pumped dye laser, *Dermatol Surg* 22:3, 1996.
344. Fitzpatrick RE: Laser treatment of scars. Presented at International Society of Laser Medicine and Surgery, Los Angeles, 1991.
345. Castro DJ, Abergel RP, Meeker CA et al: Effects of the Nd:YAG laser on DNA synthesis and collagen production in human skin fibroblast cultures, *Am Plast Surg* 22:214, 1983.
346. Abergel RP, Meeker CA, Dwyer RM et al: Non-thermal effects of Nd:YAG laser in biological functions of human skin fibroblasts in culture, *Lasers Surg Med* 3:279, 1984.
347. Abergal RP, Dwyer RM, Meeker CA et al: Laser treatment of keloids: a clinical trial and an in vitro study with Nd:YAG laser, *Lasers Surg Med* 4:291, 1984.
348. Ginsbach G, Kohnel W: The treatment of hypertrophic scars and keloids by argon laser: clinical data and morphological findings, *ASPRS-EF-ASMS Plast Surg Forum* 1:61, 1978.
349. Henderson DL, Cromwell TA, Mes LG: Argon and carbon dioxide laser treatment of hypertrophic and keloidal scars, *Lasers Surg Med* 3:271, 1984.
350. Peacock BE Jr, van Winkle W Jr: *Surgery and wound repair,* Philadelphia, 1970, Saunders.
351. Leung KS et al: Microcirculation in hypertrophic scars after burn injury, *J Burn Care Rehabil* 10:436, 1989.
352. Page RE, Robertson GA, Pettigrew NM: Microcirculation in hypertrophic burn scars, *Burns Incl Therm Inj* 10:64, 1983.
353. Ehrlich HP, White BS: The identification of alpha-A and alpha-B collagen chains in hypertrophic scars, *Exp Mol Pathol* 34:1, 1981.
354. Hering TM, Marchant RG, Anderson JM: Type V collagen during granulation tissue development, *Exp Mol Pathol* 39:219, 1983.

355. Zhang K, Garner W, Cohen L et al: Increased types I and III collagen and transforming growth factor-b1 mRNA and protein in hypertrophic burn scar, *J Invest Dermatol* 104:750, 1995.
356. Peltonen J, Hsiao LL, Jaakkola S et al: Activation of collagen gene expression in keloids: co-localization of type I and VI collagen and transforming growth factor beta-1 mRNA, *J Invest Dermatol* 97:240, 1991.
357. Baur PS, Latson DL, Stice Tr et al: Ultrastructural analysis of pressure-treated human hypertrophic scars, *J Trauma* 16:958, 1976.
358. Alster TS, Williams CM: Treatment of keloid sternotomy scars with 585 nm flashlamp-pumped pulsed-dye laser, *Lancet* 345:1198, 1995.
359. Topol BM, Lewis VL Jr, Benveniste K: The use of antihistamine to retard the growth of fibroblasts derived from human skin, scar, and keloid, *Plast Reconstr Surg* 68:231, 1981.
360. Alster TS: Improvement of erythematous and hypertrophic scars by the 585-nm flash-lamp-pumped pulsed dye laser, *Ann Plast Surg* 32:186, 1994.
361. Goldman MP, Fitzpatrick RE: Laser treatment of scars, *Dermatol Surg* 21:685, 1995.
362. Tran N-L T, Clark RE, Jimenez-Acosta J et al: Pulsed dye laser treatment of keloids. Poster presented at the Annual Meeting of the American Academy of Dermatology, Washington, DC, December 1993.
363. Alster TS, McMeekin TO: Improvement of facial acne scars by the 585 nm flashlamp-pumped pulsed dye laser, *J Am Acad Dermatol* 35:79, 1996.
364. Kilmer SL, Chotzen VA: Pulse dye laser treatment of old burn scars, *Lasers Surg Med Suppl* 9:34, 1997.
365. Reiken SR, Wolfort SF, Berthiaume F, et al: Control of hypertrophic scar growth using selective photothermolysis, *Lasers Surg Med* 21:71, 1997.
366. Zheng P, Lavker RM, Kligman AM. Anatomy of striae, *Brit J Dermatol* 112:185, 1985.
367. Arem AJ, Kischer CW: Analysis of striae, *Plast Recontr Surg* 65:22, 1980.
368. Tsuji T, Swabe M. Elastic fibers in striae distensae, *J Cutan Pathol* 15:215, 1988.
369. McDaniel DH, Ash K, Zukowski M: Treatment of stretch marks with the 585-nm flash-lamp-pumped pulsed dye laser, *Dermatol Surg* 22:332, 1996.
370. Narurkar V, Haas A: The efficacy of the 585nm flash lamp pumped pulsed dye laser on striae distensae at various locations and etiologic factors, *Lasers Surg Med Suppl* 9:35, 1997.
371. Engel A, Johnson ML, Haynes SG: Health effects of sunlight exposure in the United States: results from the first national health and nutrition examination survey, 1971-1974, *Arch Dermatol* 124:72, 1988.
372. Sadick NS: Treatment of varicose and telangiectatic leg veins and hypertonic saline: a comparative study of heparin and saline, *J Dermatol Surg Oncol* 16:24, 1990.
373. Duffy DM: Small vessel sclerotherapy: an overview. In Callen JP et al, editors: *Advances in dermatology,* St Louis, 1988, Mosby.
374. Weiss RA, Weiss MA: Resolution of pain associated with varicose and telangiectatic leg veins after compression sclerotherapy, *J Dermatol Surg Oncol* 16:333, 1990.
375. Goldman MP, Kaplan RP, Duffy DM: Postsclerotherapy hyperpigmentation: a histologic evaluation, *J Dermatol Surg Oncol* 13:547, 1987.
376. Ouvry PA, Davy A: The sclerotherapy of telangiectasia, *Phlebologie* 35:349, 1982.
377. Tretbar LL: The origin of reflux in incompetent blue reticular/telangiectasia veins. In Davy R, Stemmer R, editors: *Phlebologie '89,* London, 1989, Libby Eurotext.
378. de Faria JL, Moraes IN: Histopathology of the telangiectasias associated with varicose veins, *Dermatologia* 127:321, 1963.
379. Wokalek H et al: Morphology and localization of sunburst varicosities: an electron microscopic and morphometric study, *J Dermatol Surg Oncol* 15:149, 1989.
380. Merelen JF: Telangiectasies rouges, telangiectasies bleues, *Phlebologie* 23:167, 1970.
381. Somjen GM:Anatomy of the superficial venous system, *Dermatol Surg* 21:35, 1995.
382. Weiss RA, Weiss MA: Doppler ultrasound findings in reticular veins of the thigh and subdermic lateral venous sytem and implications for sclerotherapy, *J Dermatol Surg Oncol* 19:947, 1993.
383. Sommer A, Van Mierlo PLH, Neumann HAM et al: Red and blue telangiectasia; differences in oxygenation? *Dermatol Surg* 23:55, 1997.
384. Bohler-Sommeregger K, Karmel F, Schuller-Petrovic S et al: Do telangiectases communicate with the deep venous system? *J Dermatol Surg Oncol* 18:403, 1992.

385. Thibault P, Bray A: Cosmetic leg veins: evaluation using duplex venous imaging, *J Dermatol Surg Oncol* 16:612, 1990.
386. Curri GB, Lo Brutto ME: Influenza dei mucopolisaccaridi e dei loro costituenti sulla neoformazione vascolare, *Rev Pat Clin Sper* 8:379, 1967.
387. Miller SS: Investigation and management of varicose veins, *Ann R Coll Surg Engl* 55:245, 1974.
388. Mullane DJ: Varicose veins of pregnancy, *Am J Obstet Gynecol* 63:620, 1952.
389. Goodrich SM, Wood JE: Peripheral venous distensibility and velocity of venous blood flow during pregnancy or during oral contraceptive therapy, *Am J Obstet Gynecol* 90:740, 1964.
390. Keates JS, Fitzgerald DE: An interim report on lower limb volume and blood flow changes during a normal menstrual cycle. Presented at 5th European Conference on Microcirculation, Gothenburg, 1968.
391. Davis LT, Duffy DM: Determination of incidence and risk factors for postsclerotherapy telangiectatic matting of the lower extremity: a retrospective analysis, *J Dermatol Surg Oncol* 16:327, 1990.
392. Braverman IM: Ultrastructure and organization of the cutaneous microvasculature in normal and pathologic states, *J Invest Dermatol* 93:2S, 1989.
393. Miami A, Rubertsi U: Collecting venules, *Minerva Cardioangiol* 41:541, 1958.
394. Braverman IM, Keh-Yen A: Ultrastructure of the human dermal microcirculation. IV. Valve-containing collecting veins at the dermal-subcutaneous junction, *J Invest Dermatol* 81:438, 1983.
395. Bodian EL: Sclerotherapy, *Semin Dermatol* 6:238, 1987.
396. Goldman MP: *Sclerotherapy: treatment of varicose and telangiectatic leg veins,* ed 2, St Louis, 1995, Mosby.
397. Apfelberg DB et al: Study of three laser systems for treatment of superficial varicosities of the lower extremity, *Lasers Surg Med* 7:219, 1987.
398. Frazzetta M, Palumbo FP, Bellisi M et al: Considerations regarding the use of the CO_2 laser: personal case study, *Laser* 2:4, 1989.
399. Lanthaler M et al: Laser therapy of venous lakes (Bean-Walsh) and telangiectasias, *Plast Reconstr Surg* 73:78, 1984.
400. Apfelberg DB, Maser MR, Lash H et al: Use of the argon and carbon dioxide lasers for treatment of superficial venous varicosities of the lower extremity, *Lasers Surg Med* 4:221, 1984.
401. Corcos L, Longo L: Classification and treatment of telangiectases of the lower limbs, *Laser* 1:22, 1988.
402. Tan OT, KerschmannR, Parrish JA: Effect of skin temperature on selective vascular injury caused by pulsed laser irradiation, *J Invest Dermatol* 85:441, 1985.
403. Adrian RM: Treatment of leg telangiectasias using a long-pulse frequency-doubled neodymium:YAG laser at 532 nm, *Dermatol Surg* 24:19, 1998.
404. Polla LL et al: Tunable pulsed dye laser for the treatment of benign cutaneous vascular ectasia, *Dermatologica* 174:11, 1987.
405. Ashton N: Corneal vascularization. In Duke-Elder S, Perkins ES, editors: *The transparency of the cornea,* Oxford, 1960, Blackwell.
406. Folkman J, Klagsbrun M: Angiogenic factors, *Science* 235:442, 1987.
407. Ryan TJ: Factors influencing the growth of vascular endothelium in the skin, *Br J Dermatol* 82 (suppl 5):99, 1970.
408. Dvorak HF: Tumors: wounds that do not heal. Similarities between tumor stroma generation and wound healing, *N Engl J Med* 315:1650, 1986.
409. Majewski S et al: Angiogenic capability of peripheral blood mononuclear cells in psoriasis, *Arch Dermatol* 121:1018, 1985.
410. Nakagawa H, Tan OT, Parrish JA: Ultrastructural changes in human skin after exposure to a pulsed laser, *J Invest Dermatol* 84:396, 1985.
411. Tan TT, Carney JM, Margolis R et al: Histologic responses of port-wine stains treated by argon, carbon dioxide, and tunable dye lasers: a preliminary report, *Arch Dermatol* 122:1016, 1986.
412. Goldman MP et al: Pulsed dye laser treatment of telangiectasia with and without subtherapeutic sclerotherapy: clinical and histologic examination in the rabbit ear vein model, *J Am Acad Dermatol* 23:23, 1990.

413. Goldman MP, Fitzpatrick RE: Pulsed-dye laser treatment of leg telangiectasia: with and without simultaneous sclerotherapy, *J Dermatol Surg Oncol* 16:338, 1990.
414. Fajardo LF et al: Hyperthermia inhibits angiogenesis, *Radiat Res* 114:297, 1988.
415. Hsia J, Lowery JA, Zelickson B: Treatment of leg telangiectasia using a long-pulse dye laser at 595 nm, *Lasers Surg Med* 20:1, 1997.
416. Lee PK, Lask GP: Treatment of leg veins by long pulse dye laser (Sclerolaser), *Lasers Surg Med Suppl* 9:40, 1997.
417. Anderson AR et al: The optics of human skin, *J Invest Dermatol* 77:13, 1981.
418. Schroeter CA, Wilder D, Reineke T et al: Clinical significance of an intense, pulsed light source on leg telangiectasias of up to 1mm diameter, *Eur J Dermatol* 7:38, 1997.
419. Goldman MP, Eckhouse S et al: Photothermal sclerosis of leg veins, *Dermatol Surg* 22:323, 1996.
420. Weiss RA, Weiss MA: Intense pulsed light revisited: progressive increase in pulse durations for better results on leg veins. Presented at 11th Annual Meeting of the North American Society of Phlebology, Palm Desert, Calif, November 1997.
421. Weiss RA, Weiss MA: Photothermal sclerosis of resistant telangiectatic leg and facial veins using the PhotoDerm VL. Presented at Annual Meeting of the Mexican Academy of Dermatology, Monterey, Mexico, April 1996.
422. Weiss RA, Weiss MA: Combination intense pulsed light and sclerotherapy: a synergistic effect. Presented at 11th Annual Meeting of the North American Society of Phlebology, Palm Desert, Calif, November 1997.
423. West TB, Alster TS: Comparison of the long-pulse dye (590-595 nm) and KTP (532 nm) lasers in the treatment of facial and leg telangiectasias, *Dermatol Surg* 24:221, 1998.
424. Bean WB, Walsh JR: Venous lakes, *Arch Dermatol* 74:459, 1956.
425. Pasyk KA: Case 5.27: venous lake at the lower lip. In Apfelberg DB, editor: *Atlas of cutaneous laser surgery,* New York, 1992, Raven.
426. Orenstein A: Case 5.28: venous lake of the lip. In Apfelberg DB, editor: *Atlas of cutaneous laser surgery,* New York, 1992, Raven.
427. Neumann RA, Knobler RM: Venous lakes (Bean-Walsh) of the lips: treatment experience with the argon laser and 18 months follow-up, *Clin Exp Dermatol* 15:115, 1990.
428. Alcalay J, Sandbank M: The ultrastructure of cutaneous venous lakes, *Int J Dermatol* 26:645, 1987.
429. Rosio TJ: Case 7.31: venous lake. In Apfelberg DB, editor: *Atlas of cutaneous laser surgery,* New York, 1992, Raven.
430. Rowson KEK, Mahy BWJ: Human papova (wart) virus, *Bacteriol Rev* 31:100, 1967.
431. Lever WF, Schaumberg-Lever G: Diseases caused by viruses. In WF Lever, editor: *Histopathology of the skin,* Philadelphia, 1983, Lippincott.
432. Nemeth AJ, Reyes BA: Copper vapor laser treatment of genital and body warts, *Lasers Surg Med* 10:52, 1990.
433. Webster GF, Satur N, Goldman MP et al: Treatment of recalcitrant warts using the pulsed dye laser, *Cutis* 56:230, 1996.
434. Tan OT, Hurwitz RM, Stafford TJ: Pulsed dye laser treatment of recalcitrant verrucae: a preliminary report, *Lasers Surg Med* 13:127, 1993.
435. Kauvar AB, McDanial DH, Geronemus RG: Pulsed dye laser treatment of warts, *Arch Fam Med* 4:1035, 1995.
436. Jacobsen E, McGraw R, McCagh S: Pulsed dye laser efficacy as initial therapy for warts and against recalcitrant verrucae, *Cutis* 59:206, 1997.
437. Jain A, Storwick GS: Effectiveness of the 585 nm flashlamp-pulsed tunable dye laser (PTDL) for treatment of plantar verrucae, *Laser Surg Med* 21:500, 1997.
438. Huilgol SC, Barlow RJ, Markey AC: Failure of pulsed dye laser therapy for resistant verrucae, *Clin Exp Dermatol* 21:93, 1996.
439. Ross BS, Levine VJ, Nehal K et al: Pulsed dye laser treatment of warts: a re-evaluation, *Lasers Surg Med Suppl* 9:42, 1997.
440. Stern P, Levine N: Controlled localized heat therapy in cutaneous warts, *Arch Dermatol* 128:945, 1992.
441. Diakuzono N, Joffe SN, Tajiri H et al: Laserthermia: a computer controlled contact Nd:YAG system for interstitial local hyperthermia, *Med Instrum* 21:275, 1987.
442. Pfau A, Abd-El-Raheem TA, Baumler W et al: Nd:YAG laser hyperthermia in the treatment of recalcitrant verrucae vulgares (Regensburg's technique), *Acta Derm Venereol (Stockh)* 74:212, 1994.

443. Pfau A, Abd-El-Raheem TA, Baumler W et al: Treatment of recalcitrant verrucae vulgares with Nd:Yag laser hyperthermia (Regensburg's technique): preliminary results in 31 cases, *J Dermatol Treat* 6:39, 1995.
444. Laor Y, Schwartz RA: Epidemiologic aspects of American Kaposi's sarcoma, *J Surg Oncol* 12:299, 1979.
445. Safai B, Good RA: Kaposi's sarcoma: a review and recent developments, *CA Cancer J Clin* 31:2, 1981.
446. Hymes KG, Cheurg T, Greene JB et al: Kaposi's sarcoma in homosexual men: a report of eight cases, *Lancet* 2:598, 1981.
447. Marmor M, Friedman-Kien AE, Zolla-Pazner S et al: Kaposi's sarcoma in homosexual men, *Ann Intern Med* 100:809, 1984.
448. Master SP, Taylor JF, Kyalwazi SK et al: Immunological studies in Kaposi's sarcoma in Uganda, *Br Med J* 1:600, 1970.
449. Kungu A, Gatei DG: Kaposi's sarcoma in Kenya, *Antibiot Chemother* 29:38, 1981.
450. Hoshaw RA, Schwartz RA: Kaposi's sarcoma after immunosuppressive therapy with prednisone, *Arch Dermatol* 116:1280, 1980.
451. Lo TCM, Salzman FA, Smedal MI et al: Radiotherapy for Kaposi's sarcoma, *Cancer* 45:684, 1980.
452. Solan AJ, Greenwald ES, Silvay O: Long-term complete remissions of Kaposi's sarcoma with vinblastine therapy, *Cancer* 47:637, 1981.
453. Odom RB, Goette DK: Treatment of cutaneous Kaposi's sarcoma with intralesional vincristine, *Arch Dermatol* 114:1693, 1978.
454. Krown SE, Real FX, Cunningham-Rundles S et al: Preliminary observations on the effect of recombinant leukocyte A interferon in homosexual men with Kaposi's sarcoma, *N Engl J Med* 308:1071, 1983.
455. Hiza PR: Surgical treatment of Kaposi's sarcoma, *Antibiot Chemother* 29:70, 1981.
456. Goldman L, Wilson R, Hornby P et al: Laser radiation of malignancy in man, *Cancer* 18:533, 1965.
457. Wheeland RG, Balin R, Norris MJ: Argon laser photocoagulative therapy of Kaposi's sarcoma: a clinical and histologic evaluation, *J Dermatol Surg Oncol* 11:1180, 1985.
458. Rosenfeld H: Case 6.11: Kaposi's sarcoma, upper eyelid. In Apfelberg DB, editor: *Atlas of cutaneous laser surgery,* New York, 1992, Raven.
459. Tappero JW, Grekin RC, Zanelli GA et al: Pulsed-dye laser therapy for cutaneous Kaposi's sarcoma associated with acquired immunodeficiency syndrome, *J Am Acad Dermatol* 27:526, 1992.
460. Marchell N, Alster TS: Successful treatment of cutaneous Kaposi's sarcoma by the 585-nm pulsed dye laser, *Dermatol Surg* 23:973, 1997.
461. Ciatti S, Varga J, Greenbaum SS: The 585 nm flashlamp-pumped pulsed dye laser for the treatment of telangiectases in patients with scleroderma, *J Am Acad Dermatol* 35:487, 1996.
462. Nunez M, Miralles ES, Boixeda P et al: Pulsed dye laser treatment of cutaneous vascular lesions of CREST syndrome, *J Dermatol Treatment* 5:219, 1994.
463. Nunez M, Boixeda P: Pulsed dye laser treatment of telangiectatic chronic erythema of cutaneous lupus erythematosus, *Arch Dermatol* 132:354, 1996.
464. Thornton CM, Eichenfield LF, Shinall EA et al: Cutaneous telangiectases in neonatal lupus erythematosus, *J Am Acad Dermatol* 33:19, 1995.
465. Nunez M, Boixeda P, Miralles ES et al: Pulsed dye laser treatment for lupus erythematosus telangiectoides, *Br J Dermatol* 133:1010, 1995.
466. Zachariae H, Bjerring P, Cramers M: Argon laser treatment of cutaneous vascular lesions in connective tissue diseases, *Acta Derm Venerol (Stockh)* 68:179, 1988.
467. James DG: Sarcoidosis of the skin. In Fitzpatrick TB, Wolff K, Freedberg IM et al, editors: *Dermatology in general medicine,* ed 3, New York, 1987, McGraw-Hill.
468. Shaw M, Black MM, Davis PKB: Disfiguring lupus pernio successfully treated with plastic surgery, *Clin Dermatol* 9:614, 1984.
469. Goodman MM, Alpern K: Treatment of lupus pernio with the flashlamp pulsed dye laser, *Lasers Surg Med* 12:549, 1992.
470. Mordovtsev VN, Alanova VI: Morphology of skin microvasculature in psoriasis, *Am J Dermatopathol* 11:33, 1989.
471. Folkman J: Angiogenesis in psoriasis: therapeutic implications, *J Invest Dermatol* 59:40, 1972.

472. Telner P, Fekete Z: The capillary responses in psoriatic skin, *J Invest Dermatol* 36:225, 1961.
473. Sackstein R, Falanga V, Streilein JW et al: Lymphocyte adhesion to psoriatic dermal endothelium is mediated by a tissue-specific receptor/ligand interaction, *J Invest Dermatol* 91:423, 1988.
474. Creamer D, Allen MH, Sousa A et al: Localization of endothelial proliferation and microvascular expansion in active plaque psoriasis, *Br J Dermatol* 136:859, 1997.
475. Bolton S, editor: *Pharmaceutical statistics: practical and clinical applications,* New York, 1990, Marcel Dekker.
476. Zelickson BD, Mehregan DA, Wendelschfer-Crabb G et al: Clinical and histologic evaluation of psoriatic plaques treated with a flashlamp pulsed dye laser, *J Am Acad Dermatol* 35:64, 1996.
477. Ros AM, Garden JM, Bakus AD: Psoriasis response to the pulsed dye laser, *Lasers Surg Med* 19:331, 1996.
478. Alster TS, Nanni CA: Successful treatment of porokeratosis with 585 nm pulsed dye laser irradiation, *J Am Acad Dermatol,* 1998.
479. Goltz RW, Peterson WC, Gorlin RJ et al: Focal dermal hypoplasia, *Arch Dermatol* 86:708, 1962.
480. Temple IK, MacDowall P, Baraitser M et al: Focal dermal hypoplasia (Goltz syndrome), *J Med Genet* 27:180, 1990.
481. Boothroyd AE, Hall CM: Radiological features of Goltz syndrome: focal dermal hypoplasia: a report of two cases, *Skeletal Radiol* 17:505, 1988.
482. Alster TS, Wilson F: Focal dermal hypoplasia (Goltz's syndrome): treatment of cutaneous lesions with the 585-nm flashlamp-pumped pulsed dye laser, *Arch Dermatol* 131:143, 1995.
483. Imperial RH, Helwig EB: Angiokeratoma: a clinicopathological study, *Arch Dermatol* 95:166, 1967.
484. Occella C, Bleidl D, Rampini P et al: Argon laser treatment of cutaneous multiple angiokeratomas, *Dermatol Surg* 21:170,1995.
485. Altman J, Mehregan AH: Inflammatory linear verrucose epidermal nevus, *Arch Dermatol* 104:385, 1971.
486. Alster TS: Inflammatory linear verrucous epidermal nevus: successful treatment with the 585 nm flashlamp-pumped pulsed dye laser, *J Am Acad Dermatol* 31:513, 1994.
487. Lever WF, Schaumburg-Lever G: *Histopathology of the skin,* ed 7, Philadelphia, 1990, Lippincott.
488. Orenstein A, Nelson JS: Treatment of facial vascular lesions with a 100-μm spot 577-nm pulsed continuous wave dye laser, *Ann Plast Surg* 23:310, 1989.
489. Hoffman SJ, Walsh P, Morelli F: Treatment of angiofibroma with the pulsed tunable dye laser, *J Am Acad Dermatol* 29:790, 1993.
490. Arndt DA: Adenoma sebaceum: successful treatment with the argon laser, *Plast Reconstr Surg* 70:91, 1982.
491. Pasyk KA, Argenta LC: Argon laser surgery of skin lesions in tuberous sclerosis, *Ann Plast Surg* 20:426, 1988.
492. Janniger CK, Goldberg DJ: Angiofibromas in tuberous sclerosis: comparison and treatment by carbon dioxide and argon laser, *J Dermatol Surg Oncol* 16:317, 1990.
493. Wheeland RG, Bailin PL, Kantor GR et al: Treatment of adenoma sebaceum with carbon dioxide laser vaporization, *J Dermatol Surg Oncol* 11:861, 1985.
494. Weston J, Apfelberg DB, Maser MR et al: Carbon dioxide laserabrasion for treatment of adenoma sebaceum in tuberous sclerosis, *Ann Plast Surg* 15:132, 1985.
495. Spenter CW, Achauer BM, Vander Kam VM: Treatment of extensive adenoma sebaceum with a carbon dioxide laser, *Ann Plast Surg* 20:586, 1988.
496. Kaufman AJ, Grekin RC, Geisse JK et al: Treatment of adenoma sebaceum with the copper vapor laser, *J Am Acad Dermatol* 33:770, 1995.
497. Mills CM, Lanigan SW: Treatment of multiple angiofibromata with the pulsed dye laser, *J Dermatol Treat* 6:237, 1995.
498. Chun SI, Ji HG: Kimura's disease and angiolymphoid hyperplasia with eosinophilia: clinical and histopathologic differences, *J Am Acad Dermatol* 27:954, 1992.
499. Cheney ML, Googe P, Bhatt S, Hibberd PL: Angiolymphoid hyperplasia with eosinophilia (histiocytoid hemangioma): evaluation of treatment options, *Ann Otol Rhinol Laryngol* 103:303, 1993.

500. Nelson DA, Jarratt M: Angiolymphoid hyperplasia with eosinophilia, *Pediatr Dermatol* 1:210, 1984.
501. Bunse T, Kuhn A, Groth W, Mahrle G: Angiolymphoid hyperplasia with eosinophilia, *Hautarzt* 44:225, 1993.
502. Lertzman BH, McMeekin T, Gaspari AA: Pulsed dye laser treatment of angiolymphoid hyperplasia with eosinophilia lesions, *Arch Dermatol* 133:920, 1997.
503. Jones EW, Orkin M: Tufted angioma (angioblastoma), *J Am Acad Dermatol* 20:214, 1989.
504. Frenk E, Vion B, Merlot Y et al: Tufted angioma, *Dermatologica* 181:242, 1990.
505. Bernstein EF, Kantor G, Howe N et al: Tufted angioma of the thigh, *J Am Acad Dermatol* 31:307, 1994.
506. Drosner M, Vogt HJ: Xanthelasma palpebrarum: Behandlug mit dem Argonlaser, *H G* 67:144, 1992.
507. Schonermark MP, Raulin C: Treatment of xanthelasma palpebrarum with the pulsed dye laser, *Lasers Surg Med* 19:336, 1996.
508. Kilmer SL, Chotzen VA: Pulse dye laser treatment of rhytids, *Lasers Surg Med Suppl* 9:44, 1997.

CHAPTER three

Treatment of Benign Pigmented Cutaneous Lesions

Suzanne Linsmeier Kilmer, Mitchel P. Goldman, and Richard E. Fitzpatrick

Patients consider a number of benign pigmented cutaneous lesions objectionable because of their color, size, number, or location. Epidermal pigmented lesions include lentigines, café-au-lait macules, ephelides, junctional nevi, nevi spilus, and seborrheic keratoses. Dermal pigmented lesions include blue nevi, nevi of Ota or Ito, traumatic and decorative tattoos (see Chapter 4), and postsclerotherapy hyperpigmentation. Some pigmented lesions, such as melasma, postinflammatory hyperpigmentation, Becker nevi, and compound nevi, have both an epidermal and a dermal component.

The most common treatment approach for many epidermal lesions is to use a destructive modality to remove the epidermis containing the unwanted lesion. Cryosurgery with liquid nitrogen is frequently used successfully to treat individual lesions. A mild acid, such as trichloroacetic acid (TCA), is often employed to peel larger epidermal lesions. Although satisfactory results typically occur, these treatments are problematic because of possible resultant hypopigmentation, hyperpigmentation, atrophy, scarring, and frequent recurrence. Chemical depigmenting agents, such as hydroquinone, which produces reversible inhibition of the enzymatic oxidation of tyrosine to dopa in melanocytes, can induce epidermal depigmentation, which unfortunately can be permanent and might not remain localized to the lesion.

Treatment of dermal lesions by destructive agents frequently causes scarring, and thus they have not been amenable to treatment except by surgical excision. Because treatment of these pigmented lesions is often done for cosmetic reasons, it must be effective and also free from the adverse sequelae of scarring and permanent dyspigmentation as much as possible. Therefore selectively targeting of the pigment-containing cells is preferable.

MECHANISM OF ACTION: SELECTIVE PHOTOTHERMOLYSIS

Selective destruction of human epidermis with lasers using melanin as the target chromophore was first demonstrated by Goldman and colleagues[1,2] in the early 1960s using a normal-mode ruby laser (wavelength 694 nm, pulse width 500 μsec). Subsequent studies by this same group using a Q-switched ruby laser with a 50-nsec pulse width showed the threshold radiant exposure to be 10 to 100 times lower, suggesting a more selective effect of the shorter pulse width.[3] For the next 20 years this work was largely ignored, with attention focused primarily on argon and carbon dioxide (CO_2) lasers. Successful treatment of pigmented lesions was reported using the argon laser[4] (488 and 514 nm, continuous wave [CW]), the CO_2 laser[5]

(10,600 nm, CW), and the neodymium:yttrium-aluminum-garnet (Nd:YAG) laser[6] (1064 nm, CW) as a form of thermal cautery, with melanin an absorptive target (argon) or interacting in a nonspecific manner (CO_2 and Nd:YAG).

When Anderson and Parrish[7] elucidated their theory of selective photothermolysis, they redirected attention to the concept of treating a *specific* target with *specific* laser parameters: wavelength, pulse width, and energy level. Wavelength is chosen to limit absorption to a specific target chromophore. Thermal damage is then confined to that target by limiting the pulse width to less than the thermal relaxation time of the target chromophore to avoid thermal diffusion beyond the intended target (Figures 3-1 and 3-2; see also Figure 2-1). Once laser energy is confined to the specific target, threshold energy levels can be determined to achieve a desired effect.

Melanin, which is most concentrated in the basal layer of the epidermis, has a broad absorption spectrum, being most intense in the ultraviolet (UV) range, then dropping off through the visible to the near-infrared (IR) spectra. Melanin is densely packed within melanosomes, which are found within melanocytes and keratinocytes. Selective injury to melanosomes and pigmented cells occurs with high-intensity pulsed light at various wavelengths across this spectrum: 351, 355, 435, 488, 504, 530, 532, 560, 590, 625, 694, 720, 750, and 1064 nm.[8,15] Across this wide range of wavelengths, melanosomal alterations are qualitatively similar but different in threshold dose and depth of penetration into the dermis. Shorter wavelengths require less energy to damage the pigment cell, whereas greater energy is required for longer wavelengths because the absorption coefficient (μa) for melanin decreases as the wavelength increases (0.12 J/cm^2 at 351 nm, 0.3 J/cm^2 at 694 nm). Longer wavelengths penetrate more deeply and more effectively target pigmented cells at greater dermal depths. Wavelengths in the 351- to 532-nm range are also absorbed by hemoglobin and therefore induce purpura in superficial capillaries.

With endogenous pigmented epidermal lesions the target is the *melanosome,* the cellular organelle containing the pigment melanin. The melanosome measures approximately 1×0.5 to 0.75 μm in diameter and has a thermal relaxation time estimated to be 10 to 100 nsec.[8,16-20] One study demonstrated that any pulse width less than 1 μsec is capable of causing selective melanosomal damage,[9] and femtosecond pulses[8,10,21-23] are required to produce ultraselective melanosomal injury without cytoplasmic or nuclear damage. Watanabe et al[22] evaluated the histologic effect of 694-nm, 630-nm, and 532-nm wavelengths in various pulse widths as short as 6.5×10^{-14} sec on albino and black guinea pig skin. They found melanosomal injury to be independent of pulse width at these wavelengths as long as the pulse width is below 1 μsec. Therefore 1 μsec appears to be the effective thermal relaxation time of the melanosome. However, the shorter the pulse width, the more localized is the damage. When the pulse width approaches the melanosome's thermal relaxation time, greater radiant exposures are necessary for its rupture. Melanosomal injury leads to degeneration and lysis of the cells containing this organelle, the melanocytes and keratinocytes.[8]

When the pulse width significantly exceeds the thermal relaxation time of the melanosome, no ultrastructural evidence indicates melanosomal disruption even at exposure levels that cause gross injury. Instead, generalized damage occurs to surrounding organelles and cells, presumably secondary to the dissipation of heat from melanosomes during the long 400-μsec pulses used.[9,23,24] In addition, threshold radiant exposures were found to increase when the pulse width exceeded the thermal relaxation time of melanosomes[22]; to achieve the same peak temperatures, longer pulse widths require deposition of more energy to make up for heat diffusing into the surrounding tissue. Conversely, when the pulse width is less than 1 μsec, melanosome damage is thought to occur from heat absorption, as well as shock waves or cavitation from the rapid thermal expansion.[11,25,26] The degree of injury at higher exposures correlates with pigment content.[22] In contrast, the pigment cell's

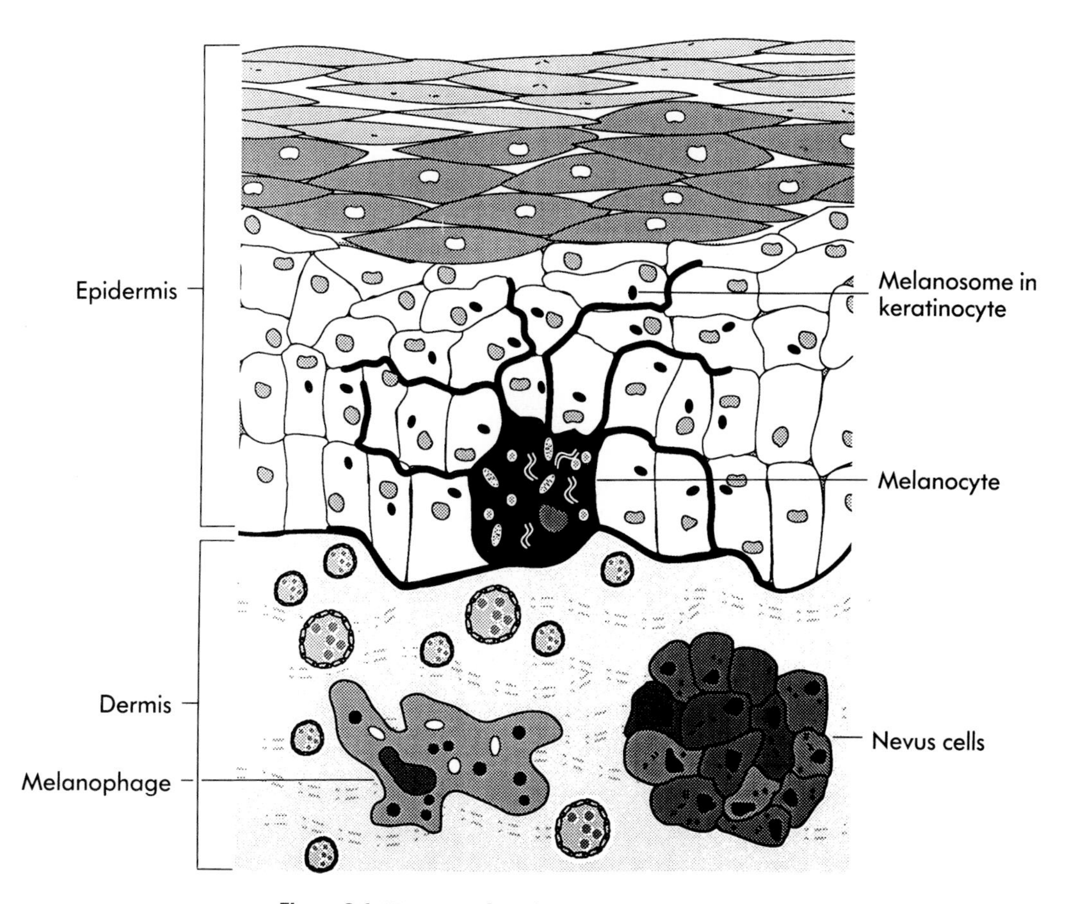

Figure 3-1 Nonvascular pigment targets in cutis.

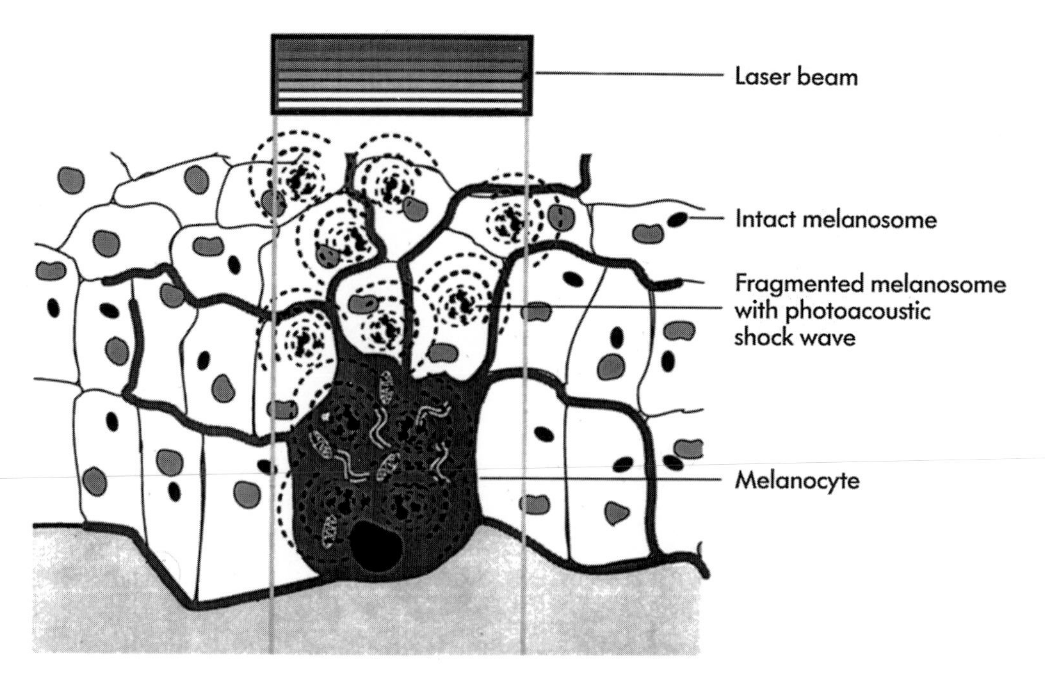

Figure 3-2 Vaporization/fragmentation of melanosome-containing melanocyte and epidermal cells.

damage threshold varies inversely with the pigment content,[12] and interestingly, subthreshold energy may result in pigment stimulation.[10-12,21-26]

In addition, the extent of pigment incontinence from laser treatment is correlated with pulse duration. Pulse durations of 500 nsec result in more marked, deeper, and aggregated pigment granules than 100-nsec pulse durations.[27,28] Pigment incontinence at these longer pulse durations may be caused by macrophage stimulation, phagocytizing disrupted melanosomes and migrating to the dermis.[28] The lowest pulse duration studied (100 nsec) produced the least amount of pigment incontinence. Therefore the ideal[27] pigment lesion dye laser (PLDL) for superficial lesions would have a wavelength of about 504 nm and a pulse duration of 100 to 150 nsec or shorter. Deeper lesions require longer wavelengths to aid penetration into the dermis but also require greater fluences to make up for the lower absorption coefficient.

The immediately observable clinical effect of laser interaction with a pigmented lesion treated at the proper threshold irradiance is whitening of the lasered tissue. This represents a sudden increase in light scattering secondary to the thermal and mechanical events associated with energy deposition in the melanosome[9] (Figure 3-3). Kilmer et al[29] infer that the scattering is secondary to cavitation followed by nitrogen gas bubble formation, which slowly dissipates back into tissue,[30] similar to "the bends" phenomenon associated with scuba diving.

When energies greater than the clinical threshold for immediate whitening are used, pinpoint bleeding and epidermal exfoliation are seen clinically. This produces damage to pigment and epidermal cells, resulting in epidermal sloughing followed by transient hypopigmentation with healing. Repigmentation occurs from residual melanocytes in adnexal structures and from migration of undamaged epidermal melanocytes peripheral to the treatment site.[14] Interestingly, repigmentation occurs faster at wavelengths above 435 nm,[13-15,30] supporting the theory that deeper penetration by longer wavelengths may stimulate follicular melanocytes to repopulate and pigment the healing epidermis.[14] In addition, direct melanocytic stimulation has been demonstrated to occur at subthreshold exposure doses in experimental animals[13,14] and humans.[31] Subthreshold and near-threshold exposures of 1.5 to 2.5 J/cm^2 appear to mildly stimulate melanogenesis in humans, especially with untanned skin. More

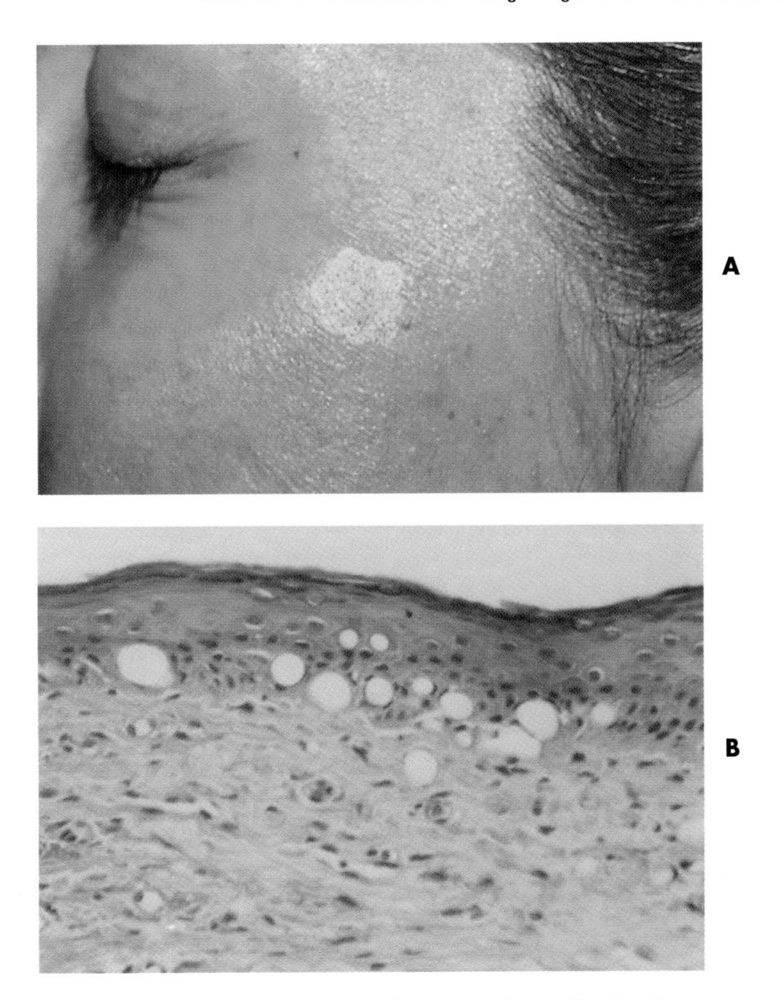

Figure 3-3 **A,** Lentigo simplex in 30-year-old woman immediately after treatment with PLDL at 2.25 J/cm². **B,** Histologic examination demonstrates vacuolization of pigmented cells throughout epidermis, primarily at dermal-epidermal junction and most superior aspect of superficial dermis. Adjacent superficial dermal capillaries, as well as remaining epidermal and dermal structures, appear unaltered. (Hematoxylin-eosin; ×400.)

often noted when treating melasma, lentigines, and café-au-lait macules with the PLDL at fluences of 2.25 J/cm², melanogenesis has not been seen with subthreshold radiant exposures for tattoo treatments with the Q-switched ruby, Nd:YAG, and alexandrite lasers. "Laser tanning" has been hypothesized to result from interference with feedback inhibition of melanogenesis, stimulation of tyrosinase activity, or release of intracellular or extracellular melanocyte-stimulating factors. This phenomenon is independent of postinflammatory hyperpigmentation.

Histologic evaluation of PLDL-treated lesions confirms the principle of selective photothermolysis.[21] At fluences of 2.5 J/cm² and lower, selective vacuolization of melanin-containing cells occur with displacement of melanin to the cell periphery, producing ring cells[10,14] (Figure 3-3). At energies of 2.0 to 2.5 J/cm², nonpigmented epidermal keratinocytes are selectively spared, and only neighboring melanocytes appear vacuolated. With increasing energy the number of vacuoles increases, eventually forming vesicles. Laser energies above 2.5 J/cm² may result in suprabasilar separation (Figure 3-4) and even epidermal necrosis, but no evidence of dermal necrosis has been noted.[21]

As noted previously, the laser targets melanocytes and keratinocytes. Even if damage is restricted to the melanosome, the entire melanocyte is killed in the process.

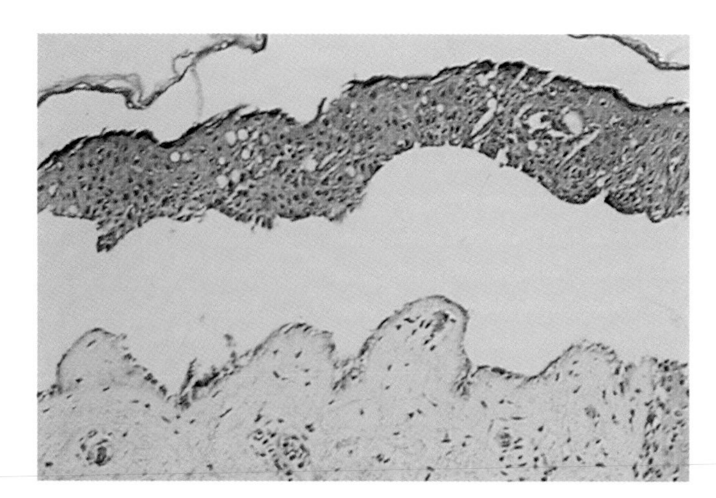

Figure 3-4 Becker nevus on right lateral cheek of 22-year-old Asian man treated with PLDL at 3 J/cm^2. Biopsy was done immediately after treatment. Note complete separation of epidermis at dermal-epidermal junction. No significant epidermal or dermal necrosis is seen. Superficial epidermal capillaries appear unaltered. Some vacuolization has occurred in pigmented epidermal cells.

Keratinocytes contain most of the melanin in the epidermis and are also easily destroyed. In fact, the melanocytes may be completely devoid of pigment, having transferred all their pigment granules to the overlying keratinocytes, which may explain a lesion's recurrence, because the cells synthesizing the pigment are still viable.

Low fluences are useful in maximizing the selectivity of lasers with a strong hemoglobin absorbance (e.g., PLDL, fd Nd:YAG) by reducing purpura but still result in complete removal of lesions. Increasing the fluence to 3.5 J/cm^2 leads to more purpura but with more epidermal necrosis, allowing lesions with a thick epidermal component, such as seborrheic keratoses, to be more effectively treated. In this situation one can wipe off the thickened epidermis with saline-saturated gauze and retreat the lesion if persistent keratosis remains.

The remainder of this chapter discusses the various pigmented entities amenable to laser treatment. Lesions are grouped according to their location in the epidermis, dermis, or in both.

EPIDERMAL LESIONS

Epidermal lesions are amenable to treatment with multiple modalities because of their superficial location; virtually all injuries confined to the epidermis heal without scarring. The PLDL, Q-switched ruby, frequency-doubled (fd) Nd:YAG (532 nm), and alexandrite lasers are often used when more conservative treatment modalities are unsuccessful (Figure 3-5). Even though less penetrating, the shorter wavelengths are particularly useful because their greater melanin absorption best targets the superficial pigment containing keratinocytes and melanocytes. Thus the 510-nm (PLDL), 532-nm (fd Nd:YAG), and 694-nm (ruby) wavelengths are best suited, followed by the 755-nm (alexandrite) and, least effective, the 1064-nm wavelength.

Lentigines

Lentigines are small, irregular but sharply marginated brown macules that may occur on any cutaneous surface, including mucous membranes. They usually average a few millimeters in diameter but can enlarge to a few centimeters.

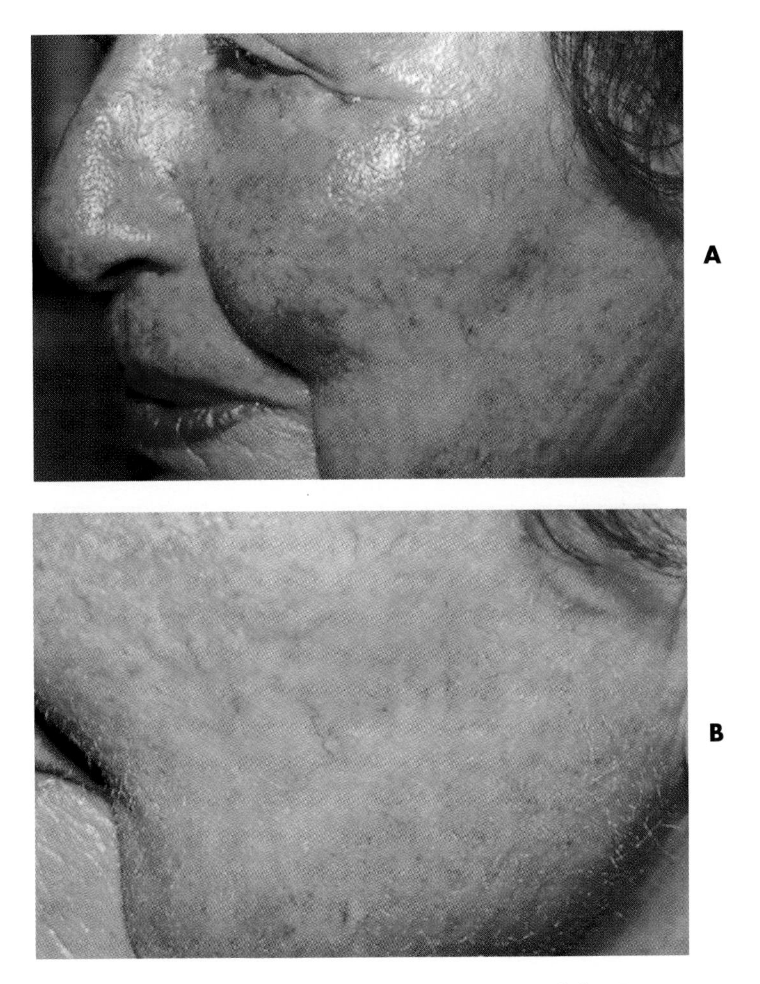

Figure 3-5 Lentigo on cheek of 72-year-old woman persisted despite treatment with liquid nitrogen, 35% trichloroacetic acid (TCA) medium-depth peeling, and combination of liquid nitrogen and 35% TCA. **A,** Before laser treatment. **B,** Eight weeks after treatment with PLDL at 2.5 J/cm^2.

Lentigo simplex is the common form of lentigo. It often arises in childhood without a predilection for sun-exposed skin. Pigmentation is usually uniform throughout the lesion, varying from light brown to black. Histologically these lesions have elongated rete ridges that extend into the underlying papillary dermis. The basal cell layer of the epidermis often shows hypermelanosis with an increased number of basal melanocytes.[32]

Solar lentigo (lentigo senilis) is an acquired lentigo resulting from sun exposure. These lesions increase in number with advancing age and are usually related to the extent of past sun exposure. Their histologic appearance is similar to that of lentigo simplex. They are not premalignant.

Lentigines can also be a component of different cutaneous syndromes, including lentiginosis profusa, Peutz-Jeghers syndrome, Moynahan syndrome, and leopard (multiple lentigines) syndrome. In these syndromes the histology of the lentigo is identical to a normal lentigo simplex or slightly different, with the finding that basal melanocytes are not always increased in number as with other lentigines. In addition, in Peutz-Jeghers syndrome the melanosomes are deeply melanized. Giant macromelanosomes are found in the cells of the leopard syndrome.

With one PLDL (510 nm) treatment on 29 patients with 432 lentigines, using an average fluence of 2.1 J/cm^2, 48% completely cleared (Figure 3-6), 33% were improved by 75% or more, and the remaining 19% were approximately 50% lighter

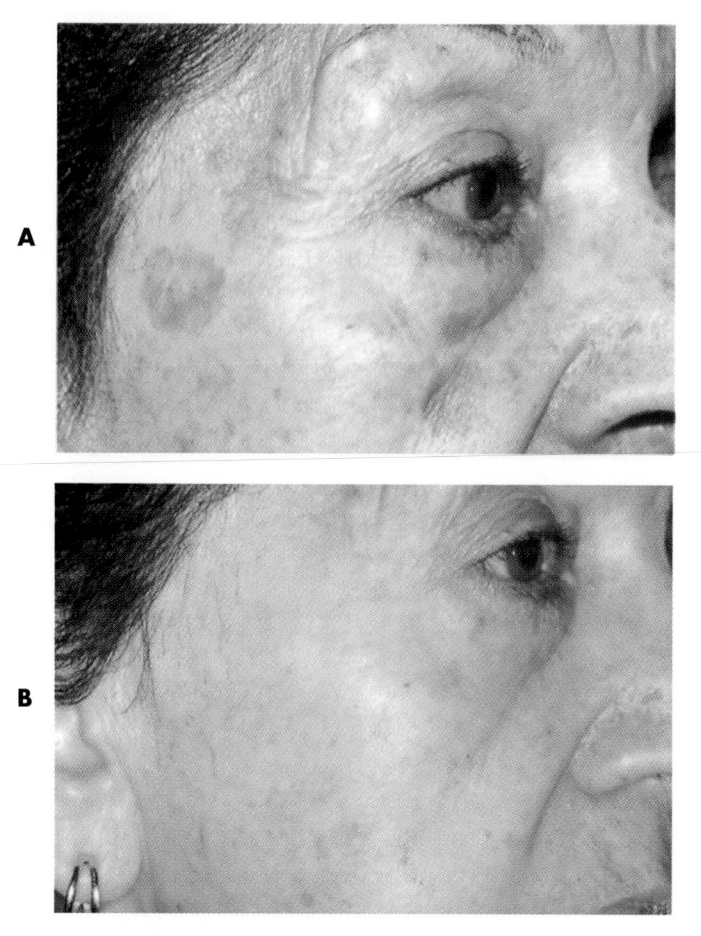

Figure 3-6 **A,** Multiple lentigo simplex on face of 70-year-old woman did not respond to previous liquid nitrogen cryotherapy and 30% TCA chemical peeling. **B,** After three separate treatments with PLDL at 2.25 J/cm^2 × 29 pulses, 2.5 J/cm^2 × 40 pulses, and 2.75 J/cm^2 × 30 pulses. Treatments were 1 month apart.

than their original color. All lesions cleared, usually with two treatment sessions, and no adverse responses were noted. Tan et al[33] treated 29 lentigines with the PLDL at fluences 2.0 to 3.5 J/cm^2 and noted that 2.2 to 2.5 treatments were required for complete clearing. Grekin et al[34] report a similar experience, with 58% to 89% of lesions clearing in one to four treatments with PLDL treatment at fluences ranging from 2.0 to 3.75 J/cm^2. Interestingly, they noted an increased efficacy of treatment of face and hand lesions compared with arm and truncal lentigines, and those on the leg did not uniformly respond to PLDL treatment even at fluences of 4.0 J/cm^2.[34,35]

Q-switched ruby[36-38] and fd Nd:YAG[29] lasers provide excellent results with only transient hypopigmentation. The latter is associated with purpura and more erythema, secondary to its absorption by hemoglobin. Both provide excellent results, usually with a single treatment. Use of longer-pulsed ruby[39] and alexandrite lasers for hair removal has been associated with removal of lentigines and freckles in the treatment area. Further studies with these lasers are underway.

Kilmer et al[29] demonstrated equivalent efficacy with the fd Q-switched Nd:YAG laser (532 nm, 5-10 nsec) in treating epidermal lesions, and many cleared with a single treatment. The ruby laser also successfully treats lentigines. Although only 33% (4 of 12) of lesions improved at a fluence of 20 to 40 J/cm^2 with a pulse duration of 2 msec,[40] the Q-switched ruby laser is more efficacious, clearing labial lentigines in one or two treatments with a fluence of 10 J/cm^2 and a pulse duration of

40 nsec.[41] Several recent articles attest to its excellent ability to target superficial as well as deeper lesions.[38] The alexandrite laser is similarly effective.

Labial Melanotic Macules

Labial melanotic macules (LMMs) occur in up to 3% of normal persons but predominantly in young women on the lower lip.[42] Most often seen as isolated lesions, they may be part of the Langier-Hunziker syndrome, which is associated with oral mucosal melanotic macules and melanonychia striata.[43] Lesions appear as uniform or irregularly pigmented brown macules.

The differential diagnosis of these lesions includes lentigo maligna, superficial spreading malignant melanoma, ephelides, melanocytic nevi, venous lake, dental amalgam tattoo, or, as a component of Peutz-Jeghers syndrome, Addison disease, Albright syndrome, or neurofibromatosis.[44]

Histologically, parakeratosis and rarely hyperkeratosis is present, overlying pigmented and nonpigmented portions of the lesion. Epithelial acanthosis may also occur. The rete ridges are not elongated as in other forms of lentigines. Although nevoid melanocytes and cellular atypia are absent,[45] melanin is significantly increased in the basal layer, and melanophages may be found in the dermal papillae.[46] Immunohistochemical studies support their benign nature.[44]

Similar to lentigines found on sun-exposed skin, labial lentigines respond to one or two treatments with any of the Q-switched lasers.

Ephelides

The ephelis, or freckle, is a common, small, tan-brown macule that occurs on sun-exposed skin and increases in color in response to sunlight. It is not found on mucous membranes. Ephelides appear early in childhood and increase in number during the summer (Figure 3-7). Their incidence decreases with age. Freckles are more prominent in people of Celtic descent, especially those with red hair. Axillary freckling, the only type that appears in non-sun-exposed skin, is seen in von Recklinghausen disease (neurofibromatosis).

Histologically an ephelis shows normal epidermis without elongation or branching of the rete ridges, as occurs in lentigines. Hypermelanization is generally confined to the basal cell layer. The total number of basal melanocytes does not increase, but melanosomes and melanocytes are larger and more active.[47,48]

Treatment of ephelides usually consists of sunscreen application and sun avoidance. Alpha-hydroxy acids and tretinoin can also diminish freckling if applied regularly. When requested for cosmetic purposes, the PDPL, Q-switched ruby, alexandrite, and fd Nd:YAG[29] lasers would be expected to treat these lesions as well. Reexposure without adequate sun protection stimulates recurrence and new ephelides.

Seborrheic Keratoses

Seborrheic keratoses are common benign epidermal proliferations that may appear unsightly and at times become irritated by clothing or physical activity. They may also itch independent of trauma. There appears to be an inherited autosomal dominant pattern in 50% of patients.[49]

Clinically, seborrheic keratoses evolve from light-yellow, smooth macules to verrucous pigmented papules or plaques. They increase in width and depth with time. Several histopathologic variants of seborrheic keratoses occur. The *acantholytic* type

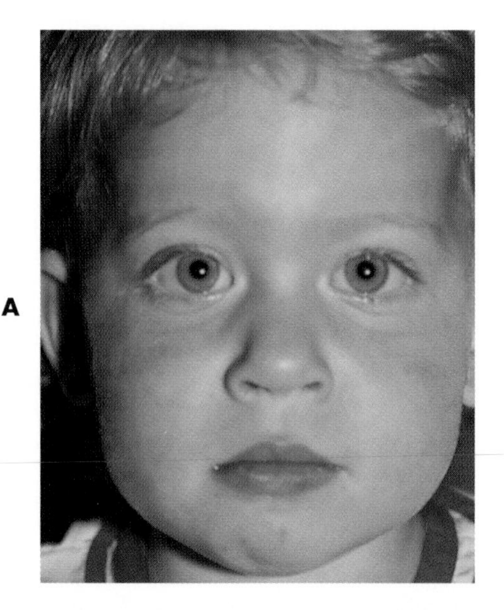

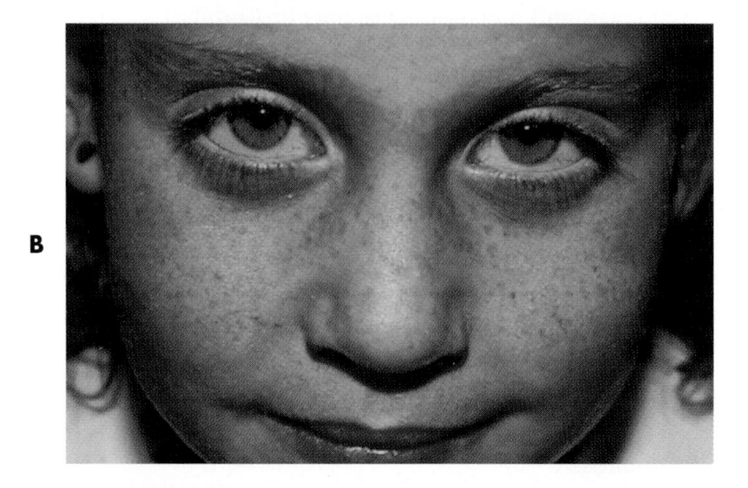

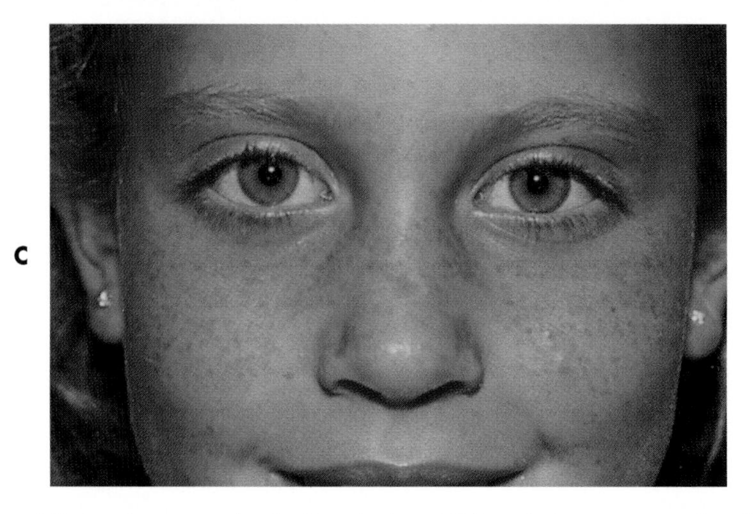

Figure 3-7 Development of ephelides during childhood. **A,** At 19 months of age. No evidence of ephelides. **B,** At 7 years of age, in January. Note extensive number of ephelides. **C,** Nine months later after summer sun exposure, even with daily application of SPF (sun protection factor) 29 sunscreen. Note only slight increase in number of ephelides, which are slightly darker in appearance.

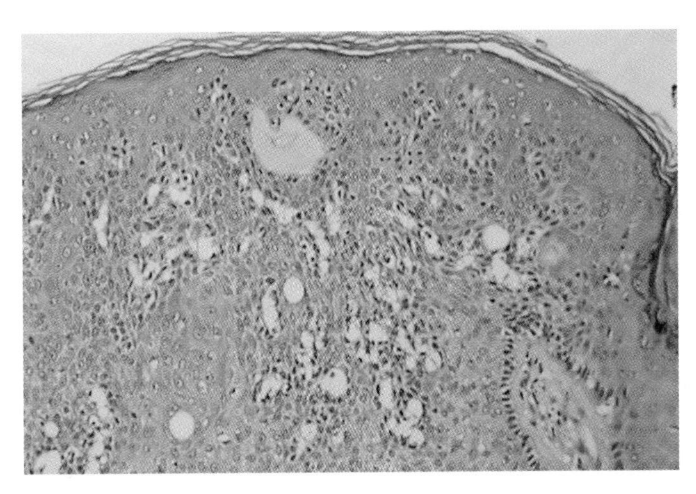

Figure 3-8 Biopsy specimen from patient with seborrheic keratosis immediately after treatment with PLDL at 2.5 J/cm^2. Note vacuolization of cells, or ring cells, throughout entire thickness of the lesion. (Hematoxylin-eosin; ×200.)

is most common, consisting of interweaving bands of keratinocytes associated with variable amounts of increased epidermal pigmentation. The *hyperkeratotic* type has elongated dermal papillae with pigmentation throughout the lesion's epidermal cells. The adenoid type may arise from lentigines and is usually flat in appearance.[50]

Because seborrheic keratoses do not spontaneously regress and may regrow after incomplete removal, patients seek treatment, especially for lesions in areas of cosmetic significance or when traumatized by clothing. Treatment usually consists of light electrodesiccation, liquid nitrogen cryosurgery, superficial curettage, or shave excision. All these treatment modalities may result in pigmentary changes, especially hypopigmentation. Rarely, hypertrophic scarring may result, as with any superficial surgical procedure. Seborrheic keratoses respond similarly to the lasers discussed for lentigines, but thicker lesions may require additional treatments. Histologic examination after PLDL treatment showed vacuolization of melanin-containing cells to at least 1 mm in depth (Figure 3-8). After two treatments, 75% of the lesions were completely clear and the remaining 25% were more than 75% clear. No scarring occurred, but 33% developed a shadowlike hyperpigmentation that resolved within 4 to 6 months.

The normal-mode ruby laser used at 20 to 40 J/cm^2 with a pulse duration of 2 msec cleared 9 of 12 of seborrheic keratoses.[40] An additional report with the ruby laser at 4 J/cm^2 demonstrated complete clearance after three treatments, but with hypopigmentation.[51] The argon laser at 1.7 W, 1-mm spot diameter, and 0.02-sec pulses is also effective but produces hypopigmentation.[52]

Café-au-lait Macules

Café-au-lait macules (CALMs) are light-tan to brown hypermelanotic flat lesions, 2 to 20 cm in diameter, that are sharply demarcated from surrounding normal skin.[53] Found in up to 13.8% of the population, CALMs may appear at birth or soon thereafter and increase in number over the first two decades of life.[54] This lesion may be found in several syndromes, including von Recklinghausen disease, Albright syndrome, and Marfan syndrome, and may be present in a greater percentage of patients with juvenile xanthogranulomas.[55]

Histologically, hypermelanosis is present in the basal layer of the epidermis in melanocytes and keratinocytes. Giant melanosomes, present in keratinocytes and basal melanocytes of CALMs in patients with neurofibromatosis, have not been

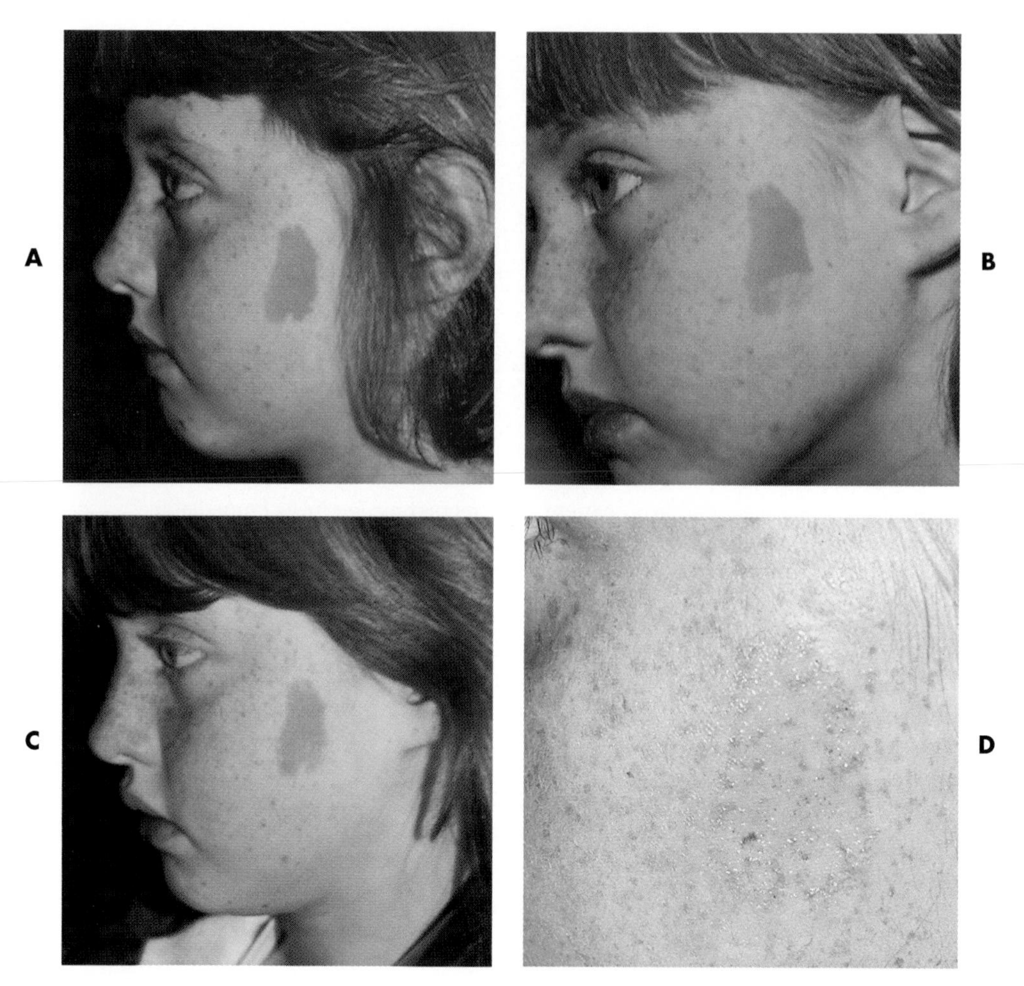

Figure 3-9 Café-au-lait macule on lateral aspect of cheek of 6-year-old girl. **A,** Before treatment. **B,** Three weeks after partial treatment with 15 laser impacts with PLDL at 2.25 J/cm^2. Note complete clearing. **C,** Repigmentation 3 months later. **D,** Further treatment with Q-switched ruby laser at 6 J/cm^2 resulted in complete clearance.

reported in other CALMs patients.[55] Because these lesions have no malignant potential, their removal would be for cosmetic reasons only.

The PLDL cleared most CALMs, with an average fluence of 2.3 J/cm^2 (Table 3-1).[10] Pigmentary changes gradually normalized over 4 to 6 months without scarring.

Melanocytic stimulation may occur at subthreshold laser energies, supporting the use of higher fluences. It is recommended to treat the entire lesion at each session because partial treatment resulted in repigmentation (Figure 3-9). Tan et al[33] treated 18 patients with the PLDL at fluences of 2.0 to 3.5 J/cm^2 for an average of 3.3 (1-7) treatments to achieve clearing. Grekin et al[34] reported that 50% of facial and 17% of truncal CALMs responded to PLDL treatment with greater than 75% improvement, although 6 of 14 patients had no improvement. Alster[56] published excellent results, with 100% clearing after an average of 8.4 treatments with similar fluences.

The Q-switched ruby laser (5.0-6.5-mm spot size with 5-8 J/cm^2) and fd Q-switched YAG lasers (3-4-mm spot size with 1-4 J/cm^2) have been used to treat CALMs as well.[29,57] In addition, the argon laser coupled to the Hexascan is reported to produce an excellent result.[57,58]

Table 3-1
Results of Treatment for Café-au-lait Macules (CALMs)

No. of Treatments	Total Patients	100% Clear	75% Clear	50% Clear	25% Clear	0% Clear	Hyperpigmentation	Hypopigmentation	Scar
1	16/16	3	1	7	2	0	3	1*	0
2	10/16	0	6	4	0	0	0	0	0
3	5/16	5	0	0	0	0	0	0	0
	16/16	8	2	5	1	0	2	1*	0

From Fitzpatrick RE, Goldman MP, Ruiz-Esparza J: *J Dermatol Surg Oncol* 18:341, 1993.
*Patient with hypopigmentation cleared 100%. Fluence 2 to 3 J/cm^2 (average 2.3 J/cm^2).

CALMs may recur within a few weeks of complete clearance; however, retreatment results in rapid clearing. This variable behavior of treated lesions implies a subset of lesions with unique biologic behavior. Repigmentation may occur from surrounding normal melanocytes, from abnormal but inactive melanocytes free of melanin at the time of treatment, or from a dermal signal that stimulates melanocytic activity to reconstitute the lesion.

Nevi Spilus

Nevus spilus is a lesion in which "darker pigmented macules or papules lie within a typical CALM."[59] Estimated to occur in 2.3% of patients (male and female equally) visiting a dermatology practice, nevi spilus seem to be concentrated on the trunk and lower extremities.[60] Although nevus spilus is generally not considered to be a precursor of malignant melanoma, several studies have reported cutaneous melanomas within these nevi.[59-65]

Histologically, these lesions are composed of a lentiginous elongation and hyperpigmentation of rete ridges with an increase in melanocytes. Often a nesting of nevus cells occurs within the lesion. The clinically darker speckled areas are either junctional nevi or compound nevi.[62,66-68]

Although reports of nevus spilus undergoing malignant degeneration suggest exercising caution when treating them, many report a good response to PLDL and fd Nd:YAG, Q-switched ruby, and alexandrite lasers.[34,35,69] Unfortunately, some patients respond poorly,[34] and complete resolution may require four or more treatments. The underlying biology may explain the poor responders; all involved melanocytes may not be targeted (insufficient melanin).[70] The histology of these lesions reveals nothing that would further explain those with a poor response.

DERMAL-EPIDERMAL LESIONS

Becker Nevus

Becker nevi usually appear in childhood or early adult life on any cutaneous area as a light-to-medium brown patch ranging in size from 2 to 40 cm in diameter. Lesions are variably hyperkeratotic, with an increase in coarseness of hair occurring during puberty. Incidence has been calculated to be 0.5% of the population.[71] Histologically, these lesions show rete ridge elongation and basal layer hyperpigmentation with variable amounts of acanthosis and hyperkeratosis. Although no nevus cells are found, melanocytes appear to be increased, and the dermis tends to be thickened. In addition, hypertrophied sebaceous glands and bundles of smooth muscle fibers and enlarged pilar apparatus may be present. Therefore this lesion is more correctly considered an *organoid hamartoma*.[72,73]

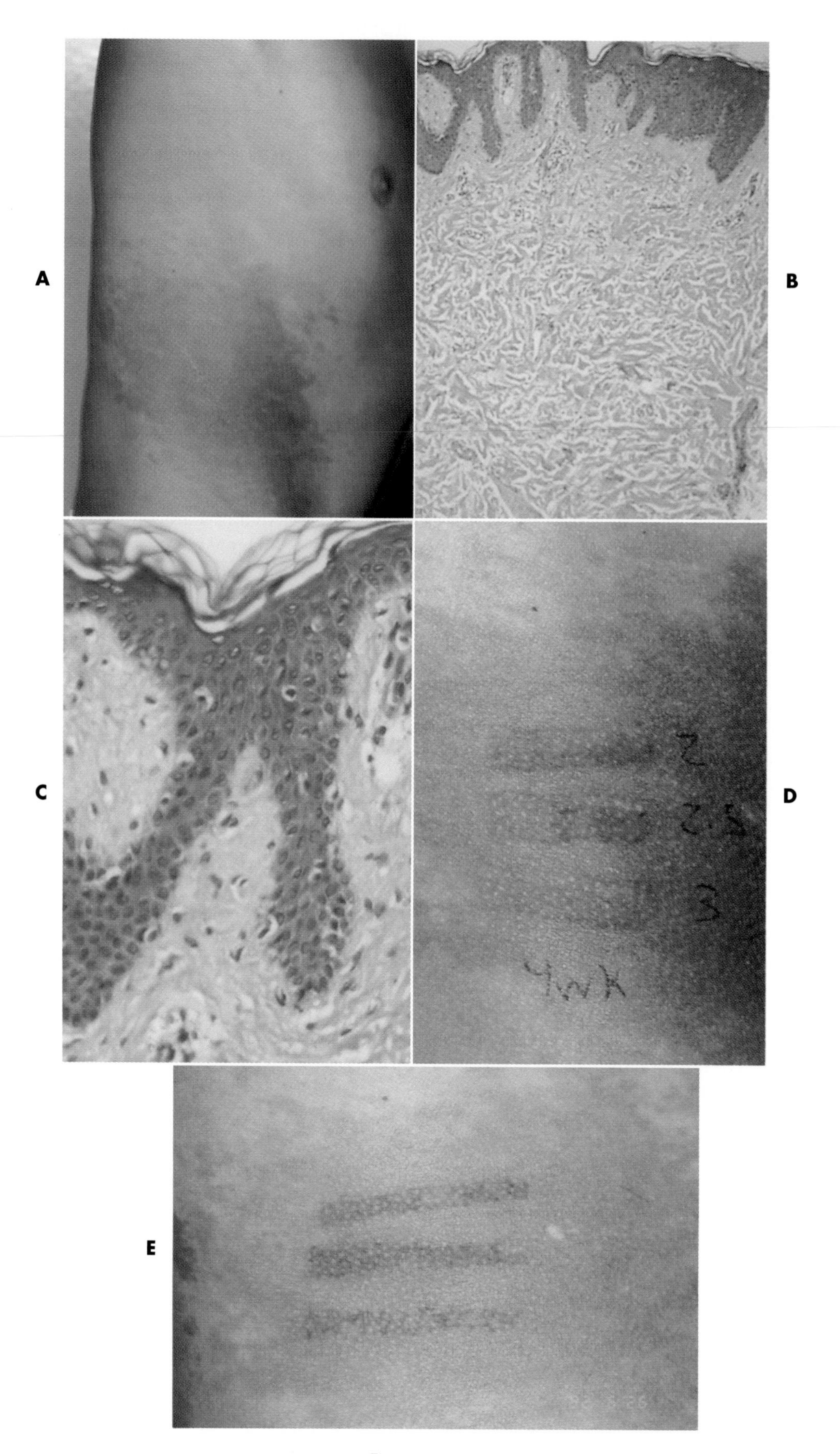

Figure 3-10

Figure 3-10 **A,** Becker nevus before treatment in 16-year-old boy. **B,** Histologic appearance demonstrating elongation of rete ridges with basal hyperpigmentation. Dermis is thickened with hypertrophied bundles of smooth muscle. (Hematoxylin-eosin; ×100.) **C,** High-power examination of same patient demonstrating increased number of melanocytes with basal cellular hyperpigmentation. **D,** Posttreatment hyperpigmentation 4 weeks after treatment with PLDL at 2, 2.5, and 3 J/cm^2. **E,** Four weeks after treatment with Q-switched alexandrite laser at 4, 5, and 6 J/cm^2 overlapping previously treated area. Note hyperpigmentation, which persisted despite two additional treatments with alexandrite laser at 6 and 6.5 J/cm^2.

Becker nevi are notoriously difficult to clear, possibly because of their hamartomatous pathophysiology (Figure 3-10). Several studies have reported limited success with a variety of lasers. The normal-mode ruby laser has shown success in treating three of five Becker nevi,[40] and Tan et al[33] reported on the successful treatment of Becker nevi with the PLDL in two patients, who cleared after two to six treatments. The Q-switched ruby, alexandrite, and fd Nd:YAG lasers can effectively target the increased pigmentation in Becker nevi, but recurrence is common. The long-pulsed ruby and alexandrite lasers may offer more permanent cleaning of both the pigmentation and the increased hair growth.

Melasma

Melasma is an acquired, usually symmetric, light-to-dark brown facial hypermelanosis that develops slowly. It may be idiopathic or more often associated with pregnancy or ingestion of oral contraceptives. This disorder, with a reported incidence of 50% to 70% in pregnant women, usually occurs in the second and third trimesters. It has an incidence of 8% to 29% in women taking oral contraceptives.[74,75] The etiology and pathogenesis of melasma are unknown. However, a genetic predisposition is supported by a 21% familial occurrence in one series.[74]

Two types of melasma exist on histologic examination. In the *epidermal* type the major sites of melanin deposition are in the basilar and suprabasilar layers. The melanocytes have been found to contain highly melanized melanosomes.[74] The *dermal* type is characterized by melanophages in the superficial and deep dermis in addition to the epidermal hyperpigmentation. A simple clinical differentiation between the two types uses the long-wave UV Wood light examination, which shows enhancement of pigmentation in the epidermal type and not in the dermal type. Clinically, lesions with a prominent epidermal component have very sharp borders because of the superficial location of the increase in pigment, whereas those with dermal predominance tend to have more vague borders, representative of the deeper pigment location.

Based on the histologic appearance, one would assume that melasma would be amenable to treatment with a number of different laser systems, including the Candela PLDL and the Q-switched alexandrite, ruby, and YAG lasers. Unfortunately, although results are initially encouraging, repigmentation is very common.

Lack of permanent improvement is most likely caused by failure in stopping the pathoetiologic mechanism for the hypermelanosis. Theoretically, pretreatment and posttreatment administration of high concentrations of hydroxyquinones should effectively prevent repigmentation, particularly in combination with tretinoin. In Grekin et al's series of 10 patients treated with the PLDL, only two patients had minimal lightening even after three treatments with fluences up to 4 J/cm^2.[34]

Although long-term studies regarding hydroxyquinone treatment have not yet been performed, patients are strongly counseled to avoid sun exposure and apply appropriate UVA- and UVB-blocking sunscreens. Test sites help to predict which patient will respond to Q-switched laser treatment. Those with a more superficial component are more likely to respond to the shorter wavelengths, and those with a dermal component respond better to longer wavelengths. In addition, some patients can worsen, further supporting use of test site before a larger area is treated.

Postinflammatory Hyperpigmentation

Any tissue injury site can heal with epidermal postinflammatory hyperpigmentation. Whether this postinflammatory melanosis results from an increased number of active melanocytes or from basal cell layer hyperpigmentation without melanocytic hyperplasia is uncertain, because little or no microscopic information is available on pigmented scars. Pigment incontinence and melanophages laden with pigment may contribute a dermal component. Depending on the etiology of the initiating trauma, hemosiderin may also be present.

Hydroquinone and a broad-spectrum sunscreen are essential. Test sites with any of the available Q-switched lasers may be beneficial, as with melasma, to help predict a patient's response to treatment. Again, failure to improve occurs too often (Figure 3-11).

Figure 3-11 **A,** Postinflammatory hyperpigmentation after abrasion. **B,** Three years after one treatment with PLDL at 3 J/cm².

DERMAL LESIONS

Nevocellular Nevi

Common acquired nevi

Common acquired nevi appear after the first 6 to 12 months of life and enlarge with body growth, reaching a peak average count in the third or fourth decade.[61] Although the exact factors that influence the natural history of common nevi are not yet fully understood, a relationship exists between sun exposure and the number of nevi. The number of nevi increases with a greater concentration in sun-exposed areas.[76] In addition, environmental factors, such as a propensity to burn rather than tan, a history of sunburn, a tendency to freckle, and a life-style involving increased sun exposure, are also related to the number of benign pigmented nevi in children.[77]

Unfortunately, the increased prevalence of benign melanocytic nevi in certain subgroups is a major predictor of malignant melanoma, with relative risks of 10 or more reported.[78-81] In addition, small nevi, present from birth or in early childhood, may give rise to malignant melanomas, with approximately 44% of melanomas in the under-30 age group developing within a nevus of this type.[82] Therefore any treatment of common acquired nevi without histologic evaluation should be undertaken cautiously.

The efficacy of Q-switched laser treatment of nevi is variable.[83-86] Smaller nevi respond better, and all three Q-switched laser systems are effective with minimal side effects. Unfortunately, many nevi recur or only partially respond (Figure 3-12).

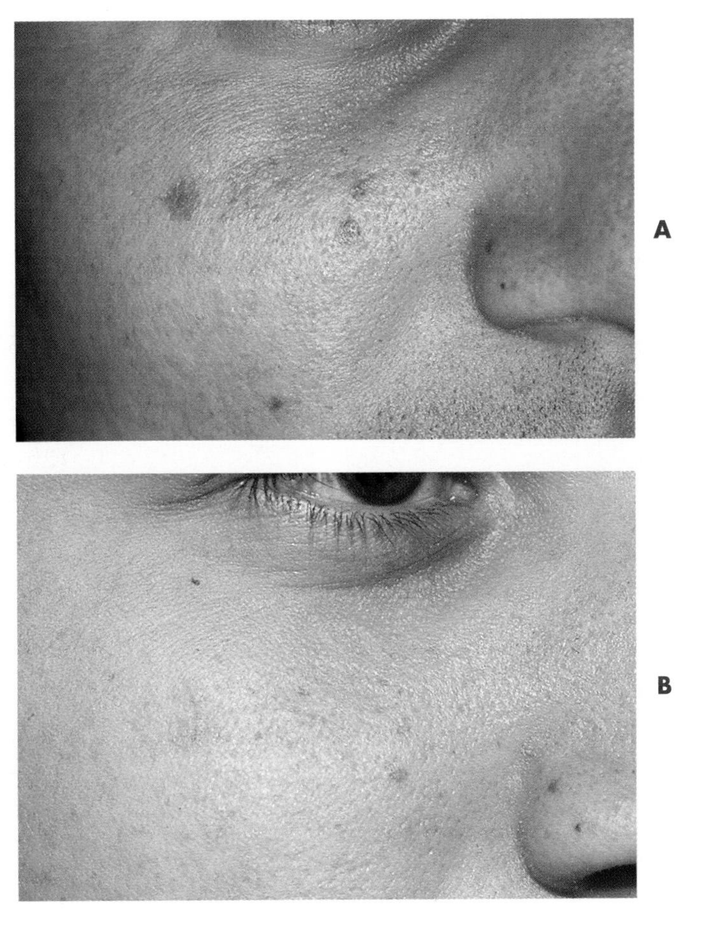

Figure 3-12 **A,** Junctional nevus on cheek of 24-year-old man before treatment. **B,** Two months after second treatment with Q-switched ruby laser at 8 J/cm^2.

Congenital nevocellular nevi

The prevalence of congenital nevocellular nevi ranges from 1% to 2.5% of newborns.[87-89] Although melanoma is rare before puberty, it can occur.[61,90] The relative risk of melanoma associated with very large congenital nevocellular nevi has been estimated to be at least 17-fold, with a lifetime risk of 6.3%.[61,91] Unfortunately, small congenital nevi are also infrequent precursors of melanoma.[61,90-94] The proportion of melanomas reported to develop in association with small congenital nevi ranges from 3% to 15% and thus is several orders of magnitude greater than the expected rate based on chance occurrence.

It is still unknown whether laser treatment will increase or decrease the risk for malignant degeneration. Arguments that irritation of melanocytes leads to increased risk of melanoma formation are countered by the decreased melanocytic load possibly decreasing this risk. In either case, removal of the superficial component may leave a deeper dermal component that may be changed, hidden, or not pigmented, making routine surveillance difficult. Therefore many recommend that small congenital nevi should be excised rather than undergo laser therapy whenever possible to prevent melanoma.[95] Larger lesions, especially in cosmetically difficult areas, may be more amenable to treatment.

With these cautions and background information, many patients choose to have common acquired nevi removed for cosmesis. The ruby laser has been shown to be effective in removing only 12% (9 of 74) of pigmented nevi in a Japanese population.[40] In an effort to find reasons for this reported lack of efficacy, biopsies of 62 pigmented nevi were performed before and after laser treatment.[96] Histologic examination demonstrated nevocellular nests in the middermis in all the nonresponding lesions and junctional nests in all successfully treated lesions. Although multiple treatments were not performed, lesions unresponsive to a single treatment might have lightened with additional therapy.

Similarly, a 5-year-old boy with a 1-cm congenital nevus on the medial right cheek was treated with the PLDL at 3 J/cm², with 50% to 75% resolution after one treatment. Unfortunately, 4 months after treatment the mole completely repig-

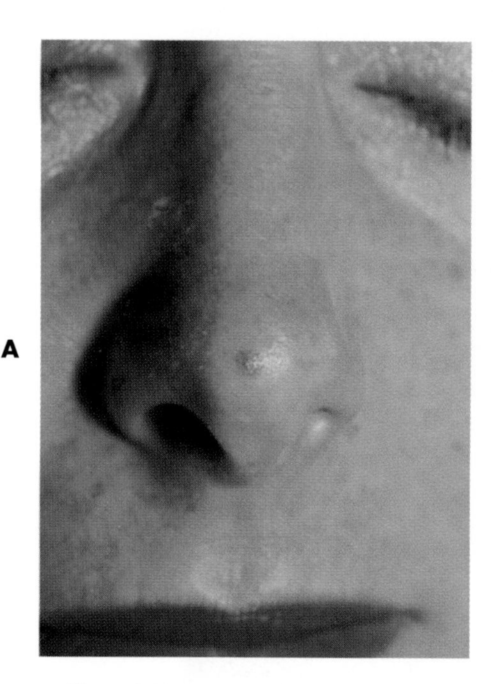

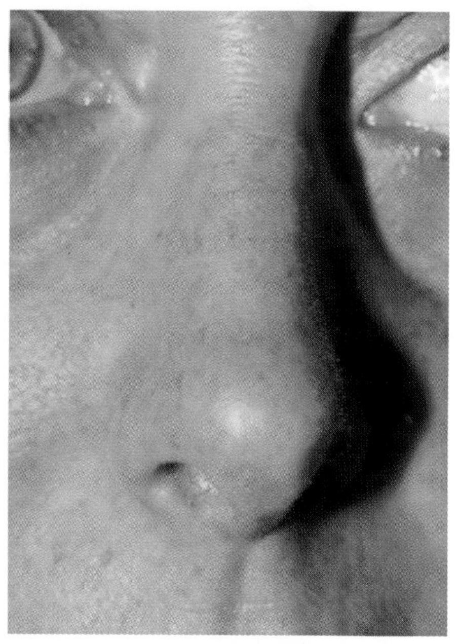

Figure 3-13 **A,** Nasal tip nevi on 39-year-old woman before treatment. **B,** Fourteen months after treatment with PLDL at 2.5 J/cm² for 5 pulses.

mented. Further treatment (four sessions) resulted in the lesion becoming thinner in depth and lighter in color (approximately 50%) but with residual lesion persisting, probably because of the short, less deeply penetrating wavelength used. In contrast, an acquired 3 mm nevus on the nasal tip of a 39-year-old woman cleared completely with one PLDL treatment at 2.5 J/cm^2 without recurrence for 14 months (Figure 3-13). Similar results have been reported by others using the Q-switched ruby, alexandrite, and Nd:YAG lasers.[97] Normal-mode ruby lasers are effective, as noted in several reports,[40,97] and long-pulsed ruby and alexandrite lasers may offer further benefit.

Because congenital nevocellular nevi extend into the deepest reticular dermis in an estimated 37% of patients, it is unlikely that treatment even with a Q-switched ruby or alexandrite laser at 694 or 755 nm would destroy all these cells[54] (Figures 3-14 and 3-15). A similar comparison would be the treatment of giant congenital nevi with dermabrasion. This technique, although improving the cosmetic appearance, does not remove most nevus cells and thus is not recommended as an effective treatment for the prevention of melanoma in these lesions.[98] Laser treatment of congenital nevi, similar to dermabrasion,[95] likely removes only the superficial pigment-bearing nevus cells, leaving residual dermal, subcutaneous, and even fascial nevus cells. Some physicians accept laser removal

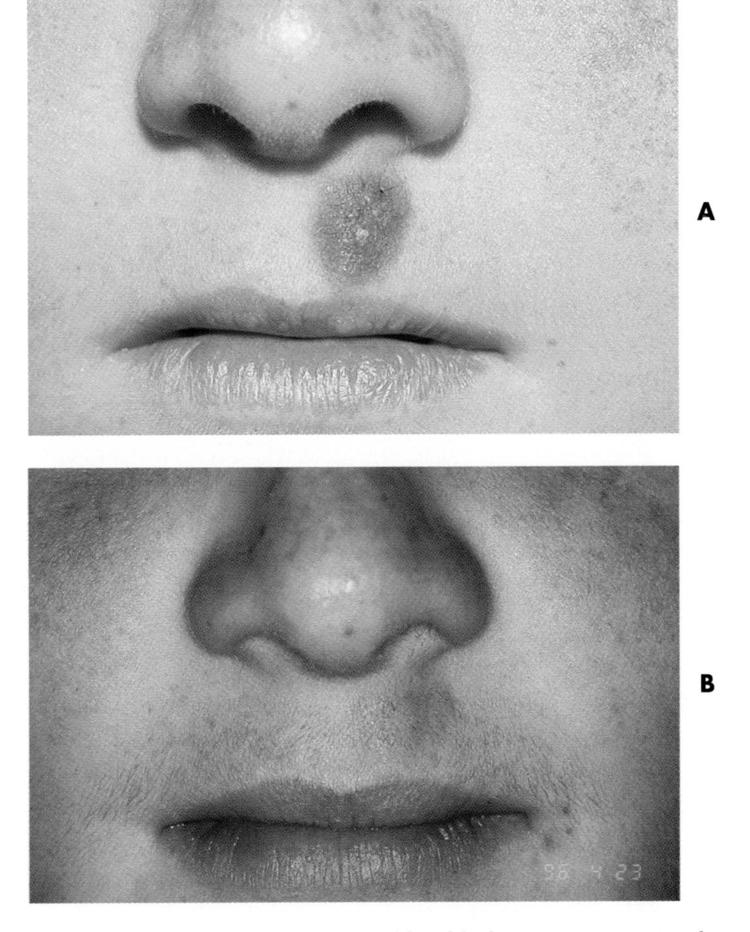

Figure 3-14 **A,** Congenital nevus on 6-year-old girl before treatment. **B,** After five treatments at monthly intervals with PLDL (3 J/cm^2), Q-switched alexandrite (8 J/cm^2), Q-switched ruby at 10 J/cm^2, and Q-switched Nd:YAG at 10 J/cm^2, the nevus persisted. The lesion was then resurfaced with ultrapulse CO_2 laser. Appearance 4 months after resurfacing.

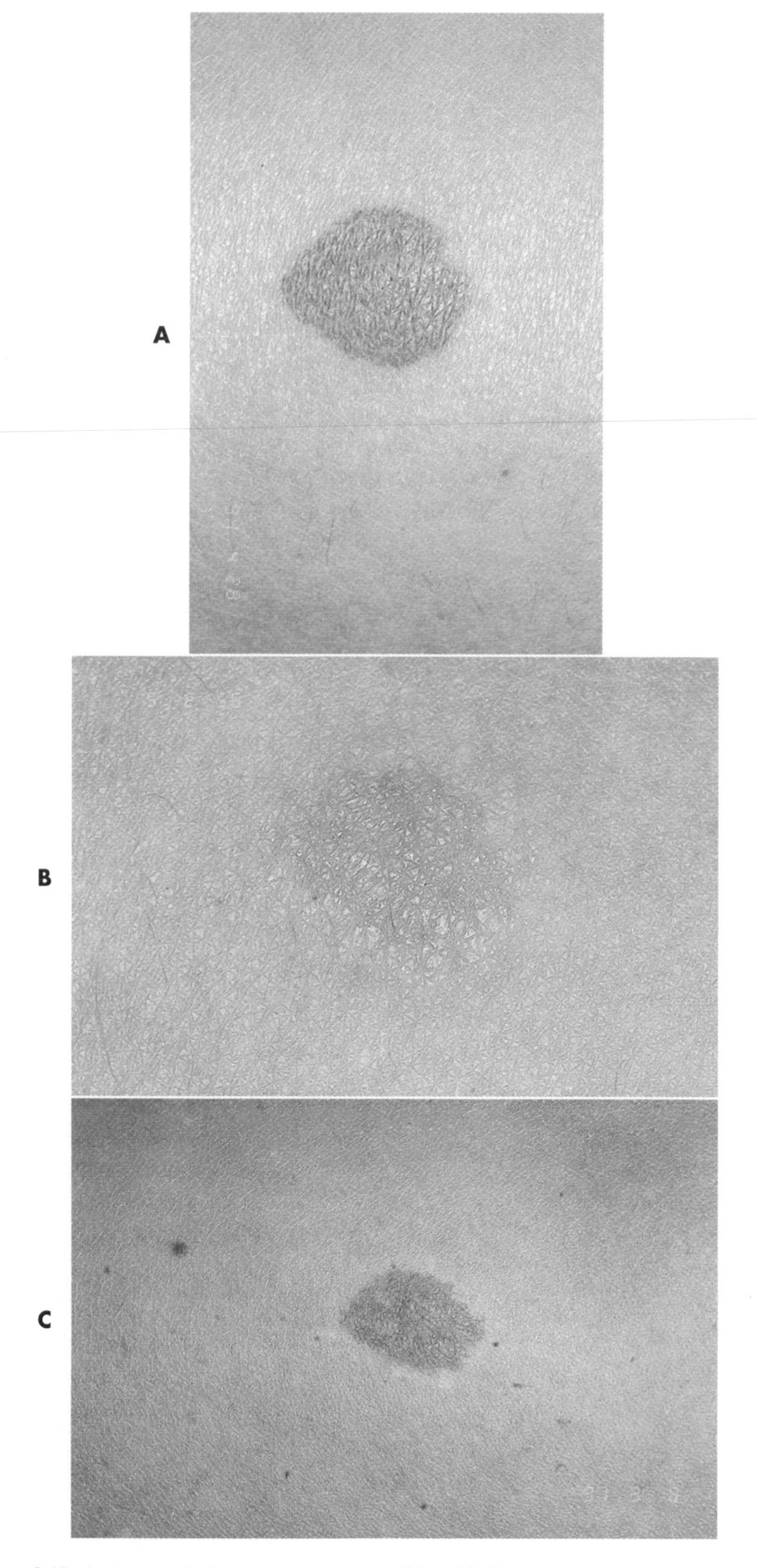

Figure 3-15 **A,** Congenital nevus on 5-year-old girl before treatment. **B,** Apparent complete clearance after four treatments with Q-switched alexandrite laser (8 J/cm^2), followed 2 months later by Q-switched ruby laser (8 J/cm^2), then followed 2 months later by Q-switched Nd:YAG laser (8 J/cm^2) and repeated 2 months later. **C,** Complete regrowth 2 years later.

of the superficial layer of nevus cells in congenital nevi not amenable to surgical excision because they believe removing a percentage of the potential precursors proportionately reduces risk of melanoma and improves cosmetic appearance. This remains controversial, however, because other physicians are concerned that repeated laser injury to residual nevus cells may predispose them to malignant change, and laser-induced thermal scarring may conceal changes occurring deeper in the dermis. Cases must be reviewed on an individual basis with consideration of these factors.

Nevus of Ota

Nevus of Ota represents a persistent, bluish gray macular lesion that typically appears on the facial skin and is limited to the area innervated by the first and second divisions of the trigeminal nerve. It is frequently associated with ipsilateral ocular pigmentation. This nevus is most often found in Asians and blacks and has a strong predilection for females. Incidence in the Japanese population is estimated at 1% to 2%.[99]

The etiology and pathogenesis of nevus of Ota are unknown. The clinical appearance resembles a powder blast, showing multiple deep-colored small spots on a fainter blue-brown background. Lesions vary in color from light brown to a dark black-purple and are always macular. The edge of discoloration is usually not sharply demarcated but blends gradually with adjacent normal skin.

Histologic examination shows bipolar long, slender dermal melanocytes scattered largely in the upper half of the dermis. The normal dermal collagen architecture is well preserved. Although the epidermis is generally normal, focal basal hyperpigmentation may also be seen. The lesions are usually benign, but rare associations have been reported with the development of malignant melanoma.[100]

Treatment is discussed in conjunction with nevus of Ito because the lesions are similar histologically and in their response to treatment.

Nevus of Ito

Nevus of Ito is a persistent, grayish blue discoloration with the same histologic characteristics of nevus of Ota. It is generally present on the shoulder or upper arm in the area innervated by the posterior supraclavicular and lateral brachial cutaneous nerves. The lesion is much rarer than nevus of Ota, and the exact incidence is unknown. It is largely confined to the Japanese population.

Treatment of nevi of Ota and Ito is undertaken predominantly for cosmetic concerns. Cryosurgery with either liquid nitrogen or CO_2 "snow" has been the usual treatment method. Although satisfactory results have occurred in 90% of patients,[101] complications include hypertrophic scarring and hypopigmentation. A newer microsurgical treatment reportedly yields satisfactory clinical postoperative results, although the surgical technique appears technically demanding and somewhat risky.[102]

The argon laser (0.2-1.0-mm spot, 0.5-1.5 W, 1-2-sec pulse) was reported to resolve a nevus of Ota without skin texture changes but with hypopigmentation.[103] Non–Q-switched (normal-mode) ruby laser treatment at 10 J/cm^2 partially cleared this lesion without significant adverse sequelae.[40,104]

Because the nevus of Ota is primarily a dermal lesion, treatment with the Q-switched ruby,[105-107] alexandrite,[108] and Nd:YAG[38] lasers is efficacious because their longer wavelengths target deeper melanin (Figure 3-16) and their nanosecond pulse width minimizes thermal injury to surrounding collagen (Figure 3-17). Geronemus[105] reported treating 15 patients with nevus of Ota present for 6 to 52 years with the Q-switched ruby laser at 40 nsec. Complete clearing was noted in 4 of 15 patients, with a minimum of 50% lightening in the remaining 11.

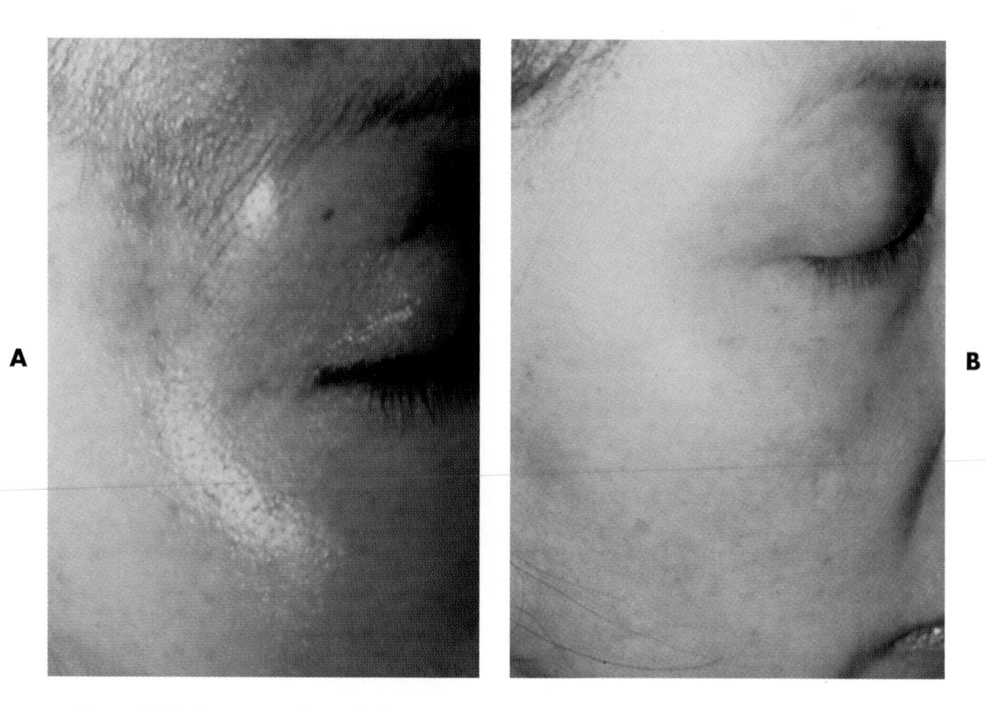

Figure 3-16 **A,** Nevus of Ota before treatment. **B,** Two months after two treatments with Q-switched ruby laser at fluence of 10 J/cm². (Courtesy Nicholas Lowe, MD.)

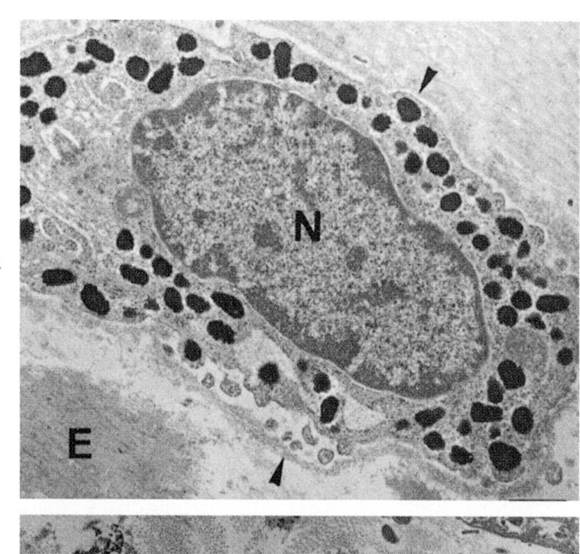

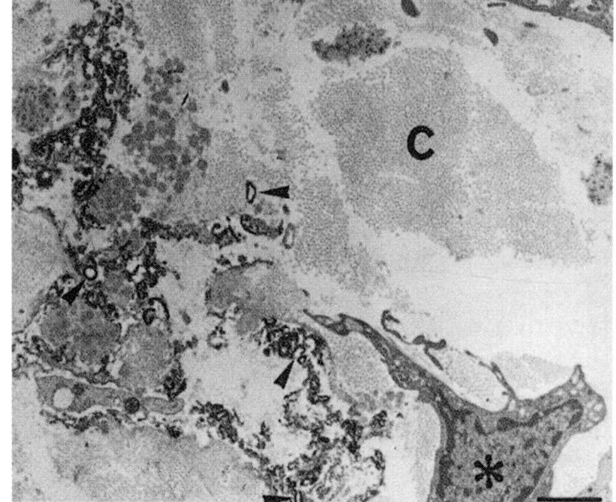

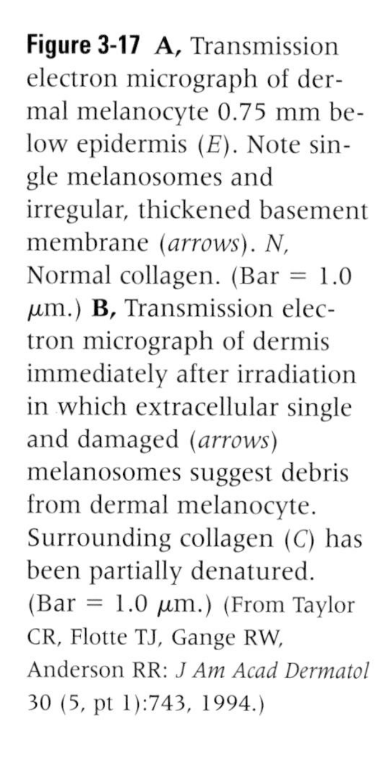

Figure 3-17 **A,** Transmission electron micrograph of dermal melanocyte 0.75 mm below epidermis (*E*). Note single melanosomes and irregular, thickened basement membrane (*arrows*). *N,* Normal collagen. (Bar = 1.0 μm.) **B,** Transmission electron micrograph of dermis immediately after irradiation in which extracellular single and damaged (*arrows*) melanosomes suggest debris from dermal melanocyte. Surrounding collagen (*C*) has been partially denatured. (Bar = 1.0 μm.) (From Taylor CR, Flotte TJ, Gange RW, Anderson RR: *J Am Acad Dermatol* 30 (5, pt 1):743, 1994.)

The energy fluence ranged from 6 to 10 J/cm^2, with one to seven treatments. Energies of 9 to 10 J/cm^2 were found to cause the most significant tissue lightening. No scarring occurred, and only two patients had transient hyperpigmentation or hypopigmentation.

New commercial Q-switched ruby lasers use a shorter pulse width (20-28 nsec), which results in higher peak energies. Time must be allowed for macrophage engulfment of pigment and gradual clearing of lesions over several months. Conflicting reports of fluences necessary for treatment as well as the necessary number of treatments and treatment intervals probably result from the variability in lesions and spot size used. Using the Q-switched ruby laser at 28 nsec, Lowe et al[106] reported 50% or better improvement in 16 patients with nevus of Ota after four treatments with energy fluences of 7.5 to 10 J/cm^2. Treatments were given at 6- to 8-week intervals. No adverse sequelae were noticed.

The Q-switched alexandrite laser (wavelength 755 nm, pulse 100 nsec) at a fluence of 6 J/cm^2 provided an excellent cosmetic result (Figure 3-18), with two to six treatments generally required to produce a near-100% resolution of the lesion. The Q-switched Nd:YAG laser provides similar results. The optimal treatment interval remains to be eludicated for all these lasers.

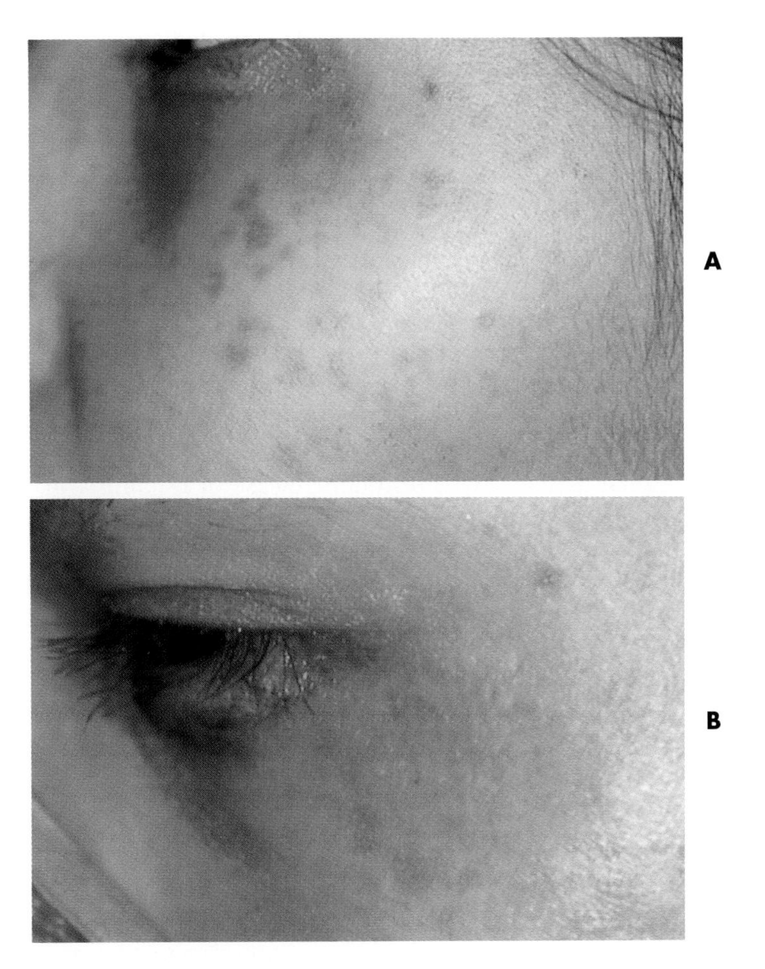

Figure 3-18 **A,** Melasma and nevus of Ota at left lateral canthus of 32-year-old Filipino woman. Circular brown pigmentation represents postinflammatory hyperpigmentation from PDPL treatment of melasma 4 months previously. **B,** Three months after treatment with alexandrite laser at 6 J/cm^2 to both lentigo and postinflammatory hyperpigmentation. Note complete resolution of nevus of Ota and significant lightening of pigmentation. Black component of nevus of Ota on temple was not treated.

Blue Nevus

Blue nevi are usually solitary, discrete, well-circumscribed papules 1 to 8 mm in diameter that arise spontaneously, most often in children and young adults. The male/female ratio is approximately 2:1.[109,110] The melanin-producing cells are deep within the dermis, and their blue-black color results from the Tyndall light-scattering effect of the overlying tissues.

Histologic examination shows an extensive number of spindle-shaped, elongated, bipolar melanocytes within the middle and lower dermis, occasionally extending into the fat. These cells may be grouped in fascicles between collagen bundles and tend to aggregate around adnexal structures, nerves, and blood vessels. Melanophages may also be present within the lesion. The epidermis is usually unremarkable, with relative sparing of the nevoid process in the superficial papillary dermis.

Because of their benign nature, blue nevi are usually removed for cosmetic reasons. Although extremely rare, malignant blue nevi have been reported.[111] The primary method of removal of these lesions is local excision. Similar to treatment of nevi of Ota and Ito, the Q-switched ruby,[112] alexandrite, and Nd:YAG lasers should also be effective in removing these deep dermal melanocytes, as long as the lesion does not extend into the subcutaneous fat.

The only mode of treatment mentioned in the literature is with the Q-switched ruby laser or Candela PDPL,[56] although all three Q-switched lasers should be efficacious, similar to their use with nevi of Ota and Ito. Again, the longer-pulsed ruby and alexandrite lasers may prove helpful.

Postsclerotherapy Hyperpigmentation

Cutaneous pigmentation typically occurs after sclerotherapy of varicose and telangiectatic leg veins. The incidence may be correlated with the type of sclerosing solution used, as reported in 30% of patients treated with sodium tetradecyl sulfate (STS) and hypertonic saline (HS)[113,114] and 10.7% of patients treated with polidocanol (POL).[115]

Pigmentation most likely reflects hemosiderin deposition, which is probably secondary to extravasation of red blood cells (RBCs) through damaged endothelium.[116-118] Endothelial damage with resultant release of inflammatory mediators may increase endothelial contraction and thus venular permeability. This contraction causes the formation of intercellular gaps large enough for RBCs to extravasate.[119,120] Endothelial contraction also occurs because of histamine release from stimulated or damaged perivascular mast cells.[121,122]

Postsclerotherapy hyperpigmentation is secondary to hemosiderin deposition and not melanin incontinence; thus bleaching agents that primarily affect melanocytic function are usually ineffective. Exfoliants such as TCA can hasten the apparent resolution of this pigmentation by decreasing the superficial cutaneous pigmen-

Table 3-2
Treatment response and pigmentation depth in postsclerotherapy hyperpigmentation

Patients	Response (%)	Depth of Pigmentation (mm)
6	100	0.3-1.4
11	0	0.2-2.8
13	75	0.3-1.5

From Goldman MP: *J Dermatol Surg Oncol* 18:417, 1992.

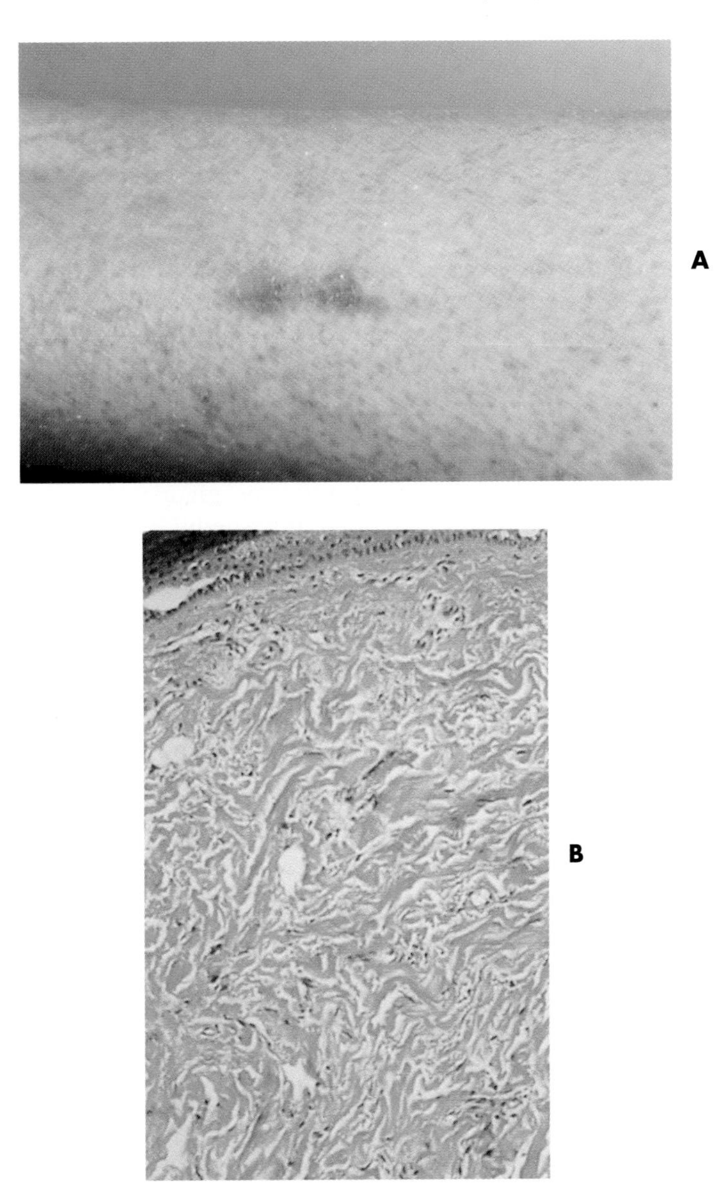

Figure 3-19 **A,** Clinical appearance of postsclerotherapy hyperpigmentation of anterior aspect of calf from injection of morrhuate sodium 7 years earlier. **B,** Immediately after treatment with PLDL at 2 J/cm². Note vacuolization of epidermal melanocytes and dermal hemosiderin-laden macrophages. Depth of pigmentation measured 2.8 mm. (Hematoxylin-eosin; ×200.)

tation, but risks of scarring, permanent hypopigmentation, and postinflammatory hyperpigmentation exist.

The CW copper vapor laser and the PLDL have resulted in significant resolution of hemosiderin pigmentation in about 70% and 45% of patients, respectively.[123,124] The effectiveness of these lasers probably results from the depth of penetration and absorption characteristics of hemosiderin. Depth of hemosiderin pigmentation ranged from 0.2 to 2.8 mm from the granular layer in nine biopsy specimens from pigmented areas after sclerotherapy (Figure 3-19). Treatment response correlated somewhat with the depth of pigmentation. Two superficial lesions responded with 75% to 100% lightening (Table 3-2).

Hemosiderin has an absorption spectrum that peaks at 410 to 415 nm, followed by a gradually sloping curve throughout the remainder of the visible spectrum[125,126] (Figure 3-20). The copper vapor laser has greater selectivity for hemosiderin than either epidermal structures or blood vessels at 511 nm. The PLDL has an almost identical wavelength of 510 nm. However, the two lasers have extremely different pulse characteristics. The copper vapor laser has a 20-nsec pulse delivered at a repetition rate of 15,000 Hz and a pulse energy of 2.4 mJ/pulse, whereas the PLDL has a 300-nsec pulse, repetition rate of 1 Hz, and pulse energy of 785 mJ/pulse (at a setting of 4 J/cm^2). Hemosiderin particles are approximately the same diameter (1-5 μm)[125,126] as tattoo granules. Therefore, as demonstrated by laser treatment of tattoo granules (see Chapter 4), a pulse of 10 to 100 nsec would be ideal in producing a selective photothermal effect. This may explain the relative enhanced efficacy of the copper vapor laser in treating hemosiderin deposits.

The effect of Q-switched ruby lasers on tattoo pigment may result from mechanical or photoacoustic waves generated in tissue by high-energy pulses rather than from a purely thermal effect.[127] These waves seem to fragment pigment granules, which are later removed by dermal phagocytes. Because the wavelengths of the copper vapor laser and PLDL allow only minimal dermal penetration, this may limit the effectiveness of treatment to the more superficially located hemosiderin. However, the shock waves generated by laser interaction may effectively disperse hemosiderin at a depth greater than that reached by the laser light itself. Removal of dermal hemosiderin by the PDPL was demonstrated both histologically and clinically.[124]

Patients with postinflammatory hyperpigmentation in various body areas have been treated with the PDPL (Table 3-3). The average lesion improved by more than

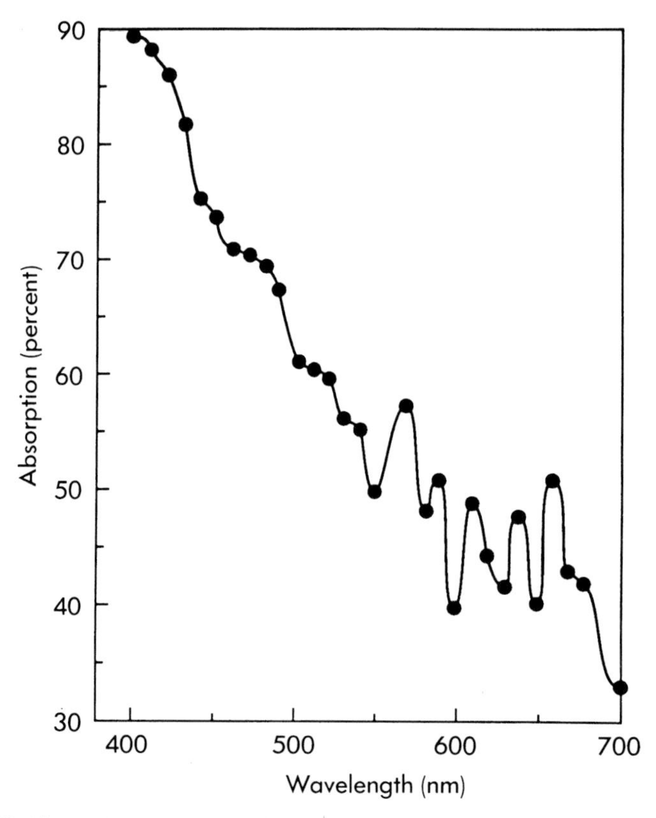

Figure 3-20 Absorption spectrum of oxygenated hemoglobin. (From Wells CI, Wolken JJ, *Nature* 193:977, 1962.)

Table 3-3
Patient and treatment characteristics in postinflammatory hyperpigmentation

Type	Scar age (yr)	Location	Fluence (J/cm²)	Treatments	Outcome (%) Improvement
Excision	4	Thigh	2	2	75
Excision	1	Arm	2	1	25
Excision	1	Abdomen	2.5	1	50
Excision	4	Abdomen	2	2	100
Excision	1	Cheek	2.5	1	100
Excision	1	Breast	2	2	100
Excision	1	Abdomen	2	2	75
Ulceration	1	Medial malleolus	2.25	1	100
Ulceration	3	Thigh	2, 2.25	2	50
Abrasion	10	Leg	2	1	100
Abrasion	1-2	Thigh	2	1	75
AVERAGE				1.45	77

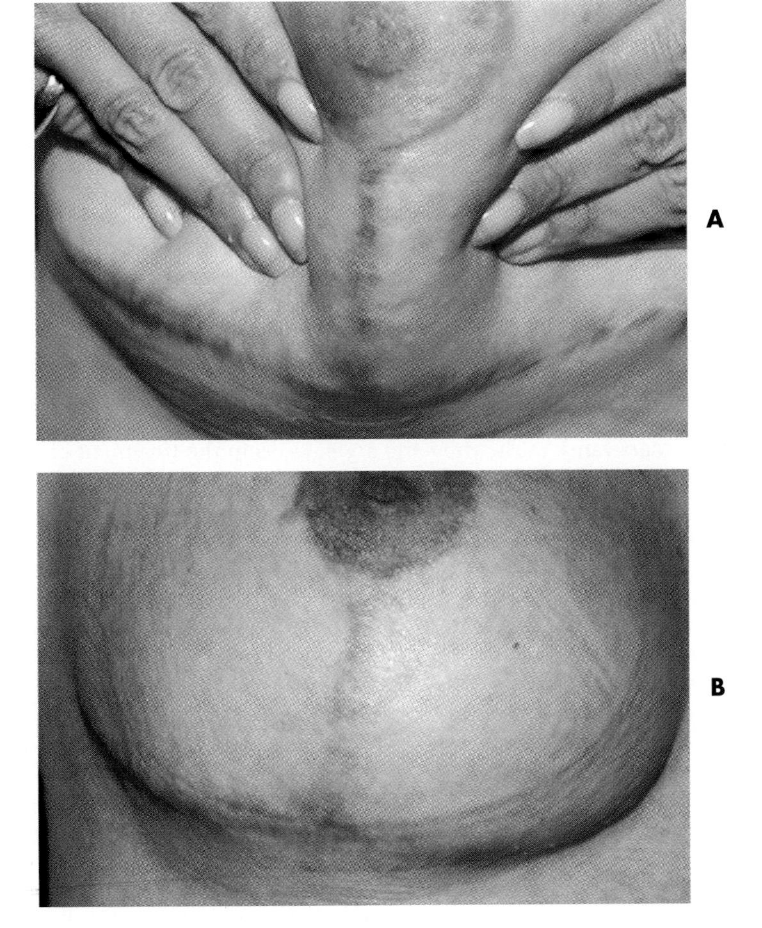

Figure 3-21 **A,** Postinflammatory hyperpigmentation in 42-year-old woman before treatment. **B,** Eight weeks after second treatment with Candela PLDL at 2 J/cm².

75%, and five lesions completely cleared after two treatment sessions. Further treatment would be expected to result in continued resolution of the remaining pigment.

The response to PDPL treatment in postinflammatory hyperpigmentation was not significantly altered by the fluence of laser energy, with lesions just as likely to respond to 2 J/cm^2 as to 2.5 J/cm^2. The number of treatments necessary for complete resolution was either one or two, but no patients received more than two. No relationship was seen between age of the lesion and efficacy of treatment (Fig. 3-21).

With pigmented scars the laser target is the epidermal melanin pigment; therefore all pigment-specific lasers should be effective. One case report[128] shows an excellent response of posttraumatic hyperpigmentation in an Asian woman with the Q-switched ruby laser at 3 J/cm^2. Clearance was also reported with the fd Nd:YAG[29] and alexandrite lasers. Shorter wavelengths (510 and 532 nm) result in enhanced absorption by epidermal melanin, thereby decreasing the risk of denudal reaction,[15] which may be important in some cases of hypertrophic scars.

SUMMARY

Most benign pigmented lesions respond fairly well to laser treatments. Those located more superficially can be treated with the shorter wavelengths of 510 and 532 nm as well as 694 and even 755 nm. Deeper lesions require the longer wavelengths of 694, 755, and 1064 nm for better depth of penetration. Larger spot sizes also enhance the penetration depth.[129] Unfortunately, pigmented lesions respond variably to lasers, and for any individual it is difficult to predict treatment outcome. The optimizing of laser parameters, refined techniques, and a better understanding of the underlying biology may further help clinicians to treat these lesions more effectively.

REFERENCES

1. Goldman L et al: Radiation from a Q-switched ruby laser: effect of repeated impacts of power output of 10 megawatts on a tattoo of man, *J Invest Dermatol* 44:69, 1965.
2. Goldman L et al: Laser treatment of tattoos: a preliminary survey of three years' clinical experience, *JAMA* 201:841, 1967.
3. Goldman L: Optical radiation hazards to the skin. In Sliney D, Wolbarsht M, editors: *Safety with lasers and other optical sources: a comprehensive handbook,* New York, 1983, Plenum.
4. Ohshiro T, Maruyama Y: The ruby and argon lasers in the treatment of naevi, *Ann Acad Med Singapore* 12:388, 1983.
5. Dover JS et al: Low-fluence carbon dioxide laser irradiation of lentigines, *Arch Dermatol* 124:1219, 1988.
6. Goldman L et al: High-power neodymium-YAG laser surgery, *Acta Derm Venereol* (Stockh) 53:45, 1987.
7. Anderson RR, Parrish JA: Selective photothermolysis: precise microsurgery by selective absorption of pulsed irradiation, *Science* 220:524, 1983.
8. Murphy GF, Shepard RS, Paul BS et al: Organelle-specific injury to melanin-containing cells in human skin by pulsed laser irradiation, *Lab Invest* 49:680, 1983.
9. Polla LL, Margolis RJ, Dover JS et al: Melanosomes are a primary target of Q-switched ruby laser irradiation in guinea pig skin, *J Invest Dermatol* 89:281, 1987.
10. Fitzpatrick RE, Goldman MP, Ruiz-Esparza J: Laser treatment of benign pigmented epidermal lesions using a 300 nsec pulse and 510 nm wavelength, *J Dermatol Surg Oncol* 18:341, 1993.
11. Ara G, Anderson RR, Mandel KG et al: Irradiation of pigmented melanoma cells with high intensity pulsed radiation generates acoustic waves and kills cells, *Lasers Surg Med* 10:52, 1990.
12. Hruza GJ, Dover JS, Flotte TJ et al: Q-switched ruby laser irradiation of normal human skin, *Arch Dermatol* 127:1799, 1991.

13. Anderson RR, Margolis RJ, Watanabe S et al: Selective photothermolysis of cutaneous pigmentation by Q-switched Nd:YAG laser pulses at 1064, 532 and 355 nm, *J Invest Dermatol* 93:28, 1989.
14. Margolis RJ, Dover JS, Polla LL et al: Visible action spectrum for melanin-specific selective photothermolysis, *Lasers Surg Med* 9:389, 1989.
15. Sherwood KA, Murray S, Kurban AK et al: Effect of wavelength on cutaneous pigment using pulsed irradiation, *J Invest Dermatol* 92:717, 1989.
16. Anderson RR, Parrish JA: The optics of human skin, *J Invest Dermatol* 77:13, 1981.
17. Vassiliadis A: Ocular damage from laser radiation. In Wolbarsht M, editor: *Laser applications in medicine and biology,* New York, 1971, Plenum.
18. Kurban AK, Scearbo ME, Morrison P et al: Pulse duration effects on cutaneous pigment ablation, *Lasers Surg Med Suppl* 2:213A, 1990.
19. Parrish JA, Anderson RR, Harrist T et al: Selective thermal effects with pulsed irradiation from laser: from organ to organelle, *J Invest Dermatol* 80:755, 1983.
20. Kurban AK, Morrison PR, Trainor S et al: Pulse duration effects on cutaneous pigment, *Lasers Surg Med* 12:282, 1992.
21. Tong AKF, Tan OT, Boll J et al: Ultrastructural effects of melanin pigment on target specificity using pulsed dye laser (577 nm), *J Invest Dermatol* 88:747, 1987.
22. Watanabe S, Anderson RR, Brorson S: Comparative studies of femtosecond to microsecond laser pulses on selective pigmented cell injury in skin, *J Photochem Photobiol* 53:757, 1991.
23. Dover JS, Polla LL, Margolis RJ et al: Pulsewidth dependence of pigment cell damage at 694 nm in guinea pig skin. In Scott RS, Parrish JA, Jaffe N, editors: *Lasers in medicine, Proc SPIE,* 1986.
24. Watanabe S, Flotte T, Margolis R et al: The effects of pulse duration on selective pigmented cell injury by dye lasers, *J Invest Dermatol* 88:523A, 1987.
25. Mainster MA, Sliney DW, Blecher D et al: Damage mechanisms, instrument design, and safety, *Ophthalmology* 99:973, 1983.
26. Carome EF, Clark NA, Moeler CE: Generation of acoustic signals in liquids by ruby laser-induced thermal stress transients, *Appl Phys Lett* 4:95, 1964.
27. Kurban AK, Morrison PR, Trainot SW et al: Pulse duration effects on cutaneous pigment, *Lasers Surg Med* 12:282, 1992.
28. Yasuda Y, Tan OT, Kurban AK et al: Electron microscopic study on black pig skin irradiated with pulsed dye laser (504 nm). In Tan OT, White RA, White JV, editors: *Lasers in dermatology and tissue welding, Proc SPIE* 1422:50, 1991.
29. Kilmer SL, Wheeland RG, Goldberg DJ, Anderson RR: Treatment of epidermal pigmented lesions with the frequency-doubled Q-switched Nd:YAG laser: a controlled, single-impact, dose-response, multicenter trial, *Arch Dermatol* 130:1515, 1994.
30. Dover JS, Margolis RJ, Polla LL et al: Pigmented guinea pig skin irradiated with Q-switched ruby laser pulses: morphologic and histologic findings, *Arch Dermatol* 125:43, 1988.
31. Hruza G, Dover JS, Flotte TJ et al: Q-switched ruby laser irradiation of normal human skin, *Arch Dermatol* 127:1799, 1991.
32. Braun-Falco O, Schoefinias HH: Lentigo senilis, *Hautarzt* 22:277, 1971.
33. Tan OT, Morelli JG, Kurban AK: Pulsed dye laser treatment of benign cutaneous pigmented lesions, *Lasers Surg Med* 12:538, 1992.
34. Grekin RC et al: 510-nm pigmented lesion dye laser: its characteristics and clinical uses, *J Dermatol Surg Oncol* 19:380, 1993.
35. Goldman MP, Fitzpatrick RE: Unpublished observations, 1993.
36. Taylor CR, Anderson PR: Treatment of benign pigmented epidermal lesions by Q-switched ruby laser, *Int J Dermatol* 32:908, 1993.
37. Goldberg DJ: Benign pigmented lesions of the skin: treatment with the Q-switched ruby laser, *J Dermatol Surg Oncol* 19:376, 1993.
38. Tse Y, Levine VJ, McClain SA, Ashinoff R: The removal of cutaneous pigmented lesions with the Q-switched ruby laser and the Q-switched neodymium: yttrium-aluminum-garnet laser: a comparative study, *J Dermatol Surg Oncol* 20:795, 1994.
39. Goldberg DJ: Laser treatment of pigmented lesions, *Dermatol Clin* 15(3):397, 1997.
40. Ohtsuka H et al: Ruby laser treatment of pigmented skin lesions, *Jpn J Plast Reconstr Surg* 44:615, 1991.

41. Ashinoff R, Geronemus RG: Q-switched ruby laser treatment of labial lentigos, *J Am Acad Dermatol* 27:809, 1992.
42. Ficarra G, Shillitoe EJ, Adler-Storthz K et al: Oral melanotic macules in patients infected with human immunodeficiency virus, *Oral Surg Oral Med Oral Pathol* 70:748, 1990.
43. Laugier P, Hunziker N: Pigmentation melanique lenticulaire essentielle de la muqueuse jugale et des levres, *Arch Belg Dermatol Syphilol* 26:391, 1970.
44. Ho KK-L, Dervan P, O'Loughlin S et al: Labial melanotic macule: a clinical histopathologic and ultrastructural study, *J Am Acad Dermatol* 28:33, 1993.
45. Weathers DR, Corio RL, Crawford BE et al: The labial melanotic macule, *Oral Surg* 42:196, 1976.
46. Spann CR, Owen LG, Hodge SJ: The labial melanotic macules, *Arch Dermatol* 123:1029, 1987.
47. Breathnach AS: Melanocyte distribution in forearm epidermis of freckled human subjects, *J Invest Dermatol* 29:253, 1957.
48. Breathnach AS, Wyllie LM: Electronmicroscopy of melanocytes and melanosomes in freckled human epidermis, *J Invest Dermatol* 42:398, 1964.
49. Goldes JA: Seborrheic keratoses. In Demis DJ, editor: *Clinical dermatology,* ed 19, Philadelphia, 1992, Lippincott.
50. Mehregan AH: Lentigo senilis and its evolutions, *J Invest Dermatol* 65:429, 1975.
51. Miyasaka M, Tanino R, Morita T: Case 8.31: seborrheic keratosis of anterior part of the left ear. In Apfelberg DB, editor: *Atlas of cutaneous laser surgery,* New York, 1992, Raven.
52. Pasyk KA: Case 5.49: seborrheic keratosis. In Apfelberg DB, editor: *Atlas of cutaneous laser surgery,* New York, 1992, Raven.
53. Crowee FW, Scnull WJ: Diagnostic importance of café-au-lait spot in neurofibromatosis, *Intern Med* 91:758, 1953.
54. Stenn KS, Arons M, Hurwitz S: Patterns of congenital nevocellular nevi: a histologic study of 38 cases, *J Am Acad Dermatol* 9:388, 1983.
55. Duray TH: Café-au-lait spots. In Demis DJ, editor: *Clinical dermatology,* ed 19, Philadelphia, 1992, Lippincott.
56. Alster TS: Complete elimination of large café-au-lait birthmarks by the 510-nm pulsed dye laser, *Plast Reconstr Surg* 96(7):1660, 1995.
57. Nelson JS: Case 8.24: epidermal melanosis secondary to café-au-lait spot. In Apfelberg DB, editor: *Atlas of cutaneous laser surgery,* New York, 1992, Raven.
58. McDaniel DH: Case 8.21: café-au-lait lesion. In Apfelberg DB, editor: *Atlas of cutaneous laser surgery,* New York, 1992, Raven.
59. Rhodes A, Mihm MC Jr: Origin of cutaneous melanoma in a congenital dysplastic nevus spilus, *Arch Dermatol* 126:500, 1990.
60. Kopf AW, Levine LJ, Rigel DS et al: Congenital nevus-like nevi, nevi spili, and café-au-lait spots in patients with malignant melanoma, *J Dermatol Surg Oncol* 11:275, 1985.
61. Rhodes AR: Neoplasms: benign neoplasma, hyperplasias, and dysplasias of melanocytes. In Fitzpatrick TB, Eisen AZ, Wolff E et al, editors: *Dermatology in general medicine,* ed 3, New York, 1987, McGraw Hill.
62. Vion B, Belaich S, Grossin M et al: Les aspects evolutifs du naevus sur naevus, *Ann Dermatol Venereol* 112:813, 1985.
63. Wagner RF, Cottel WI: In situ malignant melanoma arising in a speckled lentiginous nevus, *J Am Acad Dermatol* 20:125, 1989.
64. Stern JB, Haupt HM, Aaronson CM: Malignant melanoma in a speckled zosteriform lentiginous nevus, *Int J Dermatol* 29:583, 1990.
65. Rutten A, Goos M: Nevus spilus with malignant melanoma in a patient with neurofibromatosis, *Arch Dermatol* 126:539, 1990.
66. Cohen HJ, Minkin W, Frank S: Nevus spilus, *Arch Dermatol* 102:433, 1970.
67. Stewart DM, Altman J, Megregan AH: Speckled lentiginous nevus, *Arch Dermatol* 114:895, 1978.
68. Brufau C, Moran M, Armijo M: Naevus sur naevus, *Ann Dermatol Venereol* 113:409, 1986.
69. Grevelink JM, Gonzalex S, Bonoan R et al: Treatment of nevus spilus with the Q-switched ruby laser, *Dermatol Surg* 23(5):365, 1997.
70. Miyasaka M, Tanino R, Morita T et al: Case 8.29: nevus spilus of the cheek; and case 8.30: nevus spilus of the left knee. In Apfelberg DB, editor: *Atlas of cutaneous laser surgery,* New York, 1992, Raven.

71. Tymen R, Forestier JF, Boutet B et al: Nevus tardiaf de Becker, *Ann Dermatol Venereol* 108:41, 1981.
72. Chapel TA, Tavafoghi V, Mehregan AH: Becker's melanosis: an organoid hamartoma, *Cutis* 27:405, 1981.
73. Haneke E: The dermal component in melanosis naeviformis Becker, *J Cutan Pathol* 6:53, 1979.
74. Sanchez NP, Pathak MA, Sato S et al: Melasma: a clinical, light microscopic, ultrastructural and immunofluorescent study, *J Am Acad Dermatol* 4:698, 1981.
75. Resnick S: Melasma induced by oral contraceptive drugs, *JAMA* 199:95, 1967.
76. Kopf AW, Lazar M, Bart RS et al: Prevalence of melanocytic nevi on the lateral aspect and medial aspect of the arms, *J Dermatol Surg Oncol* 4:153, 1987.
77. Pope DJ, Sorhan T, Marsden JR et al: Benign pigmented nevi in children: prevalence in associated factors: the west midlands, United Kingdom mole study, *Arch Dermatol* 128:1201, 1992.
78. Beral V, Evans S, Shaw H et al: Cutaneous factors related to the risk of malignant melanoma, *Fr J Epidemiol* 109:162, 1983.
79. Sorahan T, Grimley RP: The aetiological significance of sunlight and fluorescent lighting in malignant melanoma: a case-control study, *Br J Cancer* 52:765, 1985.
80. Green A, Bain C, McLennan R et al: Risk factors for cutaneous melanoma in Queensland, *Recent Results Cancer Res* 102:77, 1986.
81. Osterlind A, Tucker MA, Hou-Jensen K et al: The Danish case-control study of cutaneous malignant melanoma. 1. Importance of host factors, *Int J Cancer* 42:200, 1988.
82. Mackie RM, Watt D, Doherty V et al: Malignant melanoma occurring in those aged under 30 in the west of Scotland, 1979-1986: a study of incidence, clinical features, pathological features, and survival, *Br J Dermatol* 124:560, 1991.
83. Rosenbach A, Williams CM, Alster TS: Comparison of the Q-switched alexandrite (755 nm) and Q-switched Nd:YAG (1064 nm) lasers in the treatment of benign melanocytic nevi, *Dermatol Surg* 23(4):239, 1997.
84. Vibhagool C, Byers HR, Grevelink J: Treatment of small nevomelanocytic nevi with a Q-switched ruby laser, *J Am Acad Dermatol* 36(5, pt 1):738, 1997.
85. Grevelink JM, van Leeuwen RL, Anderson RR, Byers HR: Clinical and histological responses of congenital melanocytic nevi after single treatment with Q-switched lasers, *Arch Dermatol* 133(3):349, 1997.
86. Waldorf HA, Kauvar AN, Geronemus RG: Treatment of small and medium congenital nevi with the Q-switched ruby laser, *Arch Dermatol* 132(3):301, 1996.
87. Alper J, Holmes LB, Mihm MC: Birthmarks with serious medical significance, *J Pediatr* 95:696, 1979.
88. Walton RG, Jacobs AH, Koch AJ: Pigmented lesions in newborn infants, *Br J Dermatol* 95:389, 1976.
89. Kopf AW, Levine LJ, Rigel DS et al: Prevalence of congenital-nevus-like nevi, nevi spili, and café-au-lait spots, *Arch Dermatol* 121:766, 1985.
90. Trozak DJ, Rowland WD, Hu F: Metastatic melanoma in prepubertal children, *Pediatrics* 55:191, 1975.
91. Rhodes AR, Weinstock MA, Fitzpatrick TB et al: Risk factors for cutaneous melanoma: a practical method of recognizing predisposed individuals, *JAMA* 258:3146, 1987.
92. Illig L, Weidner F, Hundeiker M et al: Congenital nevi < 10 cm as precursors to melanoma: 52 cases, a review, and a new conception, *Arch Dermatol* 121:1274, 1985.
93. Rhodes AR, Sober AJ, Day CL et al: The malignant potential of small congenital nevocellular nevi: an estimate of association based on a histologic study of 234 primary cutaneous melanomas, *J Am Acad Dermatol* 6:230, 1982.
94. Rhodes AR, Melski JW: Small congenital nevocellular nevi and the risk of cutaneous melanoma, *J Pediatr* 100:219, 1982.
95. Rhodes AR: Congenital nevi: should these be excised? *JAMA* 262:1696, 1989.
96. Nakoaka H, Ohtsuka H: Ruby laser treatment of pigmented nevi: a histological analysis of ineffective cases, *Jpn J Plast Surg* 35:25, 1992.
97. Ueda S, Imayama S: Normal-mode ruby laser for treating congenital nevi, *Arch Dermatol* 133(3):355, 1997.
98. Zitelli JA, Grant MG, Abell E et al: Histologic patterns of congenital nevocitic nevi and implications for treatment, *J Am Acad Dermatol* 11:402, 1984.

99. Kudo S, Irao R: Nevus of Ota. In Nishiyama S, Shimao S, Hori Y, editors: *Current treatment of skin diseases,* Tokyo, 1987, Nankodo.
100. Dorsey CS, Montgomery H: Blue nevus and its distinction from Mongolian spot in the nevus of Ota, *J Invest Dermatol* 22:225, 1954.
101. Ihm C-W: Nevus of Ota and nevus of Itō. In Demis DJ, editor: *Clinical dermatology,* ed 19, Philadelphia, 1992, Lippincott.
102. Kobayashi T: Microsurgical treatment of nevus of Ota, *J Dermatol Surg Oncol* 17:936, 1991.
103. Apfelberg DB: Case 4.50: nevus of Ota. In Apfelberg DB, editor: *Atlas of cutaneous laser surgery,* New York, 1992, Raven.
104. Miyasaka M, Tanino R, Morita T et al: Case 8.28: nevus of Ota of the left eyelid. In Apfelberg DB, editor: *Atlas of cutaneous laser surgery,* New York, 1992, Raven.
105. Geronemus RG: Q-switched ruby laser therapy of nevus of Ota, *Arch Dermatol* 128:1618, 1992.
106. Lowe NJ, Wieder JM, Sawcer D, Burrows P: Nevus of Ota: treatment with the high energy fluences of the Q-switched ruby laser, *J Am Acad Dermatol* 29(6):997, 1993.
107. Taylor CR, Flotte TJ, Gange RW, Anderson RR: Treatment of nevus of Ota by Q-switched ruby laser, *J Am Acad Dermatol* 30(5, pt 1):743, 1994.
108. Alster TS, Williams CM: Treatment of nevus of Ota by the Q-switched alexandrite laser, *Dermatol Surg* 21:592, 1995
109. Spielvogel RL: Blue nevus. In Demis DJ, editor: *Clinical dermatology,* ed 19, Philadelphia, 1992, Lippincott.
110. Rodriguez HA, Ackerman LV: Cellular blue nevus: clinicopathologic study of 45 cases, *Cancer* 21:393, 1968.
111. Rubenstein N, Kopolovic J, Wexler MR et al: Malignant blue nevus, *J Dermatol Surg Oncol* 11:921, 1985.
112. Milgraum SS, Cohen ME, Auletta MJ: Treatment of blue nevi with the Q-switched ruby laser, *J Am Acad Dermatol* 32:307, 1995.
113. Tournay PR: Sclerosing treatment of very fine intra or subdermal varicosities, *Soc Fran Phlebo* 19:235, 1966.
114. Bodian EL: Techniques of sclerotherapy for sunburst venous blemishes, *J Dermatol Surg Oncol* 11:696, 1985.
115. Cacciatore E: Experience of sclerotherapy with aethoxysklerol, *Minerva Cardioangiol* 27:255, 1979.
116. Cuttell PJ, Fox JA: The etiology and treatment of varicose pigmentation, *Phlebologie* 35:387, 1982.
117. Goldman MP, Kaplan RP, Duffy DM: Postsclerotherapy hyperpigmentation: a histologic evaluation, *J Dermatol Surg Oncol* 13:547, 1987.
118. Goldman MP: Complications and adverse sequelae of sclerotherapy. In Goldman MP, editor: *Sclerotherapy treatment of varicose and telangiectatic leg veins,* St Louis, 1991, Mosby.
119. Simionescu N, Simionescu M, Palade GE: Open junctions in the endothelium of the postcapillary venules of the diaphragm, *J Cell Biol* 79:27, 1978.
120. Heltinau C, Simionescu M, Simionescu N: Histamine receptors of the microvascular endothelium revealed in situ with a histamine-ferritin conjugate: characteristic high-affinity binding sites in venules, *J Cell Biol* 93:357, 1982.
121. Bjork J, Smedegard G: The microvascula of the hamster cheek pouch as a model for studying acute immune-complex-induced inflammatory reactions, *Int Arch Allergy Appl Immunol* 74:178, 1984.
122. Fox J, Galey F, Wayland H: Action of histamine on the mesenteric microvasculature, *Microvasc Res* 19:108, 1980.
123. Thibault P, Wlodarczyk J: Postsclerotherapy hyperpigmentation: the role of serum iron levels and the effectiveness of treatment with the copper vapor laser, *J Dermatol Surg Oncol* 18:47, 1992.
124. Goldman MP: Post-sclerotherapy hyperpigmentation: treatment with a flashlamp-excited pulsed dye laser, *J Dermatol Surg Oncol* 18:417, 1992.
125. Shoden A, Sturgeon P: Hemosiderin. 1. A physio-chemical study, *Acta Haematol* 23:376, 1960.
126. Wells CI, Wolken JJ: Biochemistry: microspectrophotometry of haemosiderin granules, *Nature* 193:977, 1962.

127. Scheibner A, Kenny G, White W et al: A superior method of tattoo removal using the Q-switched ruby laser, *J Dermatol Surg Oncol* 16:1091, 1990.
128. Nelson JS: Case 8.23: epidermal melanosis secondary to post-traumatic hyperpigmentation. In Apfelberg DB, editor: *Atlas of cutaneous laser surgery,* New York, 1992, Raven.
129. Kilmer SL, Farinelli WE, Tearney G, Anderson RR: Use of a larger spot size for treatment of tattoos increases clinical efficacy and decreases potential side effects, *Lasers Surg Med Suppl* 6:51, 1994.

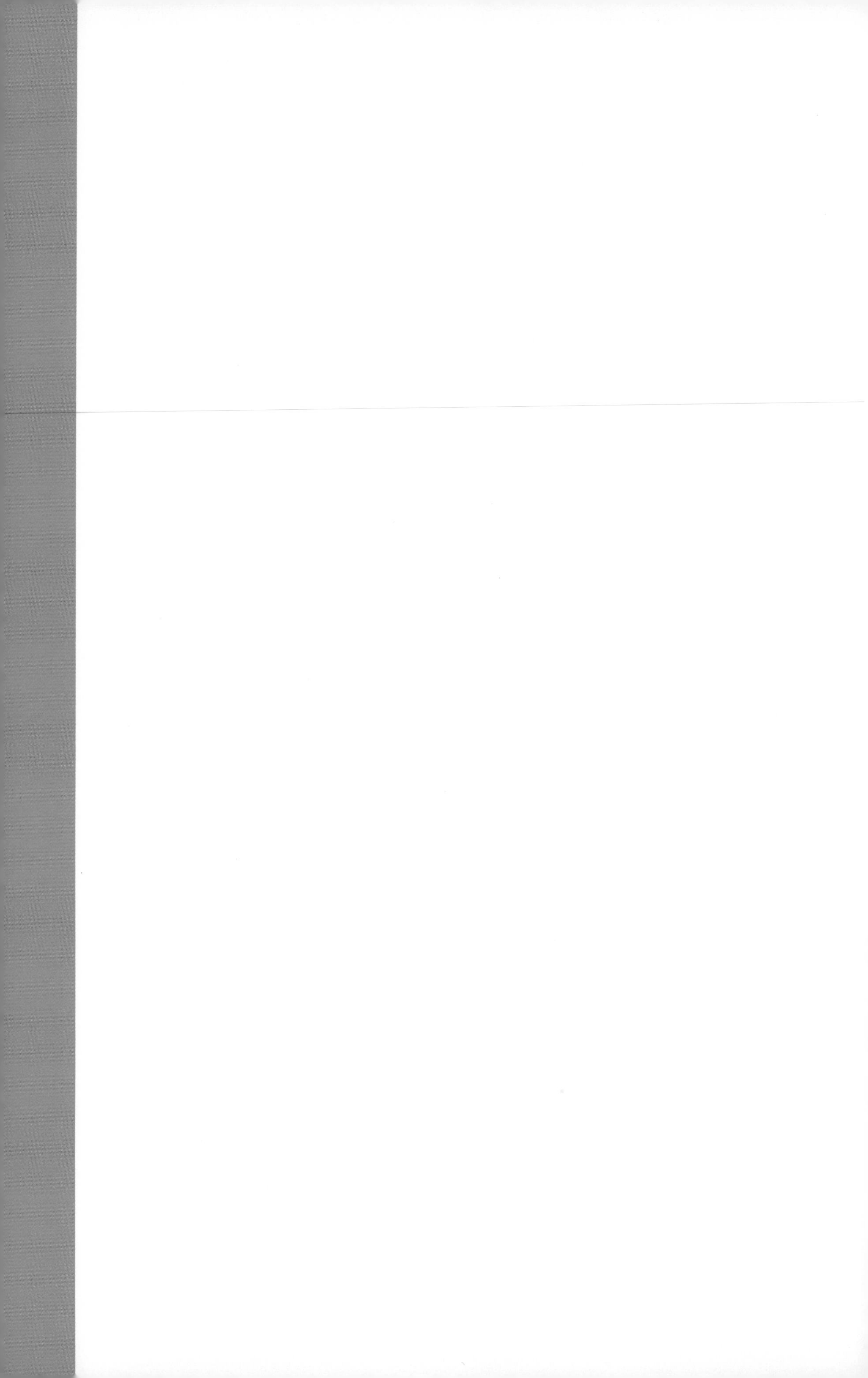

CHAPTER four

Treatment of Tattoos

Suzanne Linsmeier Kilmer, Richard E. Fitzpatrick, and Mitchel P. Goldman

OVERVIEW

Tattooing is an ancient art whose origins have been traced as far back as the Stone Age (12,000 BC).[1] Primitive humans slashed their skin during bereavement ceremonies and rubbed ash into the cuts as a sign of grief. Decorative tattooing has been traced to the Bronze Age (8000 BC) by the circumstantial evidence of crude needles and pigment bowls found in caves in France, Spain, and Portugal.[2] People of this age decorated animal skins worn for warmth with ochre and plant pigments. This may have led to decorative tattooing of their own skin, because mummies dating from 4000 BC had crude tattoos.[3] Tattooing thrived as well throughout ancient China, Japan, and North Africa, areas isolated by geography and absence of communication, suggesting that tattooing represents a response to an inherent human need.

Although most psychologic studies of persons with tattoos have been restricted to psychiatric inpatients,[4-6] prisoners in correctional institutions,[4-9] and military personnel,[10-12] and as such reflect only specific populations, one common conclusion of these studies is that, of all the various motives for obtaining a tattoo, the quest for personal identity is central. The skin serves as a useful canvas to portray statements of individuality, sexuality, belonging, machismo, frustration, boredom, and anger. The average age of acquisition of a professional tattoo is 18 years[13] and that of a self-inflicted amateur tattoo 14 years.[14-16] However, one's quest for identity at ages 14 to 18 is often irrelevant or embarrassing at age 40, and 50% or more of individuals regret their tattoos.[5,12] Even Egyptian mummies from 4000 BC show evidence of attempts at tattoo removal.[17] Because most people live in the present rather than in anticipation of future endeavors, however, tattoos remain popular; 9% to 11% of adult men in the United States have tattoos (Candela Laser Corporation, unpublished data, 1991), and 50,000 to 100,000 women actively pursue tattooing as body art each year.[18] In a recent study of professional women with tattoos, 94% were pleased with the tattoo,[18] although a potential bias exists in that those who were pleased may have been more likely to respond; 55% had friends with tattoos, a known influential factor. Despite this bias and stated satisfaction, 38% mentioned significant problems with having a tattoo and 28% were considering tattoo removal. In general, tattoos are not well received by the public and often are a barrier to employment. Tattooed individuals are perceived as antisocial, aggressive, or immature and as unable to accept controls and authority.

HISTOLOGY

Very little is known regarding the natural history of an intradermally placed tattoo. A report of serial biopsy examinations of tattoos placed 24 hours; 1, 2, and 3 months; and 40 years previously has given some insight into this process,[19] as has an electron microscopic study of tattoos treated with the Q-switched ruby,[20] argon, and tunable dye lasers.[21] Initially, ink particles are found within large phagosomes in the cytoplasm of both keratinocytes and phagocytic cells, including fibroblasts, macrophages, and mast cells.[22-24] The epidermis, epidermal-dermal junction, and papillary dermis appear homogenized immediately after tattoo injection. At 1 month the basement membrane is reforming, and aggregates of ink particles are present within basal cells. In the dermis, ink-containing phagocytic cells concentrate along the epidermal-dermal border below a layer of granulation tissue closely surrounded by collagen. Pigment is not seen within mast cells, endothelial cells, pericytes, Schwann cells, in the lumina of blood and lymphatic vessels, or extracellularly. At 1 month, transepidermal elimination of ink particles through the epidermis is still in progress, with ink particles present in keratinocytes, macrophages, and fibroblasts.

Reestablishment of an intact basement membrane prevents further transepidermal loss. In biopsies obtained at 2 to 3 months and 40 years, ink particles are found only in dermal fibroblasts, predominantly in a perivascular location beneath a layer of fibrosis, which had replaced the granulation tissue.[25] Rabbit studies support that the fibroblast is responsible for the stable intracutaneous life span of the tattoo.[24] Ink particle aggregates were usually surrounded by a single membrane, suggesting they were partially free in the dermis; however, they were not found free in several studies[19,20,24] and in one study[21] were present both extracellularly as well as within fibroblasts. The interpretation of free extracellular tattoo pigment may be a consequence of the difficulty in detecting the single membrane seen by some investigators.[19,20,24] Tattoo pigment has been reported both intracellularly and extracellularly[26-32] and with mild fibrosis and occasional foreign body giant cell reactions,[25] allergic granulomas,[26,27] and sarcoid reactions.[25,33,34]

Tattoo particles are initially dispersed diffusely as fine granules in the upper dermis as well as in vertical foci at sites of injection but aggregate to a more focal concentrated appearance between 7 and 13 days.[19,24] Black ink granules have a mean diameter of 4.42 ± 0.72 μm[19] as compared to a mean particle diameter of 4.024 ± 0.76 μm when embedded in agar. Taylor and colleagues[20] found black pigment granules in tattoos to be polymorphous, varying 0.5 to 4.0 μm in diameter. Turquoise and red pigment particles are approximately twice as large as black granules. In both amateur and professional tattoos, pigment ink depth and density are highly variable, although greater variability of size, shape, and location is noted with amateur tattoos. However, despite the diverse origins of tattoo pigment, the light and electron microscopic appearances of all pigments are remarkably similar, except for their color (Figure 4-1).

Tattoo pigment granules are composed of three kinds of loosely packed particles, ranging 2 to 400 nm in diameter,[20] most often 40 nm, much less often 2 to 4 nm and slightly more electron dense, and least frequently 400 nm and very electron dense with a crystalline structure. A study of freshly implanted eyeliner tattoo ink revealed particle size in the extracellular matrix to be 0.1 to 1.0 μm, even though the average particle size in the pigment vial before implantation was 0.25 μm.[35] A prominent network of connective tissue surrounds each of the fibroblasts containing ink particles, effectively entrapping and immobilizing the cell. The life span of these fibroblasts is unknown and may persist for the individual's life.

Although these studies give considerable detail regarding the architectural morphology and physiology, they do not fully explain the natural history of dermal tattoo ink. It is common to observe that a tattoo becomes duller, bluer, more indistinct, and blurred with time, presumably a consequence of ink particles moving deeper into the dermis, by the action of mobile phagocytic cells. Indeed, random biopsies of older tattoos demonstrate pigment in the deep dermis as opposed to a more superficial location of newer tattoos.[36] Eventually tattoo ink appears in regional lymph nodes of tattooed patients.[36,37]

Tattoo ink is remarkably nonreactive histologically, even though many different pigments, often of unknown purity and identity, are used by tattoo artists (Box 4-1).[5,35,37-39] Amateur tattoo inks consist of simple carbon particles from burnt wood,

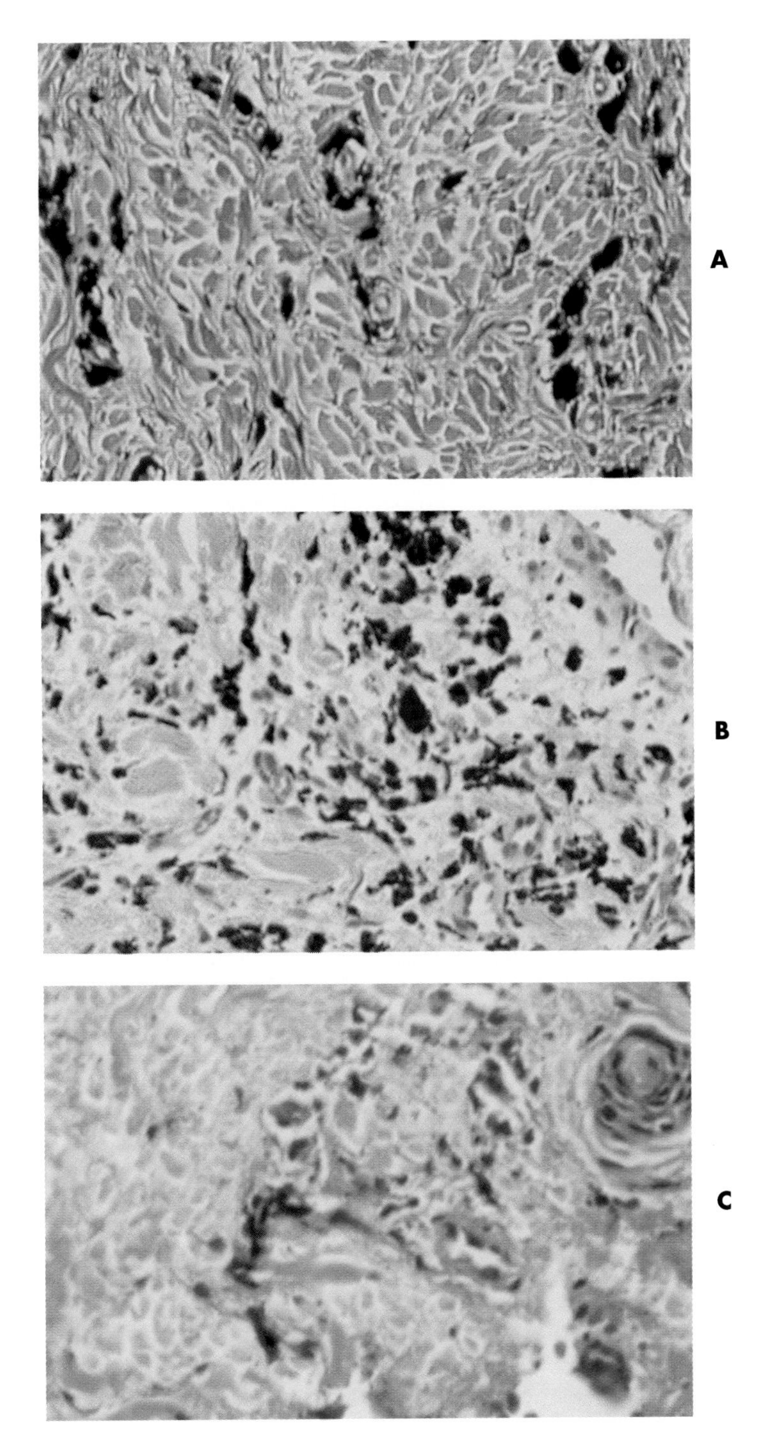

Figure 4-1 **A,** Black tattoo ink in dermis. **B,** Red tattoo ink in dermis. **C,** Green tattoo ink in dermis. (All magnification ×40.)

cotton, plastic, or paper or from a variety of inks, including India ink, various pen inks, and even vegetable matter. Although rare, red (mercury),[30,31,38,40,41] yellow (cadmium),[37,42-44] green (chromium),[38,41,44,45] and blue (cobalt)[46] tattoo pigments have elicited a persistent localized allergic or photoallergic dermatitis, and, more rarely, systemic reactions.[47-50] Interestingly, the colors most often involved in allergic reactions (red and yellow) often spontaneously disappear from a tattoo, even without any clinical signs of reaction[42] (Figure 4-2).

Box 4-1 Pigments used by tattoo artists

Black
Carbon
Iron oxide
Logwood (extract from logwood tree)

Blue
Cobaltic aluminate (azure blue)

Green
Chrome oxide (Casalis green)
Hydrated chromium sesquioxide (Guignet green)
Malachite green
Lead chromate
Ferro-ferric cyanide
Curcumin green
Phthalocyanine dyes (copper salts with yellow coal tar dyes)

Red
Mercury sulfide (cinnabar)
Cadmium selenide (cadmium red)

Red—cont'd
Sienna (ochre: ferric hydrate and ferric sulfate)

Yellow
Cadmium sulfide (cadmium yellow)
Ochre
Curcumin yellow

Brown
Ochre

Violet
Manganese violet

White
Titanium dioxide, zinc oxide

Flesh
Iron oxides (variant of ochre)

Data from Everett MA: Tattoos: abnormalities of pigmentation. In *Clinical dermatology,* Hagerstown, Md, 1980, Harper & Row; and Rosfenberg A, Brown RA, Caro MR: *Arch Dermatol Syph* 62:540, 1950.

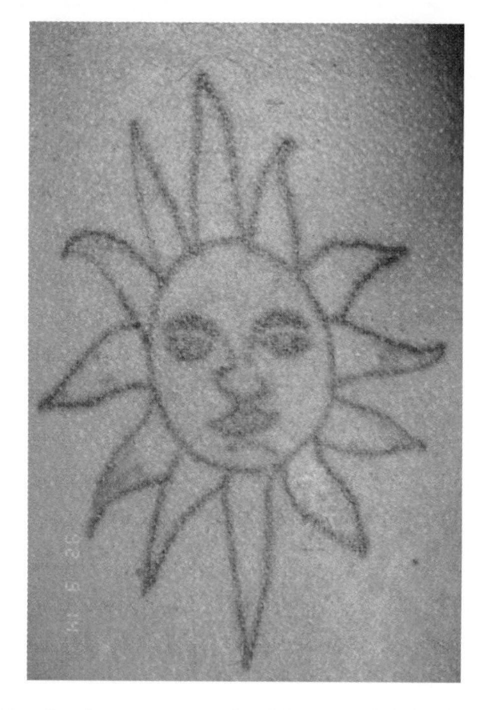

Figure 4-2 This tattoo has been present for 20 years. Original tattoo consisted of red "flames" from sun with yellow tips. Over the years the yellow has faded completely and the red has faded away greater than 95%.

Tattoo Removal Techniques

Over the centuries, many different methods for tattoo removal have been explored. The earliest documented report of tattoo removal was by Aetius, a Greek physician, who described salabrasion in 543 AD.[16] Older tattoo removal techniques involve destruction or removal of the outer skin layers by mechanical, chemical, or thermal means, accompanied by inflammation. Transepidermal elimination of pigment occurs through denuded skin[51-54] and via an exudative phase that allows tattoo pigment to migrate to the wound surface to be absorbed into the dressing. The inflammatory response may also promote macrophage activity with increased phagocytosis, enabling additional pigment loss during the healing phase.

MECHANICAL TISSUE DESTRUCTION

The primary method of mechanical tissue destruction is *dermabrasion.* To remove as much of the tattoo pigment as possible, a rapidly spinning diamond fraise wheel or a wire brush abrades skin that has usually been frozen with a skin refrigerant such as Frigiderm to produce a hard surface.[51,54] This tends to be bloody with tissue and blood particulates of a size that can access the pulmonary and mucosal surfaces, aerosolized in the operative suite,[55] with potentially infectious agents.

Subsequent scarring is worse if complete pigment removal is attempted in one session by creating a deep wound to the full depth of the tattoo pigment. Removing tissue only to the depth of the papillary dermis[52] (Figure 4-3) minimizes scarring but leaves significant tattoo pigment, requiring additional procedures, thereby increasing the potential for scarring. To enhance the efficacy of the procedure, gentian violet[56,57] or tannic acid and silver nitrate[52] have been applied to the superficially abraded surface, and exposed pigment has been curetted[58] or removed with fine tweezers.[59,60] Other mechanical treatments include linear incisions, scratches, punctures,[56] and a grid of crisscross abrasions followed by application of a caustic chemical.[59]

Salabrasion, the oldest method of physical tissue destruction, involves abrading the superficial dermis past the point of bleeding with coarse granules of common table salt and a moist gauze pad.[16] Salt is then applied to the wound surface and left in place under the surgical dressing for 24 hours. Although some authors are very enthusiastic about this procedure,[61-65] residual tattoo pigment often remains after the wound heals.

The primary disadvantage of all these mechanical destructive modalities is the high risk of *scarring;* hypertrophic scars are very common when the removal of tissue is performed deeply in an attempt to remove all tattoo pigment. In addition, residual tattoo pigment is common (Figure 4-4), and postoperative pain can be significant.

Surgical excision of skin containing tattoo pigment is also common but often results in incomplete tattoo removal, tissue distortion, and scarring because of limitations in wound closure and healing (Figure 4-5). Small tattoos located in areas of adequate skin laxity allowing primary closure without excessive tension can be removed very satisfactorily with simple excision.[64] However, this situation does not occur often, and complex wound closures,[56,63] skin grafting,[56,66] multistage excision,[54,56,59,64,67] and the use of tissue expanders[66] are often necessary to repair the tissue defect created by excision of the tattoo. These techniques typically result in scarring and tissue changes that are unacceptable to the patient. Split-thickness tangential excision without grafting has been reported as well[68] but has the same limitations as dermabrasion.

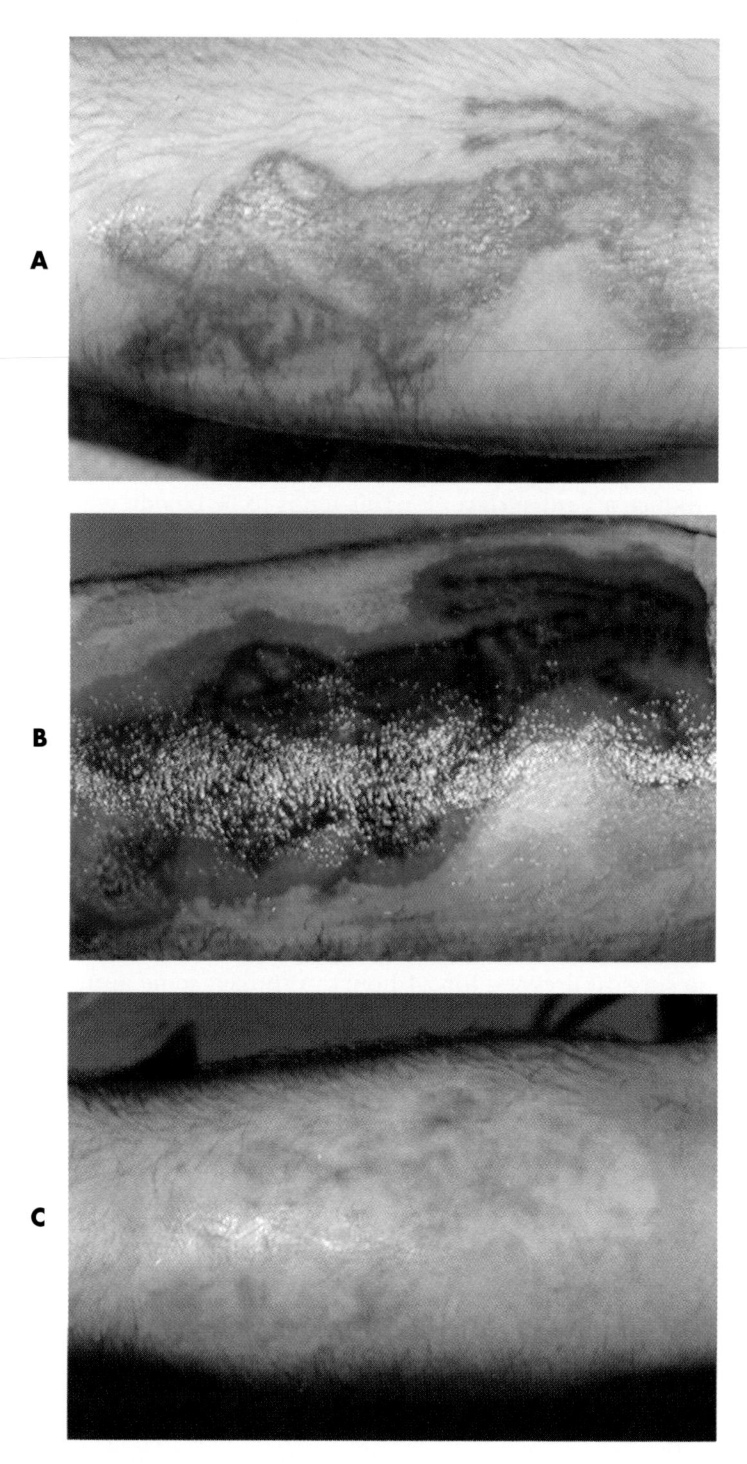

Figure 4-3 **A,** Tattoo of forearm 1 month after one session of superficial dermabrasion. **B,** Immediately after dermabrasion session number two. **C,** Scarring and residual tattoo are evident 6 months after fourth dermabrasion session.

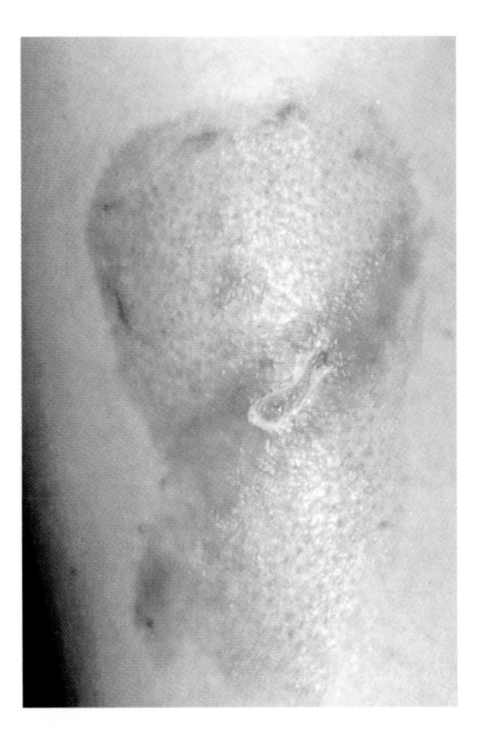

Figure 4-4 Hypertrophic scar is present in central aspect of this tattoo, as well as residual pigment at superior aspect 1 month after dermabrasion.

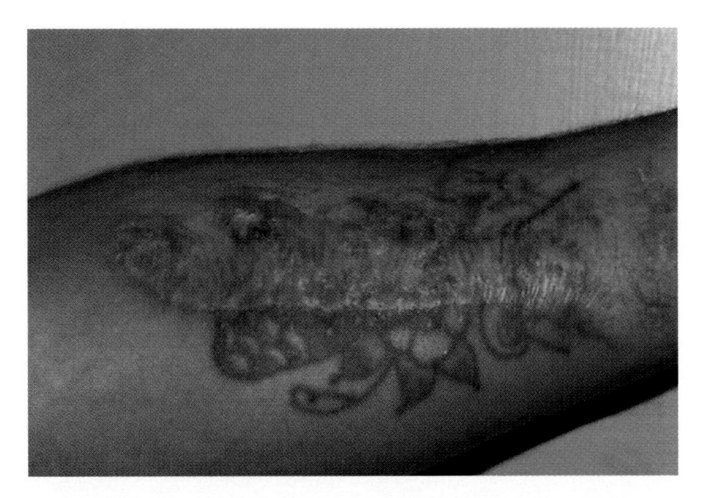

Figure 4-5 Staged linear excisions of this tattoo had been planned but were abandoned because of difficulty in wound closure. Incomplete tattoo removal and widely stretched unsightly scar are end result of procedure performed.

Chemical Tissue Destruction

Variot first described the use of caustic chemicals (tannic acid and silver nitrate) after disruption of the skin surface with punctures and incisions in 1888.[69] This technique, known as the *French method,* results in a less coarse scar than that which would occur from the application of more destructive chemicals[59] but often has variable amounts of residual tattoo. A combination of superficial dermabrasion and application of tannic acid also resulted in hypertrophic scarring in 34% of patients and residual tattoo in cases with deep tattoo pigment.[70]

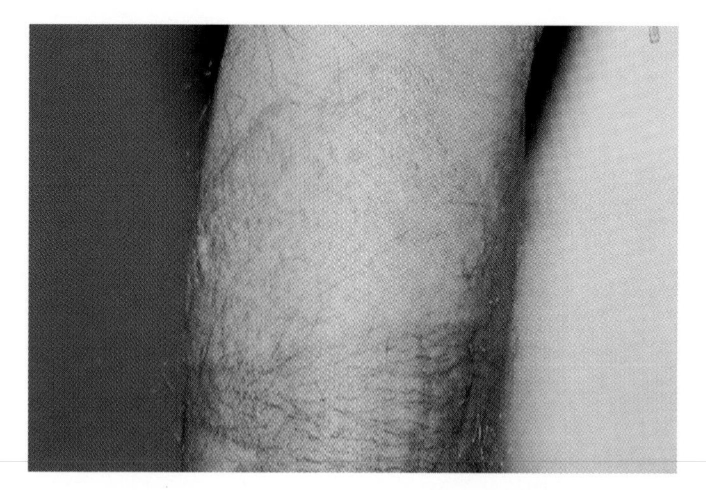

Figure 4-6 Upper portion of this tattoo was removed by injection of tannic acid into skin by a tattoo needle, which induced tissue necrosis and slough followed by hypertrophic scarring.

Intradermal injection of tannic acid with the use of reciprocating needles results in epidermal and superficial dermal slough and has the same risks as other destructive modalities[16] (Figure 4-6). Phenol solution, used in the same manner as for facial peels,[63] and trichloroacetic acid (TCA) used in a 95% solution[71,72] have been used to remove tattoos but result in hypopigmented scars. Repeat application is hazardous and may result in a full-thickness burn requiring skin grafting.

Thermal Tissue Destruction

Thermal injury, via fire, hot coals, and cigarettes, has been used for centuries in an attempt to remove unwanted tattoos, usually with significant scarring. Thermal cautery, with the use of a glowing soldering iron or an electrical spark for electrodesiccation or electrocautery, is equally crude and unpredictable (Figure 4-7).

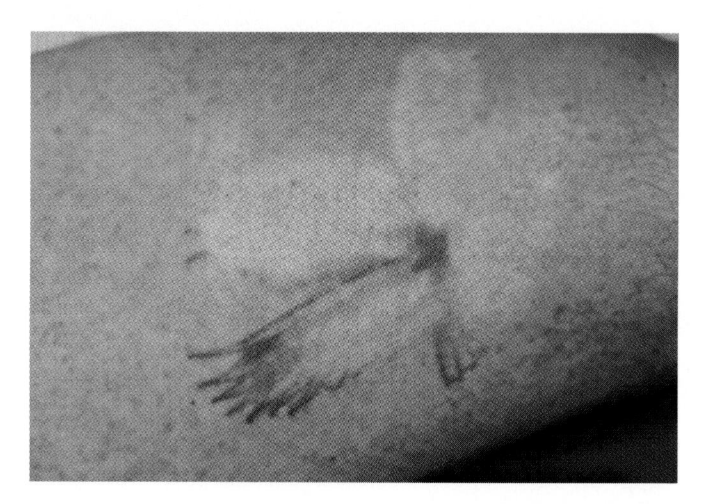

Figure 4-7 Patient attempted to remove this tattoo from his arm by heating a butter knife with a cigarette lighter flame and applying the hot knife blade to his skin. Resultant scarring and tattoo removal are comparable to other nonspecific tissue-destructive treatment modalities.

The *infrared coagulator,* developed in West Germany in 1979, delivers a noncoherent, multispectral light with preset pulses triggered by an electronic timer. This instrument is used in an attempt to produce a more controlled cutaneous thermal injury[73] for treatment of cutaneous vascular lesions[74-76] and tattoos.[76-79] A tungsten halogen light is used as the energy source and emits light with wavelengths of 400 to 2700 nm and a maximum emission near the infrared (IR) range at 900 to 960 nm. The primary tissue chromophores at this range are water and oxygenated hemoglobin (see Chapters 2 and 3), but when exogenous black and blue tattoo pigments predominate as target chromophores, a nonspecific thermal burn from heat absorption and diffusion into tissue would be expected. Pulse duration can be varied from 0.8 to 1.5 sec; pulses of 1.25 and 1.5 sec have been reported,[77-80] with use of a 1.125-sec pulse achieving coagulation to a depth of 1 mm.[80] These pulse durations are far in excess of the thermal relaxation time of tattoo particles, blood vessels, and other dermal structures and thus produce nonspecific damage. A quartzlike guide is used to transmit light to a 6-mm sapphire tip, which is placed on the skin surface. This technique has little advantage over the other nonspecific methods reviewed, because scarring is inevitable, and incomplete tattoo removal is common. Amateur tattoos have been more responsive than professional tattoos, particularly those on the fingers.[80]

Although the use of liquid nitrogen (−196° C) to destroy superficial cutaneous lesions is commonly used in general dermatology,[81,82] it has not proved very useful in tattoo removal because the nonspecific destruction leads to prolonged healing and unpredictable results.[56,67,83] However, successful treatment has been described,[84-86] particularly the use of two 30-sec freeze-thaw cycles for the treatment of digital tattoos.[86]

Thermal Tissue Destruction with Lasers

Early on, it was hoped that lasers would provide a precise means of inducing predictable thermal necrosis to tattoo-containing tissue in a manner that would eliminate scarring. Tattoo removal with the ruby and argon laser was first proposed by Goldman et al in 1963,[87] and a relatively enthusiastic report of the normal-mode ruby laser[87] was soon followed by one using the Q-switched ruby laser.[89] Goldman's initial report of successful tattoo removal using ruby (694 nm) and neodymium:yttrium-aluminum-garnet (Nd:YAG) (1060 nm) lasers appeared in 1967.[90] A study of Q-switched ruby laser interaction with tattoo pigment appeared the same year,[91] and further studies[92,93] confirmed this specific laser-tissue interaction. Unfortunately, these early reports were largely ignored for 15 years, and attention was focused on the newly emerging field of laser surgery using the argon and carbon dioxide (CO_2) lasers.

Argon Laser

The first report of the use of the argon laser for tattoo removal in 28 patients appeared in 1979.[94] Although hypertrophic scarring occurred in 21% and half of the patients had residual tattoo pigment, the complete removal of tattoo pigment in eight patients (29%) with acceptable cosmetic results (reported as excellent, without scarring) led the authors to recommend this laser enthusiastically for tattoo removal. In their subsequent study, 20 of 60 patients had complete removal of tattoo pigment without scarring, with amateur tattoos responding slightly better than professional tattoos (42% versus 29%).[95] However, hypertrophic scarring occurred in 35% of patients, and residual tattoo pigment remained in 67%. Biopsy studies showed obliteration of the dermis to a depth of 1 mm, and the authors stressed the preservation of adnexal structures to aid wound healing and avoid scarring.[94-96]

The initial use of the argon laser for treatment of tattoos was based on selective absorption of energy with vaporization from its 488- and 514-nm wavelengths by complementary tattoo pigment colors.[95,97] However, the clinical usefulness of this factor is severely limited by melanin and hemoglobin absorption of laser energy, resulting in unwanted thermal damage to tissue.[21,97] It was also originally thought that selective heating of tattoo pigments and their immediate surroundings would elicit an inflammatory response and help remove or obscure the pigment. Although nonspecific heat absorption resulted in diffuse tissue necrosis, this was thought to be necessary for successful pigment removal.[21]

A histologic study was performed to determine if it was possible to oxidize or fragment tattoo pigment, confining thermal necrosis to a zone immediately adjacent to tattoo particles and thus avoiding widespread thermal necrosis of the dermis.[21] The argon laser was used with powers ranging from 1.0 to 3.5 W and shuttered pulses of 0.2 sec and 50 msec in addition to a continuous beam, using a 1-mm spot size. At 48 hours, subepidermal blisters overlying necrotic papillary dermal collagen appeared with all treatment parameters. At 3 months, fibrosis was present in the papillary and upper reticular dermis. Pigment-laden macrophages were present at the junction of fibrotic and nonfibrotic dermis, with pigment present at a deeper level within the dermis. Thus, even though these authors were able to demonstrate somewhat selective absorption of laser energy by tattoo pigment (the threshold be-

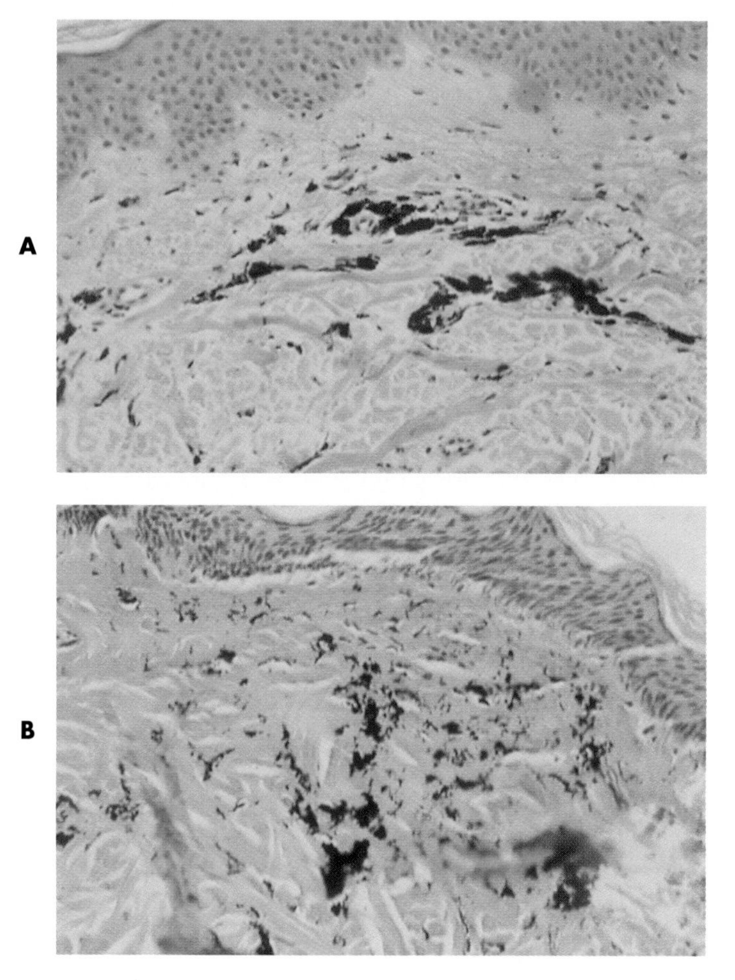

Figure 4-8 Nonspecific thermal damage of dermis and epidermis after treatment of tattoo using the argon laser at 1.2 W with a continuous beam. (×40.) **A,** Before treatment. **B,** After treatment.

ing 6.25 J/cm^2 for black and red tattoos, compared with 20 J/cm^2 for injury to normal skin), the 50- to 200-msec pulses allowed extensive diffusion of heat from all absorbing chromophores, resulting in nonselective thermal destruction. The inflammatory response was found to be a minor factor; clinical improvement depended on widespread necrosis removing pigment and resultant fibrosis altering light transmission through the dermis to obscure underlying residual pigment. Fitzpatrick et al[98] confirmed these results and the lack of a specific laser-induced change in tattoo pigment particles as a result of argon laser therapy (Figure 4-8). Although Apfelberg and colleagues[99] reported the argon laser to be comparable to the CO_2 laser for tattoo removal, the relatively low power emission of the argon laser results in inefficient removal of tattoo pigment, requiring multiple treatment sessions, and a high incidence of hypertrophic scarring (Figure 4-9).

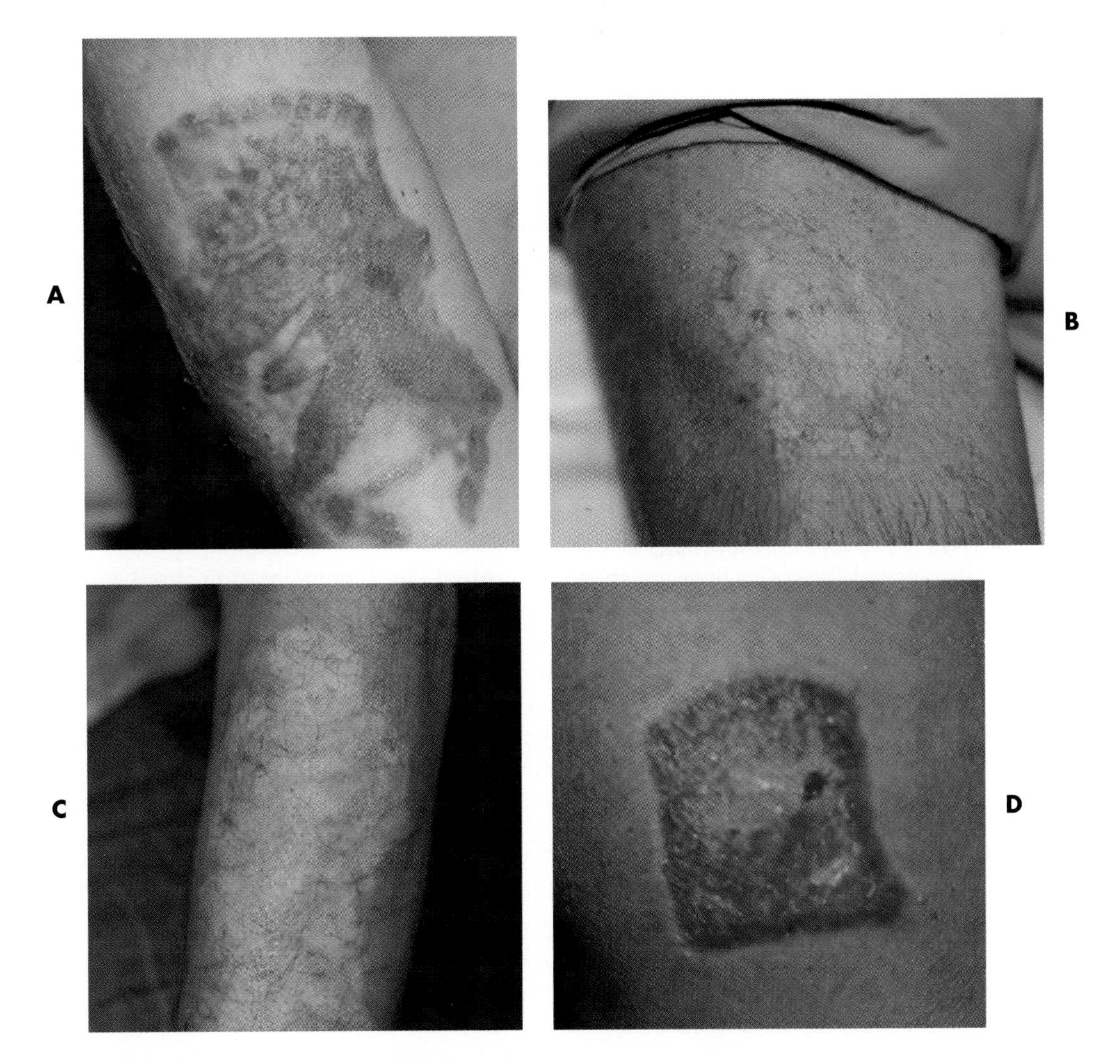

Figure 4-9 Spectrum of results of tattoo removal using argon laser. **A,** Incomplete tattoo removal 1 month after single treatment session. **B,** Mild scarring and minimal residual tattoo 1 year after third treatment session with argon laser. **C,** Atrophic scarring, hypopigmentation, and residual pigment 6 months after seven treatment sessions with argon laser. **D,** Hypertrophic scar and residual tattoo pigment after treatment with argon laser.

Carbon Dioxide Laser

Initial reports of the successful removal of tattoos with the CO_2 laser appeared in 1978,[97,100,101] and other reports followed soon thereafter.[102-105] The CO_2 laser emits a continuous beam at 10,600 nm, a wavelength completely absorbed by water, limiting penetration to a depth of 0.1 to 0.2 mm. Instantaneous transfer of heat from laser absorption by tissue (cellular) water results in immediate vaporization. The physics of this interaction were initially misinterpreted to imply that this always results in confinement of thermal damage to the 30- to 50-μm layer of laser impact. In reality, thermal diffusion can be quite extensive when a continuous beam is used. Even with pulses of 50 to 200 msec, great caution must be used to avoid unwanted thermal necrosis (see Chapter 6).

The original objective in CO_2 treatment of tattoos was to vaporize tissue containing tattoo pigment, using visual control to remove all tattoo pigment in one treatment session. Attempts were made to confine the depth of tissue vaporization to the precise level of tattoo pigment, which often varies from one portion of the tattoo to another, resulting in a variable wound depth. Histologic evaluation of the created wounds revealed loss of dermis and subcutaneous tissue up to a depth of 5 mm.[102] Because of the slow healing time (4.5 ± 1.5 weeks)[97] and resultant thick, unsightly scars, most did not attempt complete pigment removal in one session and instead treated more conservatively, relying on macrophage engulfment and transepidermal removal of tattoo pigment during the healing phase.[102] Residual pigment is re-treated after healing is complete. Recently applied tattoos respond more readily to treatment with the CO_2 and argon lasers, presumably because pigment is more uniformly superficial in the papillary dermis, lying free rather than within dermal fibroblasts, particularly during the first month after application (Figure 4-10).

Originally used as a continuous beam, repetitive pulses of 50 to 200 msec or superpulsed CO_2 lasers became more acceptable, with reports of good results in 29 of 30 tattoos after an average of 2.4 treatments. Although only a 7% incidence of hypertrophic scarring was noted, vaporization confined to the tattoo may result in a scar in its original shape; therefore feathering into normal tissue is recommended. Power settings of 8 to 25 W were common for repetitive treatments, with higher powers more rapidly vaporizing tissue.

Because of the common occurrence of residual tattoo pigment after more superficial CO_2 laser vaporization, together with the increasing risk of hypertrophic scarring with subsequent treatments, methods to improve the results of a single treatment were explored. Although the concomitant use of 2% gentian violet to prolong the exudative phase following superficial CO_2 laser vaporization did not increase efficacy, 50% urea paste did improve results,[106] as previously reported in conjunction with the argon laser.[107] Tissue is vaporized only to the papillary dermis. A generous application of 50% urea in hydrophilic ointment is applied to the wound and covered with a nonstick dressing. The dressing is changed daily with reapplication of the urea ointment for 1 to 2 weeks, until tattoo pigment is no longer seen on the bandage. This usually removes more than 95% of the tattoo pigment in a single treatment. Hypertrophic scarring depends more on anatomic location than operative technique (25% incidence for deltoid and chest areas, 10% for other locations), and although excellent results can be obtained, the cosmetic results are unpredictable and some scarring usually occurs.

In summary, the CO_2 laser removes tattoo pigment in much the same way as the argon laser, although with higher fluences, tissue vaporization with the CO_2 laser is significantly more efficient. Tattoo pigment is removed by direct tissue vaporization, as well as by thermal necrosis of adjacent tissue and through loss of pigment in the exudative healing phase. Dermal tissue is reconstituted by fibrosis and scar tissue.

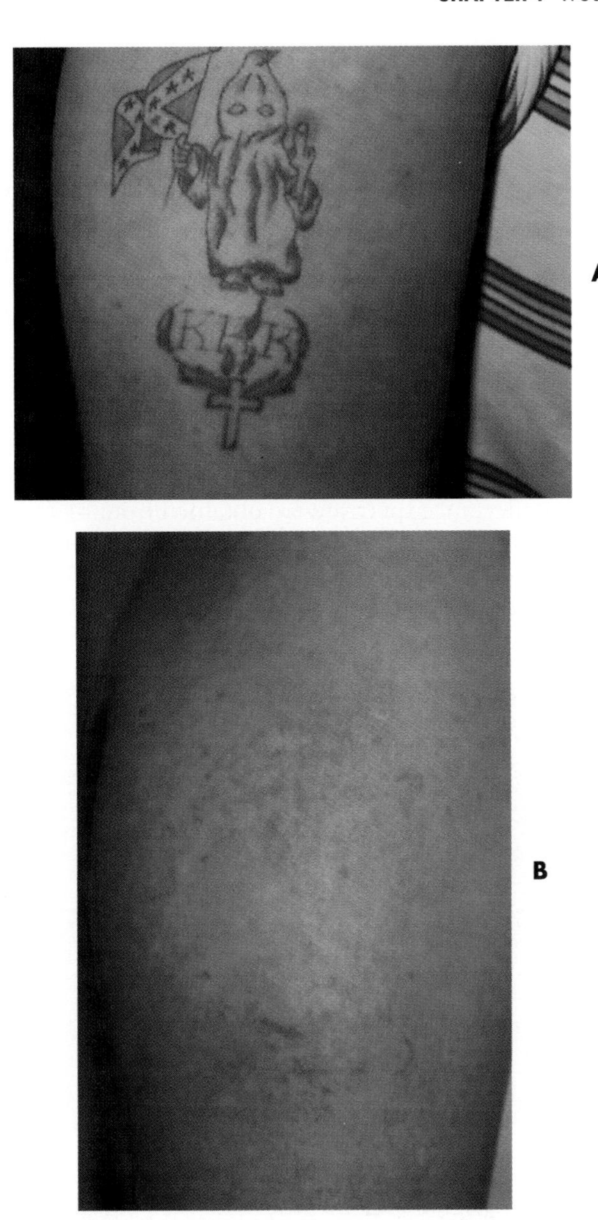

Figure 4-10 Complete removal of tattoo present less than 72 hours with two treatments of argon laser. **A,** Before treatment. **B,** Six months after second argon laser treatment.

PULSED LASER TREATMENT OF TATTOOS

Anderson and Parrish's principle of *selective photothermolysis* revolutionized the treatment of tattoos.[108] They proposed that if a wavelength was well absorbed by the target and the pulse width was equal to or shorter than the target's thermal relaxation time, the heat generated would be confined to the target. To target tattoos specifically, laser wavelength and pulse duration must be appropriately chosen. In one of the earliest studies, Diette et al[21] examined the effects of a tunable dye laser at three wavelengths (505, 577, and 680 nm) using a 1-μsec pulse to remove black, blue, red, and white tattoo pigment. They found that the threshold dose to induce the same histologic changes was much less than that required for the argon laser, and that each wavelength reacted only with complementary colors of tattoo pigment. However, despite the short 1-μsec pulse, widespread tissue necrosis was observed, and tattoo lightening occurred only as a result of significant dermal necrosis and resultant fibrosis. The authors postulated that an even shorter pulse in the nanosecond domain would interact best with the micrometer-sized pigment granule's approximate thermal relaxation time.

To destroy tattoo ink selectively, the best wavelength is chosen to achieve selective absorption for that ink color while minimizing the nonspecific thermal effects from the primary endogenous chromophores, hemoglobin and melanin. Black ink is by far the most common color seen in tattoos, followed by blue, green, red, then yellow and orange. More recently applied tattoos have an even greater range of colors, including various shades of pink, brown, purple, and even flourescent colors. Reflectance spectra data for tattoo ink colors may aid in choosing the best available wavelength.[109,110]

Because of difficulties with absorption spectroscopy, diffuse reflectance spectroscopy was studied to model dermal tattoo ink using 17 different tattoo ink colors and six different variants of black tattoo ink mixed with gelatin (Candela, unpublished data, 1991). Reflectance spectra were obtained from 450 to 1000 nm for each pigment and used to provide information on their absorption properties.

Figures 4-11 and 4-12 illustrate that black pigment would be expected to be absorptive at all wavelengths (having minimal reflectance), and that competition from

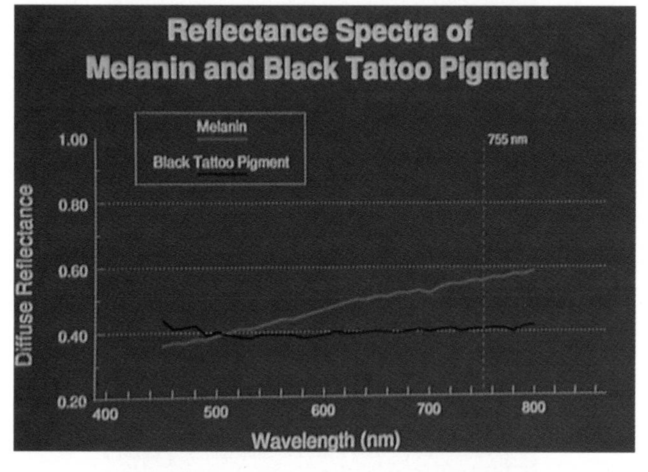

Figure 4-11 Diffuse reflectance spectra of black tattoo pigment and melanin. (Courtesy Candela Laser Corp.)

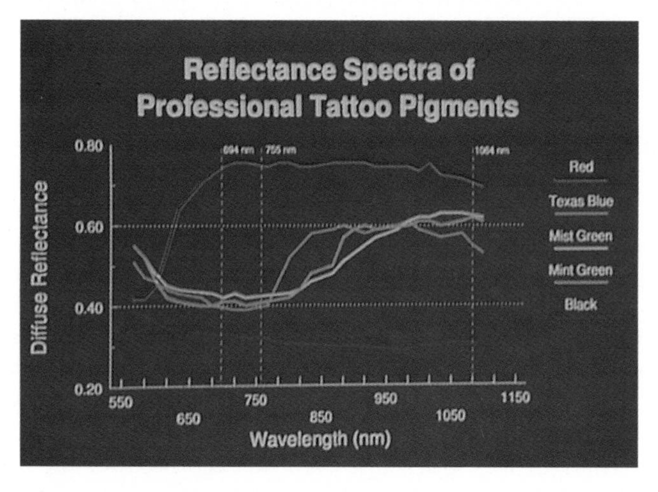

Figure 4-12 Diffuse reflectance spectra of black, blue, green, and red tattoo pigments. (Courtesy Candela Laser Corp.)

melanin absorption in the epidermis decreases gradually as wavelength increases. Absorption for blue and green is greatest for wavelengths of 625 to 755 nm, whereas red absorbs best below 575 nm (Figures 4-12 and 4-13). Yellow is primarily reflective above 520 nm, orange above 560 nm, and violet is very similar to red in its absorption and reflectance properties (Figure 4-13). Tan pigment is most absorptive below 560 nm and flesh-colored pigment below approximately 535 nm (Figure 4-14). These observations for optimal wavelength absorption for different tattoo ink colors were corroborated by Kilmer et al[109] and Hodersdal et al.[110]

Many tattoo inks are mixtures of colors having a wide range of tint (blues, greens, violets, oranges) and are difficult to classify as a single pigment. When a color is a mixture of two or more pigments (one of which is reflective and one absorptive), some of the reflected light from nonabsorbing pigment will reach the absorbing pigment, causing plasma formation. The resultant reaction may be adequate to affect both pigments because of the proximity of the two pigments in the mixture.

The differing composition of amateur (elemental carbon) and professional (organic dyes mixed with metallic elements) tattoos may in part explain why the latter respond less favorably. However, the primary difference between amateur and professional tattoos may simply be the former's usual paucity of pigment granules.[111] Of

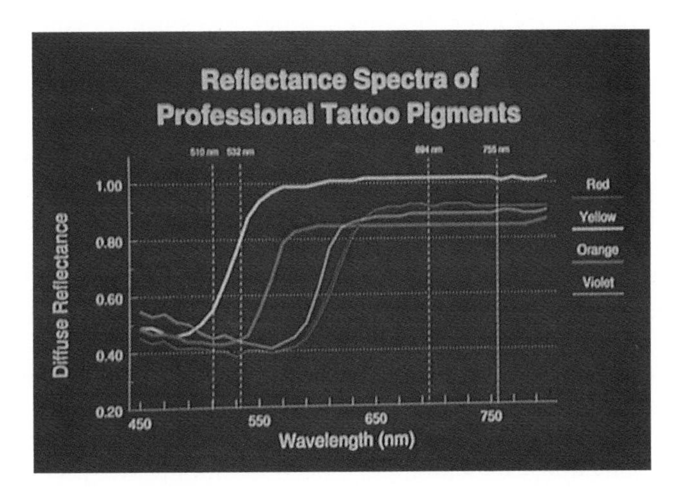

Figure 4-13 Diffuse reflectance spectra of yellow, red, violet, and orange tattoo pigments. (Courtesy Candela Laser Corp.)

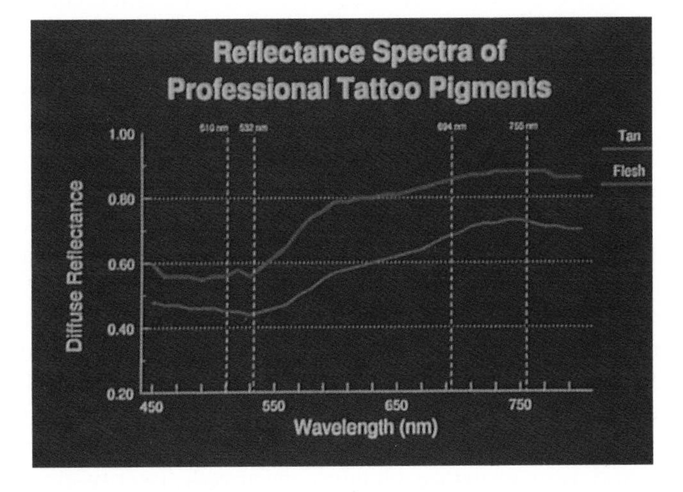

Figure 4-14 Diffuse reflectance spectra of tan and flesh-colored tattoo pigments. (Courtesy Candela Laser Corp.)

25 tattoos studied, five of eight amateur tattoos were among the 10 having the lowest volume of pigment granules and cleared rapidly, and overall, tattoos responded according to their total pigment volume.

Q-switched Ruby Laser

The earliest reports of tattoo-pigment interaction with short-pulsed lasers were by Goldman et al in 1965.[88,89] They compared the reaction of a dark-blue tattoo to a Q-switched ruby laser having nanosecond pulses with a microsecond-pulsed ruby laser and found nonspecific thermal necrosis with microsecond impacts, whereas nanosecond impacts only produced transient edema accompanied by a peculiar whitening of the impact area, lasting about 30 minutes. No thermal necrosis was present, but tattoo fragments remained in the dermis. The mechanism of this reaction was unknown but was not thought to be thermal because of normal measurements taken with a thermistor. Because of the reported retention of tattoo pigment, this modality was originally interpreted as a failure. Goldman, however, followed the patient's progress and noted continued fading of the treated area. Unable to continue this work because his engineer was fatally electrocuted, Goldman abandoned the project. Only 3 years later, however, other investigators confirmed and expanded these results,[92,93] using a Q-switched ruby laser (694 nm, 20 nsec) to remove blue and black tattoo pigment successfully without tissue damage. Biopsies performed after 3 months showed absence of tattoo pigment and no evidence of thermal damage. These effects were dose dependent, with fluences of 5.6 J/cm^2 or less showing absence of thermal damage but incomplete pigment removal. Higher fluences lead to subepidermal blisters similar to a second-degree burn and dermal fibrosis at 3 months, although pigment removal was more complete. Subsequent studies[112,113] concluded that this treatment modality was impractical because of the small target areas and the risk of coagulation necrosis of tissue surrounding the tattoo pigment.

Reid and co-workers[114] continued to study the Q-switched ruby laser and in 1983 published an additional report on removal of black pigment in professional and amateur tattoos. They reported good results, particularly with amateur tattoos, but noted several disadvantages, including the need for multiple treatments, often six or more, for complete pigment removal. They also reported scarring in two patients and emphasized the need to use relatively low powers (but above the threshold to produce immediate tissue whitening) and the importance of the treatment interval. At least 3 weeks between treatments was necessary for tissue healing and pigment removal by macrophages. In vitro tests showed an immediate reaction in ink that could be explained only by a chemical reaction. Biopsy specimens revealed evidence of fragmentation of ink into smaller particles, which were then phagocytized by macrophages. These two phenomena correspond with the clinical observations of an immediate reduction in pigment observable the first week after treatment, followed by gradual fading over the next several weeks without further therapy.

Stimulated by studies of the Q-switched ruby laser preferentially damaging melanized cells in animal skin[115,116] and the tattoo studies previously cited, researchers at the Wellman Laboratories of Photomedicine at Harvard Medical School completed a detailed dose-response study of Q-switched ruby laser in 1990.[117] Using a 40- to 80-nsec pulse, they treated 41 tattoos five times at doses of 1.5 to 4.0 J/cm^2. Of 27 amateur tattoos, eight cleared by more than 75% (all of which had been treated at 4 J/cm^2) in an average of 2.6 treatments. None of the 14 professional tattoos reached this level of clearing within five treatment sessions, and frequent purpura and rare punctate bleeding occurred. Twenty-eight tattoos with residual pigment were treated an additional five sessions at fluences of 5 to 8 J/cm^2 with more tissue damage, frequent purpura, and occasional superficial erosions noted. At the completion of this phase an additional 10 amateur tattoos cleared over 75%, requiring an average of an additional 3.5 treatments. Three professional tattoos achieved this degree of clearing after an additional single high-dose treatment at 7 J/cm^2. Overall results were excellent in 78% of amateur tattoos, but only 23% of professional tattoos.

Despite these rather discouraging statistics, the authors were optimistic that the Q-switched ruby laser would develop into a preferred treatment for tattoos, because of the rare scarring. In addition, the authors stressed the competitive absorption by melanosomes leading to vacuolization of melanocytes and keratinocytes, with hypopigmentation noted in 39% (low fluences) to 46% (higher fluences) of cases. Normal pigmentation was progressively reestablished over a 4- to 12-month period; however, 4 of 10 tattoos examined 1 year after treatment still had confetti-like hypopigmentation.

The authors agreed with previous investigators that the immediate whitening seen represents rapid localized heating with steam or gas formation resulting in dermal and epidermal vacuolization. They noted an unexplained brief emission of white light as the laser pulse struck the tattoo pigment. Interestingly, histologic persistence of altered tattoo pigment in areas of clinical clearing was noted, suggesting a change in the optical properties of the tattoo pigment.

This study was not able to establish an optimal treatment interval. Although the mean interval was 3 weeks, intervals of 1 to 5 weeks were used, and no statistical difference in responses was noted. Blue and black pigments were most responsive, whereas green and yellow responded less well, and red was poorly responsive if at all. Purpura and punctate bleeding most likely represent indirect vascular injury from photoacoustic waves generated by laser interaction with tattoo pigment.

A study by Scheibner and co-workers[118] reported preliminary results of treatment of 101 amateur and 62 professional tattoos using fluences of 2 to 4 J/cm^2 with a 40-nsec pulse width, spot sizes of 5 and 8 mm, and a treatment interval of 5 to 6 weeks. Although details of response are lacking, after an average of four treatments, 87% of amateur tattoos were greater than 80% clear, whereas of 62 professional tattoos, only 11% were greater than 80% clear. Treated areas required 10 to 14 days to heal and remained erythematous for an additional 1 to 3 weeks, and most patients developed hypopigmentation lasting 2 to 6 months. Skin textural changes resolved over 6 to 8 weeks, with no scarring reported. Tattoos of the face and neck responded sooner but were more sensitive to tissue damage, necessitating the use of lower fluences. Interestingly, better response was noted with older professional tattoos and blue inks in comparison to other colors.

As stated earlier, Taylor and colleagues[20] reported on light and electron microscopic analysis of Q-switched ruby laser–treated tattoos. After irradiation, all three previously described particle types could still be found, in addition to round, lamellated, electron-lucent particles measuring 25 to 40 nm and more often in the deeper dermis and even into the subcutaneous fat. These altered particles are thought to originate from the 40-nm particle. After treatment, pigment granules measured approximately 1 μm (compared with their original 4-μm size) and were loosely packed. Those granules in the papillary dermis measured 0.2 to 0.4 μm and were very densely packed. Again, clinical clearing poorly correlated with histologic clearing, because tattoos responding well often had residual pigment.

The mechanism of action of the Q-switched ruby laser is through photon absorption by tattoo pigment within fibroblasts. During the 40-nsec pulse, temperatures exceeding 1000° C can occur. Gaseous products of pyrolysis or pores created by superheated steam may account for the lamellated appearance of the granules after laser exposure. The reduction in pigment particle size and fragmentation of pigment-containing cells probably result from rapid thermal expansion, shock waves, and potentially localized cavitation. Fluence-dependent thermal damage to collagen immediately surrounding the irradiated tattoo pigment also occurs.

Newer ruby lasers with a shorter pulse duration (approximately 25 nsec), higher fluences (8-10 J/cm^2), and better beam quality more rapidly clear tattoos.[119,120] Lowe et al[121] reported similar results using 10 J/cm^2 at 6- to 8-week intervals and after five treatment sessions reported 22 of 28 professional tattoos as having excellent results (greater than 75% improvement) (Figure 4-15). Levins and co-workers' preliminary report was similar, with excellent results and minimal side effects.[122]

Kilmer and Anderson[123] initiated treatment at a fluence of 6 to 8 J/cm^2 with a 40- to 80-nsec pulse width and reported black and green ink to be most responsive, with other colors requiring significantly more treatments. Amateur tattoos usually required four to six treatment sessions and professional tattoos six to ten sessions, but in some instances up to 20 treatment sessions were needed. The authors noted several trends; professional, distally located, recently placed, or deeply placed tattoos may be difficult to remove, requiring more treatment sessions to eradicate them completely. Acceptable clearing varied greatly from patient to patient, with some individuals more accepting of vague residual pigment.

In summary, the Q-switched ruby laser is remarkably effective in removing tattoos with minimal scarring, although multiple treatment sessions are necessary (Figure 4-16). Hypopigmentation is common (more than 50% of patients), and although usually transient (2 to 6 months), it may be permanent[123] (Figure 4-17). Transient hyperpigmentation is also common and seems to be related more to skin type than laser treatment (Figure 4-18). Scarring and textural changes occur more rarely. The risk of adverse tissue response and speed of clearing both appear to be fluence and pulse width related, with higher fluences and shorter pulses being more effective but causing more nonspecific tissue damage as well. These high-energy short pulses cause a pressure shock wave that ruptures blood vessels and aerosolizes tissue with potentially infectious particles, requiring the use of a protective barrier or a plastic tube to protect the operator from tissue and blood contact. The use of

A

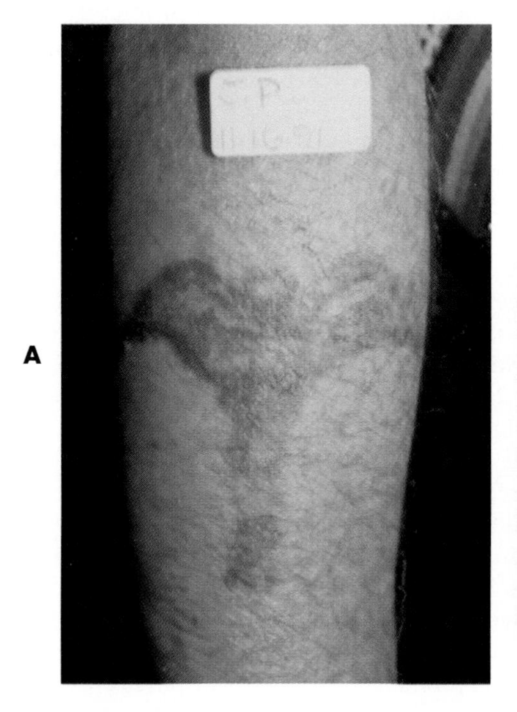

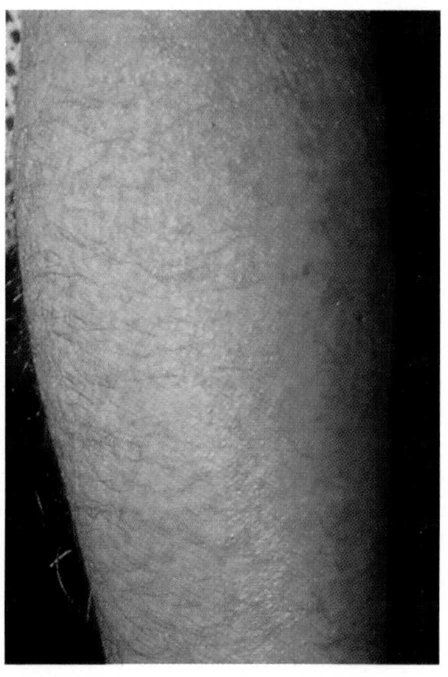

B

Figure 4-15 Virtually complete tattoo pigment removal after two treatments with ruby laser at 10 J/cm^2 with 8 weeks between treatments. **A,** Before treatment. **B,** Approximately 6 months after second treatment. (Courtesy Dr. Nicholas Lowe, Santa Monica, Calif.)

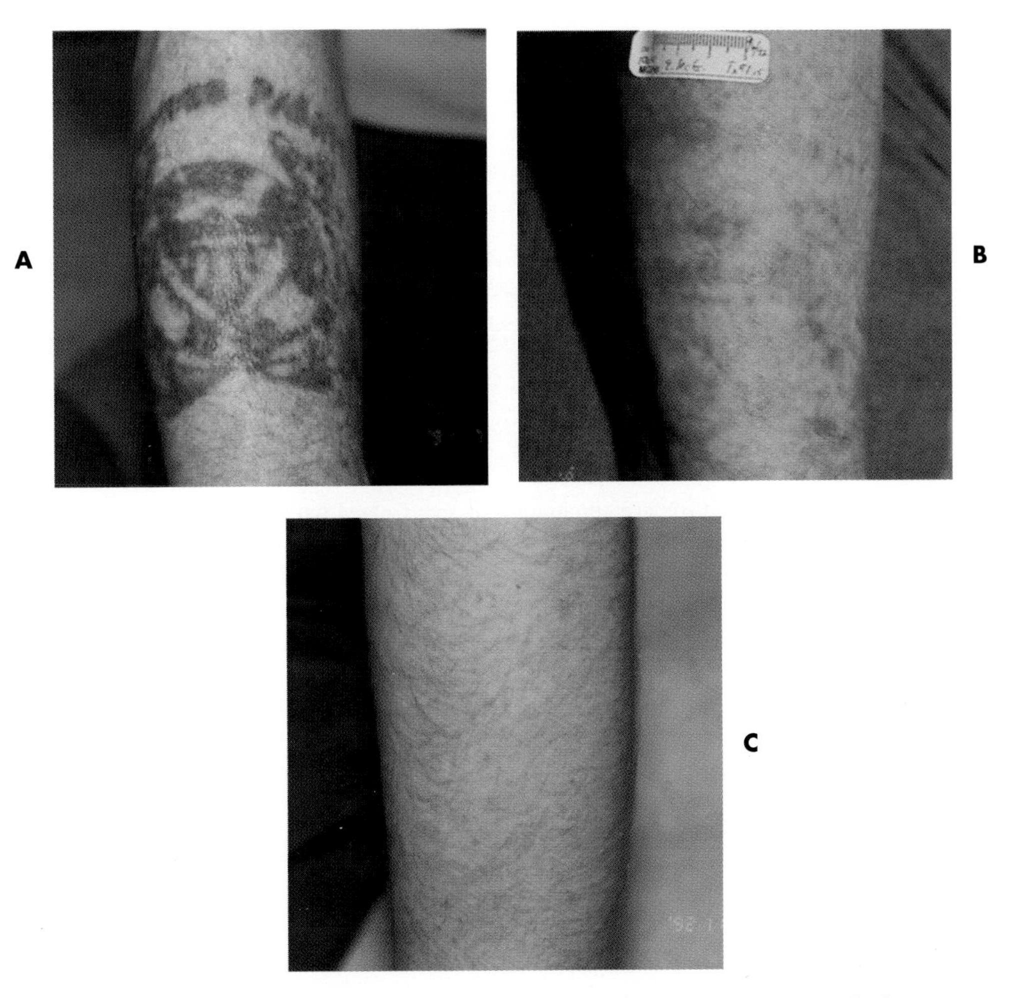

Figure 4-16 **A,** Tattoo before treatment. **B,** Tattoo after four treatments with the ruby laser. **C,** Tattoo after five treatments with ruby laser. Green pigment remains. (Courtesy Dr. Joop Grevelink, Massachusetts General Hospital Laser Center.)

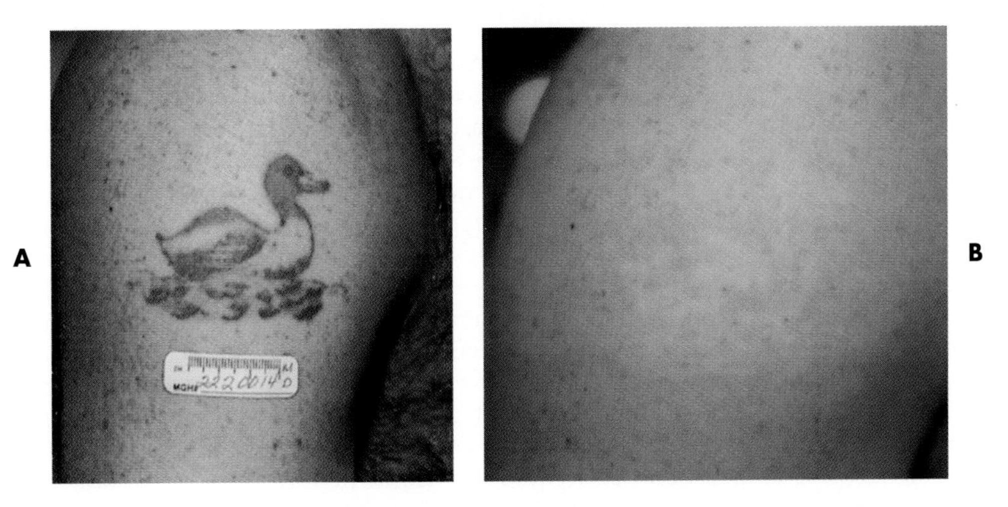

Figure 4-17 **A,** Tattoo before treatment. **B,** Tattoo after eight treatments with ruby laser. Mild hypopigmentation and persistence of some green pigment are visible. (Courtesy Dr. Joop Grevelink, Massachusetts General Hospital Laser Center.)

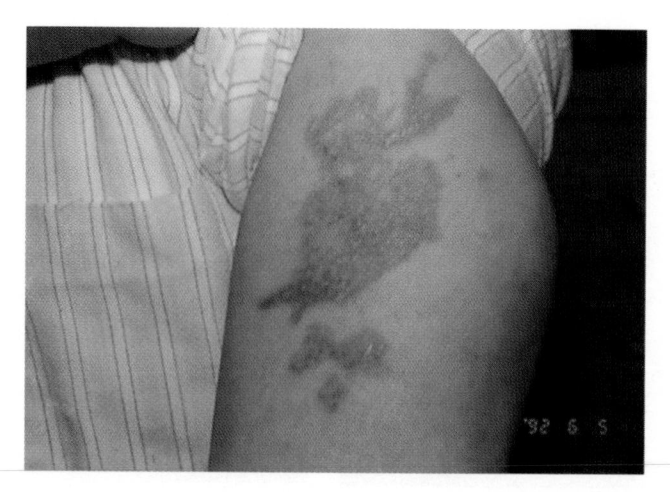

Figure 4-18 Transient hyperpigmentation of area treated with Q-switched ruby laser. (Courtesy Dr. Joop Grevelink, Massachusetts General Hospital Laser Center.)

lower fluences eliminates this problem to a large degree but results in the need for more treatment sessions. The occurrence of scarring or tissue textural changes has also been attributed to hot spots within the beam and pulse-to-pulse variability. The ruby laser is very effective for removing black, blue-black, and green ink; green ink can be difficult, even though reflectance spectra predict that it should respond to a 694-nm wavelength. Other colors are poorly responsive. The ruby laser has a repetitive rate of 1 pulse every 1 to 2 sec, but no aiming beam to assist in proper alignment. Bleeding and tissue splatter can be cumbersome, but use of cone devices protect the operator from exposure.

Q-switched Nd:YAG Laser

The Q-switched Nd:YAG laser was then explored in anticipation that its longer wavelength (1064 nm) would increase dermal penetration and decrease melanin absorption (Figure 4-11), improving the response of ruby laser–resistant tattoos and avoiding pigmentary changes. An initial report of 20 professional and three amateur tattoos in four treatment sessions showed the Nd:YAG laser to be equal to the ruby laser in removal of blue-black tattoos at 6 J/cm^2. Hypopigmentation and skin texture change were more common with the ruby laser. Green and red pigment were not removed with the Nd:YAG laser, whereas some green pigment was removed with the ruby laser.[124]

The ability of the Q-switched Nd:YAG laser (1064 nm, 10 nsec, 5 Hz) to remove pigment in ruby laser–resistant tattoos was assessed in the treatment of 28 tattoos (23 professional, five amateur) using fluences of 6 to 12 J/cm^2 with a 2.5-mm-diameter spot size. In most cases, greater than 50% lightening of residual tattoo ink was noted with the first treatment, with the greatest improvement seen with higher fluences.[125] Unfortunately, the higher fluences (12 J/cm^2) and shorter pulses (10 nsec) resulted in more tissue debris and bleeding, necessitating the use of a plastic shield to promote laser operator safety.

Kilmer et al[126] investigated both ruby laser–resistant and untreated tattoos in a prospective, blinded, dose-response study using the Q-switched Nd:YAG laser (2.5-mm spot size). Twenty-five professional tattoos and 14 amateur tattoos were treated in quadrants using 6, 8, 10, and 12 J/cm^2. Four treatment sessions were performed at 3- to 4-week intervals. Greater than 75% ink removal was seen in 77% of black tattoos and over 95% ink removal in 28% of tattoos (11 of 39) treated at 10 to 12 J/cm^2. There was no significant difference in the response of previously untreated tattoos and ruby laser–resistant tattoos. Treatment at the highest fluence (12 J/cm^2) proved to be significantly more effective ($p < 0.01$) at removing black tattoo ink than the lower doses of 6 and 8 J/cm^2. Green, yellow, white, and red inks were virtually resistant to treatment and cleared 25% or less after four treatment sessions. Purple and orange inks responded minimally. Although textural changes were noted during the course of treatment, these cleared with time, and only 2 of 39 tattoos were graded as having trace textural changes. No hypopigmentation and a single case of hyperpigmentation were noted. These results were similar to those reported by Ferguson and August.[127]

Biopsy of treated tattoos revealed fragmentation of black ink particles up to 1.5 mm below the surface. There was little if any fibrosis in the superficial dermis. In addition, biopsies demonstrated that even with clinical clearing of the tattoo, ink remained in the dermis, as reported with the Q-switched ruby laser.[20]

Kilmer et al[126] noted that the lack of scarring both clinically and histologically, despite the increased bleeding and tissue splatter seen, is most likely caused by the lack of thermal injury to collagen. The dermis and epidermis sustain mechanical injury from the photoacoustic wave, but this trauma is apparently highly reparable. Textural changes generally resolve within 4 to 6 weeks, suggesting an optimal treatment interval of 6 weeks or longer.

The authors[126] also noted a bright flash of white light from the tattoo during laser exposure, as mentioned with the ruby laser. Because 1064-nm light is not visible, this flash must result from either laser-stimulated plasma or incandescence of tattoo ink particles. These both imply extreme temperatures greater than 500° C.

The Q-switched Nd:YAG laser has a great advantage for treating darker-skinned patients (Figure 4-19). Both Jones et al[128] and Grevelink et al[129] demonstrated effective tattoo removal with minimal hypopigmentation or hyperpigmentation. This provides a significant benefit over the Q-switched ruby laser for darker-skinned patients in whom melanin absorption is a hindrance. In addition, the smaller spot size available with most Q-switched Nd:YAG lasers (1.5-mm diameter) allows for more accurate distinction of tattoo in sensitive areas (Figures 4-20 and 4-21).

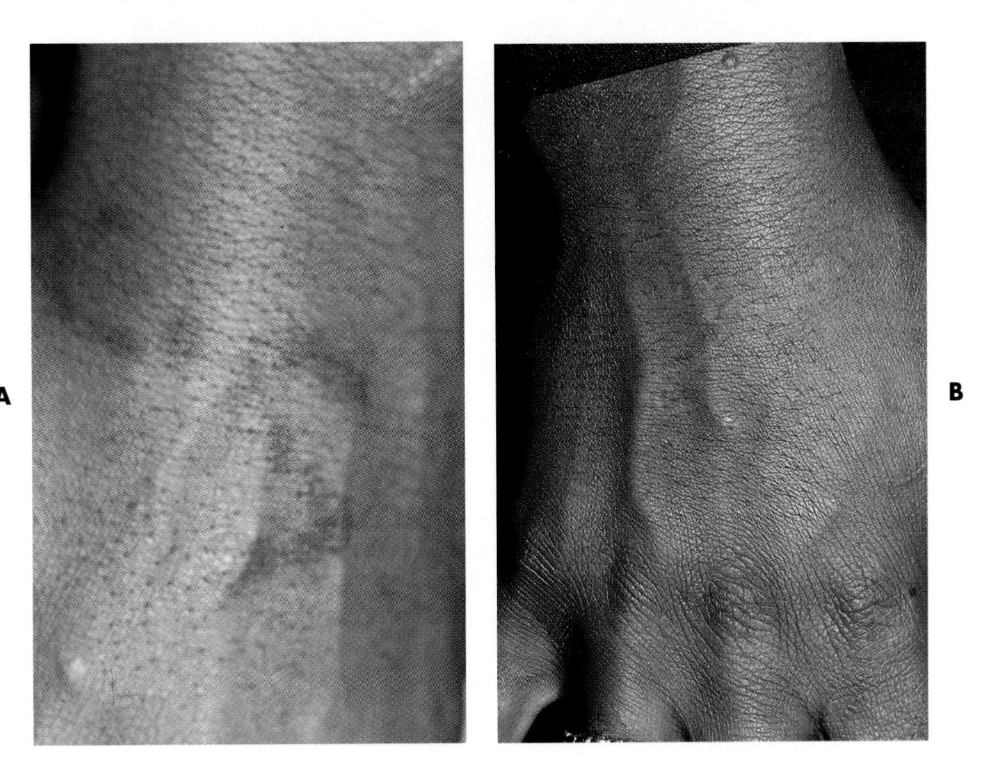

Figure 4-19 **A,** Amateur tattoo on dorsal palm of 40-year-old black male for more than 20 years. **B,** Six months after second treatment with Nd:YAG laser using 3-mm-diameter spot size at 6 to 7 J/cm^2.

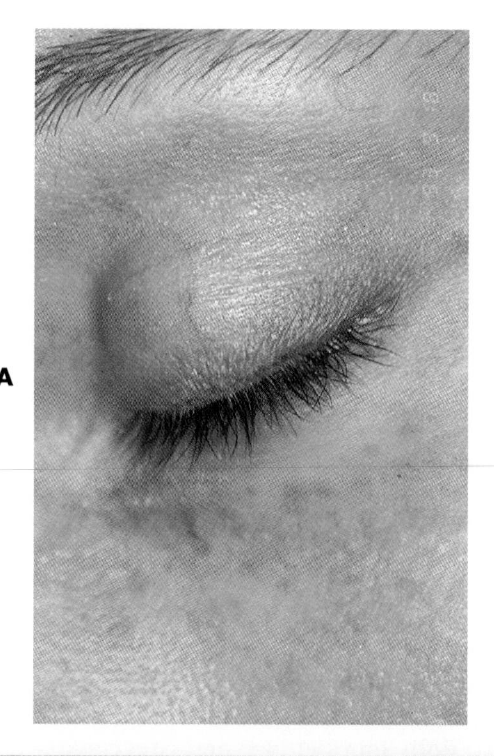

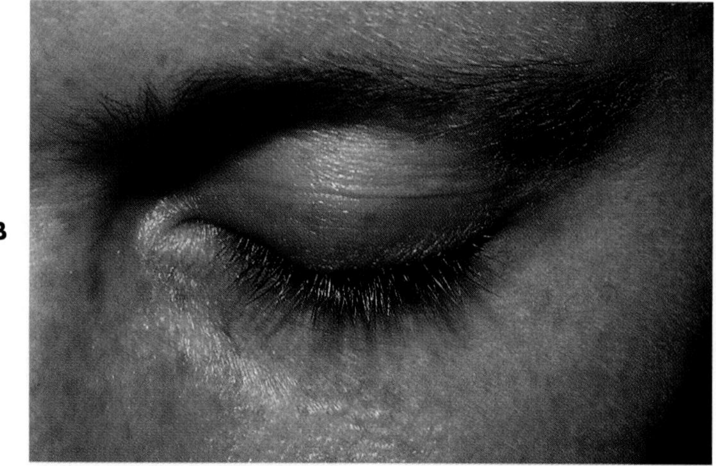

Figure 4-20 **A,** Misplaced tattoo eyeliner. **B,** Complete removal 3 weeks after single treatment with Nd:YAG laser at 10 J/cm^2 through 1.5-mm-diameter spot.

In summary, the Q-switched Nd:YAG laser has proved to be somewhat more effective in removal of black ink with rare textural changes and almost no hypopigmentation (Figures 4-22 and 4-23). These improvements are attributed to the longer wavelength, higher fluence, and shorter pulse width. These same factors cause more bleeding and tissue splatter during treatment, making the treatment itself more cumbersome. However, the faster repetition rate (1-10 Hz) shortens the treatment session, although this is somewhat counterbalanced by the use of a smaller beam size (2-4 mm versus 5-6.5 mm for the ruby laser). Larger spot sizes up to 6 mm are now available with new, higher-powered Nd:YAG laser systems, enabling deeper penetration and more effective treatment of deeper, denser tattoos.[130] Better beam profiles have minimized epidermal damage, decreasing bleeding, tissue splatter, and transient textural changes. Often, little wound care is needed.

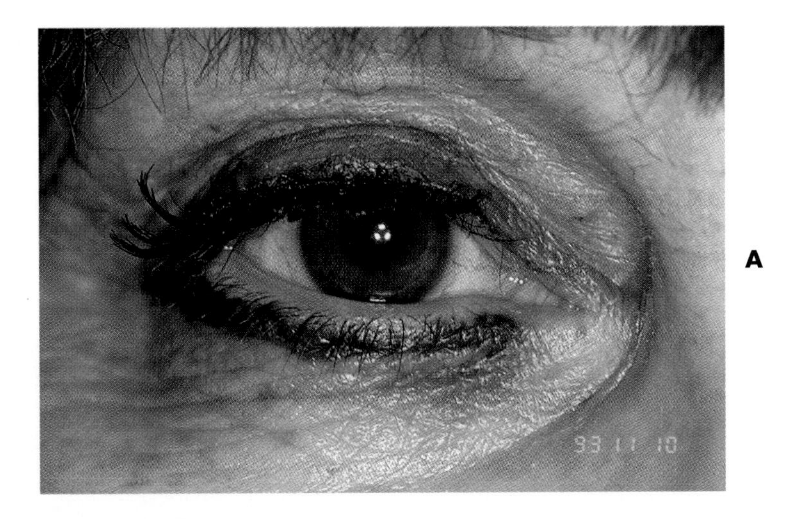

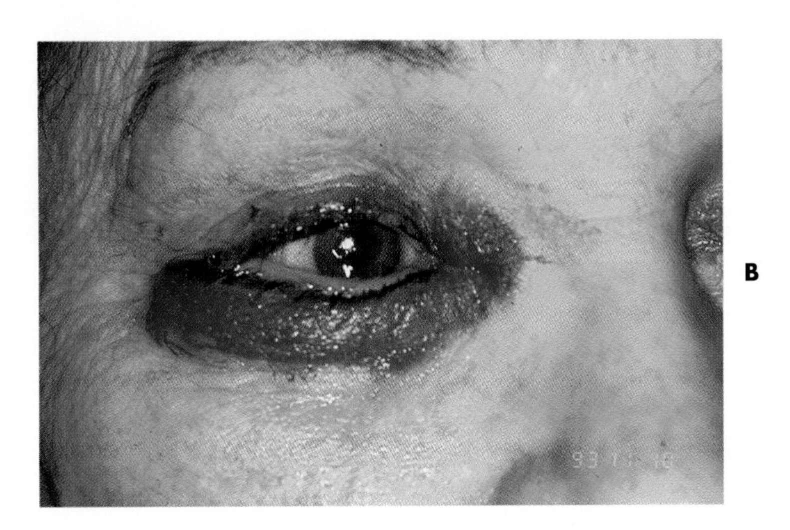

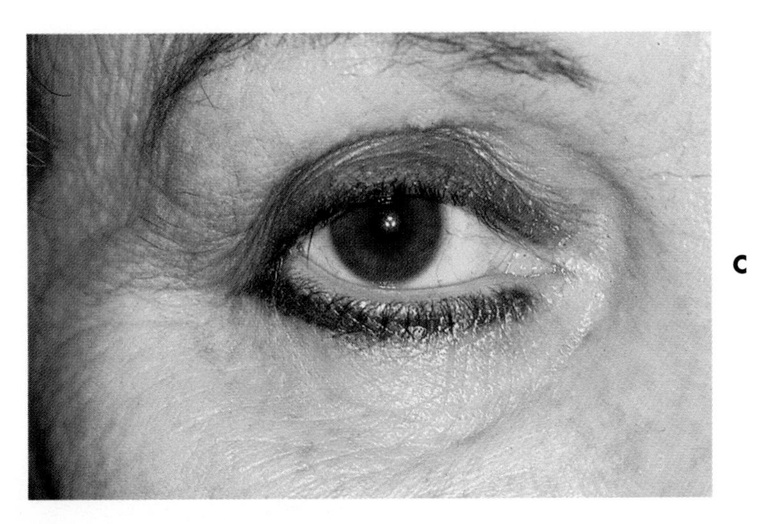

Figure 4-21 **A,** Spread of tattoo pigment 1 month after placement. **B,** Immediately after treatment with Nd:YAG laser using 2-mm-diameter spot at 10 J/cm^2. **C,** Five months after single treatment showing tattoo the patient wanted to receive.

The primary disadvantage of 1064 nm is its limited color range, basically restricted to black and dark-blue/black tattoo pigment. However, a frequency-doubling crystal is a feature of this laser, which allows the use of the 532-nm wavelength to treat red ink effectively. Greater than 75% removal of red ink has been reported with three treatment sessions, and orange and some purples respond almost as well; however, yellow ink responds poorly, presumably because of its dramatic drop in absorbance between 510 and 520 nm, as do green and blue inks, where absorption is greater at 600 nm or longer.[109]

A 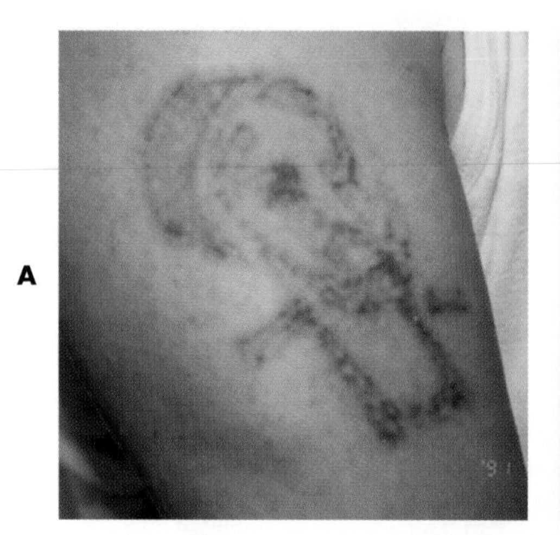

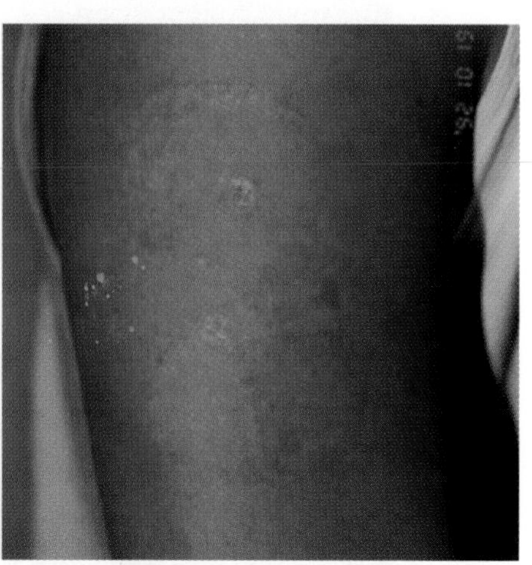 B

Figure 4-22 **A,** Amateur tattoo after 10 Q-switched ruby laser treatments. **B,** Near-complete removal after five treatments with Q-switched Nd:YAG laser. Treatment sessions were performed using 10 J/cm² and with 3 to 4 weeks between treatments.

A 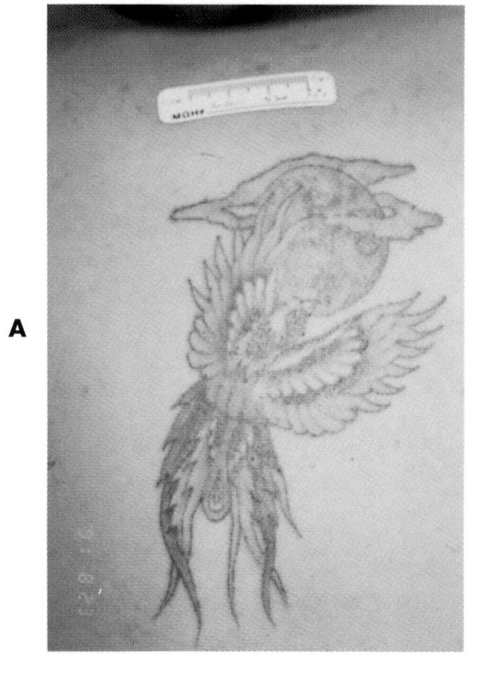

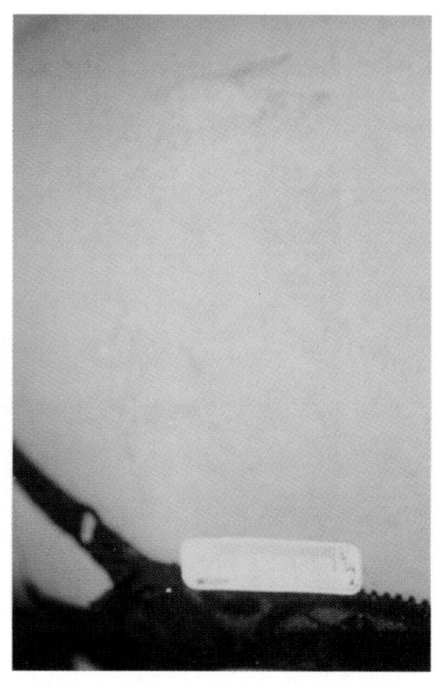 B

Figure 4-23 **A,** Professional multicolored tattoo before treatment with Nd:YAG laser. **B,** After four treatment sessions using 1064-nm wavelength and four treatment sessions using 532-nm wavelength, only small amount of blue pigment persists.

Because of absorbance of 1064-nm light by melanin and hemoglobin, blistering and purpura frequently occur.

Q-switched Alexandrite Laser

The third Q-switched laser developed for the treatment of tattoos, the alexandrite laser, has a wavelength of 755 nm, a pulse width of 100 nsec (50 nsec available in newer models), and a repetition rate of 1 Hz.[131-134] The 3-mm-diameter beam is delivered via a fiberoptic system or an articulated arm. Reflectance studies at 755 nm suggest excellent absorption by black pigment, good absorption by blue and green, and poor absorption by red pigments (Figures 4-11 to 4-13), as confirmed by preliminary studies performed on tattooed Yucatan minipigs. One treatment session provided excellent results in removal of black ink, good results with blue and green, and poor results with red ink. Efficacy was fluence related; 8 J/cm^2 was more effective than 6 J/cm^2, which was more effective than 4 J/cm^2, and 2 J/cm^2 was ineffective.[98]

In contrast to previous reports using the Q-switched ruby and Nd:YAG lasers, histologic clearing correlated with clinical clearing. Similar to reports with the other Q-switched lasers, fragmentation of tattoo pigment was followed by macrophage engulfment and gradual clearing of the pigment, but with clinically clear tattoos devoid of ink histologically. Interestingly, tattoo pigment became progressively altered during this process, initially appearing as very sharp-bordered grains of pigment in clumps and taking on a progressively more amorphous form and lighter color within the macrophages (Figure 4-24). No clinical or histologic reaction in collagen, scarring, or atrophy was seen in laser-treated sites.

The Q-switched alexandrite laser was initially studied with 30 tattoos using fluences of 4.5 to 8.0 J/cm^2. Test sites using three fluences up to 6 J/cm^2 were evaluated at 4 weeks. The appropriate fluence was then selected and treatment begun. A second test was done if none of the previous fluences revealed significant lightening. Fluences of 6 J/cm^2 or higher were used once the tattoo had lightened by 20% to 50%. Approximately 25% clearing of tattooed pigment required 1.7 treatments, 50% clearance 2.8 treatments; 75% clearance 5 treatments, 90% clearance 6.4 treatments, and total clearance 10.4 treatments (range 4 to 16) (Figure 4-25). Professional tattoos cleared as well as amateur tattoos, although the latter were more rapidly responsive, requiring approximately three fewer treatments to reach complete clearance (Figure 4-26), although some professional tattoos responded rapidly as well.[111]

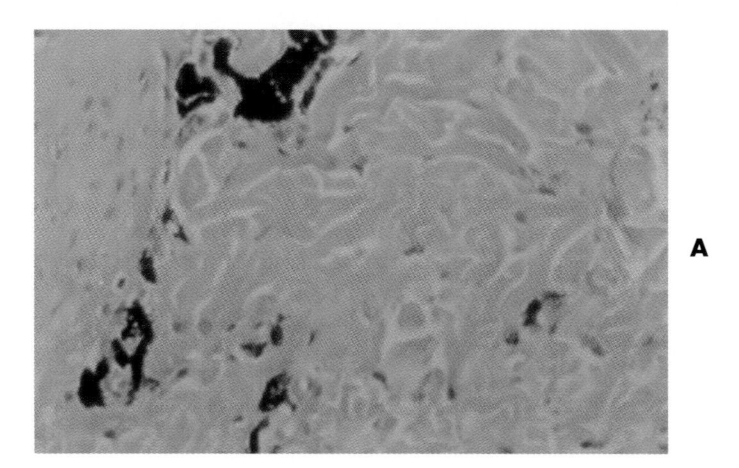

Figure 4-24 **A,** Tattoo granules present in dermis before treatment.

Continued

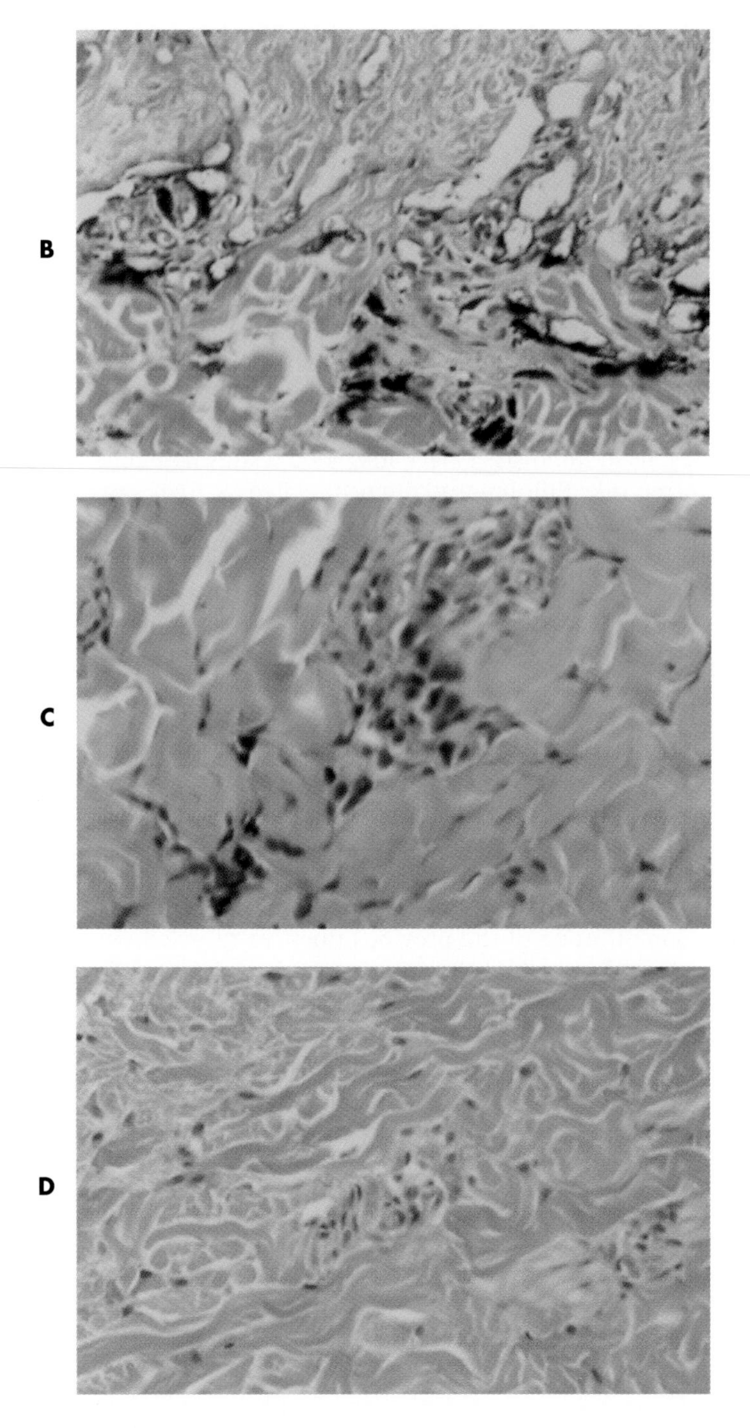

Figure 4-24, cont'd **B,** Tattoo pigment fragmentation and dermal lacunae formation 1 hour after treatment with alexandrite laser. **C,** One week after treatment, tattoo pigment is intracellular within macrophages. **D,** One month after treatment, total amount of pigment present is greatly decreased and much more amorphous within macrophages. (**A,** from Fitzpatrick RE, Goldman MP, Ruiz-Esparza J: *J Am Acad Dermatol* 28:745, 1993.)

Transient hypopigmentation is common (50% of patients), but often is not apparent until after five to seven treatment sessions, and usually resolves gradually over 1 to 12 months (Figure 4-27). As with the other Q-switched lasers, hyperpigmentation is more dependent on skin type and clears with hydroquinone and sunscreen. Transient surface textural changes have been noted in about 10%

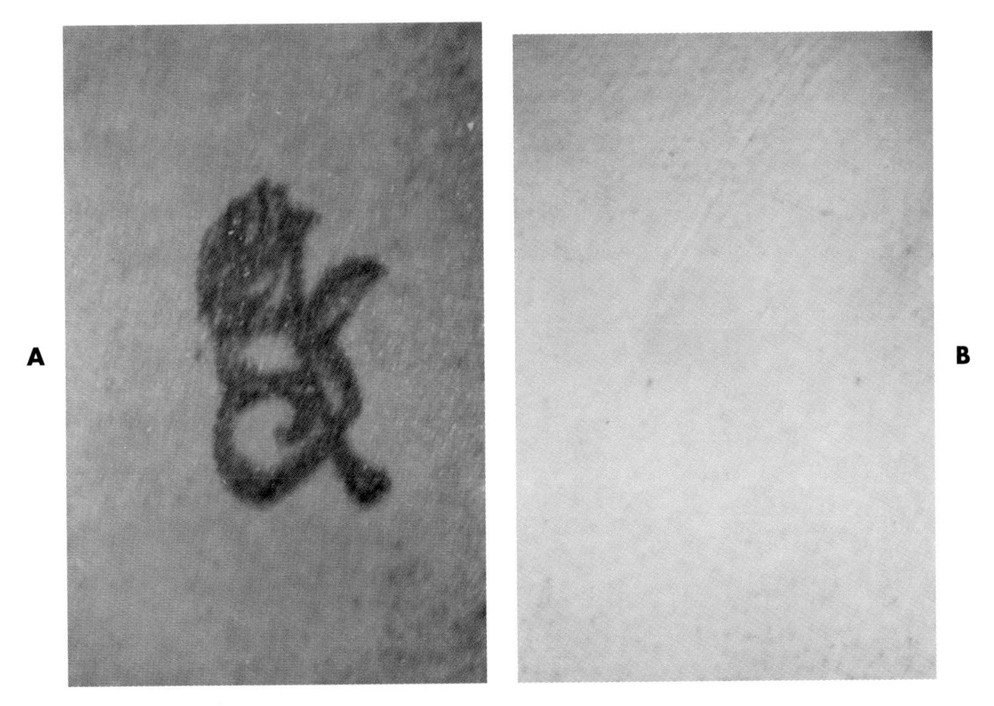

Figure 4-25 **A,** Tattoo before treatment. **B,** Complete clearance after six treatment sessions with alexandrite laser.

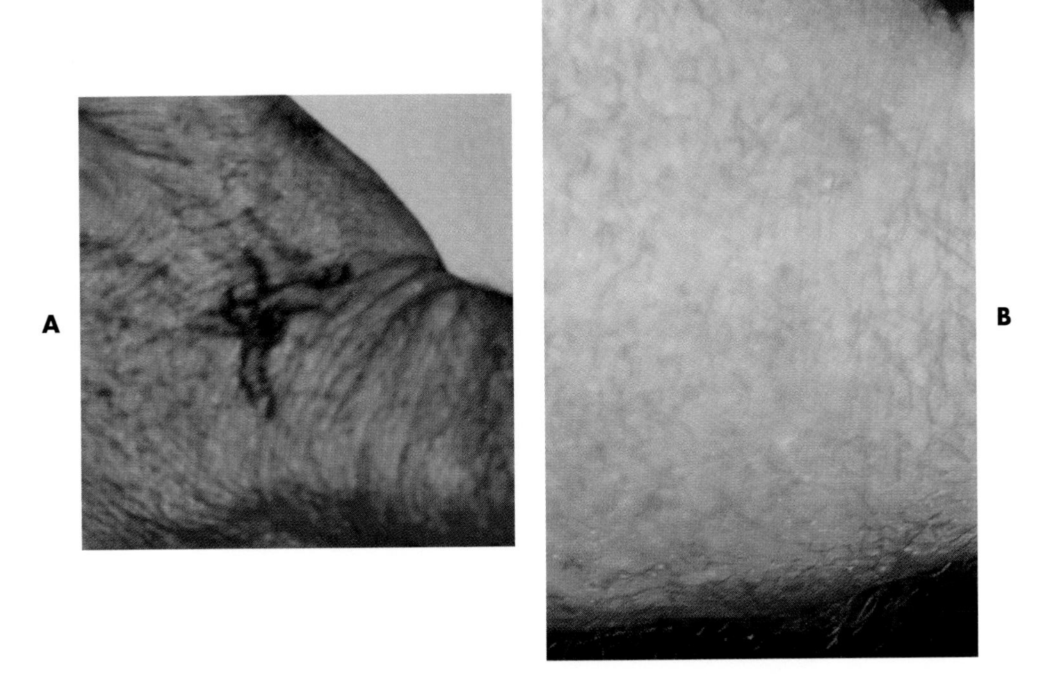

Figure 4-26 **A,** Amateur tattoo before treatment. **B,** Almost complete clearing after two treatment sessions with alexandrite laser.

of patients, but all resolved within 3 to 9 months, although one patient developed a small scar (2 × 7 mm) secondary to excoriating a treated area.

On laser impact the immediate flash of white light from the tattoo is followed by epidermal whitening and slight edema, as seen with both the Q-switched ruby and the Q-switched Nd:YAG lasers. When higher fluences are used, purpura is noticed, and pinpoint bleeding may occur. Tissue splatter and erosions were not seen at any of the fluences used with the 100-nsec pulse width, but the shorter 50-nsec pulse width, which reportedly increases tattoo clearance, is associated with more epidermal debris. Therefore it is suggested to increase the fluence up to the maximum available without causing pinpoint bleeding to prevent the problems of working in a bloody field and possible tissue trauma.

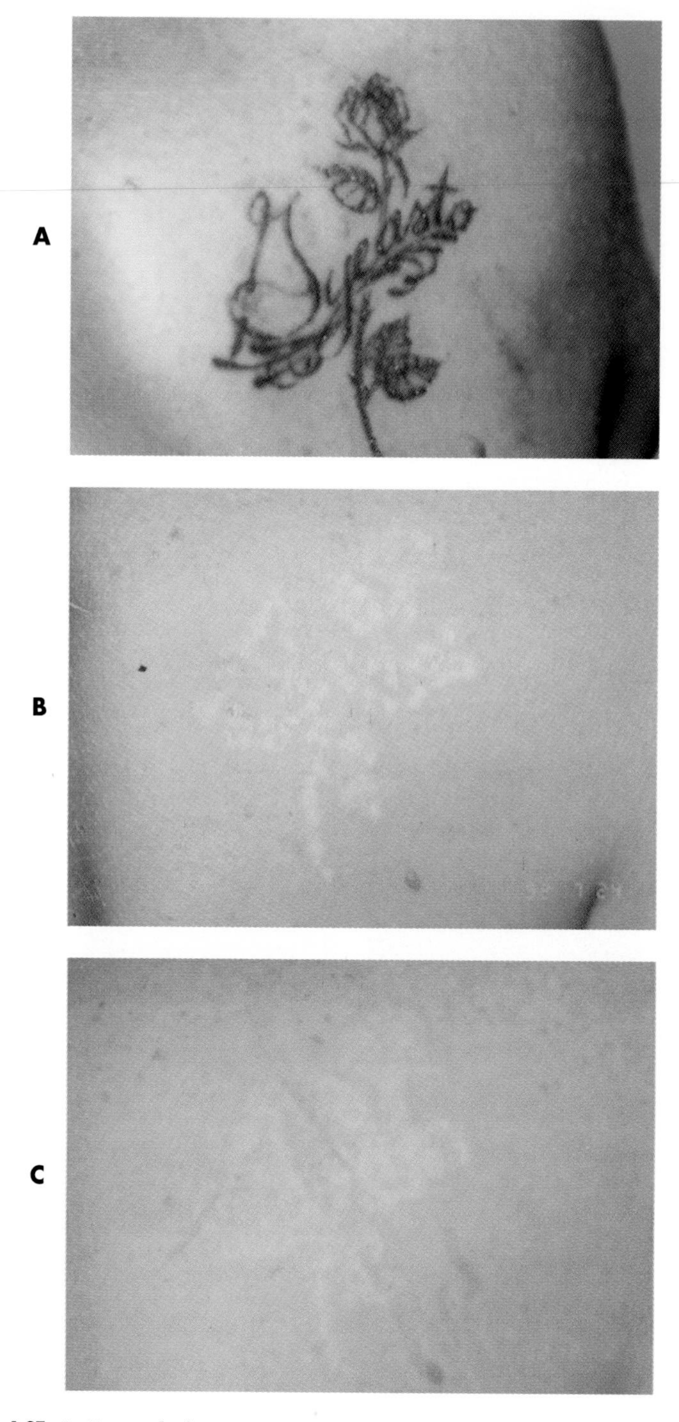

Figure 4-27 **A,** Tattoo before treatment. **B,** Hypopigmentation of treated area after nine treatment sessions. **C,** Gradual improvement of hypopigmentation after additional 3 months of healing.

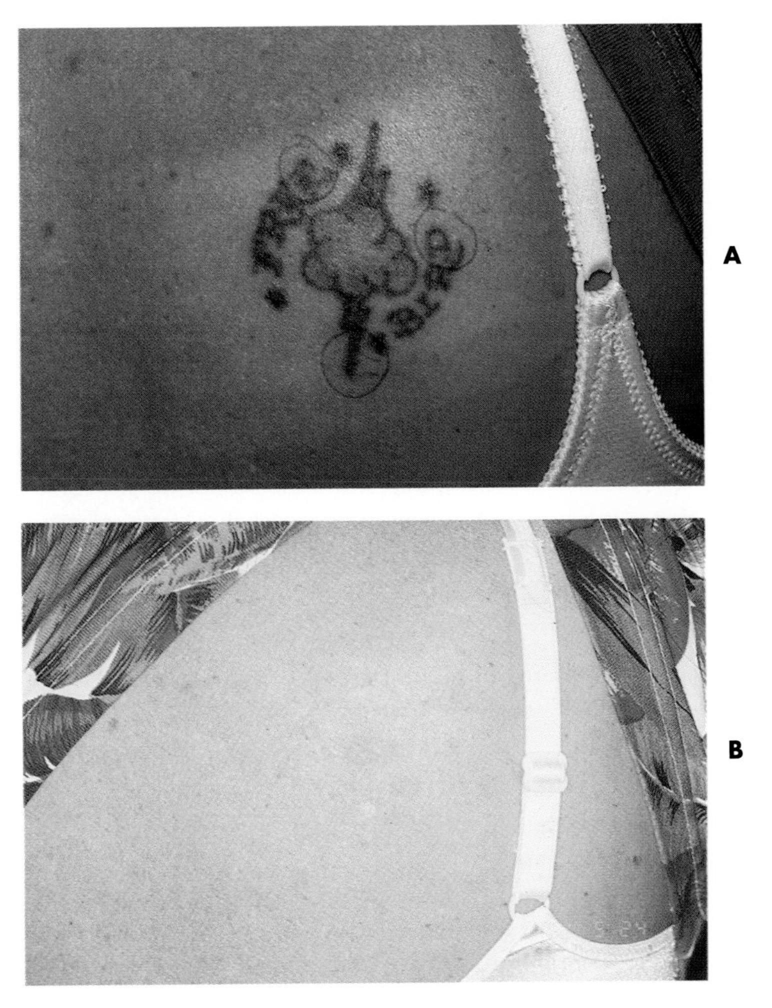

Figure 4-28 **A,** Black, blue, and red tattoo before treatment. **B,** Six months after total of 25 monthly treatments with Q-switched alexandrite laser at 8.0 J/cm^2 with 3-mm spot size. Complete clearing of all pigments was achieved without textural change in skin.

In summary, the Q-switched alexandrite laser is effective and safe for removing blue, black, and green tattoo pigment (Figure 4-28). Four to 10 treatments performed at 1- to 2-month intervals usually clears the tattoo without scarring; however, half of patients develop transient hypopigmentation.

Flashlamp-pumped Pulsed Dye Laser (510 mm, 300 nsec)

The flashlamp-pumped pulsed dye (FLPD) laser (510-nm pulse width of 300 ± 100 nsec) was developed as a companion to the Q-switched alexandrite laser for treatment of epidermal melanocytic lesions (see Chapter 3). This wavelength is also well absorbed by red pigment, and the pulse width is short enough to fragment ink granules. Successful clearing without scarring usually occurs in three to seven treatments performed at 1-month intervals using 3 to 3.75 J/cm^2[2,135] (Figure 4-29). Purple, orange, and yellow pigments required an average of five treatments for complete ink removal. No hypopigmentation, textural change, or scarring was noted. Histologically, fragmentation of red pigment particles is observed followed

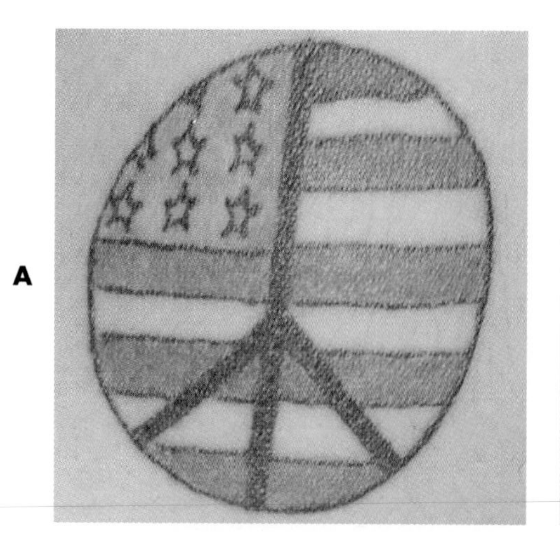
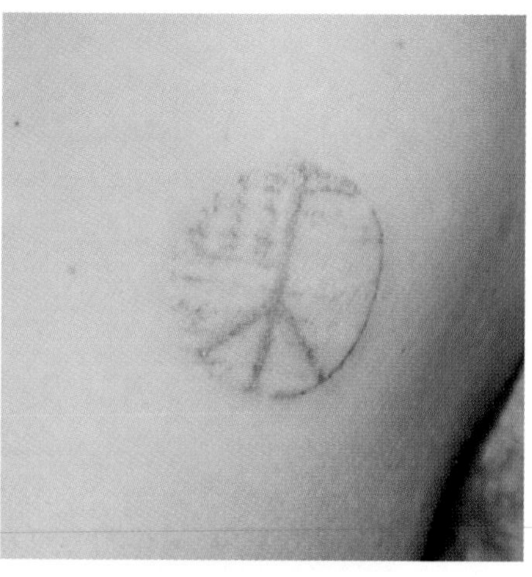

Figure 4-29 **A,** Tattoo before treatment. **B,** Removal of red tattoo pigment after three treatment sessions with 510-nm, 300-nsec, flashlamp-pumped pulsed dye laser (FLPD laser).

by macrophage engulfment. In addition, because of the epidermal absorption of this laser, transepidermal ink loss occurs.

Q-switched Laser Treatment in General

Treatment intervals

In early studies of Q-switched lasers, patients were treated every 4 weeks. In the alexandrite study, of the four patients unable to return for their scheduled treatment, two went 3 months and two went 5 months between treatments. Two of these four patients reported progressive and gradual clearing of their tattoo during this prolonged interval between treatment sessions, whereas two patients noticed only immediate improvement and then stabilization without further clearing. To study different treatment intervals, one group of patients received three treatments within 7 to 10 days and then no treatment for 3 months, a second group had a single treatment at 2-month intervals, and the third group had a single treatment at 1-month intervals.

Appropriate treatment interval is critical and yet poorly understood. It had been hoped that rapid fragmentation of tattoo pigment by condensing three treatment sessions within a 7- to 10-day period, followed by adequate time for macrophage activity (3 months), would result in more rapid tattoo removal with fewer total treatments required. However, the condensed treatment protocol did not enhance clearing. Treatment intervals of 1 month could interfere with macrophage activity, because the pigment-containing macrophages are laser targets as well as the stationary pigment-laden fibroblasts.[21,97] By extending the treatment interval to 2 and 3 months, essentially no difference was seen in the rate of tattoo clearing, because all three treatment intervals resulted in approximately 50% clearing after three treatment sessions. However, as the number of treatments increases, the potential for tissue reaction increases as well. Occasional rest periods or longer treatment intervals of 2 to 3 months allow recovery of melanin and normalization of any transient textural changes, which may be beneficial for avoiding unwanted adverse tissue response. Higher fluences and shorter pulse widths appear to remove tattoo pigment more rapidly but have the potential of inducing excessive shock wave tissue reaction and therefore must be balanced with the desire to remove pigment without scarring or hypopigmentation. Therefore the current recommendation is to treat at 6- to 8-week intervals unless a longer period is needed for tissue recovery.

Recommended treatment parameters

The main parameters to be chosen include pulse duration, wavelength, fluence, and spot size. All the Q-switched lasers are in the nanosecond domain, and the pulse width is predetermined by the laser used. The wavelength is chosen based on the best available wavelength for the tattoo ink color to be treated. In other words, red ink by a green wavelength (510 or 532 nm) and green ink by a red wavelength (694 or 755 nm). When melanin is present, the 1064-nm wavelength is the best choice to avoid disrupting the epidermis.

Fluence should be sufficient to produce immediate whitening, but immediate bleeding or blistering should be avoided. Larger spot sizes allow deeper penetration and should be used as long as sufficient fluence can be obtained. This will maximize distribution of laser light to the dermal pigment and minimize cutaneous injury.

It is difficult to predict the number of treatment sessions necessary for tattoo removal. Frequently the initial treatment session produces a more dramatic response than subsequent sessions. Very definite sites of clearing, corresponding to laser impacts, are often visible (Figure 4-30). Other tattoos are strongly unresponsive during early treatment phases, even though biopsies reveal fragmentation of tattoo granules. The explanation of these differences in response from one patient to another is likely to involve the efficiency of mobile macrophages in removal of fragmented tattoo pigment debris, as well as the density and amount of tattoo pigment present. The speed of the macrophage response, as well as the maximum amount of pigment removed per session, likely varies from patient to patient and to some extent from treatment to treatment.

To evaluate the effects of pigment placement and volume, treatment response in relation to (1) maximum pigment depth, (2) pigment surface area, and (3) total pigment volume (the product of these first two figures) was examined. As expected, the more superficial the tattoo pigment and the lesser the total volume of pigment, the fewer were the number of treatments necessary to remove the pigment; this was particularly apparent at the extremes (upper and lower 15% of values). When tattoo pigment was less than 0.92 mm in depth, seven treatments resulted in an average of 87.5% improvement, whereas pigment greater than 1.78 mm in depth required 9.3 treatments to achieve an average of 81.3% improvement (Table 4-1). In

A

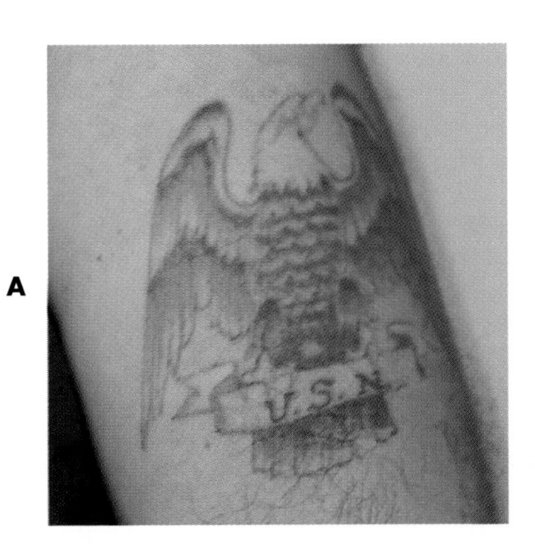

B

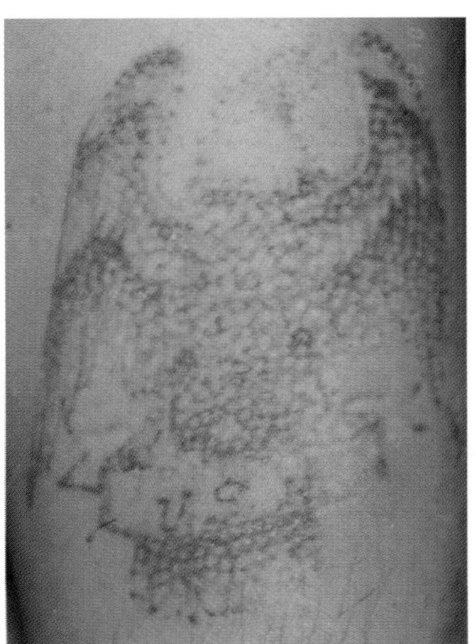

Figure 4-30 **A,** Tattoo before treatment. **B,** From 40% to 50% improvement after single treatment session with alexandrite laser.

Table 4-1
Q-switched laser treatment: tattoo pigment depth effect

Tattoo Pigment Maximum Depth (mm)	No. of Patients	Average Improvement	Average No. of Treatments
<0.92 (average 0.58)	4	87.5%	7
>1.78 (average 2.19)	4	81.3%	9.3

Table 4-2
Q-switched laser treatment: tattoo pigment surface area effect

Tattoo Pigment Surface Area (cm^2)*	No. of Patients	Average Improvement	Average No. of Treatments
<4.3 (average 2.56)	7	92.1%	7
>16.7 (average 24.7)	5	89.0%	10.4

*Mean: 10.5 ± 6.2 cm^2.

Table 4-3
Q-switched laser treatment: tattoo pigment volume effect

Tattoo Pigment Volume (mm^3)*	No. of Patients	Average Improvement	Average No. of Treatments
>2644 (average 4040)	4	91.3%	12.5
<442 (average 328)	6	90.8%	7.5

*Mean: 1543 ± 1011 mm^3.

addition, smaller (Table 4-2) and lower-volume (Table 4-3) tattoos cleared with fewer treatments. Analysis of these values reveals that response rate is a function of pigment depth and total pigment volume, as well as surface area.

In contrast to anecdotal reports with the ruby and Nd:YAG lasers, new tattoos treated with Q-switched alexandrite lasers cleared faster, possibly because of the more superficial location of a new tattoo. New tattoos have sharp lines with bright colors, whereas older tattoos are blurred with indistinct lines and duller, bluer colors presumably from the ink moving deeper into the dermis. Further studies to explore these observations are underway.

SIDE EFFECTS

In contrast to previous modalities, the Q-switched lasers are much more effective with very few side effects. *Hypopigmentation* is more a function of the wavelength used. Increased melanin absorption seen with shorter wavelengths increases the risk for hypopigmentation, which completely resolves in most patients. *Hyperpigmentation,* however, is related more to the patient's skin type. Those with darker skin are more prone to this no matter which wavelength is used. Treatment with hydroquinone and broad-spectrum sunscreens will resolve the hyperpigmentation within a few months, although in some patients it can be more prolonged. *Textural changes* or *scars* are, luckily, very rare. Transient textural changes are often noted but resolve within 1 to 2 months. If a patient is more prone to this, longer treatment intervals are recommended.

Allergic reactions to tattoo pigment after Q-switched laser treatment are possible.[136] Unlike the destructive modalities previously described, Q-switched lasers mobilize the ink and may generate a systemic allergic response. If an allergic reaction to the ink has been noted, Q-switched laser treatment is not advised.

Finally, tattoo *ink darkening* has been noted. Although this can occur with any colored ink, it is more common with red, white, and flesh-toned inks. This is a particular concern with cosmetic tattoos and is discussed at length in a later section.

COMPARATIVE STUDIES OF Q-SWITCHED LASERS

Direct comparison studies are difficult, because varying treatment parameters including spot sizes and fluences are difficult to standardize and results are therefore often inconclusive. Several comparative studies have been done using different lasers on the same tattoos. A comparison of the ruby and Nd:YAG lasers[126] found them to be equally effective in removal of black ink, but the ruby laser was more effective for green ink. A second comparison of the ruby and Nd:YAG lasers was limited to one treatment session,[137] and a similar response was noted. After 1 month the Nd:YAG was judged to cause more textural change and hyperpigmentation than the ruby laser, possibly related to the smaller spot size used and the ruby laser causing more hypopigmentation. One report comparing the Q-switched Nd:YAG laser to the alexandrite laser found the former achieved better results, whereas a comparison between the Q-switched ruby and alexandrite lasers for amateur tattoos revealed the ruby laser to remove more pigment after two sessions.[138]

In a similar study, the ruby laser removed more pigment than the alexandrite laser and resulted in more textural change, hypopigmentation, and hair loss. A comparison at two or three treatment sessions may not be optimal because only 50% to 60% of the tattoo has been removed, and speed and efficacy of tattoo removal as well as the avoidance of textural changes, scarring, hair loss, and pigment alterations must be examined. In addition, the range of colors responsive to laser systems is important. The optimum system for tattoo removal would be to combine two laser systems to take advantage of variations in pulse width and wavelength (e.g., alexandrite or ruby and Nd:YAG lasers used together).

LASER ABLATION OF FACIAL COSMETIC TATTOOS

The use of facial cosmetics for ornamental purposes and attraction of the opposite sex is an ancient art, first traced to around 3500 BC from evidence in Egyptian tombs and limestone caves.[139] The merger of this art form with tattooing occurred in 1984, when Angres[140] popularized tattoo *blepharopigmentation* (permanent eyeliner). Although originally promoted as an alternative to eyeliner application for women crippled with arthritis or other physical impairments, it has become a popular procedure for general cosmetic purposes.[141] In addition, tattooing of eyebrows, lip lines, and cheeks to simulate facial cosmetics was introduced in 1987.[142] The public's acceptance of the cosmetic use of facial tattoos to simulate makeup application has been surprising and has stirred medical controversy.[139-141] It has led to the use of the technique by estheticians, tattoo artists, and nurse practitioners, as well as physicians. In 1987 it was estimated that more than 75,000 persons had undergone various types of cosmetic dermal pigmentation procedures.[142]

Pigment Placement

The black dye used is primarily ferric oxide and is relatively inert. Tissue examined 6 weeks after blepharopigmentation revealed an absence of inflammation.[143] Carbon and titanium oxide are often present as well,[144] and numerous other metals have been detected in the dyes by x-ray microanalysis.

Many of the dyes used have been supplied by a variety of sources, some unlicensed. Fortunately, complications have been rare. One allergic granuloma has been reported,[26] as has one case of eyelid margin necrosis with loss of lashes and secondary cicatricial entropion.[145] By far the most common complication has been misapplication of the pigment[144,146] (Figure 4-31). A survey of members of the American Society of Ophthalmic Plastic and Reconstructive Surgery reported improper pigment placement in 4% of patients who had undergone blepharopigmentation.[144] Angres[142] noted an increasing number of patients who were dissatisfied with the positioning of the pigment placed during blepharopigmentation and expressed concern over the confusion among practitioners as to the ideal cosmetic result. He further commented that proper pigment placement is directly in the lash line between the base of the lash follicles and not above the lash line.

Pigment placement is accomplished with an instrument using oscillating disposable needles, which penetrate to a fixed depth of 1.2 mm. Microscopic examination of eyelid tissue previously tattooed reveals pigment granules extending to a depth of 1.5 mm in the dermis and connective tissue of the muscle fibers of the orbicular ocular muscle.[147] Virtually all implanted pigment has been shown to be within the cytoplasm of macrophages, which persist at the site of injection. Pigment migration has been reported in 5% of patients[144] and is thought to be secondary to loss of pigment placed too superficially in the epidermis. A particularly disastrous complication referred to as *pigment fanning* is thought to be the result of tattoo pigment placed so deep that it enters the tarsal fibrous tissue of the lid and spreads in this tissue plane, causing a fan-shaped pigmentation of the entire lid[146] (Figure 4-32). Fortunately, all the Q-switched lasers can effectively treat this condition.

Pigment Removal

Techniques reported for removal of permanent cosmetic tattoos include surgical excision,[148,149] scraping the pigment off with a chelation curette,[148] ablation of the tattoo with an argon laser,[139] and injection of tannic acid with a tattoo needle.[150]

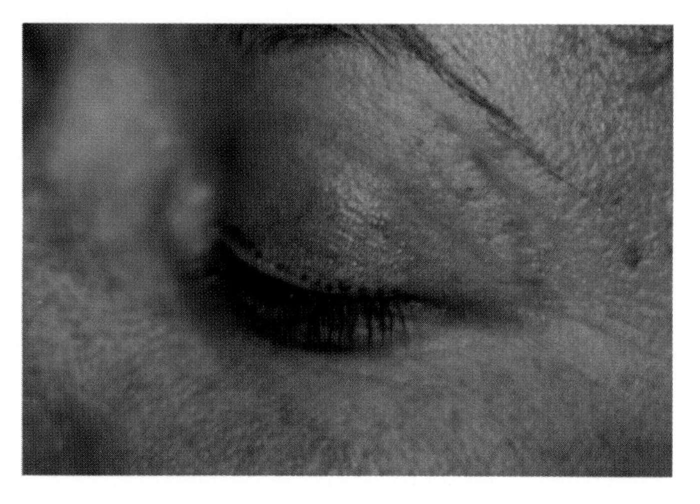

Figure 4-31 Misapplication of eyeliner tattoo pigment has been most common complication of cosmetic blepharopigmentation.

Surgical excision of a few misplaced dots is feasible and can be accomplished with a punch excision or a tiny ellipse or curettage of spots.[148] However, excision of an entire line of pigment is complicated by the presence of eyelashes within the tattoo with possible postoperative entropion or ectropion or unacceptable scarring or distortion of the vermilion border with removal of a lip line tattoo. Bleaching of unwanted tattoo pigment by injection of alcohol is suggested by the manufacturer of Accents, but this is an unproven technique in these locations and would be expected to produce inflammation, ulceration, and superficial tissue necrosis if effective, as reported with the injection of tannic acid.[150] Removal of any tattoo pigment is a difficult procedure, and most of the currently used tissue-destructive techniques are not appropriate for removal of facial cosmetic tattoos.

Vaporization of tattoo pigment with an argon laser has been successful. It is difficult, however, and thermal damage to cilial follicles results in loss of eyelashes[143] (see Chapter 5).

In one study, five different lasers were used to remove (1) midcheek rouge, (2) eyelid, (3) eyebrow, (4) lipliner, and (5) tattoos.[151] The superpulsed CO_2 laser (10,600 nm, continuous wave), a very controlled, precise instrument, provides a dry surgical field and precise removal of tattoo pigment in delicate areas such as the eyelid and eyebrow.

The superpulsed CO_2 laser was used in the SP3 under continuous mode (pulse parameters: 400 μsec, 250 Hz, 80-W peak power) and in the conventional continuous mode with a 50-msec shuttered pulse and power settings of 1 to 2 W. The beam diameter was varied between 0.1 and 1.5 mm, depending on the width of the tattoo being vaporized. When possible, individual dots of pigment were vaporized, using a beam size to correspond to the pigment dot. When the tattoo was a more uniform line, the laser was swept across the tattoo pigment, vaporizing the outer layer of skin overlying the tattoo. Repeated passes (three or four) resulted in a 1.5- to 2-mm incisional groove replacing the line of tattoo if complete removal of tattoo pigment was attempted, as in removing eyeliner tattoo. However, when the CO_2 laser was used for removal of lipliner tattoo and eyebrow tattoo, only the outer superficial tissue was vaporized, leaving an open superficial dermal wound containing tattoo pigment. As the wound healed, residual tattoo pigment would seep out onto the bandage, which was changed daily.

Before laser treatment, the skin containing tattoo pigment was infiltrated with lidocaine 1% with 1:100,000 epinephrine. During the procedure the eye was protected with a metallic scleral contact lens after instillation of topical proparacaine hydrochloride 0.5% drops in the conjunctival cul-de-sac. When vaporizing tattoo

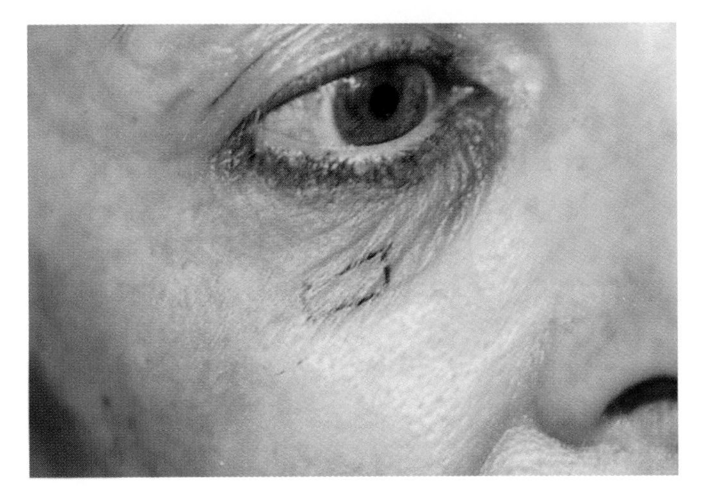

Figure 4-32 Pigment fanning after blepharopigmentation is thought to occur from tattoo pigment spreading in plane of tarsal fibrous tissue of lid.

pigment adjacent to eyelashes, the beam is pulsed in short bursts of 0.05 to 0.1 sec to achieve better control and avoid damaging the cilia follicles. Although it can be very difficult to differentiate between tattoo pigment and small fragments of charred tissue at the edges of the laser impact crater, all eyeliner tattoos cleared completely. The wounds healed by secondary intention with imperceptible scars within 6 months and no distortion of lid margins or loss of eyelashes (Figure 4-33). One

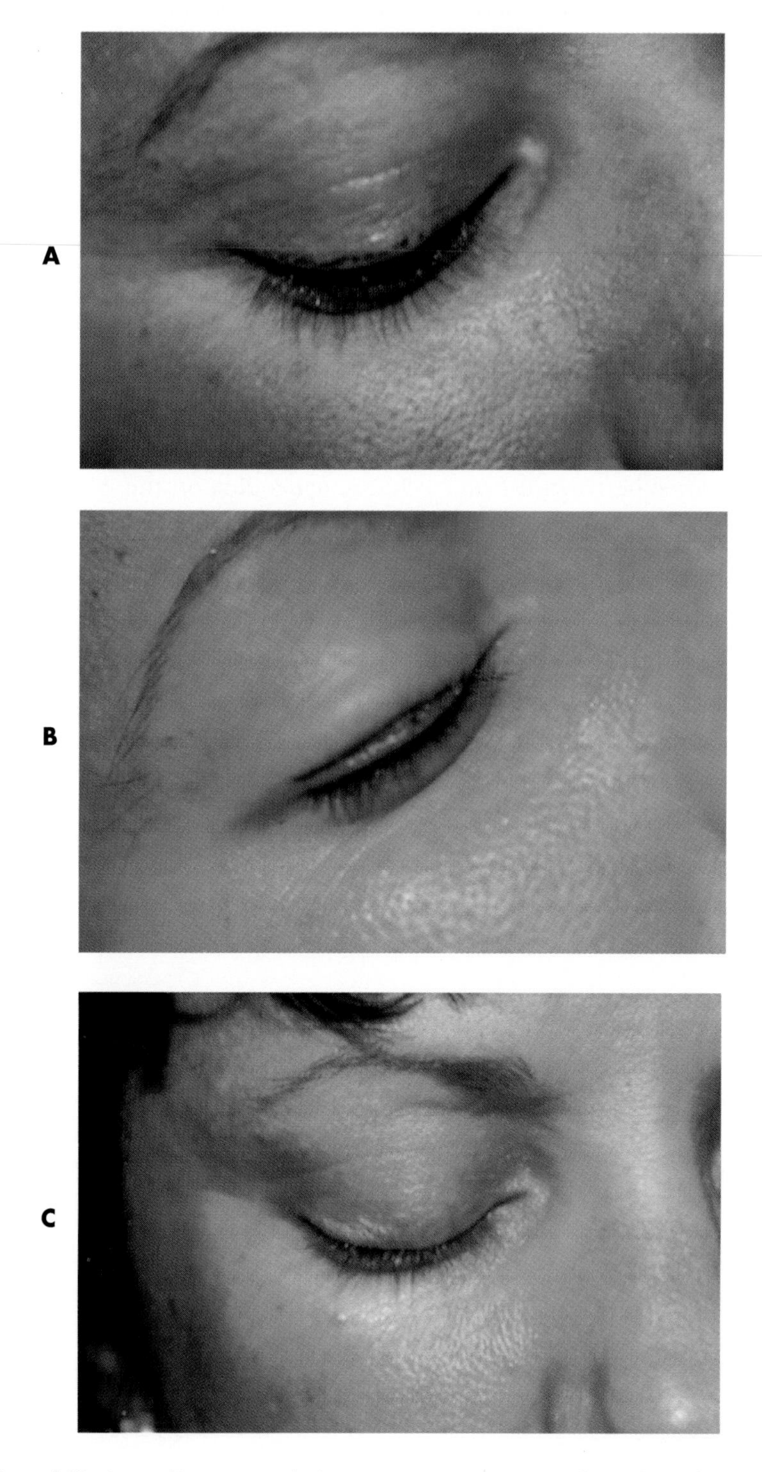

Figure 4-33 **A,** Eyeliner tattoo before treatment. **B,** Wound resulting from CO_2 laser ablation was allowed to heal by secondary intention. **C,** Final result 1 year after procedure.

eyebrow tattoo was completely removed without scarring using the CO_2 laser, but a hypopigmented scar was seen in one lipliner tattoo (Figure 4-34). The UltraPulse CO_2 ($UPCO_2$) laser further minimizes thermal damage and thereby decreases the risk of scarring and dyspigmentation.[152]

In one patient with red lipliner tattoo and one patient with cheek rouge tattoo, the FLPD laser (585 nm, 450 sec, 3- to 5-mm beam, power density of 7.5 J/cm^2, 20% overlap) was used. Both tattoos responded with 20% to 30% improvement with a single treatment. More encouraging, the FLPD laser (510 nm, 300 nsec, 5-mm spot size, energy density of 3.5 J/cm^2) completely cleared two red tattoos in five treatments at 4-week intervals without residual scarring (Figure 4-35). The frequency-doubled (fd) Nd:YAG laser (532 nm, 5 nsec) is equally effective.[153]

The argon laser with a continuous beam of 0.1 mm and power of 2.2 W (Model 1000, Coherent Medical, Palo Alto, Calif) minimally improved two lipliner tattoos. The Q-switched alexandrite and ruby lasers are also appropriate for removal of facial tattoos, as is the Q-switched Nd:YAG laser for black ink tattoos.[153]

A lipliner tattoo overtattooed with flesh tones in an attempt to cover the unwanted pigment was initially treated with the FLPD laser and irreversibly darkened to a dark slate gray (Figure 4-36). Flesh-tone, red, and white tattoo ink darkening with Q-switched ruby, Q-switched Nd:YAG, and Q-switched alexandrite laser treatment has been reported. Treatment with Q-switched lasers resulted in oxidation to a black

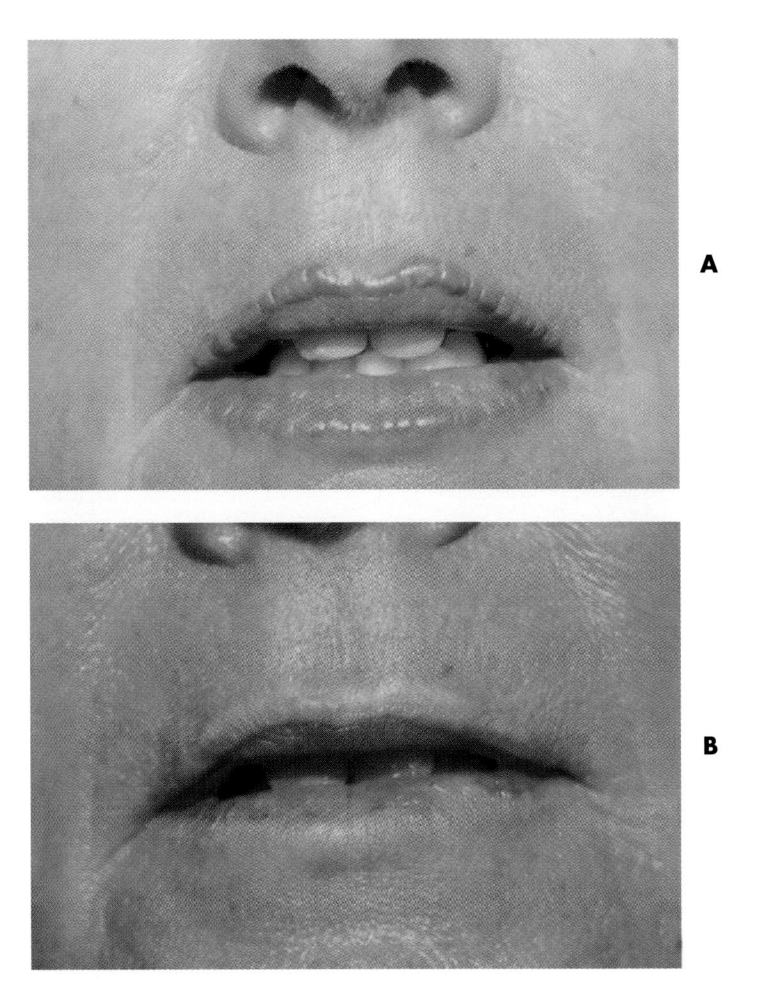

Figure 4-34 **A,** Allergic granulomatous dermatitis in red lipliner tattoo. **B,** Hypopigmented scar tissue remains after obliteration of tattoo pigment and granulomas with superpulse CO_2 laser.

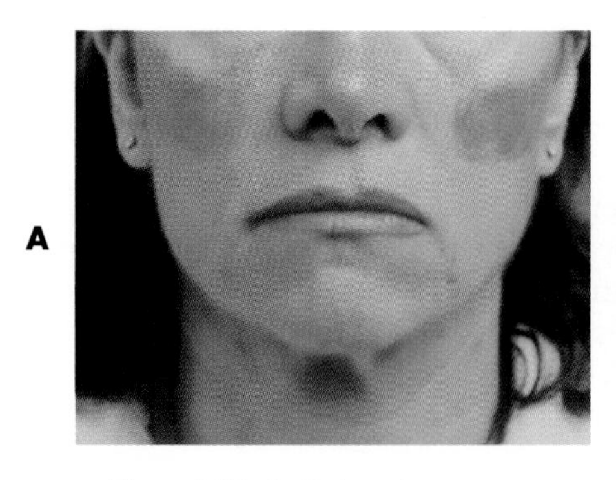

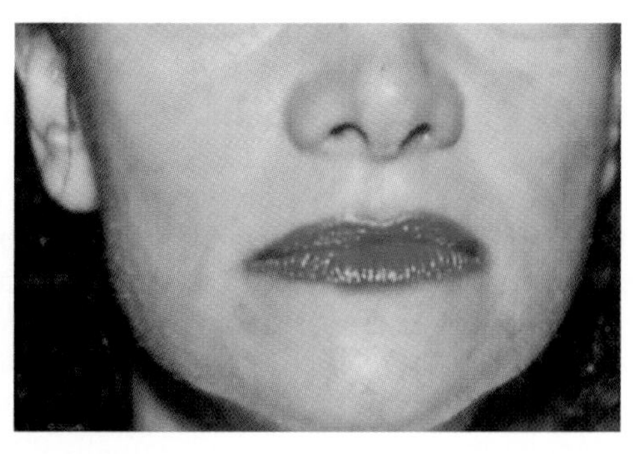

Figure 4-35 **A,** Before laser treatment, red tattoos intended to simulate rouge. **B,** Complete tattoo removal was achieved with 510-nm, 300-nsec pulsed dye laser.

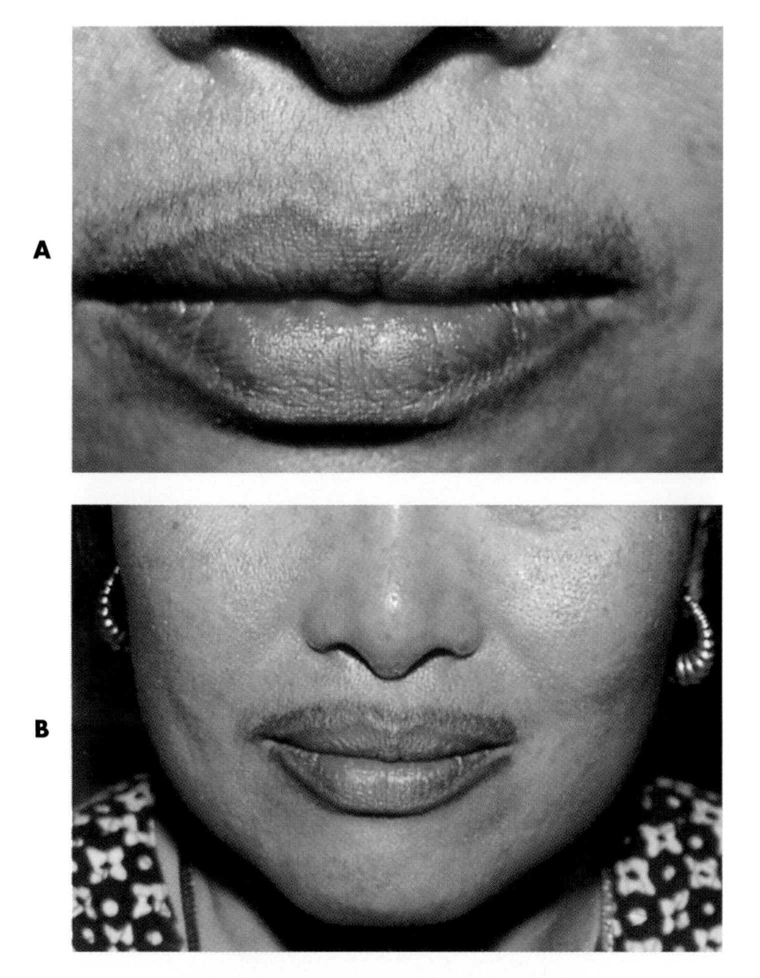

Figure 4-36 **A,** Unwanted lipliner tattoo had been overtattooed with flesh tones in attempt to cover red pigment. **B,** After single treatment with 510-nm, 300-nsec pulsed dye laser, flesh-tone pigment irreversibly changed to black.

Continued

pigment (Figure 4-37). Attempts to remove the darkened ink with further laser treatment failed in two cases, and surgical excision was necessary. In the other cases, subsequent laser treatments successfully removed the darkened ink.

In vitro tests with various tattoo pigments in agar have found that a surprising number of pigments (most containing iron oxide) will change color when irradiated

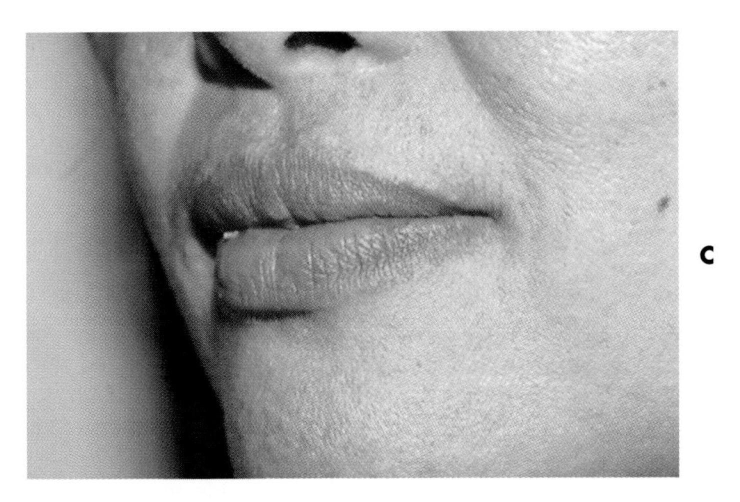

Figure 4-36, cont'd **C,** Unwanted pigment was removed after six treatments with alexandrite laser (755 nm, 100 nsec).

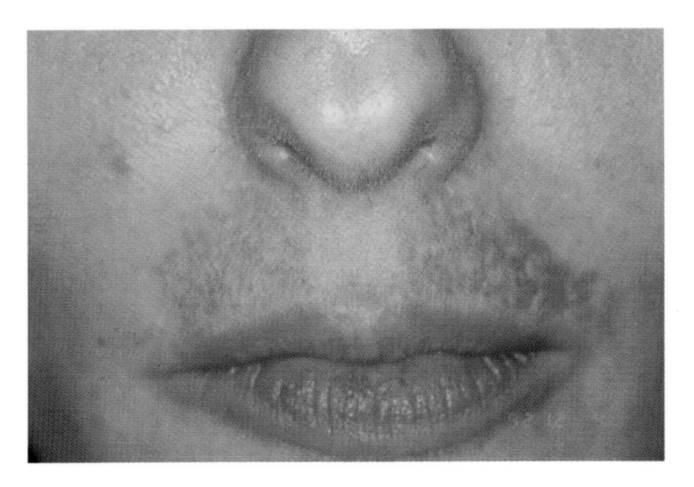

Figure 4-37 Flesh-tone tattoo applied to mask melasma of upper lip irreversibly darkened to black pigment after treatment with Q-switched ruby laser (694 nm, 40-80 nsec).

with Q-switched laser energy.[154,155] Iron oxide changes color from brown to black when raised to a temperature above 1400° C as ferric oxide is ignited.[156] In clinical practice multiple colors, including flesh tones, red, white, and brown, containing pigments (nonoxide, titanium dioxide) have been reported to change color on laser impact. Even several green and blue tattoo pigments have changed to black when irradiated with the Q-switched alexandrite laser. The chemical mechanism of tattoo ink darkening remains unknown. It likely involves the conversion of ferric oxide (Fe_2O_3) to ferrous oxide (FeO) by reduction or the strong ignition of ferric oxide above 1400° C. Crystalline ferrous oxide is unstable and tends to convert to ferric oxide or iron. Ferric oxide has a rust color and occurs in nature as the mineral hematite; ferrous oxide is black, as is Fe_3O_4, which occurs in nature as a black crystal of the mineral magnetite. The ability of each of these iron oxides to alter its composition without any structural change accounts for their ready interconvertibility.[156] These reactions may require extreme temperatures known to be generated during the very short pulse of Q-switched lasers, estimated at several hundreds to thousands of degrees Celsius.

Laser treatment of flesh-tone tattoos must be approached with caution. The resultant gray-black tattoo may be difficult to remove and is certainly more visible than a flesh tone; therefore test sites are recommend. The Q-switched lasers appear to be ideal for removal of large areas of black facial tattoos (tarsal fanning of pigment, eyebrow tattoo). However, the beam size (2-6.5 mm) may make removal of small dots of precisely confined tattoo pigment, as found in eyeliner tattoo, technically difficult without temporary or permanent hair loss from heat damage to the terminal hair. Because of the facial location of these tattoos, avoidance of scarring secondary to treatment is essential. The use of high fluences and very short pulses with the Q-switched lasers may increase the risk of tissue reaction and should be approached with caution.

In summary, the removal of unwanted facial cosmetic tattoos can be accomplished with the use of various lasers. For removal of black, red, green, or blue pigments, the appropriate Q-switched laser is best. Removal of red tattoo pigment is best accomplished with a short wavelength and a rapid pulse (510-nm, 300-nsec pigment laser) or the fd YAG laser (532 nm, 10 nsec). Treatment of cosmetic tattoos should be approached with caution because of the potential irreversible pigment darkening induced by laser interaction with iron oxide pigments or titanium dioxide. However, selected cases of eyeliner tattoo removal can be achieved with use of the $UPCO_2$ laser or other similarly engineered superpulsed CO_2 lasers because of the extreme precision obtainable.

SUMMARY

Q-switched lasers provide a dramatic improvement over previous modalities for tattoo removal. Appropriate wavelength choice will facilitate clearing of multicolored tattoos. Cosmetic tattoos should be approached with caution. Exploration into the use of picosecond lasers is underway and may further enhance our ability to treat tattoos.[153,156]

REFERENCES

1. Grumet GW: Psychodynamic implications of tattoos, *Am J Orthopsychiatry* 53:482, 1983.
2. Scutt R, Gotch C: *Art, sex and symbol: the mystery of tattooing,* Cranbury, NJ, 1974, Barnes.
3. Ebensten H: *Pierced hearts and true love,* London, 1953, Verschoyle.
4. Pers M, von Herbst T: Tatovering af umyndige, *Ugeskr Laeg* 31:973, 1965.
5. Pers M, von Herbst T: The demand for removal of tattoos: a plea for regulations against tattooing of minors, *Acta Chir Scand* 131:201, 1966.
6. Gittleson N, Wallen G, Dawson-Butterworth K: The tattooed psychiatric patient, *Br J Psychiatry* 115:1249, 1969.
7. Taylor A: A search among Borstal girls for the psychological and social significance of their tattoos, *Br J Criminol* 8:170, 1968.
8. Hamburger E, Lacovara D: A study of tattoos in inmates at a federal correctional institution: its physical and psychological implications, *Milit Med* 128:1205, 1963.
9. Roe A, Howell R, Payne I: Comparison of prison inmates with and without juvenile records, *Psychol Rep* 34:1315, 1974.
10. Lander J, Kohn A: A note on tattooing among selectees, *Am J Psychiatry* 100:326, 1943.
11. Youniss R: The relationship of tattoos to personal adjustment among enlisted submarine school volunteers, *US Naval Med Res Lab Rep No 319* 18:1, 1959.
12. Goldstein N: Psychological implications of tattoos, *J Dermatol Surg Oncol* 5:883, 1979.
13. Hellgren L: *Tattooing: the prevalence of tattooed persons in a total population,* Stockholm, 1967, Almquist & Wiksell.
14. Hamburger E: Tattooing as a psychic defence mechanism, *Int J Soc Psychiatry* 12:60, 1966.
15. Lepine A: Tattooing in approved schools and remand homes, *Health Trends* 1:11, 1969.
16. Scutt RWB: The chemical removal of tattoos, *Br J Plast Surg* 25:189, 1972.
17. Cohen M: Tattooing: some medical and psychological aspects, *Br J Dermatol* 39:290, 1927.
18. Armstrong ML: Career-oriented women with tattoos, *J Nurs Schol* 23:215, 1991.
19. Lea PJ, Pawlowski A: Human tattoo: electron microscopic assessment of epidermis, epidermal-dermal junction, and dermis, *Int J Dermatol* 26:453, 1987.

20. Taylor CR, Anderson R, Gange W et al: Light and electron microscopic analysis of tattoos treated by Q-switched ruby laser, *J Invest Dermatol* 97:131, 1991.
21. Diette KM, Bronstein BR, Parrish JA: Histologic comparison of argon and tunable dye lasers in the treatment of tattoos, *J Invest Dermatol* 85:368, 1985.
22. Patipa M, Jakobiec FA, Krebs W: Light and electron microscopic findings with permanent eyeliner, *Ophthalmology* 93(10):1361, 1986.
23. Christensen HE, Schmidt H: The ultrastructure of tattoo marks, *Pathol Microbiol Scand* 80A:573, 1972.
24. Mann R, Klingmuller G: Electron-microscopic investigation of tattoos in rabbit skin, *Arch Dermatol Res* 271: 367, 1981.
25. Goldstein AP: Histologic reactions in tattoos, *J Dermatol Surg Oncol* 5:896, 1979.
26. Yang DS, Kim SC, Lee S et al: Foreign body epithelioid granuloma after cosmetic eyebrow tattooing, *Cutis* 43:224, 1989.
27. Ravits HG: Allergic tattoo granuloma, *Arch Dermatol* 86:287, 1962.
28. Guillaume AC: Recherches sur le mechanisme du tatouage et enseignements qui en resultent au point de vue des fonctions de la peau, *Bull Med Paris* 41:1399, 1927.
29. Guillaume AC: Quelques particularites des fonctions de la peau qui sont enseignes par l'etude des tatouages, *Bull Med Paris* 41:1457, 1927.
30. Silberberg I, Leider M: Studies of a red tattoo, *Arch Dermatol* 101:299, 1970.
31. Abel EA, Silberberg I, Queen D: Studies of chronic inflammation in a red tattoo by electron microscopy and histochemistry, *Acta Dermatol Venereol (Stockh)* 52:453, 1972.
32. Olander K, Kanai A, Kaufman HE: An analytical electron microscopic study of a corneal tattoo, *Ann Ophthalmol* 15:1046, 1983.
33. Dickinson JA: Sarcoidal reaction in tattoos, *Arch Dermatol* 100:315, 1969.
34. Farzan S: Sarcoidal reaction in tattoos, *NY State J Med* 77:1477, 1977.
35. Tse T, Folberg R, Moore K: Clinicopathologic correlate of a fresh eyelid pigment implantation, *Arch Ophthalmol* 103:1515, 1985.
36. Goldstein N, Sewell M: Tattoos in different cultures, *J Dermatol Surg Oncol* 5:857, 1979.
37. Everett MA: Tattoos: abnormalities of pigmentation. In *Clinical dermatology,* vol 2, units 11-21, Hagerstown, Md, 1980, Harper & Row.
38. Rostenberg A, Brown RA, Caro MR: Discussion of tattoo reactions with report of a case showing a reaction to a green color, *Arch Dermatol Syph* 62:540, 1950.
39. Anderson RR: Tattooing should be regulated, *N Engl J Med* 326:207, 1992.
40. Ballin DB: Cutaneous hypersensitivity to mercury from tattooing: report of case, *Arch Dermatol Syph* 27:292, 1933.
41. Bonnell JA, Russell B: Skin reactions at sites of green and red tattoo marks, *Proc R Soc Med* 49:823, 1956.
42. Bjornberg A: Reactions to light in yellow tattoos from cadmium sulfide, *Arch Dermatol* 88:267, 1963.
43. Tindall JP, Smith JG Jr: Unusual reactions in yellow tattoos: microscopic studies on histologic sections, *South Med J* 55:792, 1962.
44. Loewenthal LJA: Reactions in green tattoos: the significance of valence state of chromium, *Arch Dermatol* 82:237, 1960.
45. Bjornberg A: Allergic reactions to chrome in green tattoo markings, *Acta Derm Venereal* 39:23, 1959.
46. Tazelaar DJ: Hypersensitivity to chromium in a light-blue tattoo, *Dermatologiea* 141:282, 1970.
47. Rorsman H, Dahlquist I, Jacobsson S et al: Tattoo granuloma and uveitis, *Lancet* 11:27, 1969.
48. Swinny B: Generalized chronic dermatitis due to tattoo, *Ann Allergy* 4:295, 1946.
49. Novy FG: A generalized mercurial (cinnabar) reaction following tattooing, *Arch Dermatol* 49:172, 1944.
50. Goldstein N: Complications for tattoos, *J Dermatol Surg Oncol* 5:869, 1979.
51. Boo-Chai K: The decorative tattoo: its removal by dermabrasion, *Plast Reconstr Surg* 32:559, 1963.
52. Clabaugh W: Removal of tattoos by superficial dermabrasion, *Arch Dermatol* 98:515, 1968.
53. Clabaugh W: Tattoo removal by superficial dermabrasion, *Plast Reconstr Surg* 55:401, 1975.
54. Bunke HJ, Conway H: Surgery of decorative and traumatic tattoos, *Plast Reconstr Surg* 20:67, 1957.

55. Wentzell JM, Robinson JK, Wentzell JM et al: Physical properties of aerosols produced by dermabrasion, *Arch Dermatol* 125:1637, 1989.
56. Goldstein N: Tattoo removal, *Dermatol Clin* 5:349, 1987.
57. Bailey BN: Treatment of tattoos, *Plast Reconstr Surg* 40:361, 1976.
58. Ceilley RI: Curettage after dermabrasion: techniques of removal of tattoos, *J Dermatol Surg Oncol* 5:905, 1979.
59. Goldstein N, Penoff J, Price N et al: Techniques of removal of tattoos, *J Dermatol Surg Oncol* 5:901, 1979.
60. Robinson J: Tattoo removal, *J Dermatol Surg Oncol* 11:14, 1985.
61. Crittenden FM: Salabrasion: removal of tattoos by superficial abrasion with table salt, *Cutis* 7:295, 1971.
62. Koerber WA: Price NM: Salabrasion of tattoos, *Arch Dermatol* 114:884, 1978.
63. Lindsay DG: Tattoos, *Dermatol Clin* 7:147, 1989.
64. Morgan BDG: Tattoos, *Br Med* J 3:34, 1974.
65. Strong AMM, Jackson JT: The removal of amateur tattoos by salabrasion, *Br J Dermatol* 101:693, 1979.
66. Apfelberg DB, Manchester GH: Decorative and traumatic tattoo biophysics and removal, *Clin Plast Surg* 14:243, 1987.
67. Gupta SC: An investigation into a method for the removal of dermal tattoos: a report on animal and clinical studies, *Plast Reconstr Surg* 36:354, 1965.
68. Wheeler ES, Miller TA: Tattoo removal by split thickness tangential excision, *West J Med* 124:272, 1976.
69. Variot G: Nouveau procede de destruction des tatouages, *Compte Rendu Societe Biologie (Paris)* 8:836, 1888.
70. Penoff JH: The office treatment of tattoos: a simple and effective method, *Plast Reconstr Surg* 79:186, 1987.
71. Piggot TA, Norris RW: The treatment of tattoos with trichloroacetic acid: experience with 670 patients, *Br J Plast Surg* 41:112, 1988.
72. Hudson DA, Lechtape-Gruter RU: A simple method of tattoo removal, *S Afr Med J* 78:748, 1990.
73. Colver GB, Jones RL, Cherry GW et al: Precise dermal damage with an infrared coagulator, *Br J Dermatol* 114:603, 1986.
74. Colver GB, Cherry GW, Dawber RPR et al: The treatment of cutaneous vascular lesions with the infrared coagulator: a preliminary report, *Br J Plast Surg* 39:131, 1986.
75. Colver GB, Hunter JAA: Venous lakes: treatment by infrared coagulation, *Br J Plast Surg* 40:451, 1987.
76. Dorn B, Christophers E, Kietzmann H: Treatment of port-wine stains and haemangiomas by infrared contact coagulation, *17th World Congress of Dermatology Abstracts* 2:307, 1987.
77. Groot DW, Arlett JP, Johnston PA: Comparison of the infrared coagulator and the carbon dioxide laser in the removal of decorative tattoos, *J Am Acad Dermatol* 15:518, 1986.
78. Colver GB, Cherry GW, Dawber RPR et al: Tattoo removal using infrared coagulation, *Br J Dermatol* 112:481, 1985.
79. Venning VA, Colver GB, Millard PR et al: Tattoo removal using infrared coagulation: a dose comparison, *Br J Dermatol* 117:99, 1987.
80. Colver GB: The infrared coagulator in dermatology, *Dermatol Clin* 7:155, 1989.
81. Leopold PJ: Cryosurgery for facial skin lesions, *Proc R Soc Med* 68:606, 1975.
82. Zacarian SA: Cryosurgery for cutaneous carcinoma, *Dermatol Dig* 9:49, 1970.
83. Ruiz-Esparza J, Fitzpatrick RE, Goldman MP: Tattoo removal: selecting the right alternative, *Am J Cosmetic Surg* 9:171, 1992.
84. Colver GB, Dawber RPR: Tattoo removal using a liquid nitrogen cryospray, *Clin Exp Dermatol* 9:364, 1984.
85. Dvir E, Hirshowitz B: Tattoo removal by cryosurgery, *Plast Reconstr Surg* 66:373, 1980.
86. Colver GB, Dawber RPR: The removal of digital tattoos, *Int J Dermatol* 24:567, 1985.
87. Goldman L, Blaney DJ, Kindel DJ et al: Effect of the laser beam on the skin: preliminary report, *J Invest Dermatol* 40:121, 1963.
88. Goldman L, Blaney DJ, Kindel DJ et al: Pathology of the effect of the laser beam on the skin, *Nature* 197:912, 1965.
89. Goldman L, Wilson RG, Hornby P et al: Radiation from a Q-switched ruby laser, *J Invest Dermatol* 44:69, 1965.

90. Goldman L et al: Laser treatment of tattoos: a preliminary survey of three years' clinical experience, *JAMA* 201:841, 1967.
91. Goldman L, Rockwell RJ, Meyer R et al: Laser treatment of tattoos, *JAMA* 201:163, 1967.
92. Yules RB, Laub DR, Honey R et al: The effect of Q-switched ruby laser radiation on dermal tattoo pigment in man, *Arch Surg* 95:179, 1967.
93. Laub DR, Yules RB, Arras M et al: Preliminary histopathological observation of Q-switched ruby laser radiation on dermal tattoo pigment in man, *J Surg Res* 5(8):220, 1968.
94. Apfelberg DB, Maser MR, Lash H: Argon laser treatment of decorative tattoos, *Br J Plast Surg* 32:141, 1979.
95. Apfelberg DB, Rivers J, Maser MR et al: Update on laser usage in treatment of decorative tattoos, *Lasers Surg Med* 2:169, 1982.
96. Apfelberg DB, Laub DR, Maser MR et al: Pathophysiology and treatment of decorative tattoos with reference to argon laser treatment, *Clin Plast Surg* 7:369, 1967.
97. Reid R: Tattoo removal with laser, *Med J Aust*, April 8, 1978 (letter).
98. Fitzpatrick RE, Goldman MP, Ruiz-Esparza J: The use of the alexandrite laser (755 nm, 100 μsec) for tattoo pigment removal in an animal model, *J Am Acad Dermatol* 28:745, 1993.
99. Apfelberg DB, Maser MR, Lash R et al: Comparison of argon and carbon dioxide laser treatment of decorative tattoos: a preliminary report, *Ann Plast Surg* 14:6, 1985.
100. McBurney EI: Carbon dioxide laser treatment of dermatologic lesions, *South Med J* 71:795, 1978.
101. Brady SC, Blokmanis A, Jewett L: Tattoo removal with the carbon dioxide laser, *Ann Plast Surg* 2:482, 1978.
102. Beacon JP, Ellis H: Surgical removal of tattoos by carbon dioxide laser, *J R Soc Med* 73:298, 1980.
103. Bailin PL, Ratz JL, Levine HL: Removal of tattoos by CO_2 laser, *J Dermatol Surg Oncol* 6:997, 1980.
104. Reid R, Muller S: Tattoo removal by CO_2 laser dermabrasion, *Plast Reconstr Surg* 65:717, 1980.
105. Dixon, J: Laser treatment of decorative tattoos. In Arndt KA, Noe JM, Rosen S, editors: *Cutaneous laser therapy: principles and methods,* New York, 1983, J Wiley & Sons.
106. Ruiz-Esparza J, Goldman MP, Fitzpatrick RE: Tattoo removal with minimal scarring: the chemo-laser technique, *J Dermatol Surg Oncol* 14:1372, 1989.
107. Dismukes DE: The "chemo-laser technique" for the treatment of decorative tattoos: a more complete dye-removal procedure, *Lasers Surg Med* 6:59, 1986.
108. Anderson RR, Parrish JA: Selective photothermolysis: precise microsurgery by selective absorption of pulsed irradiation, *Science* 220:524, 1983.
109. Kilmer SL, Lee MS, Anderson RR: Treatment of multi-colored tattoos with the frequency-doubled Q-switched Nd:YAG laser (532 nm): a dose-response study with comparison to the Q-switched ruby laser, *Lasers Surg Med Suppl* 5:54, 1993.
110. Hodersdal M, Bech-Thomsen N, Wulf HC: Skin reflectance–guided laser selections for treatment of decorative tattoos, *Arch Dermatol* 132:403, 1996.
111. Fitzpatrick RE, Goldman MP: Tattoo removal using the alexandrite laser (755 nm, 100 ns), *Arch Dermatol* 130:1508, 1994.
112. Goldman L: Laser surgical research, *Ann NY Acad Sci* 168:649, 1970.
113. Reid RI, Muller S: Tattoo removal with laser, *Med J Aust* 1:389, 1978.
114. Reid WH, McLeod PJ, Ritchie A et al: Q-switched ruby laser treatment of black tattoos, *Br J Plast Surg* 36:455, 1983.
115. Polla LL, Margolis RJ, Dover JS et al: Melanosomes are a primary target of Q-switched ruby laser irradiation in guinea pig skin, *J Invest Dermatol* 89:281, 1987.
116. Dover JS, Margolis RJ, Polla LL et al: Pigmented guinea pig skin irradiated with Q-switched ruby laser pulses: morphologic and histologic findings, *Arch Dermatol* 125:43, 1989.
117. Taylor CR, Gange RW, Dover JS et al: Treatment of tattoos by Q-switched ruby laser: a dose-response study, *Arch Dermatol* 126:893, 1990.
118. Scheibner A, Kenny G, White W et al: A superior method of tattoo removal using the Q-switched ruby laser, *J Dermatol Surg Oncol* 16:1091, 1990.
119. Geronemus RG, Ashinoff R: Use of the Q-switched ruby laser to treat tattoos and benign pigmented lesions of the skin, *Lasers Surg Med Suppl* 3:64, 1991.

120. Ashinoff R, Geronemus RG: Rapid response of traumatic and medical tattoos to treatment with the Q-switched ruby laser, *Plast Reconstr Surg* 91:841, 1993.
121. Lowe NJ, Luftman D, Sawcer D: Q-switched ruby laser: further observations on treatment of professional tattoos, *J Dermatol Surg Oncol* 20:307, 1994.
122. Levins PC, Grevelink JM, Anderson RR: Q-switched ruby laser treatment of tattoos, *Lasers Surg Med Suppl* 3:63, 1991.
123. Kilmer SL, Anderson RR: Clinical use of the Q-switched ruby and the Q-switched Nd:YAG (1064 nm and 532 nm) lasers for treatment of tattoos, *J Dermatol Surg Oncol* 19:330, 1993.
124. DeCoste SD, Anderson RR: Comparison of Q-switched ruby and Q-switched Nd:YAG laser treatment of tattoos, *Lasers Surg Med Suppl* 3:64, 1991.
125. Kilmer SL, Lee M, Farinelli W et al: Q-switched Nd:YAG laser (1064 nm) effectively treats Q-switched ruby laser resistant tattoos, *Lasers Surg Med Suppl* 4:72, 1992.
126. Kilmer SL, Lee MS, Grevelink JM et al: The Q-switched Nd:YAG laser (1064 nm) effectively treats tattoos: a controlled, dose-response study, *Arch Dermatol* 129:971, 1993.
127. Ferguson JE, August PJ: Evaluation of the Nd/YAG laser for treatment of amateur and professional tattoos, *Br J Dermatol* 135:586, 1996.
128. Jones A, Roddey P, Orengo I, Rosen T: The Q-switched Nd:YAG laser effectively treats tattoos in darkly pigmented skin, *Dermatol Surg* 22:999, 1996.
129. Grevelink JM, Duke D, Van Leeuwen RL et al: Laser treatment of tattoos in darkly pigmented patients: efficacy and side effects, *J Am Acad Dermatol* 34:653, 1996.
130. Kilmer SL, Farinelli WF, Tearney G, Anderson RR: Use of a larger spot size for the treatment of tattoos increases clinical efficacy and decreases potential side effects, *Lasers Surg Med Suppl* 6:51, 1994.
131. Fitzpatrick RE, Goldman MP: Tattoo removal using the alexandrite lasers, *Arch Dermatol* 130:1508, 1994.
132. Alster TS: Q-switched alexandrite laser treatment (755 nm) of professional and amateur tattoos, *J Am Acad Dermatol* 33:69, 1995.
133. Stafford TJ, Lizek R, Tan OT: Role of the alexandrite laser for removal of tattoos, *Lasers Surg Med* 17:32, 1995.
134. Garcia C, Clark RE: Tattoo removal using the alexandrite laser, *NC Med J* 56:336, 1995.
135. Grekin RC, Shelton RM, Geisse JK et al: 510-nm pigmented lesion dye laser: its characteristics and clinical uses, *J Dermatol Surg Oncol* 19:380, 1993.
136. Ashinoff R, Levine VJ, Soter NA: Allergic reactions to tattoo pigment after laser treatment, *Dermatol Surg* 21:291, 1995.
137. Levine V, Geronemus R: Tattoo removal with the Q-switched ruby laser and the Q-switched Nd:YAG laser: a comparative study, *Cutis* 55:291, 1995.
138. McMeekin TO, Goodwin DP: A comparison of the alexandrite laser (755 nm) with the Q-switched ruby laser (694 nm) in the treatment of tattoos, *Lasers Surg Med Suppl* 5:43, 1993.
139. Balsam MS, Sagarin E, editors: *Cosmetics: science and technology,* ed 2, New York, 1974, Wiley-Interscience.
140. Angres GA: Angres permalid-liner method: a new surgical procedure, *Am J Ophthalmol* 16:145, 1984.
141. Farber MG, Lamberg RC, Smith ME: A histologic study of eyelid pigment eight weeks after implantation (eyelid tattoo), *Arch Ophthalmol* 104:1434, 1986.
142. Angres GG: Blepharo and dermapigmentation techniques for facial cosmesis, *Ear Nose Throat J* 66:344, 1987.
143. Tanenbaum M, Karas S, McCord CD: Laser ablation of blepharopigmentation, *Ophthal Plast Reconstr Surg* 4:49, 1988.
144. Wilkes TD: The complications of dermal tattooing, *Ophthalmic Surg* 2:1, 1986.
145. Goldberg RA, Shorr N: Complications of blepharopigmentation, *Ophthalmic Surg* 20:420, 1989.
146. Angres FF: Blepharopigmentation procedure guidelines, *Plast Reconstr Surg* 77:338, 1986.
147. Hurwitz JJ, Brownstein S, Mishkin SK: Histopathological findings in blepharopigmentation (eyelid tattoo), *Can J Ophthamol* 23: 267, 1988.
148. Putterman AM, Migliori ME: Elective excision of permanent eyeliner, *Arch Ophthalmol* 106:1034, 1988.
149. Dedio RM, Henry WJ, Scipione CR: Surgical removal of blepharopigmentation, *Am J Cosmetic Surg* 7:93, 1990.

150. Fogh H, Wulf HC, Poulsen T et al: Tattoo removal by overtattooing with tannic acid, *J Dermatol Surg Oncol* 15:1089, 1989.
151. Fitzpatrick RE, Goldman MP, Dierickx C: Laser ablation of facial cosmetic tattoos, *Aesthetic Plast Surg* (in press).
152. Herbich GJ: Ultrapulse carbon dioxide laser treatment of an iron oxide flesh-colored tattoo, *Dermatol Surg* 23:60, 1997.
153. Kilmer SL, Fitzpatrick RE, Da Silva LB et al: Picosecond and femtosecond laser treatment of tattoo ink, *Lasers Surg Med Suppl* 8:36, 1996.
154. The transition elements. In Cotton FA, Wilkinson G, editors: *Advanced inorganic chemistry,* New York, 1972, Interscience.
155. Anderson RR, Geronemus R, Kilmer SC et al: Cosmetic tattoo ink darkening: a complication of Q-switched and pulsed-laser treatment, *Arch Dermatol* 8:1010, 1993.
156. Ross V, Naseef G, Lin G et al: Comparison of responses of tattoos to picosecond and nanosecond Q-switched neodymium:YAG lasers, *Arch Dermatol* 134:167, 1998.

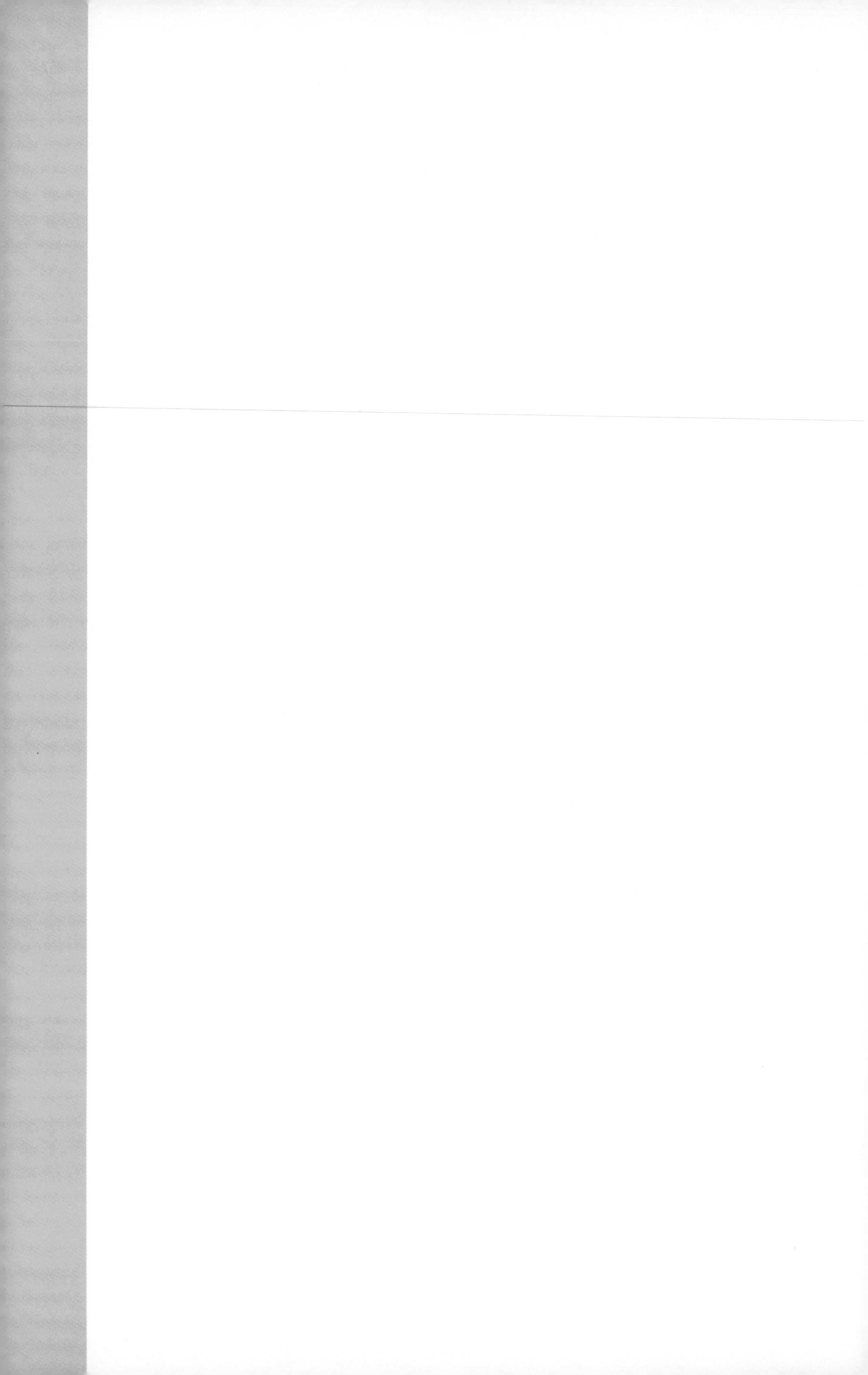

CHAPTER **five**

Hair Removal

Melanie C. Grossman

OVERVIEW

Millions of men and women compulsively remove unwanted hair daily. Cultural norms often dictate the removal of "normally distributed hair." Most North American women desire hairless legs, axillae, and inner thighs; many American men remove hair growing on their backs and shoulders. Japanese men and women also prefer the removal of body hair. Conversely, some European cultures maintain full hair growth. Medical conditions involving excess hair growth compel others to remove superfluous hair.

Individuals employ several temporary manual strategies to remove hair, including shaving, wax epilation, and chemical depilatories. Electrolysis permits the removal of single hairs. In some cases, electrolysis may be permanent, but the process remains tedious and operator dependent with occasional scarring. Pharmaceuticals provide hair growth control for some hirsute individuals.

Laser-assisted hair removal seeks to revolutionize the hair removal industry by providing efficient, reliable, long-lasting depilation over large body surface areas. However, several realities of hair growth present unique challenges, making laser hair removal a more difficult task than the removal of other dermal lesions. Human hair grows from follicles deep in the dermis. Hair growth is a dynamic process, and hair grows in cycles consisting of both growing and resting phases. The many influences on hair growth include systemic hormones and local factors, but the subtleties of hair growth remain elusive. Hair follicles also possess regenerative properties. Assuming that the destruction of hair follicles would achieve permanent alopecia, the task of achieving and documenting permanent hair removal remains challenging. Laser light must reach and destroy the growth center of the hair, and follow-up intervals must exceed the normal telogen phase.

Because laser technology is relatively new, long-term experience with most laser hair removal devices is limited. Although only one peer-reviewed study presently exists in the literature, anecdotal experience with various technologies suggests that many of these methods delay hair growth, consistent with the induction of telogen effluvium. More extensive experience over the next few years will afford a greater understanding of the mechanisms and efficacy of laser hair removal. This chapter provides a brief overview of hair biology, conditions of hair excess, and alternative hair removal techniques, as well as a discussion of current theories and knowledge of laser hair removal.

HAIR BIOLOGY

Embryology: Hair Follicle Development

Hair follicle development occurs from the ninth week through the twenty-second week of embryonic life. Embryonic hair growth of nonpigmented hairs (*lanugo*) begins at weeks 16 to 20. These hairs are shed from the thirty-sixth uterine week through the fourth month postpartum.[1]

Hair follicles form through interaction between the embryonic mesoderm and ectoderm. The *pregerm stage* consists of a cluster of nuclei in the ectodermal basal cell layer that appears with a corresponding accumulation of mesenchymal cells. The *hair germ stage* follows as the basal cell nuclei elongate and the cluster protrudes into the dermis. The ectodermal cell cluster trails the downward growth of the mesoderm, forming the *hair peg.* As maturation continues, ectodermal cells grow and multiply adjacent to the mesoderm and surround it. The result is a structure called the *bulbous hair peg,* which lies at an oblique angle to the epidermis. As it matures, the bulbous hair peg becomes a mature hair follicle. During this process, two and sometimes three "buds" of epithelial cells develop on the posterior aspect of the follicle. If three buds emerge, the superior bulb becomes the *apocrine gland* or the rudimentary apocrine gland, depending on the body location. The middle bud becomes the *sebaceous gland,* and the inferior one is the *hair bulge,* the location where the arrector pili muscle inserts. Some follicles contain only "sebaceous" and "bulge" buds. Mesenchymal cells develop at the base of the follicle and form the *Arao-Perkins body,* which is rich in elastic tissue. Hair melanocytes migrate from the neural crest and finally concentrate in the epithelial portion of the hair bulb.[1,2]

Hair Type

After lanugo hair (congenital) is shed, vellus and terminal hair replace it. *Terminal hairs* are large-diameter (approximately 60 μm), pigmented hairs that may achieve great lengths (up to 100 cm). Conversely, *vellus hairs* are small in diameter (approximately 30 μm), usually contain less pigment, and do not grow beyond 2 cm. During puberty, vellus hairs are replaced by terminal hairs in the axillary, pubic, and beard (males) regions. Eyebrows and eyelashes are considered terminal hairs despite their short length.[1,3]

Hair Anatomy

When cut in cross section, hair shafts contain a cortex comprised of cortical cells covered by a single layer of keratinized imbricated cells called the *cuticle.* Large terminal hairs also contain a central medullary zone. Melanin pigment is located in the hair cortex[1,3] (Figure 5-1).

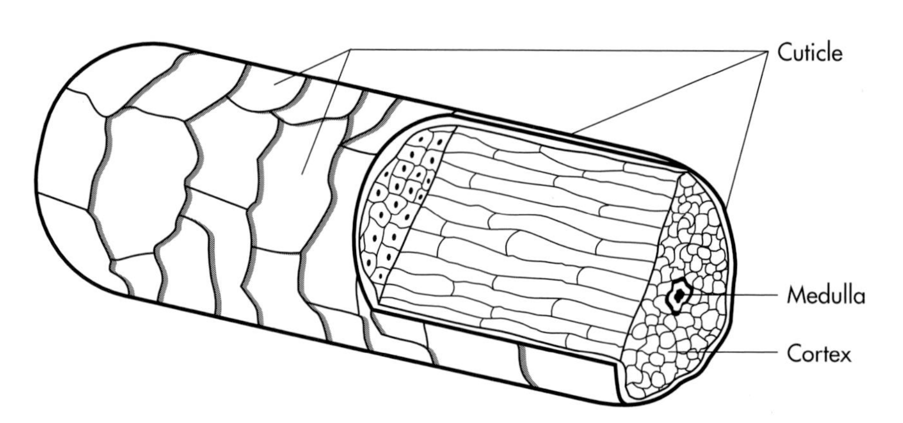

Figure 5-1 Hair shaft showing cuticle, cortex, and medulla. (From Olsen EA: *Disorders of hair growth: diagnosis and treatment,* New York, 1993, McGraw-Hill.)

Longitudinal follicular anatomy

The anagen hair follicle can be divided longitudinally into four segments. The *infundibular region,* the most superior segment, is continuous with the surrounding epidermis and terminates at the insertion of the sebaceous duct. The *sebaceous gland area* is the next deepest. The sebaceous duct is found on the posterior side of the follicle, that is, the side forming an obtuse angle with the epidermis. The *isthmus* initiates at the insertion of the sebaceous duct and ends at the insertion of the arrector pilor muscle. The *bulbar region,* the inferior segment, contains the dermal papilla, the surrounding matrix cells, and the lowest portion of the follicle (Figure 5-2).

Blood vessels and nerve fibers enter the dermal papillae at their inferior portion, which is continuous with the Arao-Perkins body on which they rest. Dermal melanocytes are primarily located interspersed among the hair matrix cells in the upper half of the bulb and are responsible for hair color. Melanocytes may also be found in the basal layer of the infundibulum in the outer and in the outer root sheath.

The two types of hair melanin are eumelanin and pheomelanin. Both pigments are formed from the precursor tyrosine through the production of an intermediate compound, dopaquinone. This reaction is facilitated by the enzyme tyrosinase (Figure 5-3). *Eumelanin* produces brown or black hair, whereas *pheomelanin* leads to red and blond hairs. Hair color is determined by the amount and distribution of melanin. Persons with dark hair have predominantly eumelanin, although some pheomelanin may be present. Patients with red hair have a high concentration of pheomelanin. Blond hair results from the production of fewer melanosomes or incompletely melanized melanosomes. White-haired individuals do not produce melanin. Gray hair results from the absence or diminished amount of melanin in the hair shaft.

Horizontal follicular anatomy

The hair follicle surrounding the hair shaft is divided into several concentric layers. The *inner root sheath* is composed of the sheath's cuticle and the Huxley and Henle layers. The Henle layer is the outermost layer of the inner root sheath; with one cell layer, it is the first to cornify. The Huxley layer is two cell layers thick and is

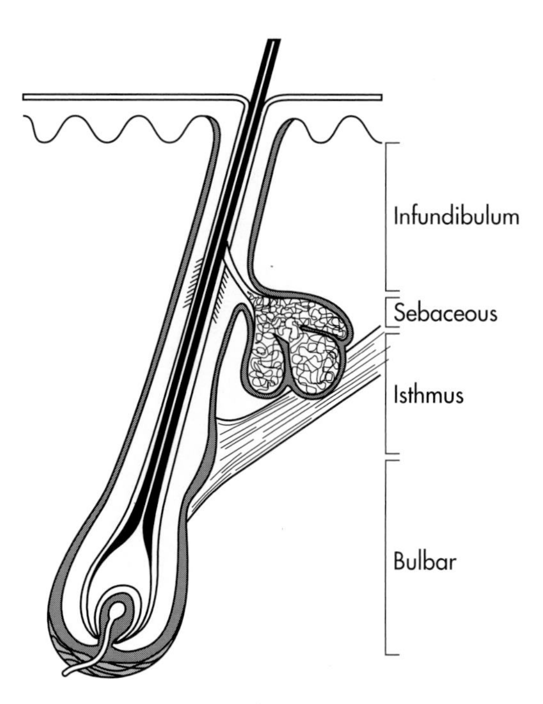

Figure 5-2 Hair follicle, longitudinal section. (From Olsen EA: *Disorders of hair growth: diagnosis and treatment,* New York, 1993, McGraw-Hill.)

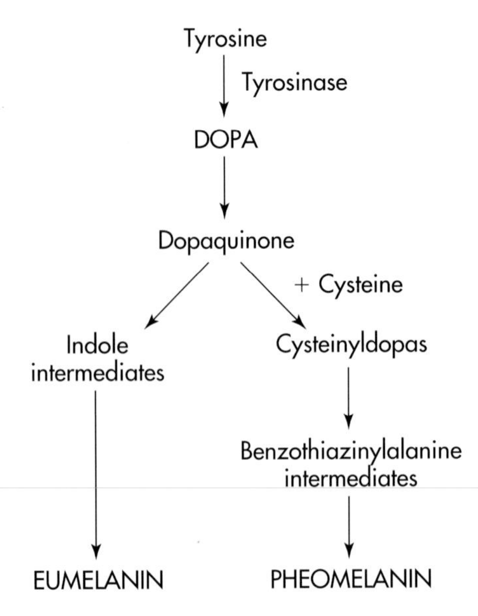

Figure 5-3 Pathway of melanin synthesis. (From Olsen EA: *Disorders of hair growth: diagnosis and treatment,* New York, 1993, McGraw-Hill.)

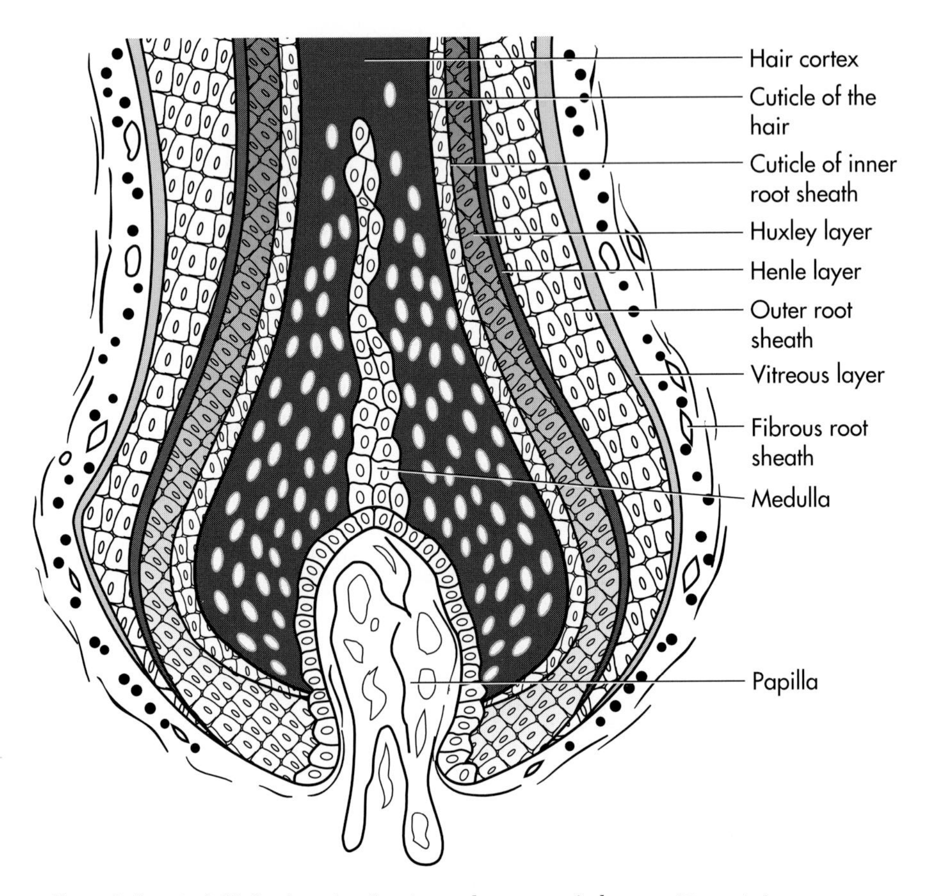

Figure 5-4 Hair follicle showing horizontal concentric layers. (From Ackerman ABA: *Histologic diagnosis of inflammatory skin diseases: a method by pattern analysis,* Philadelphia, 1978, Lea & Febiger.)

characterized by bright-eosinophilic-staining trichohyline granules. The *outer root sheath* surrounds the inner root sheath and contains epithelial cells. The *vitreous layer* lies external to the outer root sheath, is periodic acid-Schiff reaction (PAS) positive, and it is analogous to the basement membrane. The outermost layer of the hair follicle is the *fibrous root sheath,* comprised of collagen fibers and fibroblasts[1,2] (Figure 5-4).

Hair Cycle

Human hair grows in a predictable cyclic pattern consisting of growth (*anagen*), resting (*telogen*), and intermediate (*catagen*) phases. Hair growth is nonsynchronized, meaning hairs may be at different phases in the hair cycle at any given anatomic location. Morphologic and functional changes of the hair follicle characterize the periods of the growth cycle.[3]

Anagen phase

On initiation of the anagen phase, the hair papillae and matrix become metabolically active. The papillae grow in size, and the matrix cells divide. This is followed by downward growth of the hair bulb into the follicular sheath and bulb maturation. The matrix cells multiply to surround the papillae, and matrix cells differentiate into the inner and outer root sheaths as well as the hair. Melanocyte activity in the hair bulb leads to hair pigment. As hair grows, the old bulb hair is shed. This is followed by the emergence of the new anagen hair shaft. The length of the growth phase (anagen) varies at different anatomic sites and generally determines the achievable hair length of the particular site. Young patients with typical scalp hair have anagen periods lasting 2 to 8 years. Similarly, the anagen length for leg hair is 3 to 7 months, arm hair $1\frac{1}{2}$ to 3 months, and eyelash hair 1 to 6 months. Hair growth rates also vary at different anatomic sites. Scalp hair typically grows 0.37 to 0.44 mm/day and body hair 0.27 mm/day.[1,3]

Catagen phase

The catagen phase immediately follows the anagen phase. During this phase the bulbar portion of the hair follicle is degraded, hair matrix cells cease dividing, and melanin production stops in bulbar melanocytes. The degradation and shrinkage of the bulbar region of the anagen hair follicle occur through premature keratinization of the outer root sheath and apoptosis. As it shrinks, the bulbar region moves upward within the fibrous root sheath. Simultaneously, the fibrous root sheath, followed by the dermal papillae, retracts to a position adjacent to the bulge. At completion of the catagen phase, the hair papillae and resting hair matrix cells remain adjacent to the bulge, and fully formed club hair remains within the hair follicle.[1,3,4]

Telogen phase

Telogen, the resting phase, follows anagen. Throughout the telogen phase the fully formed club hair and remnants of the hair bulb remain.[1,3] The length of telogen varies according to the anatomic site. Typical telogen length for scalp hair is 3 months and for the trunk approximately 6 months.[5]

Growth cycle mechanism

Although the exact mechanism that influences local changes in cycling hairs is not known, various theories have been proposed and various growth factors and cytokines detected.

Inhibition. Because the onset of anagen may be induced by plucking of telogen hairs, a proposed explanation is the *chalone hypothesis.* An inhibitor substance (chalone) may accumulate during anagen and initiate the onset of catagen. During telogen the concentration of the chalone decreases. Plucking hair accelerates dispersal of the inhibitor. Some experimental evidence supports this theory.[6,7]

Bulge activation hypothesis. All regenerative tissues contain undifferentiated stem cells, which are slow cycling, undifferentiated cells. When stimulated, these cells can divide and give rise to *transient amplifying cells,* which are cells of limited mitotic potential that eventually become terminally differentiated. The bulge activation hypothesis proposes that the hair follicle stem cells reside in the hair bulge. According to this theory, late in telogen, when the dermal papillae lie close to the hair bulge, hair stem cells are stimulated by the dermal papillae through an unknown mechanism (perhaps a diffusable growth factor or via direct cell contact) to proliferate and give rise to active hair matrix comprised of transient amplifying cells. The new hair matrix, in association with the dermal papillae, grows downward. The matrix cells divide for a fixed period, which determines maximum hair length and length of anagen. Eventually, the matrix cells regress and retract in association with the dermal papillae adjacent to the bulge area.[8]

Environmental and systemic influences

Animals. In animals, hair growth is synchronous and controlled by environmental influences on the pineal and pituitary endocrine glands.[9-15] The pineal gland secretes *melatonin,* which induces the onset of the winter coat and suppresses growth of the summer coat. Conversely, pituitary-derived *prolactin* increases in the summer and has low levels in the winter, with effects inverse to those of melatonin. Sex and thyroid hormones also influence hair growth.

Estradiol, testosterone, and adrenal steroids delay anagen onset, whereas thyroid hormone accelerates anagen onset. Estradiol and thyroxine were also shown to shorten anagen duration. Estradiol may also decrease growth rate, but thyroxine increases it.[1,16]

Humans. In humans, seasonal effects on hair growth are subtle.[17] Several other factors are known to induce hair cycle changes. Pregnancy increases the numbers of anagen hair follicles,[18] which become telogen follicles postpartum. Several illnesses and various drugs are known to induce the onset of telogen effluvium. Common causes of telogen effluvium include anemia, hypothyroidism, nutritional deficiency, febrile illness, and hepatitis. Drugs that cause telogen effluvium include beta blockers, allopurinol, Coumadin, heparin, gold, oral contraceptives, retinoids, and vitamin A.[19]

Androgens. Follicular response to androgens varies according to body site. Androgens participate in the transformation of vellus hairs to terminal hair during puberty. They also cause baldness in some individuals. Androgens alter the size of the follicle, diameter of the hair, and duration of the hair cycle. To respond to androgens, individual follicles must contain androgen receptors.

Circulating androgens are found either bound to plasma proteins, especially sex hormone–binding globulin (SHBG), or freely circulating. Free androgens enter cells and bind to nuclear receptors,[20] resulting in upregulation of ribonucleic acid (RNA) synthesis. Androgens are thought to mediate their effects through the dermal papillae.[1] Weak androgens may be converted to potent androgens in the skin.[21]

Regenerative capabilities and importance of dermal papillae

Hair follicles contain enormous regenerative capacity. Oliver[22] demonstrated the regenerative capabilities of hair follicles through a series of experiments on rat vibrissae follicles. In one experiment the dermal papillae of multiple whisker roots were removed and hair growth ceased. Evidence of regenerating dermal papillae was seen at 8 days in the two specimens examined. Two follicles examined 10 days after removal of the original dermal papillae showed dermal papillae with fine hairs regrowing. By day 24 a fully medullated hair fiber was growing.

Another experiment demonstrated that if the entire hair bulb region (lower one third of hair follicle, including hair matrix, hair papillae, and follicular sheath) was removed, hair stopped growing. If less than one third of the follicle was removed, however, the follicle regenerated. Epithelial matrix cells regenerated from the outer root sheath, and the papillae regenerated from cells of the dermal root sheath.[22]

Furthermore, if the upper two thirds of a hair follicle remains and dermal papillae are implanted into the area from which the lower portion of the follicle was removed, the matrix cells are induced to differentiate from the outer root sheath. Hair growth resumes, suggesting that the dermal papillae is the inductive agent for hair growth and bulb formation.[23]

Papillae were found to induce hair follicle formation when transplanted to the scrotal epidermis, which is devoid of hair follicles.[24] Experiments using cultured dermal papillae cells have also shown that hair papillae cells can induce follicles in normally glaborous skin and differentiation of the epidermis. Epithelial matrix cells also appear to require dermal papillae or dermal sheath cells to proliferate.[25]

These studies illustrate the capacity for follicular regeneration and suggest that the dermal papillae play an essential role in hair regeneration.

CAUSES OF EXCESS HAIR

Hirsutism and hypertrichosis describe conditions of excess hair growth. *Hypertrichosis* signifies excessively long or dense hair for a particular individual of a certain age, gender, or race. It may be a localized, generalized, congenital, or acquired (Box 5-1).[1]

Box 5-1 Causes of hypertrichosis

Acquired
Malignancy
Drugs:
- Acetazolamide
- Cyclosporine
- Danazol
- Diazoxide
- Fenoterol
- Hexachlorobenzene
- Interferon
- Minoxidil
- Pyrimidine
- Penicillamine
- Phenytoin sodium
- PUVA*
- Sodium tetradecyl sulfate
- Streptomycin
- Topical steroids

Metabolic/Endocrine
Porphyria
- Porphyria cutanea tarda
- Variegate
- Erythropoietic protoporphyria
- Erythropoietic

Hypothyroidism
POEMS†
Anorexia nervosa

Trauma/Mechanical
Injection sites
Undercasts
Pressure
Bites
Irritants

Infection Related
Postencephalitis effect
Chronic osteomyelitis

Nervous System
Multiple sclerosis
Schizophrenia
Head injury
Denervated areas
Sympathetic dystrophy

Congenital or Hereditary
Hypertrichosis lanuginosa
de Lange syndrome
Hurler syndrome
Coffin-Siris syndrome
Gorlin (basal cell nevus) syndrome
Lawrence-Seip syndrome (total lipodystrophy)
Melanocytic nevi
Pinna
Winchester syndrome

Modified from Olsen EA: *Disorders of hair growth: diagnosis and treatment,* New York, 1993, McGraw-Hill.
*Pulsed ultraviolet actinotherapy.
†Polyneuropathy, organomegaly, endocrinopathy, M protein, skin changes

Box 5-2 Causes of hirsutism

Idiopathic hirsutism
Stein-Leventhal (polycystic ovary) syndrome
Ovarian tumors
- Unilateral benign adenoma
- Arrhenoblastoma
- Ledig cell tumor
- Hilar cell tumor
- Granular-thecal cell tumor
- Thecal cell tumor
- Luteoma

Adrenal abnormalities
- Congenital adrenal hyperplasia
- Adrenal tumor
- Idiopathic Cushing syndrome

Hyperprolactinemia
Acromegly
Oral contraceptives

From Fitzpatrick TB, et al, editors: *Dermatology in general medicine*, ed 4, New York, 1993, McGraw Hill.

Hirsutism implies hair growth in women that occurs in anatomic locations normally found at puberty in men (e.g., face, chest). *Hirsutism* may be viewed as androgen-dependent hair growth in females. Causes of hirsutism include malignancy, heredity, and drugs (Box 5-2). It may result from excess production or availability of potent or weak androgens caused by increased production, slow metabolism, or low SHBG. Hirsutism also may result from an increased end-organ ability to produce dihydrotestosterone (DHT) from weaker androgens or from increased responsiveness at the receptor. A medical workup may reveal reversible or underlying causes and should be pursued when the clinician encounters hirsute patients. Although medical strategies decrease hair growth and help some individuals with hirsutism, it is ineffective for many.[26]

NONLASER MANAGEMENT OF UNWANTED HAIR

Medical Treatment of Hirsutism

Medical therapy for hirsutism attempts to decrease androgen availability at the follicle. This may be accomplished by (1) blocking androgen receptors, (2) decreasing production of DHT, or (3) decreasing the follicle's level of exposure to androgen.

Oral contraceptives decrease androgen availability to skin primarily by suppressing ovarian androgen secretion. An additional effect results from increased production of SHBG and induction of hepatic clearance of androgens. Dexamethasone or prednisone may be prescribed to suppress adrenocorticotropic hormone (ACTH) secretion and adrenal androgen production, but this method is less effective than oral contraceptives.

Antiandrogens (e.g., spironolactone, flutamide) are androgen receptor antagonists that block androgen effects within follicles. 5α-Reductase inhibitors (e.g., finasteride) diminish intrafollicular synthesis of DHT.[1]

Temporary Management

Various methods accomplish temporary hair removal, including shaving, wax epilation, chemical depilation, and tweezing.

Shaving

Shaving with either an electric shaver or a safety razor enables inexpensive, painless hair removal. However, the well-known disadvantages include the appearance of stubble, skin irritation, and rapid hair regrowth.[27,28]

Waxing

The use of wax to remove hair remains a popular method. Both cold and hot waxes may be employed. Waxing removes hair by pulling hairs beneath the surface. Therefore regrowth is slower than with shaving or chemical depilatories, and effects last approximately 2 to 6 weeks. Hair that regrows is initially thinner, earlier-anagen hair. To wax effectively, hair must be several centimeters long. Although waxing is generally well tolerated, side effects include pain, skin irritation, and folliculitis. Waxing also contains various potential sensitizers, including beeswax, benzocaine, fragrance, and rosin.[1,27,28]

Manual hair removal

Hair plucking using tweezers may be used to remove single hairs and is therefore practiced for sparse hair removal. This method may produce ingrown hairs, cause folliculitis and scarring, and stimulate the replacement of vellus with a terminal hair. A device that manually plucks large amounts of hair (Epilady) is available to remove hair from large, hairy areas. Many find this device quite painful.[1,27,28]

Chemical depilatories

Chemicals that hydrolyze disulfide bonds and dissolve hair are available for hair removal. These compounds are applied topically and later removed. Hair removal is at the surface of the skin, and therefore the effects are comparable to shaving. Effective compounds include thioglycolates, strontium sulfide, and barium sulfide. Although many individuals can tolerate these compounds, both allergic dermatitis and irritant contact dermatitis are frequent side effects. These compounds also are malodorous and messy.[27]

Bleaching

Although technically not a method of hair removal, hair bleaching provides a means of camouflage for unwanted hair. Bleach both lightens and softens hair. The effective ingredient is hydrogen peroxide. Ammonia, water, and persulfate may be added to increase the efficacy of bleaching. Persulfate may produce severe allergic sequelae.[27,28]

Electrolysis and Thermolysis

Electrolysis employs a galvanic current to destroy hair follicles electrochemically. A low-voltage, low-amperage direct current is passed through the tissue between two electrodes. The negative electrode is the needle, and the positive electrode is placed over an uninvolved area that is not treated. Conversely, *thermolysis* uses a high-frequency, high-voltage, low-amperage current. The current is applied through a needle into the follicle. These methods are combined in "the blend" procedure. Hair regrowth is highly variable, ranging from 15% to 50%. Electrolysis is tedious and painful and should be performed by skilled clinicians to avoid scarring and other potential side effects, including infections and mechanical problems.[27]

LASER-ASSISTED HAIR REMOVAL

Continuous-wave Lasers

Initial reports using lasers for hair removal employed continuous-wave (CW) lasers to destroy hair follicles thermally. Several authors reported the use of CW lasers to treat individual hairs in trichiasis.

Gossman et al[29] used a blue-green argon laser at 1.5 W in a pulse mode (0.5 sec) and 100-μm beam diameter (spot size) to vaporize individual eyelashes. Sixty eyelids of 54 patients were treated (a total of 110 eyelashes). Follow-up intervals were at 48 hours, 1 week, and 3 months postoperatively. The authors reported a recurrence rate of 11.6%. Side effects included mild contour abnormalities and hypopigmentation.

Bartley et al[30] compared use of epilation, electrolysis, and cryotherapy with the argon blue-green laser at 1 W (diameter 50 μm, pulse duration 0.2, 0.5, and 1.0 sec) on rabbit eyelashes. Total regrowth was seen 2 weeks after epilation. Regrowth with electrolysis was variable. Cryotherapy produced "near total destruction of eyelashes." Argon laser ablation resulted in "absent or minimal regrowth." The authors concluded that the argon laser may be a suitable alternative to cryotherapy in selected patients.

Gossman et al[31] compared the carbon dioxide (CO_2) laser (2.5 W, pulse mode, 0.5-mm beam) and argon laser (1.5 W, 0.2-sec pulse, 50-μm beam) to treat trichiasis. Eyelash destruction was assessed by determining the mean eyelash recurrence. A recurrence rate of one eyelash per 3 mm of eyelid was seen for both lasers. However, side effects (e.g., notching of tarsal plate, swelling) were more severe with the CO_2 laser, suggesting that argon results were more favorable.

Other studies used lasers to remove hair from hair-bearing grafts. Kuriloff et al[32] used a CO_2 laser (5 W, 0.2 sec) to vaporize all the roots from a hair-bearing pharyngoesophageal graft. The patient had complete symptomatic relief for 1 year, but sparse hair regrowth was seen at 15 months. Finkelstein and Blatstein[33] demonstrated the use of a neodymium:yttrium-aluminum-garnet (Nd:YAG) laser in four patients to remove hair from urethral grafts. Hair was successfully removed and remained absent for at least 1 year in all patients.

Q-switched Nd:YAG and Ruby Lasers

With the advent of Q-switched lasers, delayed hair regrowth was frequently observed after multiple treatment sessions of resistant tattoos. This observation led to a small study that examined the use of Q-switched lasers for hair removal.[34] In this study, 10 patients with excess body hair on the back were treated with the Q-switched ruby (694 nm, 40 nsec, 5-mm spot, 8-10 J/cm^2) and the Q-switched Nd:YAG laser (1064 nm, 10 nsec, 3-mm spot, 3-5 J/cm^2) at six hair-bearing areas. Two control sites were used. Before treatment, each 9-mm^2 test area was photographed. Test areas received one, two, or three treatments at 4-week intervals with either Q-switched ruby or Q-switched Nd:YAG lasers at a fluence of 10 J/cm^2.

All patients were seen in follow-up at 1, 2, 3, and 4 months after the initial treatment. One patient with two sets of treatment sites had follow-up at 18 months. At the 4-month follow-up (3 months after a single treatment, 2 months after a double treatment, and 1 month after three treatments), subjects had 70%, 80%, and 90% hair reduction, respectively, after Q-switched ruby laser treatment. Hair reduction with the corresponding Q-switched Nd:YAG laser was 15%, 50%, and 60%, respectively. At the first-month follow-up visit, two test sites treated with the Q-switched ruby laser contained 50% less hair. A 40% incidence of hyperpigmentation and hypopigmentation was seen in these patients, which was transient in all but two patients. Given the high incidence of pigmentary change, unmodified Q-switched lasers used at high fluence do not provide a reasonable alternative for cosmetic hair removal. However, the study concluded that delayed hair regrowth could be achieved with the Q-switched ruby laser more effectively than with the Q-switched Nd:YAG laser.[34]

The incidence of pigmentation change in this study seems high when compared with the incidence of pigment change after tattoo treatment. This is most likely related to the high fluences used in this study. Because follow-up was only 3 months in most subjects, this study did not address the persistence of these changes.[34]

Selective Photothermolysis

Selective photothermolysis, as described by Anderson and Parrish,[35] predicts that if one chooses to destroy a target selectively within a tissue, three requirements must be met involving wavelength, pulse duration, and fluence. By choosing a wavelength preferentially absorbed by the target and limiting the light exposure to less than or equal to the thermal relaxation time, thermal confinement will be met. To destroy the target, fluences must exceed the thermal threshold.

The theoretic pulse duration necessary to destroy a target is given by the equation $t_r = d^2/gk$, with d the target dimension, k the thermal diffusivity (2×10^{-3} cm²/sec), and g the geometric factor. The thermal relaxation time (t_r) time in seconds is approximately equal to the square of the target diameter in millimeters. By this approximation the t_r for 200- to 300-μm hair follicles is about 40 to 100 msec. Pulse durations of 10 to 50 msec are probably optimal because they are greater than the epidermal t_r (3-10 msec).[36] During this time it is possible to extract heat at the epidermis, which would result in less epidermal injury while still allowing follicular damage.

Melanin provides a convenient chromophore to target hair follicles. Melanin absorbs throughout the visible and near-infrared (IR) spectra. Because hair follicles are located deep in the dermis, the choice for wavelength must be long enough to penetrate to the dermis (millimeters below the epidermis) but must have sufficient melanin absorption. The ruby laser has been shown to fulfill these criteria. An animal study showed deep selective damage to isolated pigment cells of hair follicles by the Q-switched ruby laser. In patients with darker skin types, competitive melanin absorption at the epidermis poses an additional challenge, and wavelengths with less melanin absorption and the capacity for deeper penetration may be more optimal. Theoretically, several wavelengths in the red and near-IR spectrum would be appropriate for laser hair removal.

Normal-mode Ruby Laser

In the first study employing selective photothermolysis for hair removal, a ruby laser system consisting of an optical delivery system and a normal-mode ruby laser (NMRL, 694-nm wavelength, 270-μsec pulse, 6-mm spot size) was designed to destroy a large field of hair follicles. The 694-nm wavelength was chosen because NMRL pulses were known to produce deep follicular damage in animals.[36]

The threshold fluence required to damage the follicles was determined to be about 40 to 70 J/cm² through an experiment on ex vivo black-haired dog skin. The optical delivery system designed facilitated light delivery to the deep follicles and spared the epidermis. This system contained a converging sapphire lens (a medium with a highly refractive external index) that allowed light to converge as it entered skin. The lens was cooled to 4° C to provide heat conduction from the epidermis. A large-exposure spot diameter was also used. As pulses were delivered to the skin, forceful compression eliminated blood from the dermis and reduced the distance between the surface and the hair papillae.[36]

This study examined treatment of 13 volunteers with brown or black hair and fair skin (type I-III). Six test sites received a single treatment with the NMRL at fluences of 30 to 60 J/cm². Of the six sites treated, three were wax epilated before treatment and three shaven. A shaven site and a wax epilated site were the two controls.[36]

Subjects were assessed at 1, 3, and 6 months after treatment with manual hair counts and photographic documentation (Figure 5-5). Skin biopsies were also obtained. Results showed significant delay in hair growth in all subjects at all treated sites compared with the unexposed shaven and epilated control sites (Figure 5-6). At 6 months, four subjects showed less than 50% regrowth. Fluence-dependent selective thermal injury limited to the follicular epithelium was seen histologically

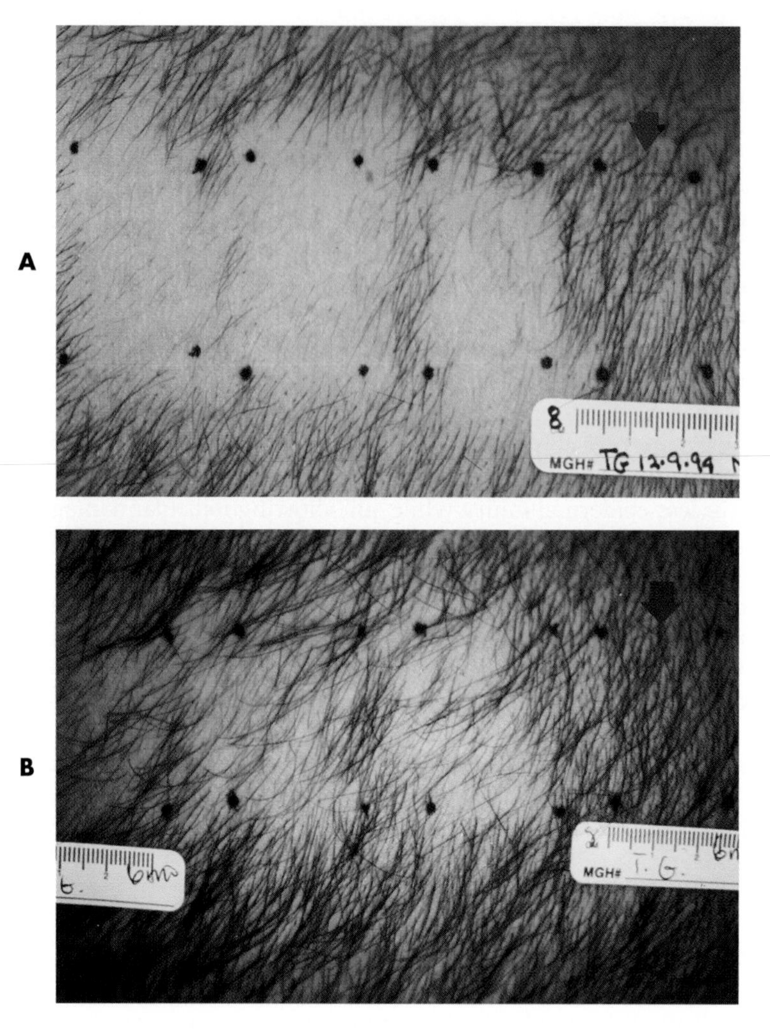

Figure 5-5 **A,** Appearance of epilated sites 3 months after single treatment with 60-, 40-, and 30-J/cm^2 long-pulsed ruby laser (*left to right*) and untreated epilated control. **B,** Same sites 6 months after single treatment. (From Grossman MC, Dierickx C, Farenelli W et al: *J Am Acad Dermatol* 35:889, 1996.)

(Figure 5-7). Patients showed transient pigmentation change (3 of 13 had hyperpigmentation, 2 of 13 had hypopigmentation) but no scarring.[36]

The conclusion was that selective photothermolysis of hair follicles with the NMRL produces growth delay consistent with prolonged telogen induction.[36] In some subjects, permanent hair removal apparently was possible. At least one subject seen up to 2 years after the initial treatment had no regrowth (unpublished data).

It is unclear which follicular target must be irreversibly destroyed to enable permanent hair removal. Both the hair bulge and the papillae are potentially important. The authors[36] hypothesized that the hairs that regrow after treatment may be at the least susceptible phase in their cycle. The location of the dermal papillae, as well as melanin production and bulge cell division, vary throughout the cycle. During telogen, dermal papillae are more superficial and therefore potentially more accessible to laser light. However, melanogenesis is more prevalent in anagen. Additionally, in late telogen, bulge cells are dividing rapidly, whereas they are relatively quiescent throughout the rest of the cycle. These conditions may render the follicles more or less susceptible to laser injury. Therefore, multiple treatments may lead to improved efficacy.[36]

Several NMRLs and an alexandrite laser were approved by the U.S. Food and Drug Administration (FDA) for laser hair removal in September 1997. Generally, when using these lasers, hair is shaven or clipped before treatment. The treatments

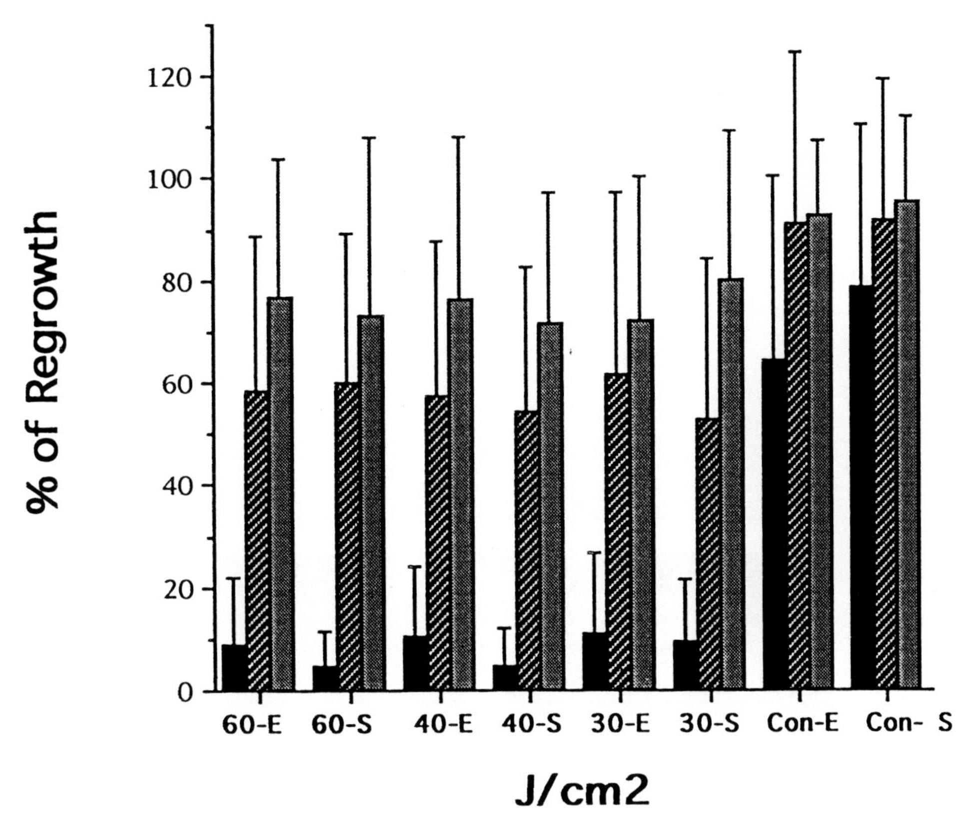

Figure 5-6 Hair regrowth for each fluence (60, 40, and 30 J/cm^2) in treated sites and control sites. 1, 3, and 6 months after treatment. *S,* Shaven sites; *E,* epilated sites; *con E, con S,* control sites. See Figure 5-5. (From Grossman MC, Dierickx C, Farenelli W et al: *J Am Acad Dermatol* 35:889, 1996.)

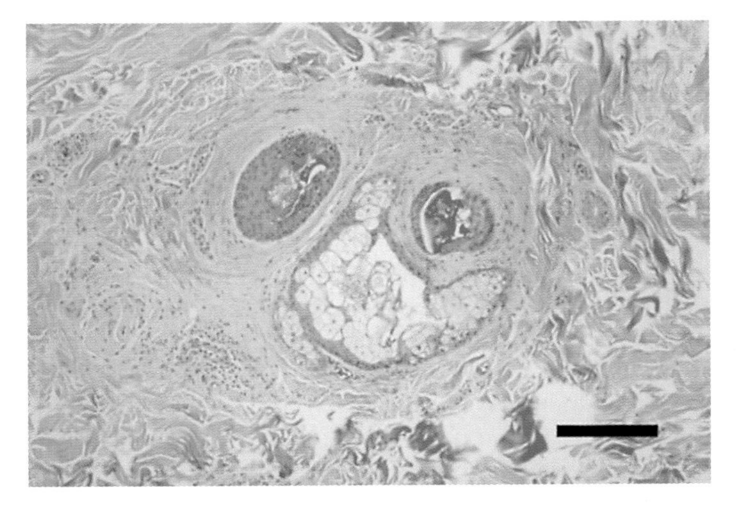

Figure 5-7 Photomicrograph of cross section of human hair follicle after 60 J/cm^2 exposure showing thermal damage of follicular epithelium and follicular rupture. Site was shaven before exposure. (Bar = 200 μm.) (From Grossman MC, Dierickx C, Farenelli W et al: *J Am Acad Dermatol* 35:889, 1996.)

are done serially because hair regrows at approximately 1 to 3 months, depending on individual patient response. Treatment fluences are chosen based on patient skin type and clinical response and vary from 10 to 50 J/cm^2.

Palomar Medical Technologies (Beverly, Mass) produces the Epilaser, which has a 3.0-msec pulse duration, 694-nm wavelength, and 1.0-cm spot size and is capable

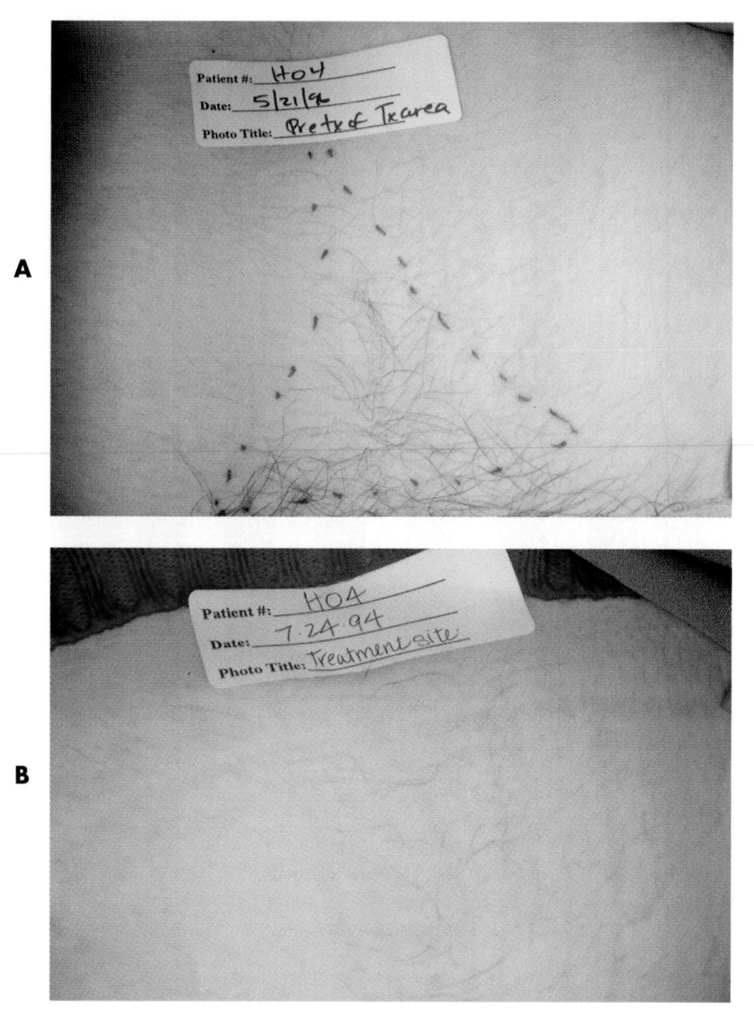

Figure 5-8 **A,** Bikini area site before treatment with long-pulsed ruby laser (694 nm, 3 msec, 7-mm spot size). **B,** Same site 2 months after treatment.

of delivering fluences of up to 50 J/cm². The laser also contains a cooling and focusing handpiece. Figure 5-8 shows treatments from a study done with this laser.

Sharplan's (Allendale, New Jersey) Epitouch (694 nm, 1 msec, 4-5 mm, 25-40 J/cm²) is used with a cooling gel. Mehl Biophile (Gainesville, Fla) produces a ruby laser (694 nm, 0.8 msec, 15 J/cm², 5-mm spot) that does not require cooling. Leaseaway (England) also produces a long-pulsed ruby laser. Cynosure (Bedford, Mass) produces a long-pulsed alexandrite laser (755 nm, 5-20 msec, 20 J/cm²). Candela Laser Corporation (Wayland, Mass) is also developing a long-pulsed alexandrite laser.

Filtered Flashlamp Pulsed Light Source

A filtered flashlamp pulsed light source (600-1000 nm) called the Epilight (Energy Systems Corp. [ESC], Yokneam, Israel) is capable of delivering single or multiple pulses to the skin surface. The pulse duration and fluence capabilities are consistent with the theory of selective photothermolysis. The spot size measures 10 × 45 mm and is designed to treat large areas. The pulse duration and pulse delay are adjustable. Typical pulse durations are 2 to 3 msec with typical fluences up to approximately 40 J/cm². Areas are shaven before treatment, and treatment is done through cooling gel.

A study is underway to determine the safety and efficacy of this device for hair removal. In a pilot study done by Gold et al at 12 weeks after a single treatment, approximately 60% of subjects had 60% to 100% less hair. Anecdotal personal experience using a similar system designed to treat leg veins led to decreased hair growth in two patients with facial hirsutism (one with axillary hair, one with inguinal hair) at 3-month follow-up. Figures 5-9 and 5-10 show clinical treatment with the Epilight and skin biopsy after treatment. Figure 5-11 shows histology after PhotoDerm VL treatment.[38]

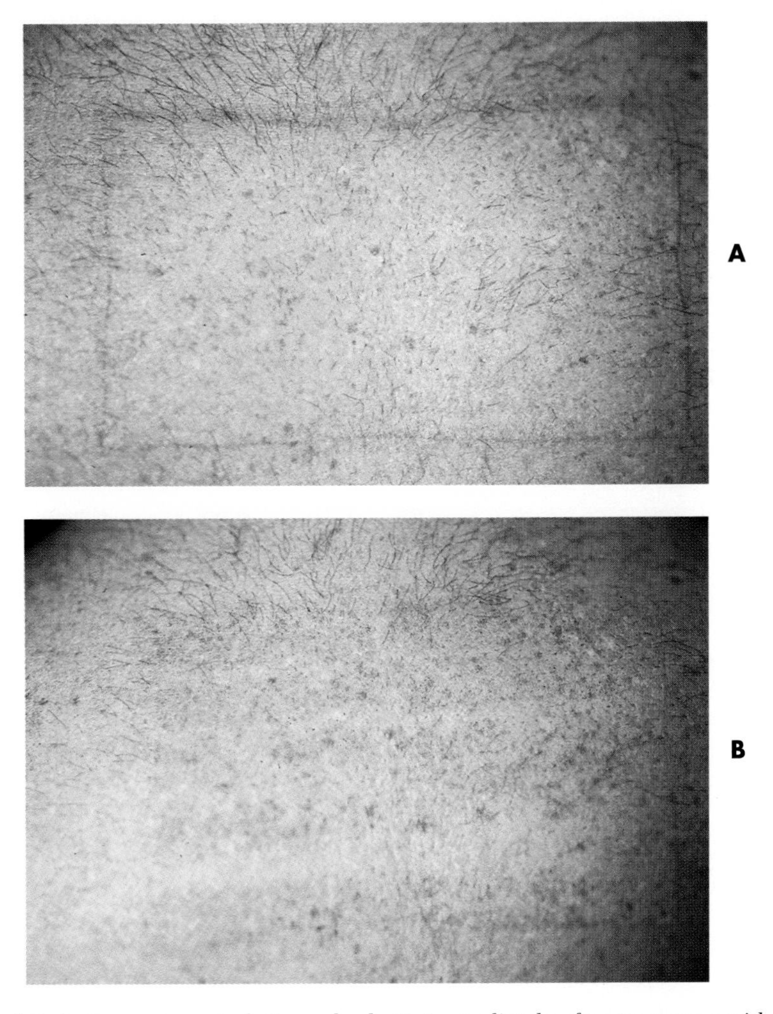

Figure 5-9 **A,** Pretreatment of site on back. **B,** Immediately after treatment with Epilight system. Both sides were treated using 645-nm cut-off filter with triple pulsing at 2.5 msec per pulse and 20-msec delay between pulses. Right side was treated at 37.5 J/cm² and left side at 42.5 J/cm².

Continued

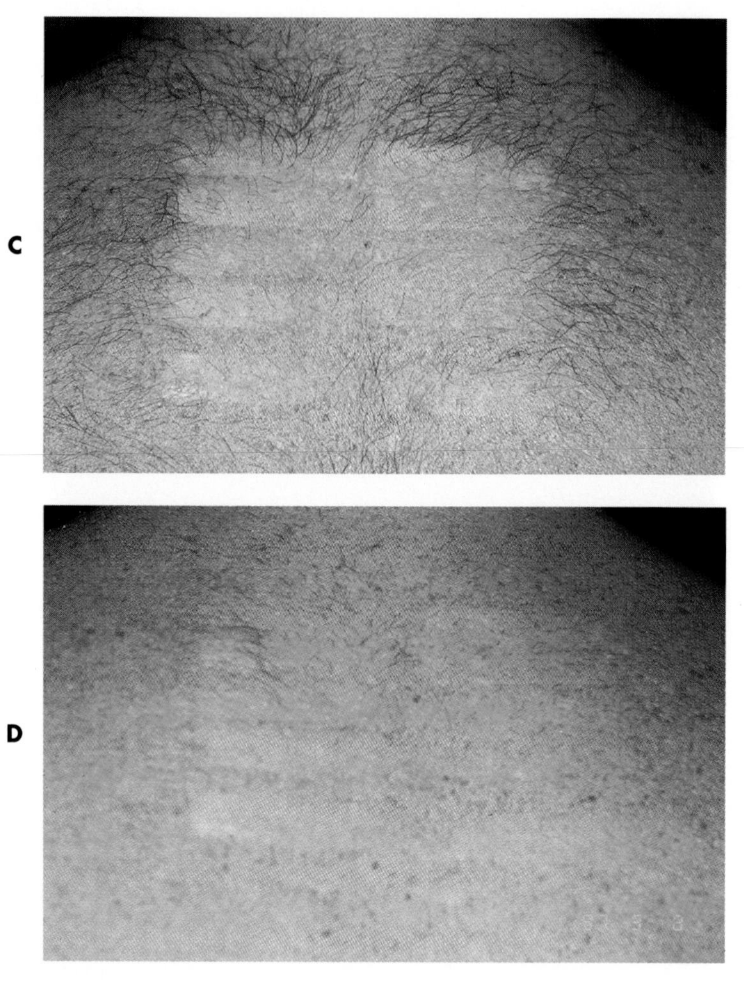

Figure 5-9, cont'd **C,** Hypopigmentation 4 weeks after treatment and lack of hair regrowth. **D,** Five months after treatment with minimal hair regrowth. (Courtesy M. Goldman, MD.)

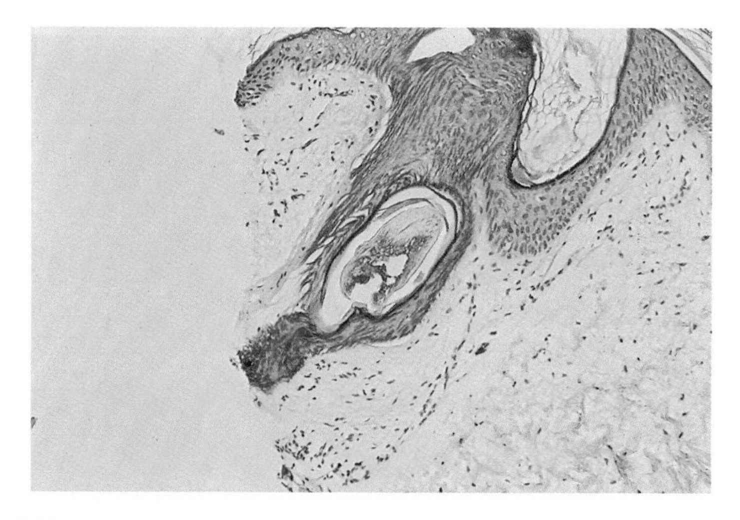

Figure 5-10 Punch biopsy taken immediately after treatment of axillary hair with Epilight system using 645-nm cut-off filter with a triple pulse setting of 2.5 msec per pulse with delay time of 20 msec between pulses and total energy of 42.5 J/cm^2. (Courtesy M. Goldman, MD.)

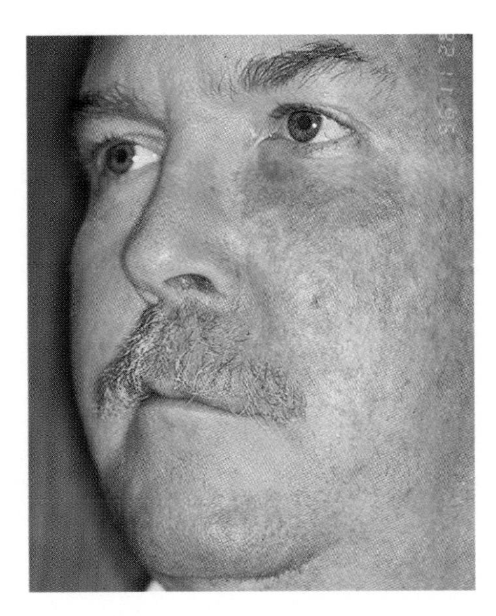

Figure 5-11 Three months after treatment with PhotoDerm VL using cut-off filter of 570 nm and fluence of 50 J/cm^2 delivered over 8 msec. Note marked resolution of port-wine stain in addition to marked alopecia of mustache area, which persisted for 20 months at last follow-up. (Courtesy M. Goldman, MD.)

Q-switched Laser and Carbon Suspension

The use of a carbon particle suspension in combination with a Q-switched Nd:YAG laser was recently developed for laser hair removal[39,40] (ThermoLase Corporation, La Jolla, CA). The system is currently available around the United States in ThermoLase Spa settings. The technology may be sublicensed and performed by physicians. Hair is removed by wax epilation before application of the carbon suspension. The carbon-containing lotion is then massaged into the skin and enters the hair follicles. A low-fluence Nd:YAG laser (1064 nm, 7-mm spot, 2-3 J/cm^2) is then used at the surface. A suction device is attached to the delivery system to remove aeorosolized carbon. Presumably, exogenous carbon particles enter the hair follicle acting as a strong chromophore, thus requiring only low-energy Nd:YAG laser treatment. Thus far, no objective studies have been published documenting the histologic presence of the carbon within the follicle.

In a recent unpublished study, 35 adults with excess facial, neck, and axillary hair were treated.[41] Subjects' hair was trimmed and topical carbon applied to the surface. Laser light was delivered using a Q-switched Nd:YAG laser (694 nm, 7-mm spot size, 10-nsec pulse duration, 2-3 J/cm^2). Subjects were evaluated at 4 weeks and 12 weeks, with 10% to 66% reduction seen at 12 weeks. Goldberg[41] concluded that this method could safely and effectively remove hair (Figure 5-12). Anecdotal experience with this method is variable. Hair seems to grow back slowly at different rates at different body sites and varies from individual to individual.

Nanni and Alster[42] examined the efficacy of this system in 12 subjects and compared four treatment conditions in each subject. Each subject received treatment in four 1.0-cm quadrants. One quadrant was treated with waxing, carbon, and laser treatment. A second was waxed and treated with the Q-switched Nd:YAG laser. A third was only laser treated and a fourth only waxed. Hair regrowth was calculated at 1, 3, and 6 months. In all laser-treated areas a growth delay was seen at 3 months, but complete regrowth was seen at all the sites at 6 months. The authors found that Nd:YAG laser–assisted hair removal is safe and effective in achieving a growth delay at 3 months and that pretreatment with wax and a carbon solution is only slightly

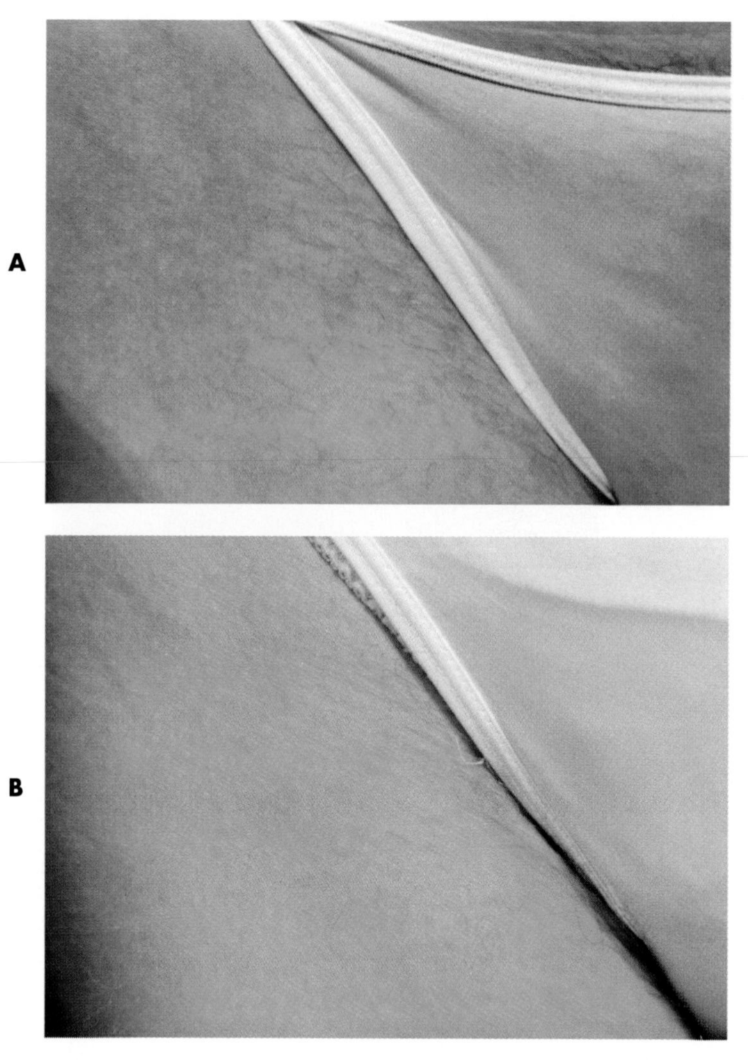

Figure 5-12 **A,** Pretreatment of bikini area. **B,** Two months after treatment with Q-switched Nd:YAG laser and carbon suspension. (Courtesy David Goldberg, MD.)

more effective than using the laser alone or in combination with waxing. Kilmer[43] also demonstrated the efficacy of the Q-switched Nd:YAG laser at achieving a growth delay, as well as follicular damage.

Recently a new carbon delivery system has been introduced for improved efficacy of the ThermoLase system. This system uses a smaller carbon particle, which is introduced through "laser propulsion" into the hair follicle using a low-energy Nd:YAG laser at 1 J/cm^2. Next, laser light at a higher fluence is delivered to the skin (2-3 J/cm^2). Skin is not waxed before this treatment. Currently, no published studies exist on the efficacy of this new method.

Photodynamic Therapy

The use of aminolevulinic acid (ALA) photodynamic therapy has been described for hair removal. This method employs topical ALA in combination with red-light exposures. In a pilot study on 12 volunteers, ALA resulted in follicular production of the photosensitizer protoporphyrin IX.[44] Six test areas in each subject were exposed to varying concentrations of ALA (10% and 20%) and varying light doses

(100 and 200 J/cm^2) with the argon-pumped dye laser (630 nm, 60 mW). Three control sites were used. A dose-dependent decrease in hair regrowth was seen at 6 months after a single treatment, with 40% less hair seen at the highest drug and light dose. Furthermore, selective damage to the follicular epithelium occurred. Transient pigmentation changes with an absence of scarring were reported. These encouraging results suggest that ALA photodynamic therapy may provide an excellent method of long-lasting hair removal.

Future Lasers

High-powered diode arrays are currently available. Laser diode systems currently under investigation include a pulsed laser diode (800 nm, 5-20 msec, 15-40 J/cm^2) made by Palomar and one by Applied Optronics Corporation (AOC) Medical Systems (South Plainfield, NJ) (690 nm, 1.2-mm spot, 10 W, epidermal scan at a 1- to 100-msec dwell time). Studies are currently underway to examine the efficacy of this technology.

SUMMARY

Tremendous potential exists for the laser industry to impact the billion-dollar hair removal industry. However, experience with this approach is limited. To date, only one peer-reviewed study using laser hair removal exists in the literature.[36] Although permanent hair removal in the few patients studied seems possible, the capacity to remove hair temporarily and induce a growth delay employing various laser-assisted methods is easier to achieve. The enormous regenerative potential of the follicle and its anatomic location continue to be challenging.

Despite the potential obstacles to achieve reliable and predictable permanent hair removal, it is likely that lasers with additional wavelengths will be developed for hair removal. It is important to understand the biology of hair growth and the potential for regeneration when assessing the efficacy of these techniques. Carefully controlled studies over long periods and follow-up (at least 6-12 months) after the last treatment should be employed to illustrate effectiveness. Through continued observation and research and a greater understanding of hair biology and the effects of laser light, reliable, safe, and permanent epilation should be possible.

References

1. Olsen EA: *Disorders of hair growth: diagnosis and treatment,* New York, 1993, McGraw-Hill.
2. Montagna W, Ellis RA, editors: *The biology of hair growth,* New York, 1958, Academic Press.
3. Montagna W, Parakkal PF: *The structure and function of the skin,* ed 3, New York, 1974, Academic Press.
4. Klingman A: The human hair cycle, *J Invest Dermatol* 33:307, 1959.
5. Ackerman ABA: *Histologic diagnosis of inflammatory skin diseases: a method by pattern analysis,* Philadelphia, 1978, Lea & Febiger.
6. Paus R, Stenn KS, Link RE: Telogen skin contains an inhibitor of hair growth, *Br J Dermatol* 122:777, 1990.
7. Frater R: Inhibition of growth of hair follicles by a lectin-like substance from rat skin, *Aust J Biol Sci* 36:411, 1983.
8. Cotsarelis G, Sun TT, Lavker RM: Label-retaining cells reside in the bulge area of pilosebaceous unit: implications for follicular stem cells, hair cycle and skin, *Cell* 61:1329, 1990.
9. Johnson E: Environmental influences on the hair follicle. In Orfanos CE, Montagna W, Stuttgen G, editors: *Hair research,* Berlin, 1981, Springer-Verlag.
10. Allain D, Rougeot J: Induction of autumn moult in mink (Mustela vison Peale and Beauvois) with melatonin, *Reprod Nutr Dev* 20:197, 1980.
11. Badura LL, Goldman BD: Prolactin-dependent seasonal changes in pelage: role of the pineal gland and dopamine, *J Exp Zool* 261:27, 1992.

12. Martinet L, Allain D, Weiner C: Role of prolactin in the photoperiodic control of moulting in the mink *(Mustela vison), J Endocrinol* 103:9, 1934.
13. Maurel D, Coutant C, Boissin J: Effects of photoperiod, melatonin implants and castration on molting and on plasma thyroxine, testosterone and prolactin levels in the European badger (*Meles meles), Comp Biochem Physiol* 93A:792, 1989.
14. Rose J, Oldfield J, Stormshak F: Apparent role of melatonin and prolactin in initiating winter fur growth in mink, *Gen Comp Endocrinol* 65:212, 1987.
15. Smale L, Dark J, Zucker I: Pineal and photoperiodic influences on fat deposition, pelage, and testicular activity in male meadow voles, *J Biol Rhythms* 3:349, 1988.
16. Maurel D, Coutant C, Boissin J: Thyroid and gonadal regulation of hair growth during the seasonal molt in the male European badger, *Meles meles L, Gen Comp Endocrinol* 65:317, 1987.
17. Randall VA, Ebling FJ: Seasonal changes in human hair growth, *Br J Dermatol* 124:146, 1991.
18. Lynfield YL: Effect of pregnancy on the human hair cycle, *J Invest Dermatol* 35:323, 1960.
19. Kligman AM: Pathologic dynamics of human hair loss, *Arch Dermatol* 35:323, 1960.
20. King RJB: The structure and function of steroid receptors, *J Endocrinol* 114:341, 1984.
21. Strauss JS, Pochi PE: The hormonal control of the pilosebaceous unit. In Toda K, Ishibashi Y, Yori Y, Morikawa F, editors: *Biology and disease of the hair,* Baltimore, 1976, University Park Press.
22. Oliver RF: Histological studies of whisker regeneration in hooded rat, *J Embryol Exp Morphol* 16:231, 1966.
23. Oliver RF: The experimental induction of whisker growth in the hooded rat by implantation of dermal papillae, *J Embryol Exp Morphol* 18:43, 1967.
24. Oliver RF: The induction of follicle formation in the adult hooded rat by vibrissa dermal papillae, *J Embryol Exp Morphol* 23:219, 1970.
25. Reynolds AJ, Jahoda CAB: Inductive properties of hair follicle cells, *Ann NY Acad Sci* 642:226, 1991.
26. Kvedar JC, Gibson M, Krusinski PA: Hirsutism: evaluation and treatment, *J Am Acad Dermatol* 12:215, 1995.
27. Wagner RF: Physical methods for the management of hirsutism, *Cutis* 45:319, 1990.
28. Richards RN, Marguerite U, Meharg G: Temporary hair removal in patients with hirsutism: a clinical study, *Cutis* 45:319, 1990.
29. Gossman MD, Yung R, Berlin AJ: Prospective evaluation of the argon laser in the treatment of trichiasis, *Ophthalmol Surg* 23:183, 1992.
30. Bartley GB, Bullock JD, Olsen TG: An experimental study to compare methods of eyelash ablation, *Ophthalmology* 94:1286, 1987.
31. Gossman MD, Brightwell JR, Huntington AC: Experimental comparison of laser and cryosurgical cilia destruction, *Ophthalmol Surg* 23:179, 1992.
32. Kuriloff DB, Finn DG, Kimmelman CP: Pharyngoesophageal hair growth: the role of laser epilation, *Otolaryngol Head Neck Surg* 98:342, 1988.
33. Finkelstein LH, Blatstein LM: Epilation of hair-bearing urethral graphs using the neodymium:YAG surgical laser, *J Urol* 146:840, 1991.
34. Kauvar ANB: Personal communication, 1998.
35. Anderson RR, Parrish JA: Selective photothermolysis: precise microsurgery by selective absorption of pulsed radiation, *Science* 220:524, 1983.
36. Grossman MC, Dierickx C, Farinelli W et al: Damage to hair follicles by normal-mode ruby laser pulses, *J Am Acad Dermatol* 35:889, l996.
38. Goldman M: Personal communication, 1998.
39. Goldberg D: Topical solution–assisted laser hair removal, *Lasers Surg Med Suppl* 7:47, 1995.
40. Goldberg D: Topical suspension assisted laser hair removal: treatment of axillary and inguinal regions, *Lasers Surg Med Suppl* 8, 1996.
41. Goldberg D: Personal communication, 1997.
42. Nanni C, Alster TA: Optimizing treatment parameters for hair removal using a topical carbon-based solution and 1064 nm Nd:YAG laser energy, *Lasers Surg Med Suppl* 9, 1997.
43. Kilmer SK: Q-switched Nd:YAG laser (1064 nm) hair removal without adjuvant topical preparation, *Lasers Surg Med Suppl* 9, 1997.
44. Grossman MC, Wimberly J, Dwyer P et al: PDT for hirsutism, *Lasers Surg Med Suppl* 7:44, 1995.

CHAPTER six

Carbon Dioxide Laser Surgery

Richard E. Fitzpatrick and Mitchel P. Goldman

The initial concept for medical lasers was to use pigmented tissue as a target for selective absorption of energy with resultant specific thermal necrosis of the targeted tissue, sparing the immediately adjacent nonpigmented tissue. In 1962 the first patient treated with a laser had a malignant melanoma; its black lesion was treated with the ruby and neodymium pulsed laser systems before excision.[1] Histologic examination showed thermal necrosis of the laser-treated areas.[1,2] This led to clinical experiments in treating patients with cutaneous melanoma metastases.[2-5] Halos of depigmentation were apparent in treated areas as thermal necrosis healed with fibrosis and scar tissue.

At first the only lasers available were those having wavelengths in the visible spectrum, so treatment was limited to pigmented lesions, particularly those having a very dark color. This requirement significantly limited the application of lasers surgically. This changed with the development of the carbon dioxide (CO_2) laser by Patel in the laboratories of the Bell Telephone Company in 1964.[6] Polanyi et al[7] demonstrated the surgical application of this laser in 1967 and developed a system for medical research.

The CO_2 laser emits a continuous beam having a wavelength of 10,600 nm, which is absorbed by biologic tissues regardless of pigmentation or vascularity because its target of interaction is water. The laser destroys tissue by rapidly heating and vaporizing intracellular water. In addition, the depth of penetration is a function of its wavelength. The *extinction length* is defined as the thickness of water that absorbs 90% of the radiant energy of the incident beam. For the CO_2 laser, this figure is approximately 30 μm.[8] This property allows the potential for very controlled tissue vaporization.

Furthermore, CO_2 laser surgery was found to seal small nerve endings, rather than leaving frayed endings as occurs with steel scalpel surgery. It is thought that this results in less postoperative pain.[9] Small lymphatics are also sealed with the CO_2 laser, resulting in less postoperative edema.[10] It is important that blood vessels 0.5 mm in diameter and smaller are photocoagulated and sealed, resulting in a relatively bloodless surgical field.[11-14]

All these properties give the CO_2 laser great potential as a surgical instrument. The beam can be used either with a very-small-diameter spot size (0.1-0.2 mm) for excisional surgery or with a broad-diameter spot (2-5 mm), increasing the area of laser-tissue interaction for destruction or vaporization of lesions. This change in spot size is accomplished by merely moving the surgical handpiece away from the tissue to be treated (Figure 6-1).

Initially the CO_2 laser was used only when mounted on an operating microscope. Because its wavelength is not visible, a coaxial red helium-neon beam is used for aiming. When used with a microscope, the aiming beam is visible through the viewing lenses and is manipulated with a joystick, with the laser activated by a foot pedal. Although these initial systems were bulky and cumbersome, they were found to be excellent for several applications, including laryngeal and gynecologic surgeries.[13-17]

The advent of the surgical handpiece and the highly articulated arm allowed much greater freedom in use and led to the development of additional surgical procedures. Because an optical fiber capable of transmitting the 10,600-nm wavelength does not exist, the delivery of the beam from the laser to the surgical site is accomplished by reflecting the beam off the surfaces of a series of mirrors. This results in the need for multiple tubular segments joined by a rotational articulation coupling containing mirrors to be able to manipulate freely the direction and orientation of the laser beam. These articulated arms have improved tremendously, with the most recent units being very comfortable to use.

The early use of the CO_2 laser in cutaneous surgery was as an excisional or destructive instrument for malignancies,[1-4,14,18-21] in the management of burns,[22,23] and for the débridement of decubitus ulcers.[24] As the availability and ease of use of the CO_2 laser increased, further applications were described. The most common dermatologic use of the CO_2 laser was simply as a replacement of the dermatologic curette and electrocautery unit.[13,21,25-28] The laser was, and still is, used to ablate cutaneous lesions in the same manner as these instruments have been used. This often did not allow the surgeon to benefit from the unique properties of the CO_2 laser but did lead to its widespread use because of the increased surgical speed, bloodless field, and reduced postoperative pain.

Although the CO_2 laser has often been referred to as the workhorse of dermatologic lasers, many practitioners in dermatology as well as other surgical specialties became disenchanted with it because of the realization that thermal damage was difficult to control. Many CO_2 lasers were virtually abandoned or their continued use questioned because of disappointing clinical results and unacceptable high rates of scarring.[29,30] These are related to the effects of heat diffusion into tissue surrounding the intended site of laser surgery and resulting in unwanted thermal necrosis. These effects are discussed in further detail in the section on laser-tissue interaction.

Laser manufacturers responded to this situation by developing pulsed CO_2 laser systems. The traditional CO_2 laser continuous beam could be electronically shuttered to produce pulses of 0.1- to 1-sec duration with consistent power, but this could not predictably prevent thermal diffusion.[31] Therefore superpulsed systems were developed with peak powers 2 to 10 times higher and pulse durations 10 to

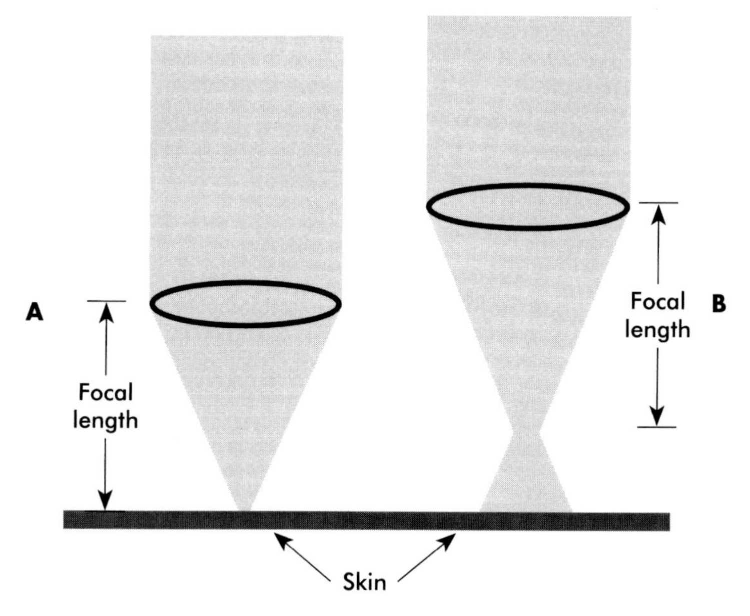

Figure 6-1 **A,** Lens of CO_2 laser allows for precise focusing on skin surface. **B,** Larger, defocused spot size can be obtained by pulling handpiece away from skin surface. (Courtesy Coherent Laser Corp., Palo Alto, Calif.)

Table 6-1
Comparison of CO_2 lasers

Feature	Ultrapulse	Superpulse	Chopped Pulse	Continuous Wave
Short-duration pulses	X	X		
High-energy pulses	X		X	
High-energy pulses, any average power	X			
Variable pulse energy	X			
High average power	X		X	X

100 times shorter than the conventional CO_2 lasers. Rapid pulses, 200 to 1000 Hz, achieve powers similar to that of a continuous-wave (CW) CO_2 laser. The basic principle of the superpulsed CO_2 laser is to use high peak powers to maximize tissue vaporization and short pulse duration to minimize thermal injury.[32] Although this modification has been shown to result in better control of thermal damage in animal models,[33-37] in human urologic surgery,[38,39] and in single laser impacts on human skin,[40] no improvement in clinical results in dermatologic surgery has been demonstrated,[41-43] other than isolated case reports.[44-47] As discussed later, by selection of proper pulse parameters, the use of the principles of selective photothermolysis can be maximized with the superpulse mode of therapy and will result in faster healing with decreased scarring if one adheres to these principles.[48,49]

Other practitioners and investigators have attempted to control unwanted thermal damage as well as the volume of ablated tissue by the use of low fluences,[50-54] but this has proved to be clinically impractical, because low power densities must be used for long exposure durations to achieve the same clinical endpoint. This results in greater time for thermal diffusion with more thermal damage to adjacent tissues, rather than decreasing this effect.

As knowledge of laser-tissue interaction has increased, the development of laser pulse parameters to minimize unwanted thermal damage in a more specific manner has become possible. Coherent Medical Lasers (Palo Alto, Calif) has introduced a new type of superpulsed CO_2 laser, the UltraPulse ($UPCO_2$), having pulse energies five to seven times higher than conventional superpulsed lasers, as well as a pulse duration less than 1 msec to correspond with the approximate thermal relaxation time of skin.[48,49] This laser has a peak pulse power of over 500 W, resulting in the ability to deliver 5 J/cm^2 per pulse, using a spot diameter of 2.5 mm. Clinical trials have proved this laser to be exceptional in its speed and efficiency, as well as its ability to avoid unwanted thermal damage (Table 6-1).

Before further discussion of the clinical uses of the CO_2 laser, it is helpful to review basic laser terminology and laser-tissue interactions. The reader is referred to Chapter 1 for a more complete understanding of laser physics.

LASER TERMINOLOGY

Misuse of terminology has resulted in confusing and sometimes bewildering situations where communication is difficult or impossible.[55] The following is a review of basic laser surgery terminology.

Energy

Energy is the capacity to do work and is expressed as force multiplied by length, or mass multiplied by velocity. The unit of measurement is a *joule* (J), which is 1 watt

(W) times 1 second (sec). Energy is usually calculated in laser surgery as power multiplied by time of application and is a dosage measurement.

Power

Power is the rate of performance, or flow, of energy; it is energy divided by the time of application. The unit of measurement is the *watt.* One watt equals 1 joule per second. Power *output* (the speed of energy emission from the laser tube) is important in limiting the severity of the laser conduction burn, but surgical control is largely a function of the power density and spot size, as well as the repetition rate.

Power Density

Power density, or *irradiance,* is the rate of energy delivery per unit of target tissue area. Power density is expressed in watts per square centimeter (W/cm^2) and is determined as the power divided by the surface area of the beam or spot size. Because the area of a circle varies with the square of its radius, any reduction in spot size will produce a fourfold increase in energy at the impact site. Increases in power output from the tube, however, result only in a corresponding linear increase in the power density. Power density is the principal determinant of the rate at which tissue is vaporized. High power densities (irradiance) vaporize tissue rapidly.

The power density is a static measurement and does not account for time. Laser *dosage* takes into account the time of delivery and is a measure of the energy delivered. The energy is a function of the number of watts of power multiplied by the delivery time and is expressed as the number of joules. Both 1 W multiplied by 1 second and 10 W multiplied by 0.1 second equal 1 J. This gives a measure of the dosage but does not describe its concentration. Fluence is a measure of energy density or concentration and combines the concepts of irradiance and dosage.

Fluence

Fluence (or the *energy density*) is the total energy divided by the cross-sectional area of the beam and is expressed as joules per square centimeter (J/cm^2). Fluence is the product of irradiance and exposure time. When the power density is greater than about 100 W/cm^2, the amount of tissue damage that occurs is proportional to the time of application of the beam, not to the irradiance (power density).[56] Whereas irradiance determines the rate at which tissue is vaporized, the volume of tissue removed is entirely a function of the amount of energy applied. A given amount of energy to vaporize a given volume of tissue can be obtained by an infinite combination of powers and times. When heat dispersion in tissue is considered, time of application is the most critical factor.

Spot Size

The spot size of the laser is controlled by focusing lenses or by simply moving the handpiece toward or away from the target tissue (Figure 6-1). It is important to realize that small variations in handpiece-to-target distance may produce dramatic alterations in the diameter of the beam or spot size and consequently in power density. The irradiance across the beam is distributed in a gaussian fashion, peaking at the center of the beam and falling off to zero at the edges. A larger spot size allows for smoother, more uniform vaporization of tissue but requires that a much higher

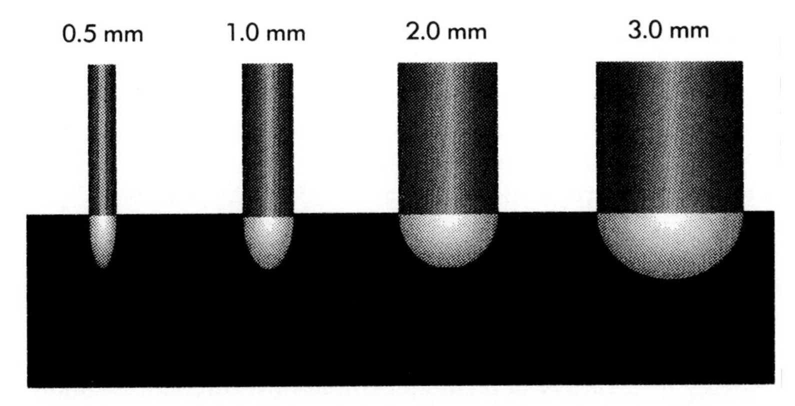

Figure 6-2 Larger spot size requires higher laser energy. As spot size increases, volume of tissue heated instantly by laser increases. This increases energy required to vaporize that volume of tissue. If laser energy is not changed, there is a decrease in thermal damage. (Courtesy Coherent Laser Corp., Palo Alto, Calif.)

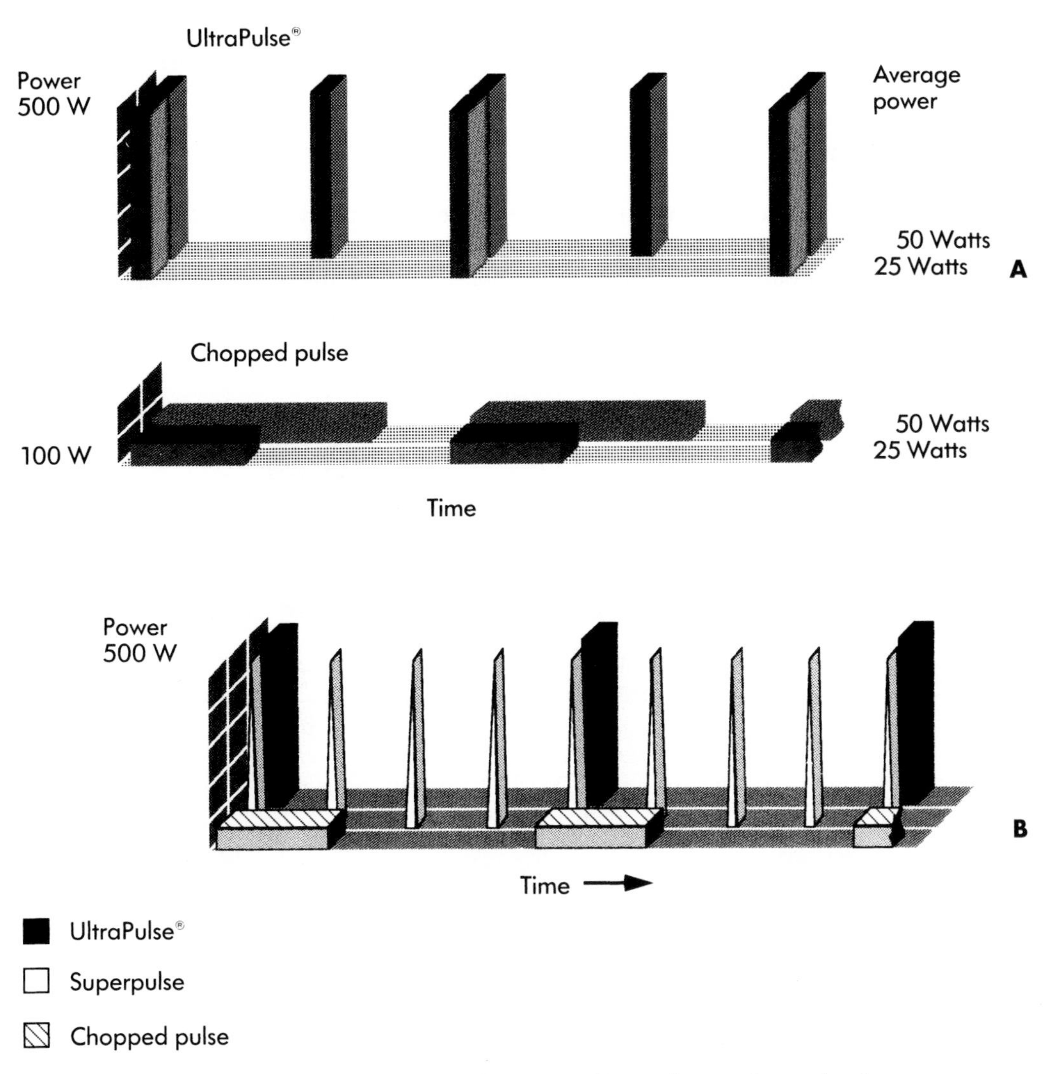

Figure 6-3 **A,** To generate identical fluence at skin surface, a chopped pulse (continuous wave) must be maintained for a longer period than with ultrapulsed or superpulsed lasers, which generate a higher peak power over a shorter time. **B,** Comparison of ultrapulse, superpulse, and chopped-pulse CO_2 laser fluence. At same average power, superpulsed laser must deliver 4 to 5 pulses for each ultrapulse. A chopped pulse is seven times longer than an ultrapulse for this same energy. (Courtesy Coherent Laser Corp., Palo Alto, Calif.)

power be used to compensate for the dilution of power density over the increased area of the larger spot size. The smaller the spot size, the greater is the tendency to create uneven ridges, furrows, and bleeding. The use of a larger spot size has been shown to result in a decrease in peripheral thermal damage as well[57] (Figure 6-2).

Laser Pulse

Laser energy from the continuous beam of the CO_2 laser can be delivered in short pulses of energy by a variety of techniques. The most common is simply mechanically shuttering the beam so that it is physically blocked for short periods, resulting in an on-off repetitive sequence of pulses. *Beam chopping* permits very-short-duration, mechanically shuttered pulses by employing a fanlike device. *Superpulsing* and *ultrapulsing* are processes of delivering very short pulses of very high peak powers by electronically pumping the laser tube. *Q-switching* employs rotating mirrors and other methods, which result in an accumulation of laser energy generating a giant pulse of very high power and extremely short duration (Figure 6-3).

Duty Cycle

When a laser is used in a repetitive pulse mode, the duty cycle refers to the time that the laser is actually on. It is the product of the pulse duration and the repetition rate expressed as a percentage. Duty cycles typically range from 2% to 50%. The average power of the laser can be increased by increasing the repetition rate. When this

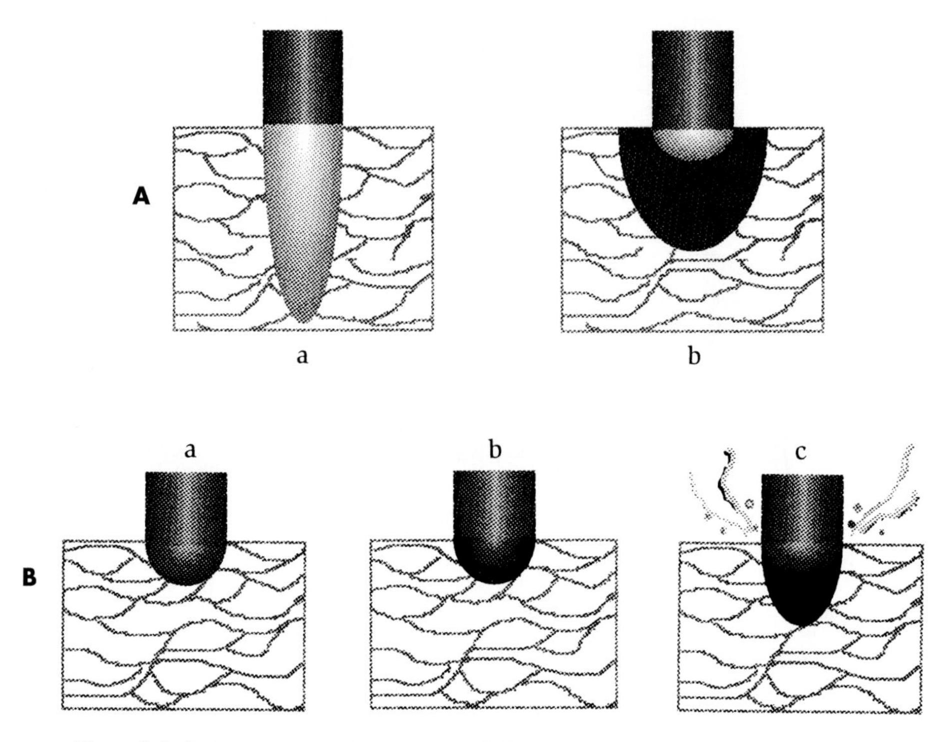

Figure 6-4 **A,** Laser energy is transmitted through skin by transmission and conduction. *a,* Laser instantly heats tissue to a depth determined by absorption length. *b,* Heat flows from region heated by laser into adjacent tissue by conduction. **B,** Laser light is absorbed by tissue. *a,* Water temperature is raised to approximately 100° C. *b,* Intercellular water boils. *c,* Heat is carried away as steam and plume. (Courtesy Coherent Laser Corp., Palo Alto, Calif.)

is done, the duty cycle is increased, but the irradiance (power density) remains the same. The power has not been turned up, but the delivery of that same power per pulse has been accelerated, resulting in a higher average power.[32] The same is true for increasing pulse width. This results in a higher average power but does not alter irradiance.

Thermal Relaxation Time

The thermal relaxation time of tissue is the time required for the heated tissue to lose 50% of its heat through diffusion. Significant thermal diffusion will not occur if the pulse duration is shorter than the time it takes the heated layer to cool. Minimal thermal damage is expected if insignificant diffusion of heat occurs during the laser pulse (Figure 6-4). The thermal relaxation time for pure water has been calculated to be 325 μsec. Calculations of values for human skin have given a figure of 695 μsec.[58] Although these are only order-of-magnitude estimates, pulse widths of 200 μsec[59] and 600 μsec[58] have been shown in animal studies to limit heat diffusion in treated skin. It is thought that a pulse width less than 950 μsec is short enough to prevent clinically significant thermal damage.

LASER-TISSUE INTERACTION

When laser energy interacts with tissue, it does so in accordance with Beer's law. This can be simplified to the statement that tissue damage at the absorption site decreases exponentially with increasing distance from the crater edge. This means that epidermal cells at the wound edge remain viable and can participate in wound healing.[60] According to *Beer's law,* laser energy heats a critical tissue volume until the tissue temperature exceeds the vaporization threshold. If fluence is sufficient to deliver adequate energy during a single laser pulse and that pulse is less than the thermal relaxation time of tissue, then one critical volume of tissue will be cleanly vaporized with each laser pulse and without thermal damage occurring beyond the impact site (Figure 6-5).

To the contrary, if the fluence used results in a pulse energy that is below the minimum necessary to vaporize tissue, tissues will coagulate, desiccate, and carbonize as heat accumulates from the additive effects of multiple pulses (or a continuous beam). Continued irradiance of carbonized tissue results in crater temperatures of more than 600° C (the temperature of red-hot coal), rather than the desired temperature of 100° C required for vaporization (the boiling point of water).[60]

When pure vaporization occurs, the temperature of the impact site of the crater is limited to 100° C. However, when tissue is heated slowly with low irradiance, burning, desiccation, and charring occur. Gross *carbonization* (Figure 6-6) is a sign that tissue temperatures exceed 300° C. Additional radiation of the black carbon creates a *heat sink,* producing tissue temperatures over 600° C.[32] This creates extensive peripheral thermal damage secondary to thermal diffusion. Conduction burns similar to those that occur with electrocautery may result. Instead of a narrow zone of thermal damage of 50 to 100 μm, lateral zones of thermal necrosis measuring 1 to 5 mm may result from thermal diffusion.

When subvaporization temperatures are reached in tissue through the use of irradiances less than approximately 4 J/cm^2, slower tissue damage occurs as a consequence of accelerated thermochemical reactions, resulting in protein denaturation, enzyme inactivation, and cytoplasmic membrane alterations, eventually causing cellular death.[61-65]

Conduction of heat in vivo takes time, and it increases with the square of the distance. The approximate time for substantial heat conduction to occur over a distance

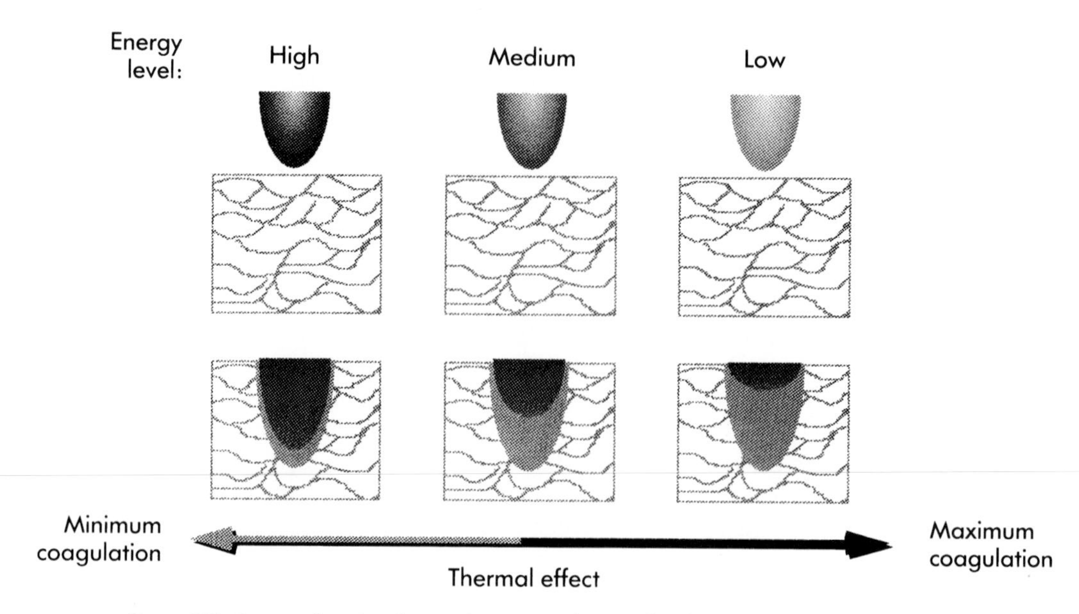

Figure 6-5 Energy density determines coagulation depth. (Courtesy Coherent Laser Corp., Palo Alto, Calif.)

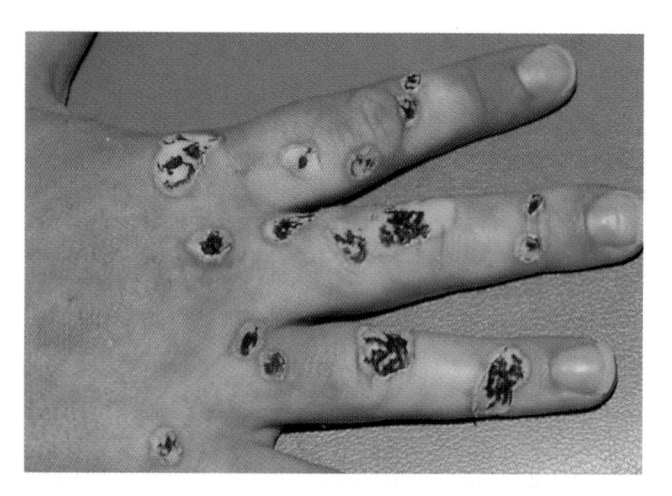

Figure 6-6 Multiple warts of dorsum of hand were treated with continuous-wave CO_2 laser at 10 watts. Obvious charring of tissue is visible immediately after treatment.

of 30 μm in tissue is about 4 msec, and for a distance of 300 μm, approximately 400 msec.[66] Thus, if after 1 second, tissue 1 mm below the surface has reached a temperature of 70° C, then tissue 2 mm below the surface will reach this temperature after 4 seconds.

Utilization of the CO_2 laser with a pulse energy above the vaporization threshold (4-5 J/cm^2) and with a pulse width less than the thermal relaxation time of skin (695-950 μsec) results in pure *steam vaporization* without additional thermal energy diffusing into adjacent tissue. However, application with lower irradiances or longer pulse widths results in a gradient of thermal damage decreasing with distance from the absorption site (Figure 6-7).

The influence of temperature on tissue is a function of time.[67,68] The lowest temperature found to cause irreversible cell damage is 44° C, but this requires an expo-

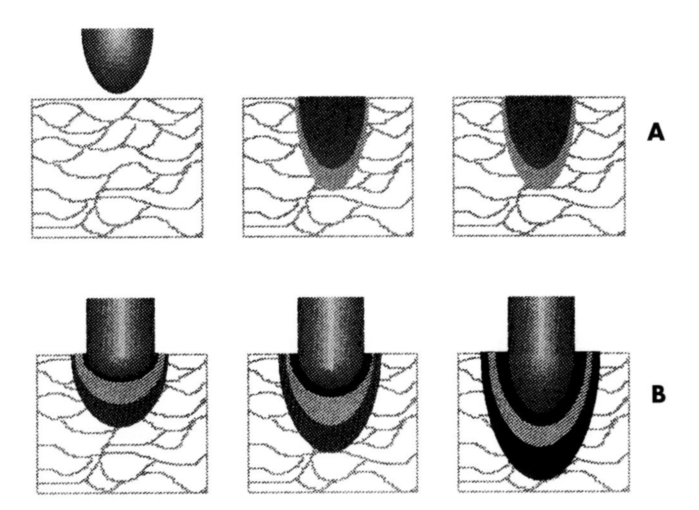

Figure 6-7 Degree of thermal damage depends on rate of vaporization. **A,** With ultrapulsed laser, thermal damage is caused by direct heating. **B,** With continuous-wave CO_2 laser, a area of char appears with thermal damage caused by direct heating of laser. Thermal damage also appears peripherally caused by heat conduction. (Courtesy Coherent Laser Corp., Palo Alto, Calif.)

sure time of 7 hours. The rate of irreversible cell injury increases dramatically as temperature increases, with complete epidermal necrosis occurring after 5 minutes at 50° C, after 5 seconds at 60° C, and after 1 second at 70° C.[67,68] When temperatures reach 100° C, vaporization of intracellular water occurs. However, cellular destruction is caused by intracellular coagulation of proteins at 60° C.[69] Other mechanisms of hyperthermal cellular injury include cell wall damage, cytoplasmic membrane alteration, ribonucleic acid (RNA) and deoxyribonucleic acid (DNA) denaturation, and enzyme inactivation.

Irradiance has been thought to be intimately related to peripheral thermal damage. However, the calculations of McKenzie[70] using a one-dimensional model show qualitative agreement but no systematic relationship of peripheral thermal damage to irradiance.[71] McKenzie's calculations show the thickness of the coagulation zone decreasing from about 500 μm at 100 W/cm^2 to 55 μm at 1000 W/cm^2 and 20 μm at 10 kW/cm^2. However, Schomacker et al[71] found almost identical damage zones with irradiances that differ by more than a factor of 40. Damage zones were found to be of the order of 80 μm for irradiances of 1 kW/cm^2 or greater. Fuller[72] and Mage et al[73] have also shown that above 800 W/cm^2, the rate of peripheral necrosis decreases, and little additional change occurs with further increases in irradiance. Thus the influence of irradiance alone on the size of the necrotic zone is minor when compared to the impact that irradiation time has on heat transfer and the thermal damage.

However, it is clear that irradiance controls the rate at which tissue is vaporized and therefore the depth of the vaporization crater. Although it is commonly advised that the highest irradiance that can be controlled should be used by the laser surgeon, this requires a rapid sweep speed with a continuous beam or a very short pulse of application. To control the depth of incision or vaporization, low power densities have been attempted. This is particularly dangerous with the airbrush vaporization technique using a continuous beam. As discussed previously, this maneuver requires an increased time of application and creates the ideal set of parameters for increasing peripheral thermal diffusion.[32,60,74]

The ideal CO_2 laser for cutaneous surgery must incise or vaporize tissue effectively and rapidly, coagulate blood vessels, and allow rapid and normal healing from adnexal structures as well as from nontreated adjacent epidermis without interfering with graft survival. The CW and mechanically shuttered CO_2 lasers have been shown to provide hemostasis and surgical speed as their only advantages over the use of conventional instrumentation.[59] The 300- to 1000-μm layer of thermal damage reported with these lasers[14,31,37,75-85] is adequate to seal automatically blood vessels 0.5 mm in diameter or smaller and may provide hemostasis of vessels as large as 2 mm in diameter.[56] However, this layer of thermal necrosis also impedes wound healing, tensile strength, and skin graft survival.

The convenience of bloodless surgical technique is a very enticing concept, and the CO_2 laser has been shown to be decidedly superior to both the electric knife and the scalpel in achieving hemostasis.[86,87] However, because this hemostasis is achieved through thermal necrosis, it is important to know its effects on wound healing as well. Early reports of the tissue effects of the CW CO_2 laser reported damage zones of 100 to 500 μm,[88,89] but later studies showed thermal damage extending as far as 2 mm beyond the incision.[86]

Skin wound healing is typically assessed by measuring the time needed to epithelialize the wound surface or by measuring the tensile strength of a wound. The CO_2 laser has been shown to result in slower epithelialization of wounds that results from a delay in onset of epidermal migration,[76,90-93] not a decreased rate of epidermal migration.[87] This delay in CO_2 laser wound epithelialization is thought to result from laser-induced thermal necrosis of the wound margin forming a firm eschar that both extends the size of the wound[91,93-95] and physically impedes epithelialization.[73,86,92,93] In addition, the recovery time needed for injured epidermal cells in the zone of reversible cellular damage adjacent to the zone of thermal necrosis delays the onset of cellular migration until after this recovery period.[94]

The *eschar* is not simply dried serosanguinous fluid, but rather a layer of tissue comprising epidermis, dermal collagen, hair follicles, and sebaceous glands.[76] Repair of the wound cannot proceed until this necrotic tissue has been removed, and interfaces with wound tensile strength as well. Early studies showed that CO_2 laser wounds healed poorly initially but rapidly after 10 days,[96] and this correlates well with removal of this necrotic tissue zone.

Tensile strength of laser incisions using a CW CO_2 laser was found to be less than that of scalpel incisions during the first 1 to 3 weeks after surgery.[76,97,98] Maximal strength for both types of wounds occurs at about 3 months and is about the same.

Increased wound infections with the use of the CW CO_2 laser have been reported as well.[90,99] Of additional significance is that the inflammatory exudate may interfere with early metabolic changes necessary for wound healing and graft survival.[14] Poor graft survival after CW CO_2 laser excision has been attributed to these factors as well as to necrotic tissue from thermal damage.[86,100-106] Delayed revascularization, increased inflammatory cell infiltrate, and accelerated and hypertrophied fibrous connective tissue formation in the graft bed were seen as a consequence of this damage.[101] When a pulsed excimer laser (193 nm, 15 nsec) was used for ablation of the graft bed, there was no detrimental effect on graft survival. Preliminary results with a pulsed CO_2 laser revealed very encouraging results in preventing interference with graft survival by controlling thermal damage.[101]

The use of pulsed CO_2 lasers has been shown to produce efficient and precise tissue ablation with decreased thermal damage to surrounding tissue.* Fluences of 4 to 19 J/cm^2 have been shown to produce precise tissue ablation (20-40 μm of tissue removed per pulse impact) while limiting peripheral thermal damage to a zone measuring less than 100 μm in thickness.[59,75,107] Although there was an initial delay in initiation of wound healing, by day 7 these laser wounds were no different from dermatome-created wounds.[75] Therefore the CO_2 laser can most effectively vaporize cutaneous lesions if used in a pulsed mode with the pulse less than the thermal

*References 32, 37, 40, 57-59, 76, 107-110.

relaxation time of skin (approximately 695-950 μsec) and irradiance of 1000 W/cm^2 or higher. Such short exposure times and high irradiances can be achieved only with a superpulsed or ultrapulsed CO_2 laser.

SUPERPULSED AND ULTRAPULSED CO_2 LASERS

Superpulsed and ultrapulsed CO_2 lasers emit a controlled train of short-duration, high-power pulses. Typically, the peak powers generated are as much as 10 times what the laser is capable of producing in the CW mode. The laser tube is pumped electronically to produce high-power pulses in repetitive short pulses. Although the repetition rate varies from laser to laser, it may be a critical parameter as well. In some lasers the repetition rate is fixed by the choice of the other parameters; in others, it may be chosen by the surgeon. Repetition rates vary over a range of 1 to 5000 Hz per second.

For most superpulsed CO_2 lasers, each pulse contains inadequate energy per single pulse to ablate tissue. In this situation the repetition rate needs to be rapid enough to avoid interpulse cooling, so a series of four or five pulses is used to accumulate enough heat to reach the tissue vaporization threshold. This creates a situation that may allow thermal diffusion beyond the intended site of treatment. This is particularly true for rapid repetition rates (>1000 Hz). In this situation the superpulsed CO_2 laser behaves essentially as a CW laser. Repetition rates as low as 10 to 100 Hz are estimated to allow slight accumulation of thermal energy.[57] However, recent calculations have suggested that the ideal repetition rate to avoid unwanted thermal damage is 93 Hz or less.[111] Additionally, repetition rates of 1 to 50 Hz allow better manual control.[59,75]

When nonablative laser irradiation was used, an analytic model predicted an upper limit for the repetition rate of a superpulsed CO_2 laser to be about 150 Hz to avoid a rise in temperature caused by multiple pulses.[108] More recent work has established that critical threshold more likely to be about 5 Hz.[109] A frequency as low as 10 Hz yields a significant accumulation of heat when conduction is the only heat transfer mechanism operative. When the CO_2 laser is used in an ablative manner, the removal of tissue removes heat as well, but the residual heat decays as per this model, and it is suggested that 5 Hz be considered the lower boundary for avoidance of heat accumulation when the spot is not moved continuously. A higher repetition rate can be used if a cooling time of 200 msec per spot is respected.[109]

Schomacker et al[71] studied the cumulative effects of multipulse versus single-pulse exposures. A single 100-msec pulse of 830 W/cm^2 resulted in a crater depth of approximately 125 μm and a layer of thermal necrosis at the base of the crater measuring 100 μm. Five repetitive pulses at 0.1 Hz (500 times the estimated tissue relaxation time) resulted in a crater depth of approximately 400 μm and a residual layer of thermal necrosis measuring 160 μm. Clearly, multiple pulses lead to increased damage. This multipulse effect explains the difference between the 100-μm damage zones typical of single 50- to 100-msec pulse exposures[71] and the 750-μm damage zones reported by Walsh et al[58] using 100 or more 50-msec pulses at 510 W/cm^2. The multipulse effect with a high repetition rate also explains the relative lack of clinically significant improved wound healing that we found in the clinical use of the Coherent Ambulase superpulsed CO_2 laser.[41,42] The superpulse parameters of this particular laser allow the choice of a repetition rate of only 250 or 500 Hz. The most significant improvement in clinical results occurred only with shuttering this superpulsed beam with a secondary pulse of 50 msec. This shuttering cuts the stream of pulses into short bursts of 10 to 12 pulses (each delivering approximately 32 mJ to tissue) that accumulate adequate energy to vaporize tissue. The "off" period protects the peripheral tissue from excessive thermal damage.

The *threshold fluence* for ablation of skin has been reported as 4.75 J/cm² based on measurements by Walsh et al[58] and 2.6 J/cm² (95% confidence interval: 1.9-3.2) based on studies by Green et al.[59] From these measurements it is estimated that the effective fluence required to ablate skin is 5 J/cm² or higher. The requirement to reach this threshold necessitates the use of a cumulative effect of multiple pulses for most superpulsed lasers. To modulate the unwanted thermal effects, as well as to add a further increment of control over the beam, a second duty cycle is superimposed on the superpulse cycle by use of a mechanically pulsed shutter. This adds additional on-off periods and cuts the train of continuous superpulse impacts into smaller groups of several pulses, separated by a longer cooling time. Typical increments of 50 msec to 0.5 sec are provided, and these repeat in cycles of 2 to 10 per second. This is an excellent means of controlling the high-irradiance superpulsed laser. Experimental data using CO_2 laser ablation of guinea pig skin suggest that less thermal damage occurs with a 50-msec pulse than with longer shuttered pulses.[31,71] We have confirmed this on human skin, both with CW CO_2 laser ablation and with superpulsed CO_2 laser ablation, using only single impacts,[40] as well as in clinical use in treatment of patients[41,42] (Figures 6-8 and 6-9).

Experimental data suggest a thermal relaxation time of 19 msec for the liquid phase that forms during laser-tissue interaction.[57,110] This *liquid tissue phase* is thought to act as a conduit of heat from the impact crater to the surrounding tissue. The shuttered pulse may be significant in controlling heat conduction through this phase. Although theoretically useful, the tissue effects of shuttered pulses shorter than 50 msec have not been reported.

Green et al[75] demonstrated normal healing of skin ablated with a mechanical scanning device using a spot size of 400 μm, pulse energy of 23 mJ, and radiant exposure of 18 J/cm² per pulse. The mechanical scanner produced a grid of overlapping pulses while moving at a speed of 25.4 mm per second. The epidermis and dermis were removed to a depth of 856 $\pm$ 230 μm, and thermal necrosis measured only 85 $\pm$ 15 μm. Healing of these wounds was compared to that caused by a dermatome and measuring 871 $\pm$ 200 μm. Healing time of the wounds was no different. The authors recognized the difficulty in reproducing these parameters clinically and suggested modification of existing laser systems to allow a larger spot size with radiant energies of 4 to 19 J/cm² and a slow repetition rate of 1 to 50 Hz.[78] The extent of

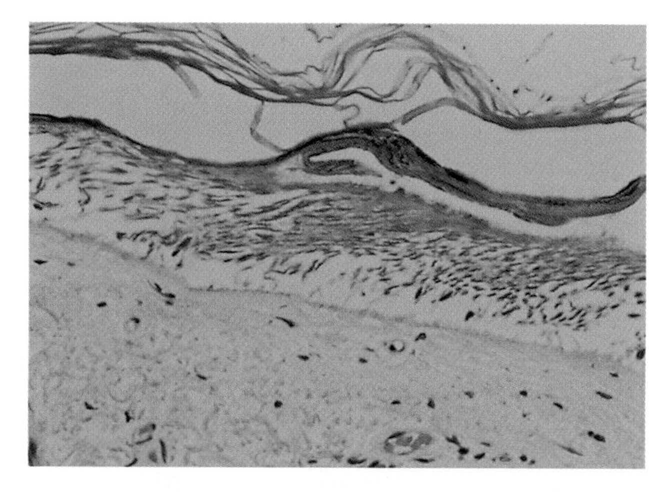

Figure 6-8 Histologic appearance of epidermis and superficial dermis in human skin after one 2-mm-diameter laser impact with Coherent Ambulase CO_2 laser at an SP1 setting of 0.1-sec pulse. Epidermis is focally detached with spindly alteration of nuclei. Dermal necrosis is less than 0.1 mm in depth. (Hematoxylin-eosin; ×40.) (From Fitzpatrick RE, Ruiz-Esparza J, Goldman MP: *J Dermatol Surg Oncol* 17:340, 1991.)

tissue damage is technique and user dependent as well. These factors also affect the ultimate clinical result. However, using ideal laser parameters minimizes the variance from operator to operator.

The introduction of the Coherent's UltraPulse CO_2 laser provided the first surgical CO_2 laser capable of vaporizing tissue in a single pulse with the use of a large spot size. This laser uses the principles of selective photothermolysis in CO_2 laser surgery of cutaneous lesions. Adherence to these principles results in improved clinical results and a decrease in adverse healing consequences. The pulse parameters of this laser are ideal for avoiding unwanted thermal damage while maximizing the ablative capacity of each laser pulse (Figures 6-10 and 6-11 and Tables 6-1 and 6-2).

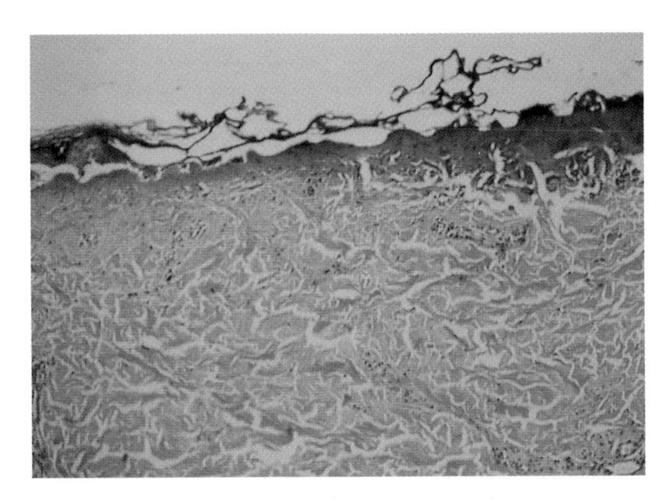

Figure 6-9 Histologic appearance immediately after laser impact with 2-mm-diameter spot from CO_2 laser at 13 W with 0.2-sec pulse. Complete loss of the epidermis has occurred, with dermal necrosis exceeding 0.2 mm in depth. (Hematoxylin-eosin; ×40.) (From Fitzpatrick RE, Ruiz-Esparza J, Goldman MP: *J Dermatol Surg Oncol* 17:340, 1991.)

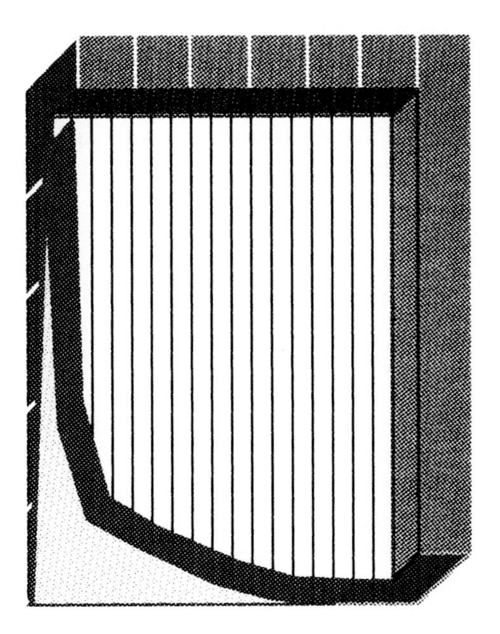

Figure 6-10 Comparison of pulse energy from ultrapulsed (*lined box*) and superpulsed (*gray*) CO_2 laser. Energy per pulse is equal to area under curve of power versus time. This graph demonstrates that ultrapulsed CO_2 laser delivers more than four times more energy per pulse. (Courtesy Coherent Laser Corp., Palo Alto, Calif.)

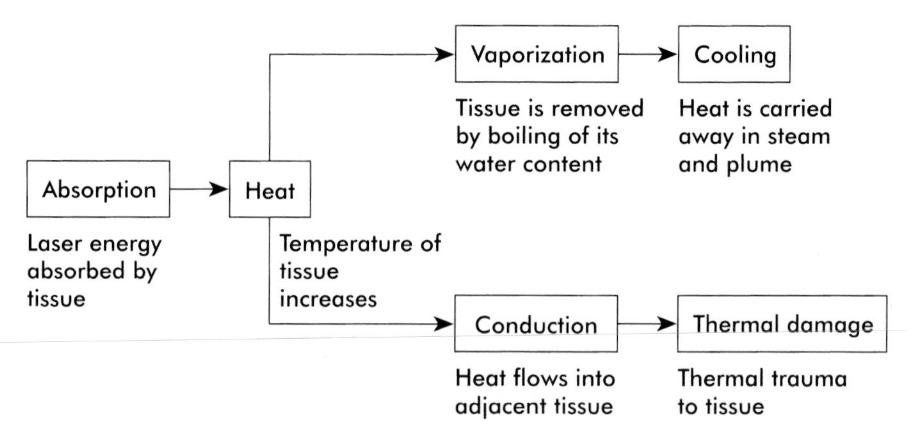

Figure 6-11

Table 6-2

Laser	Number of Patients	Failed Previous Therapy	Number of Warts	Clear	Scar	Recurrence
Continuous	22	19	121	82 (68%)	65 (54%)	39 (32%)
Superpulse	24	20	179	121 (68%)	59 (33%)	39 (22%)
Ultrapulse	24	24	150	135 (90%)	11 (7%)	15 (10%)

CLINICAL APPLICATION

The CO_2 laser can be used to cut or to vaporize tissue. These two clinical results are determined simply by the spot size and power output. Starting with the smallest spot size available in the focused mode (0.2 mm) results in the delivery of approximately 12,000 to 60,000 W/cm^2 of power density when used at 5 to 25 W of power output. Power densities of this magnitude easily cut tissue, the higher powers resulting in a deeper cut. The cut width is the same as the beam diameter, 0.2 mm. By simply moving the handpiece away from the tissue surface, the spot size enlarges, or defocuses. Typically, spot sizes of 2 to 5 mm are used for vaporization, and the power output is decreased to afford better surgical control. Using a power output of 5 W results in the delivery of approximately 50 to 150 W/cm^2 with beam diameters of 2 to 5 mm, a much smaller power density than that used for cutting with 5 W and a 0.2-mm beam (12,000 W/cm^2). The primary difference in these two situations is the rate at which tissue is vaporized. The power density (irradiance) is the determinant of the speed of vaporization. With large spot sizes, tissue can be vaporized rapidly only if the laser is capable of generating enough power to result in high power density. A spot size of 5 mm is 25 times larger than a spot size of 0.2 mm and requires 625 times the power output to cut at the same speed and depth. Power densities of 12,000 to 60,000 W/cm^2 could be generated with a 5-mm spot, and a cut 5-mm wide would be made as quickly as one now is performed with a 0.2-mm spot; however, the laser would have to deliver 3000 to 15,000 W of power instead of 5 to 25 W.

With either low or high power densities the CO_2 laser must be used with extreme care and attention. Safety glasses must be worn to protect the eyes, nonreflective surgical instruments may be useful, and nonflammable materials or wet drapes and sponges must be used in the operative field. When the laser is used to excise an exophytic growth tangentially, care must be taken to shield the area that the beam will impact once it cuts completely through the tissue. The use of smoke evacuators and high-efficiency filter masks is necessary to remove the smoke generated in the laser plume and avoid the possibility of contact with viral particles.

VAPORIZATION

When used as an instrument to vaporize tissue, the CO_2 laser has the following advantages over other therapeutic modalities: (1) the extreme precision in depth as well as in surface area that can be achieved, (2) the potential for limiting vaporization to the intended target without leaving a residual layer of unwanted thermal damage, (3) the operative speed of the procedure, (4) hemostasis during the procedure, and (5) minimal postoperative pain and edema.

The primary limitations of vaporization are (1) the clinical endpoint is achieved by visual feedback, which may have a large range of error and depends on experience, and (2) power densities and fluences may vary widely as a consequence of small variances in operative technique, particularly when one is using a continuous, nonpulsed beam. Attempts to control these variables by a more reproducible scientific approach have been cumbersome, confusing, and poorly understood; thus empiric techniques developed by individual practitioners remain the standard of practice. Therefore clinical results vary tremendously from surgeon to surgeon.

Because of these limitations and the unreliability of visual inspection as a means of determining treatment endpoints, an attempt to calibrate the CO_2 laser for vaporization of discrete cutaneous tumors was studied.[112] This approach produced reasonable results in the three patients studied, but it has been considered impractical for general use because of the large number of variables and limited data for clinical use.

Clinical use of the laser must be guided by close attention to certain parameters during the procedure. These clinical parameters and their significance with regard to depth of tissue ablation have been reported on by Reid.[60] He characterized opalescent bubbling of the skin surface accompanied by audible cracking sounds as an indication that only the epidermis had been ablated (Figure 6-12). This surface can be wiped clean with saline to reveal an intact, smooth, pink plane representing the surface of the papillary dermis (Figure 6-13). When the layer is vaporized, there is visible contraction of the tissue and the development of a yellowish, roughened appearance similar to chamois cloth (Figure 6-14). When the reticular dermis is reached, coarse collagen bundles are seen, having an appearance resembling waterlogged cotton threads (Figure 6-15). Healing of the skin down to this point will occur without scarring. To proceed deeper may increase the risk of scarring. Close attention must be paid to tissue charring. If charring occurs, thermal diffusion and unwanted tissue necrosis will occur beyond the depth of vaporization. When charring is noted, this can often be remedied by decreasing the spot size of the beam, resulting in an increased fluence but also an increased rate of tissue vaporization.

Because power density is highest at the center of the beam and lower at the periphery, it is possible to ablate cleanly with the center of the beam while producing char at the edges (Figure 6-16). This is particularly true when multiple passes are made over the same area or ablation of a deep cavity or large mass is necessary. This effect of char accumulating at the periphery can be minimized by keeping the ablation surface area as wide as possible. Less char is produced if a wide area is ablated

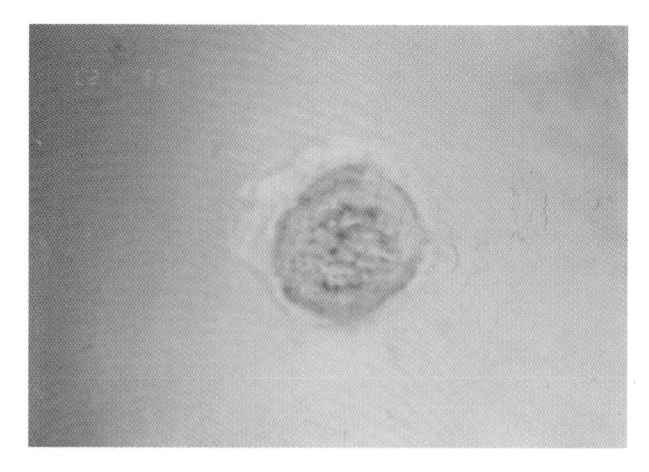

Figure 6-12 Opalescent bubbling of skin surface indicates confinement of ablation to epidermis. Note minimal charring of tissue.

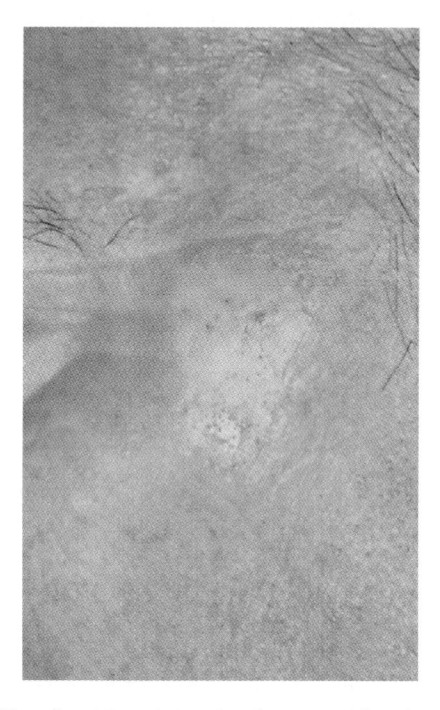

Figure 6-13 When ablated epidermis is wiped away with saline, an intact, smooth, pink plane representing papillary dermis is visible. (Vasoconstriction secondary to lidocaine with epinephrine.)

at the start and gradually increased to a greater depth, rather than starting with a narrow, deep area and ablating away the sides.[66]

When using the CO_2 laser for vaporization, one must keep in mind effects resulting from changes in the spot size. The ideal situation is to use a large spot size (2-5-mm diameter) delivered with a pulse less than 695 μsec in duration with an energy density of 4 J/cm^2 or higher. The use of a large spot allows for smoother, more uniform vaporization of tissue and has been shown to result in a decrease in peripheral thermal damage.[57,111,113] However, this must be weighed against the fact that a large spot size dilutes the power density significantly (fluence may drop as low as 0.3 J/cm^2, far below the 4 J/cm^2 ablation threshold)[42] and may lead to excessive charring and unwanted thermal damage. In this situation the risks of an uneven

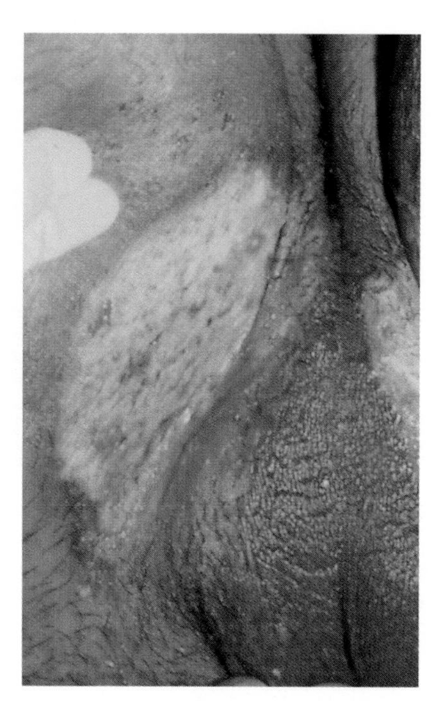

Figure 6-14 Further vaporization of papillary dermis results in immediately visible contraction of tissue and yellowish, toughened texture similar to that of chamois cloth.

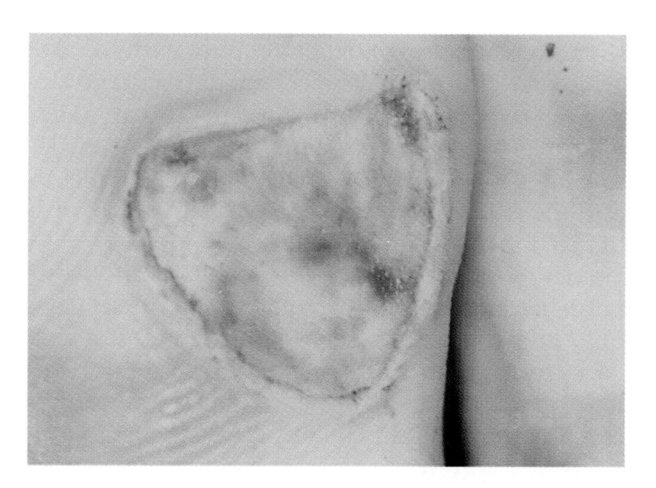

Figure 6-15 Vaporization of tissue to depth of reticular dermis reveals coarse collagen bundles similar in appearance to waterlogged cotton threads.

surface resulting from the use of a small spot must be weighed against the risk of scarring from heat accumulation and tissue charring with a large spot.

The use of low fluences to treat thin epidermal lesions has been advocated by several authors.[50-53,114] The use of the CO_2 laser in such a nonablative manner results in a situation in which conduction is the only heat transfer process. Epidermal damage induced by low-dose CO_2 laser treatment is not a laser-specific injury. It is a nonspecific thermal effect that is reproducible by sources such as a hot water bath or heated copper template.[67,68,115] The progression of visible changes observable with nonablative fluences delivered to the skin are first erythema, then whitening, and next vaporization or charring. This same sequence is producible with simple sources of heat delivery, as well as with nonablative laser heating. One study[51] showed that

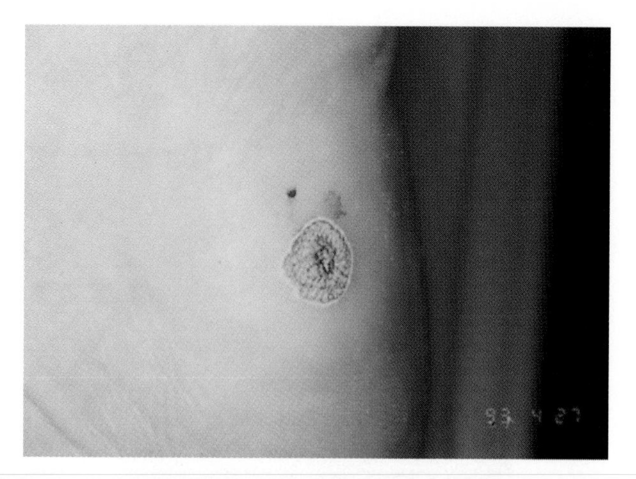

Figure 6-16 Ablation of wart with ultrapulsed laser used in concentric circles starting at periphery has resulted in char-free ablation at periphery, but charring centrally where periphery of beam overlaps with each pulse. Even though this laser is capable of char-free ablation, gaussian distribution of energy results in lower energy at periphery of beam, and heat may accumulate at this location, particularly through additional effects of multiple pulses.

the therapeutic range for this type of low-fluence CO_2 laser injury of the epidermis was very narrow (fluences between 3.7 and 4.4 J/cm^2). Higher fluences caused scarring, whereas lower fluences were ineffective, although a linear relationship has been noted between power delivered and the amount of necrosis.[116] Delivery of low fluences with such a small range of variation requires extreme precision and attention to detail. This is very difficult to achieve with a free-hand airbrush technique. Some very experienced laser surgeons have mastered this art and can use this technique with reproducible results in the same way that superficial liquid nitrogen cryosurgery can be used selectively to strip off the epidermis using cold injury. However, the use of the CO_2 laser in this manner is particularly risky because of the unseen thermal diffusion that occurs with heating of tissue.[54,74,116,117] When using a pulsed CO_2 laser in a nonablative manner, the repetition rate must be kept at about 5 Hz to avoid cumulative effects from each pulse.[109]

When epidermal growths such as seborrheic keratoses, actinic keratoses, and verruca vulgaris are treated with the CO_2 laser with vaporization as an endpoint, they may be either vaporized or superheated. When a lower fluence is used, often the central aspect of the spot will cause points of blistering or vaporization, and the periphery superheats to a gray-white color (the heat being delivered in a gaussian distribution). If the lesion is thin, the superheated area may extend to the dermal-epidermal junction with the first pass of the laser. If so, a natural split will occur at this junction, and the thermally damaged epidermis can be removed with a wipe of saline-soaked gauze. With thicker lesions, several passes are necessary to produce a dermal-epidermal cleavage plane. This should be tested by wiping the lesion after each pass to determine if it will strip off easily, rather than continuing to deliver heat and allowing char to accumulate. Studies of low-fluence CO_2 laser surgery have shown that the greatest initial histologic effects occur at the basal layer. It is thought that the structural and biologic inhomogeneity present at the dermal-epidermal junction predisposes to damage at this location.[52]

SPECIFIC APPLICATIONS

The use of the CO_2 laser offers no real advantage in some procedures, simplifies many procedures even though other approaches may be equally satisfactory, offers distinct advantages in other procedures, and is sometimes the procedure of choice. Other authors[43,118] have used a similar classification of the usefulness of the CO_2 laser. Our assessment is slightly different from theirs and reflects the use of the UltraPulse CO_2 laser as well as ideal pulse parameters.

Lesions for which CO_2 Laser Offers No Advantage

Vascular lesions (telangiectasia, port-wine stain, angioma)

Successful application of the CO_2 laser for treatment of superficial telangiectasias was reported early in its use[26,27] based on its ability to cauterize superficial vessels through intact skin on the face and extremities. A preliminary report on the use of this laser in treatment of port-wine stain (PWS) birthmarks appeared in 1982.[119] This paper reported good to excellent results in 56.8% of patients treated and hypertrophic scarring in 8.1%, figures not dissimilar to those in argon laser–treated patients.[120-124] These authors advised avoiding treatment of (1) vascular lesions of the legs because of poor response and increased risk of scarring as well as (2) prepubertal children and (3) periorbital or perioral lesions because of an increased risk of scarring.

Although many practitioners used the CO_2 laser for treatment of these vascular lesions at this time, such treatment has become controversial because of the more specific vascular targeting of the argon laser and the development of lasers more precisely targeted to vascular lesions, especially the pulsed dye laser. Authors advocating the use of the CO_2 laser for these lesions published other articles endorsing the CO_2 laser in certain circumstances,[125-128] but its use remained controversial and led to articles pointing to the limitations of the CO_2 laser for treatment of PWSs.[129,130]

The primary disadvantage of the CO_2 laser for this application is that its absorption by water requires the thermal destruction of the overlying epidermis and dermis to reach the vessels to be treated. This results in full-thickness coagulation necrosis extending at least 0.5 mm into the reticular dermis that heals with a layer of fibrosis.[131] This type of response is unavoidable because of the mechanism by which the CO_2 laser interacts with the skin. Although the majority of treated patients may heal very well, and, as pointed out by Ratz and Bailin,[127] this procedure does not differ in principle from other cosmetic resurfacing procedures such as dermabrasion or chemical peels, the primary disadvantage relates to the difficulty in controlling heat damage from thermal diffusion, and alternative treatments (e.g., pulsed dye laser therapy) do not pose this same risk (Figure 6-17).

Although the published histology of argon laser therapy of PWSs[132-134] is not very different from that of the CO_2 laser,[135] the use of short millisecond pulses[136] and epidermal cooling[130,137] optimizes the argon laser parameters and allows substantial improvement in vascular specificity, which is not possible with the CO_2 laser.

Lanigan and Cotterill[138] reported use of the CO_2 laser in treatment of PWSs that had failed to respond to argon or CW dye laser therapy or in children with pink PWSs. They reported good to excellent results in 74% of adults and 53% of children. They advise caution in treatment of children because 24% had no benefit and one (6%) developed a hypertrophic scar. The authors also noted that this laser can produce severe cutaneous damage secondary to thermal diffusion and recommend the use of a superpulsed CO_2 laser by an experienced laser surgeon to avoid this problem.

We believe the only potentially useful and safe application for the CO_2 laser in this clinical area is the vaporization of thick, hypertrophic, nodular components of mature PWS malformations. Although multiple articles have been published regarding use of the CO_2 laser in treatment of nodular components of PWSs and hemangiomas,[14,19,139-143] it is important to realize that complete vaporization of these lesions with the CO_2 laser will always result in healing with some degree of scarring. This may not be acceptable, because alternative therapies are now available that heal without scarring (e.g., pulsed dye laser). If this therapy is to be accomplished

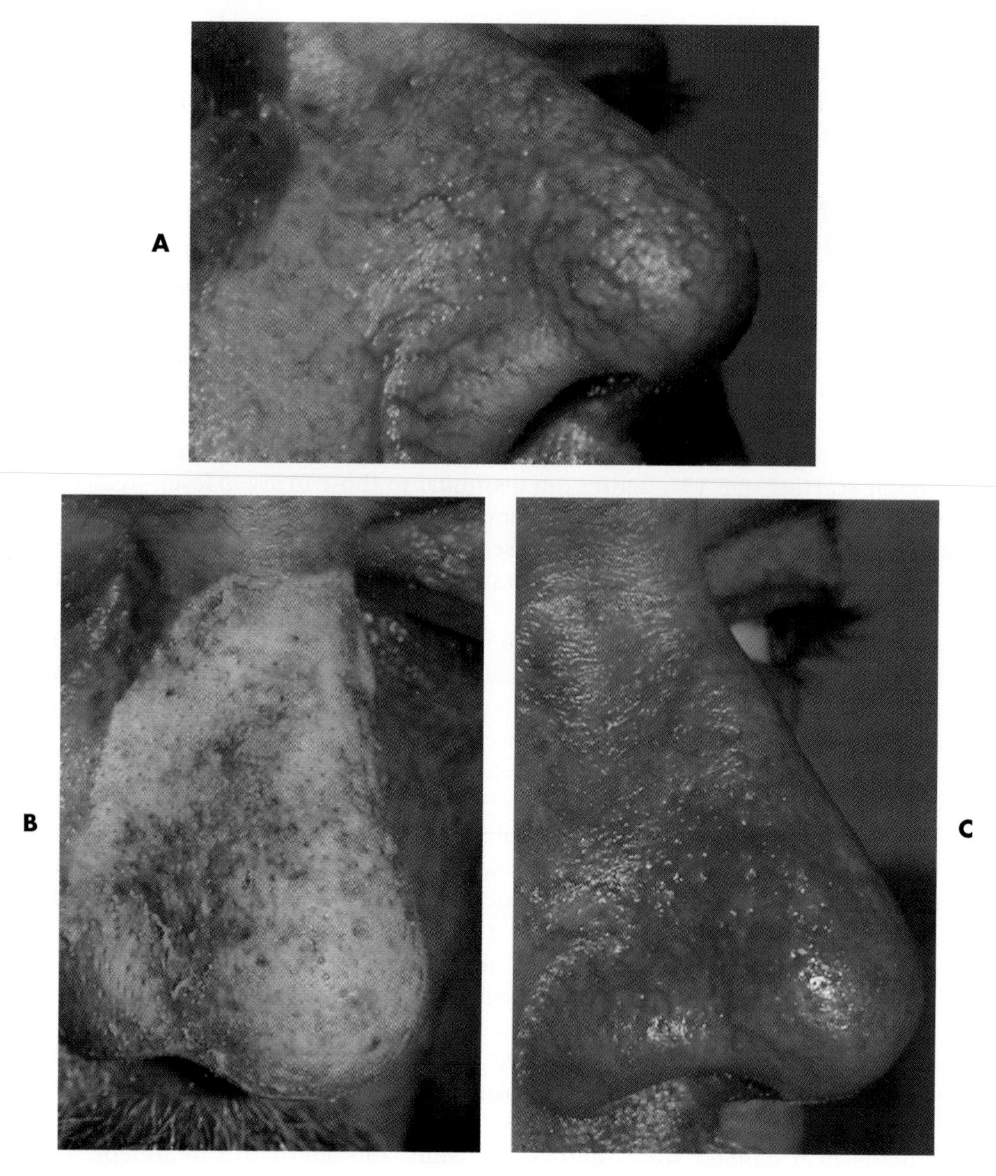

Figure 6-17 **A,** Extensive telangiectasia on nose of 49-year-old man. **B,** Immediately after CO_2 laser vaporization of telangiectasia. Coherent Ambulase CO_2 laser was used at a superpulse setting of two 0.05-sec pulses to entire nose in one pass. A second pass was performed only across individual vessels. **C,** Clinical appearance 4 months after laser treatment. Many vessels persist, with resolution of smaller vessels. No evidence of scarring is present.

with a CO_2 laser, it is important to use the appropriate pulse characteristics as well as operative techniques designed to avoid unwanted thermal damage and subsequent risk of scarring. This debulking treatment should be achieved in a superficial plane and then followed by treatment of the underlying lesion with a vascular-specific (pulsed dye) laser (Figure 6-18).

Cherry angiomas[144] and venous lakes can be treated with caution with the CO_2 laser, because these lesions are usually exophytic and have greater lesional diameter. These lesional characteristics allow avoidance of deeper thermal damage and take advantage of the more diffuse nonspecific thermal damage. However, even these lesions may be best treated with a vascular-targeted laser, such as the argon or pulsed dye, or the PhotoDerm VL.

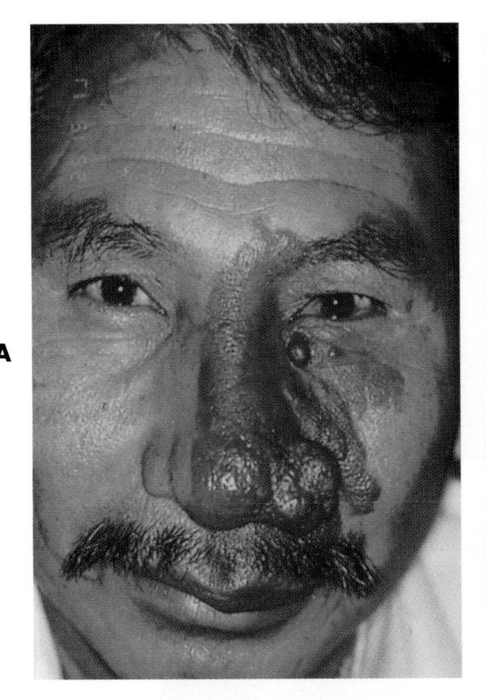

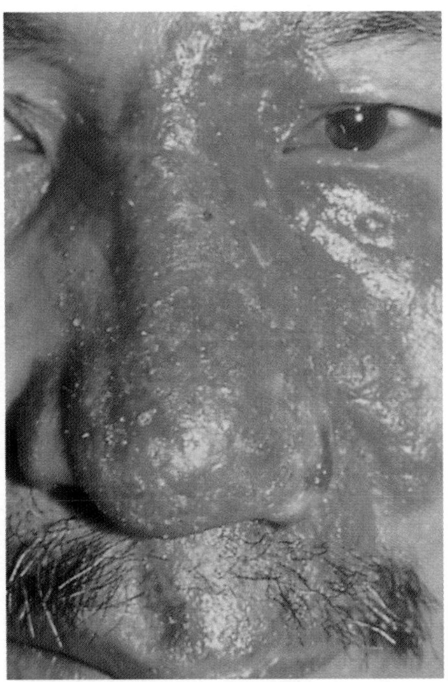

Figure 6-18 **A,** Port-wine stain (PWS) present from birth on left side of face of a 47-year-old Hispanic man. Over past 20 years lesion has grown progressively darker and developed nodular hypertrophies, especially prominent on right lateral distal aspect of nose and right inner canthus. PWS and nodular hypertrophies were treated with $UPCO_2$ laser at energy level of 250 mJ/pulse and average power of 20 W. Debulking procedure was performed using a handpiece spot size of 2-mm diameter. Tissue was cleanly ablated with overlapping pulses without charring or bleeding. CO_2 laser was then used over entire PWS in a single pass. **B,** One month after treatment, complete resolution of hypertrophic nodules and marked decrease in bluish color of lesion, which is now light pink.

In summary, although some vascular lesions can be treated successfully with the CO_2 laser, it is generally too risky for general use because the vascular-specific lasers are both more effective and safer for these applications.

Epidermal pigmented lesions

The second area where the CO_2 laser holds no therapeutic advantage is in treatment of thin epidermal pigmented lesions, such as lentigines, ephelides, and pigmented labial macules. The use of low-fluence CO_2 laser therapy has been successful in treatment of these lesions,[51,52] but the technique is fraught with difficulty, for reasons already discussed. Although labial lentigines of Peutz-Jeghers syndrome may be treated with the CO_2 laser[53] in the same manner as actinic cheilitis, treatment with pigment-specific lasers (see Chapter 3) offers more effective therapy with minimal risk of scarring and a less problematic, shorter healing time.

When evaluating our patients with lentigines treated with a CW CO_2 laser and a superpulsed CO_2 laser, we found an unacceptably high rate of scarring. Forty percent of patients treated with the CW CO_2 laser had some degree of scarring, and 28.6% of treated lesions healed with either hypopigmentation or atrophic scarring.[41,42] With the superpulse mode, poor healing with atrophic scarring also occurred in 25% of patients and 12.9% of lesions treated. These scars were minor, and patients usually did not notice or complain about them, but they were present nonetheless (Figure 6-19). When a lesion is being removed primarily for cosmetic benefit, the end result must be evaluated objectively. The presence of surface texture and pigment alterations is

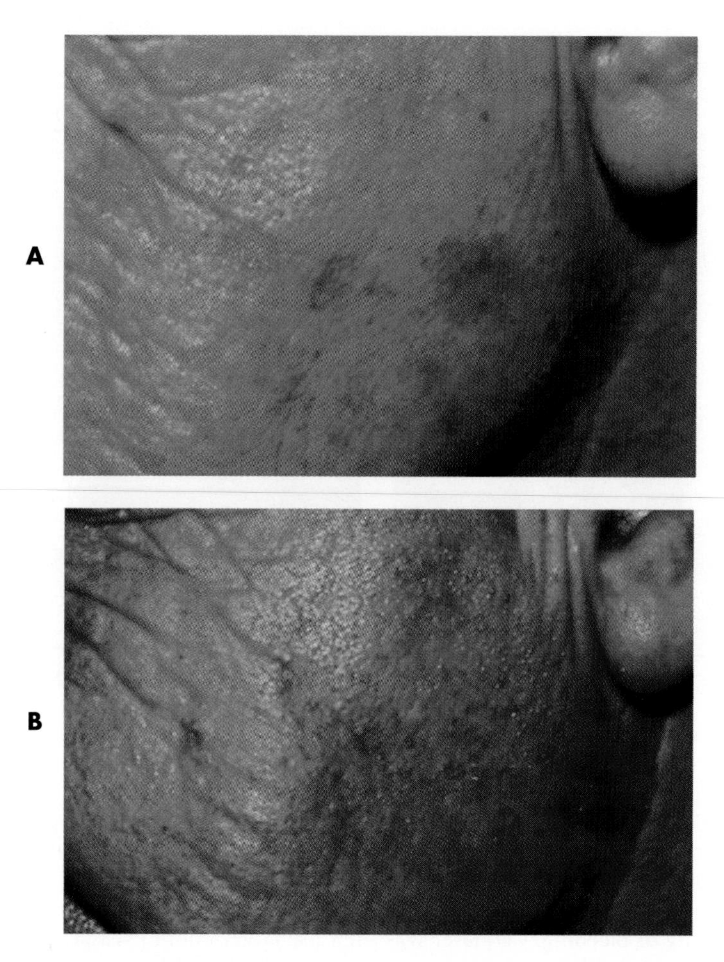

Figure 6-19 **A,** Several lentigines and actinic keratosis present on left cheek of 72-year-old man. **B,** Five months after treatment with superpulsed CO_2 laser, using 4 W, 200-μsec pulse, and 250 Hz (32 mJ/pulse). There is loss of normal skin texture as well as persistent erythema in the areas vaporized. These changes are subtle and not easily seen without close observation.

not acceptable. Although the new short-pulsed lasers have the potential of removing these lesions successfully and safely, the pigment-targeted lasers are more lesion specific and safer.

Lesions for which CO_2 Laser Simplifies Procedure

Treatment of lesions in this category may be accomplished successfully with either the CO_2 laser or other modalities, but the CO_2 laser simplifies the procedure through (1) hemostasis, (2) decreased operative time, or (3) more precise control over depth of destruction.

Decorative tattoos

The CO_2 laser offers all three advantages over other tissue-destructive modalities in treatment of decorative tattoos. The tissue-containing tattoo pigment can be precisely vaporized with a bloodless field.[145-152] The entire tattoo can be rapidly vaporized in a single treatment session with the use of high powers (15-20 W). When the entire tattoo is removed in one session, close attention to varying depths of tattoo pigment can be tissue sparing, which speeds healing and decreases scarring. However, treatment of tattoos by this method is always followed by healing with various degrees of scarring.

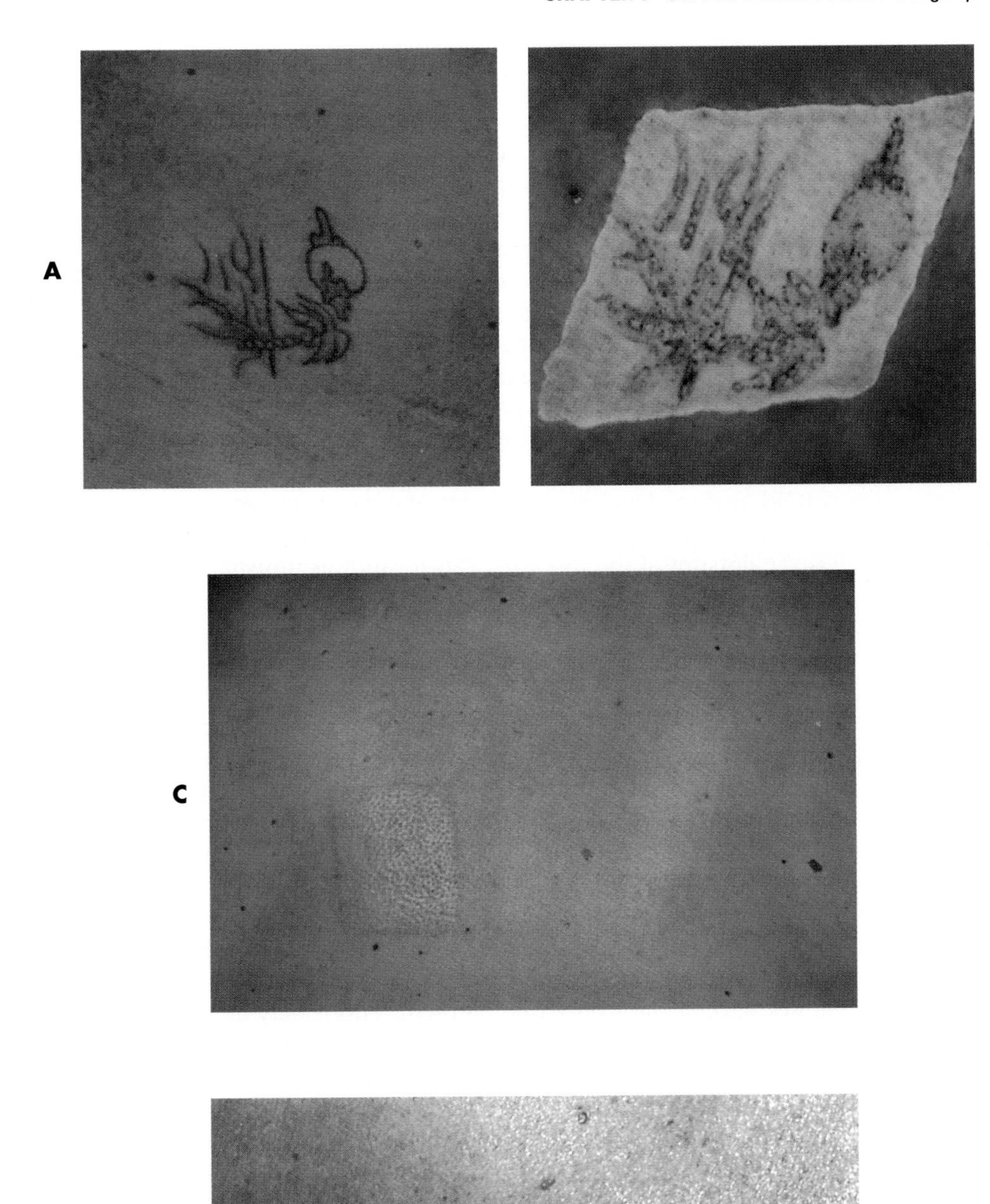

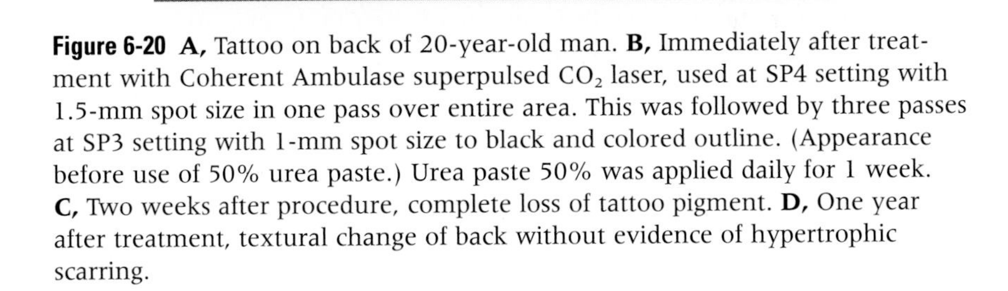

Figure 6-20 **A,** Tattoo on back of 20-year-old man. **B,** Immediately after treatment with Coherent Ambulase superpulsed CO_2 laser, used at SP4 setting with 1.5-mm spot size in one pass over entire area. This was followed by three passes at SP3 setting with 1-mm spot size to black and colored outline. (Appearance before use of 50% urea paste.) Urea paste 50% was applied daily for 1 week. **C,** Two weeks after procedure, complete loss of tattoo pigment. **D,** One year after treatment, textural change of back without evidence of hypertrophic scarring.

Hypertrophic scarring is unavoidable in a certain percentage of patients, because histologic evaluation of CW CO_2 laser wounds has revealed thermal damage as deep as 5 mm.[147] Hypertrophic scarring has been reported in 7%[150] and 16%[151] of patients. Attempts to avoid hypertrophic scarring have included the use of multiple treatment sessions,[147] combination therapy with mild acids,[152] and the use of 50% urea paste.[153] None of these alterations in technique has eliminated the risk of hypertrophic scarring. The use of 50% urea paste postoperatively has resulted in the ability to remove virtually all the tattoo pigment in one treatment session while limiting the tissue vaporization to a more superficial plane in which only 30% to 50% of the tattoo pigment is actually vaporized. This results in improved healing, decreasing the incidence of hypertrophic scarring.

Hypertrophic scarring is related in part to the degree of thermal damage and wound depth but also correlates with the anatomic location of the wound. About 25% of our patients treated with the CO_2 laser who had tattoos removed from the upper arm/deltoid region developed hypertrophic scarring, versus only 10% of those having tattoos treated in other locations. One location that tends to heal extremely well is the dorsum of the forearm. This location is unusual for the development of hypertrophic scarring (Figure 6-20; see also Figure 4-16).

The development of Q-switched lasers for tattoo treatment has made it possible to remove tattoos with minimal or no scarring[154-156] (see Chapter 4). However, these lasers require multiple treatment sessions over a prolonged period. The CO_2 laser remains an alternative treatment choice for those patients desiring tattoo removal in a single session and willing to accept healing with a scar. The high-energy, short-pulsed CO_2 lasers may be used in combination with the Q-switched lasers for more rapid tattoo removal. The pulsed CO_2 laser is used to strip away the epidermis, allowing better access to the tattoo pigment with the Q-switched lasers with less beam scattering. We found that such techniques may decrease the number of treatment sessions by 50% or more without significantly increasing the risk of scarring.

Iron-oxide flesh-colored tattoos may turn black with Q-switched laser treatment.[157] Treatment of these tattoos with pulsed CO_2 lasers is far more advantageous because it will not darken the iron-oxide pigment, and it may be the treatment of choice.[158] Generally, a series of treatments is necessary to avoid scarring.

Isolated verrucous keratoses

The second area where the CO_2 laser may be advantageous is in vaporization of isolated verruca vulgaris lesions or seborrheic keratoses. These lesions are easily and often treated with liquid nitrogen cryosurgery but may be treated equally well with the CO_2 laser. Disadvantages with this therapeutic approach are the need to use local anesthesia and the possibility of scarring through excessive vaporization depth. Advantages are the precision obtainable with the CO_2 laser and that complete removal can be achieved predictably in a single treatment session. The CO_2 laser offers a distinct advantage with its ability to vaporize a large surface area and multiple lesions rapidly in a single treatment session, as discussed later. To avoid scarring, it is important to pay attention to the cleavage plane induced by heat at the dermal-epidermal junction.[52]

Excisional surgery

The third area of potential benefit from use of the CO_2 laser is in excisional surgery, particularly some forms of cosmetic surgery. Numerous cosmetic surgeons perform blepharoplasty, mammoplasty, and "face-lift" surgery with the CO_2 laser as an incisional instrument because of its ability to control bleeding, swelling, and postoperative pain.[159]

Laser blepharoplasty was first described in 1984.[160] A study published in 1987 compared its use with cold steel surgery in 10 patients and found the CO_2 laser superior.[161] Details of surgical approach[162] and safety factors[163] were published soon thereafter. A second comparative study in 1990[164] found cold steel and CO_2

laser techniques to be comparable, with no specific benefits attributable to the CO_2 laser. A third study compared CO_2 laser surgery on one side and cold steel with electrocautery on the opposite side of 10 patients having both upper and lower blepharoplasty.[165] The authors found that the CO_2 laser provided superior surgical visibility and significantly faster operative time because of the bloodless field, as well as less bruising, swelling, and discomfort postoperatively with faster healing. An international survey of 16 physicians performing more than 4000 blepharoplasties and comparing cold steel with CO_2 laser technique found laser blepharoplasty to be faster (average 58 versus 94 minutes) and the laser patients' recovery time to be faster (average 6.3 versus 9.1 days) with less bruising, swelling, and pain.[166]

The use of the UPCO_2 laser for these cosmetic procedures is strongly recommended to achieve a char-free incision that will not interfere with wound healing. The physician needs to be not only an experienced cosmetic surgeon but also an experienced laser surgeon to combine these two fields of surgical expertise.

Lesions for which CO_2 Laser Offers Distinct Advantages

Epidermal tumors

The first area in which the CO_2 laser offers a distinct clinical advantage is in the vaporization of multiple and large epidermal tumors and low-grade superficial cutaneous malignancies that are large in surface area or are located in strategic locations that pose significant surgical problems. The development of the UltraPulse CO_2 laser has made this application particularly useful because of its decreased tendency to induce a disfiguring scar from unwanted thermal damage.

Seborrheic keratoses. Removal of large and thick seborrheic keratoses of the face, scalp, and torso has been particularly successful (Figure 6-21). The most common method of destruction of these lesions is by the use of liquid nitrogen cryosurgery. This generally requires multiple treatment sessions and often results in healing with unsightly hypopigmented scars. The pigment-targeted lasers have been used for these lesions very successfully but require multiple treatment sessions for thick lesions (see Chapter 3). This application of the CO_2 laser is particularly useful in combination with a facial chemical peel.

Multiple lesions of the torso are particularly bothersome to some patients, not only because of their cosmetic detriment, but also because of their tendency to become inflamed, irritated, and pruritic. Literally hundreds of lesions may exist, and treatment of more than 200 lesions in a single session is easily accomplished with use of the CO_2 laser. When we examined the results of treatment of 32 patients having 690 seborrheic keratoses, we found that all lesions were removed in a single surgical session.[42] However, 25% of patients treated with a CW CO_2 laser healed with at least one flat atrophic scar among the lesions treated, and 8.3% of 180 lesions healed with atrophic scarring. When the superpulse mode was used, the incidence of scarring was very similar: 25% of patients with at least one scar and 11.2% of 510 lesions treated. No hypertrophic scars were seen in either group. In contrast to lentigines and ephelides, the cosmetic significance of these atrophic scars may be different, even though they are very similar in appearance.

The cosmetic results achieved with CO_2 laser treatment of seborrheic keratoses are superior to the original lesion, as well as superior to the results obtained by other treatment modalities, with the possible exception of multiple treatment sessions with the new pigment-targeted lasers. In contrast, the results achievable with the pigment-targeted lasers in treatment of ephelides and lentigines are superior in their complete avoidance of scarring (see Chapter 3). The use of the UltraPulse CO_2 laser in treating seborrheic keratoses of the torso and face has allowed removal of multiple lesions virtually scar free because of the enhanced ability to control thermal damage below the lesion (Figures 6-22 and 6-23).

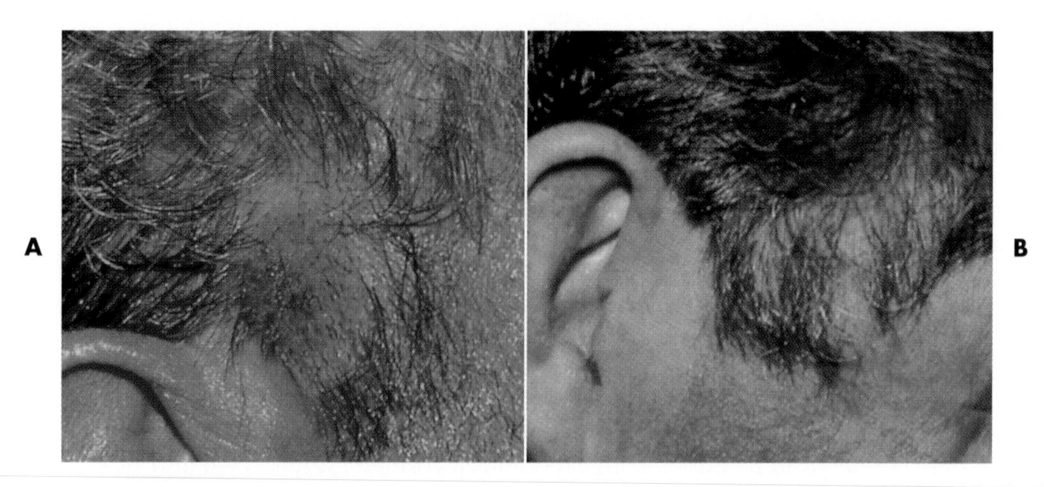

Figure 6-21 **A,** Large, thick, inflamed seborrheic keratosis in scalp just anterior to ear in 45-year-old man. **B,** Six months later, lesion is completely resolved after single treatment with superpulsed CO_2 laser (12 W, 200 μsec, 250 Hz). Note complete preservation of hair in the area treated.

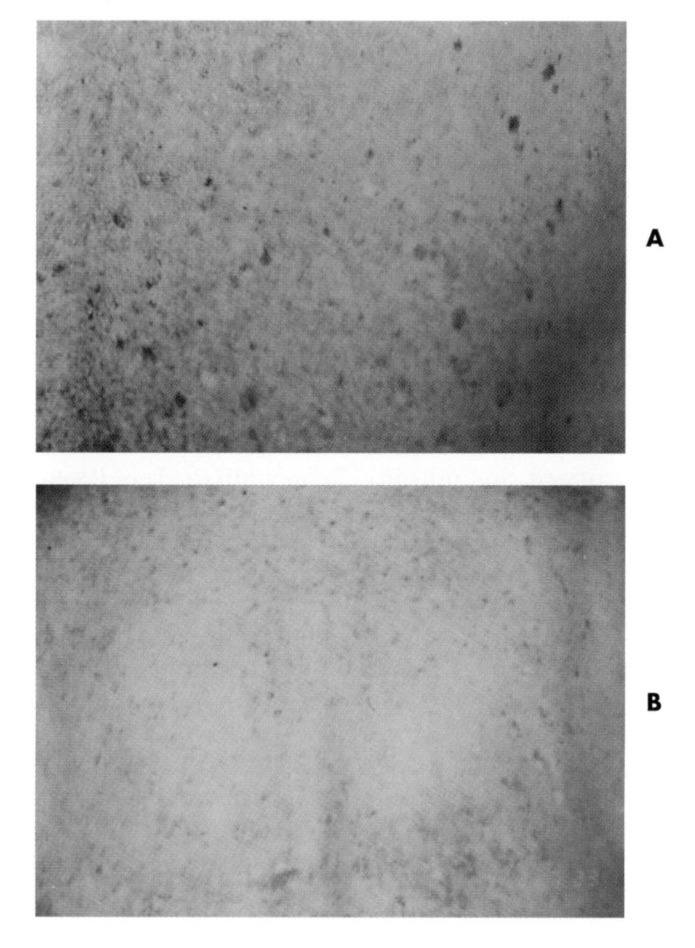

Figure 6-22 **A,** Numerous seborrheic keratoses on back of 68-year-old woman. **B,** Six months after vaporization of the larger lesions using $UPCO_2$ laser (4-10 Watts, 250 mJ/pulse, 40 Hz, 690 μsec), no scars or pigment alterations have resulted from surgery.

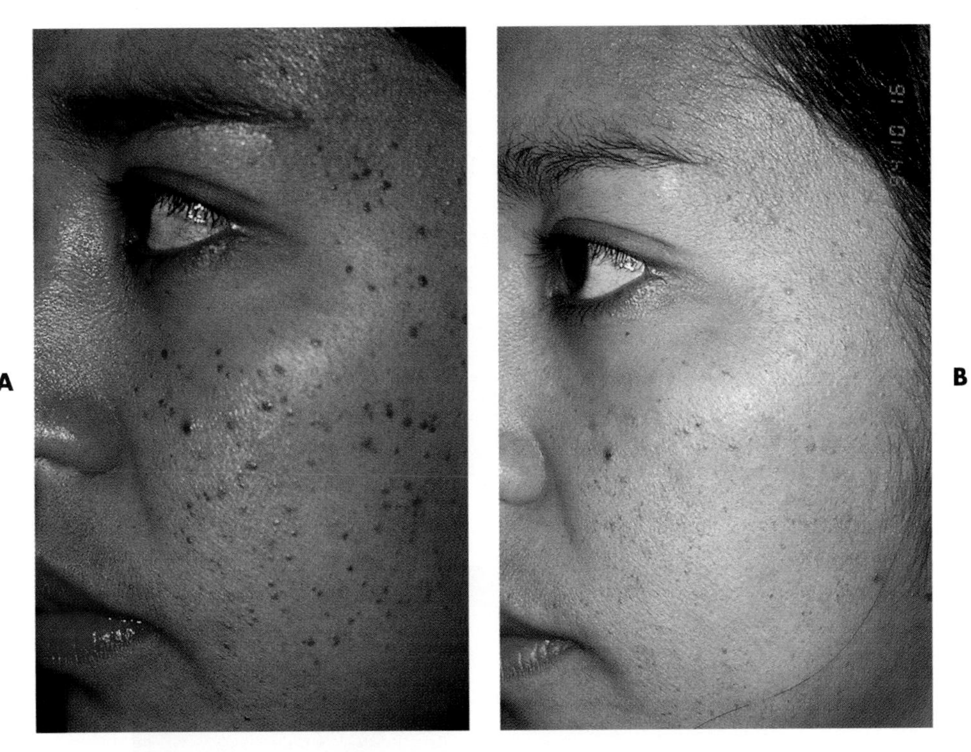

Figure 6-23 **A,** Young Philippino woman with dermatosis papulosa nigra before treatment. **B,** Nine months after one treatment with UPCO_2 laser using 0.05-sec pulse at 500 J/cm^2 with 3-mm-diameter spot size. Each lesion was vaporized with 2 to 4 pulses. After each laser pulse, charred tissue was wiped clean with normal saline.

Warts. In treatment of multiple, large, and recalcitrant warts, particularly periungual warts, plantar warts, and condylomata acuminata, the CO_2 laser has proved to be advantageous because of the precision of vaporization and the capability of full treatment in a single session. Cure rates of 32% to 96% have been reported.[42,167-174] All commonly used destructive treatment modalities, including various acids, electrocautery, liquid nitrogen cryosurgery, and intralesional bleomycin, result in imprecise tissue destruction and cure rates of 45% to 84%.[175] This imprecision may result in a high incidence of scarring or inadequate treatment with lesion recurrence.

The precise vaporization achievable with the CO_2 laser allows destruction of lesional tissue with much greater accuracy and improved clinical results. Because wart virus has been demonstrated in normal perilesional epidermis as far away from the clinical wart as 1 cm, and because this latent virus is considered the source of many recurrences,[176] consideration can be given to selective ablation of the adjacent epidermis without risk of dermal necrosis in this area by controlled use of the CO_2 laser. This cannot be achieved with other modalities typically used for treatment of warts without adding a significant risk of scarring or prolonged healing. Successful treatment generally involves vaporizing a perilesional border of 1 to 5 mm of what appears to be normal[39,167-170,177] (Figure 6-24).

The use of the CO_2 laser as an initial therapeutic modality in treatment of warts in general and plantar warts in particular has resulted in cure rates of 81%,[172,173] 94.7%,[170] and 96.3%.[171] Treatment of condylomata in 119 men with the CO_2 laser resulted in complete clearance of lesions with a recurrence rate of only 9.2% over 14 weeks postoperatively. Five of these 11 recurrences were at sites unconnected to the original treatment site.[168] Successful treatment of urethral condylomata without adverse sequelae has been reported as well.[39]

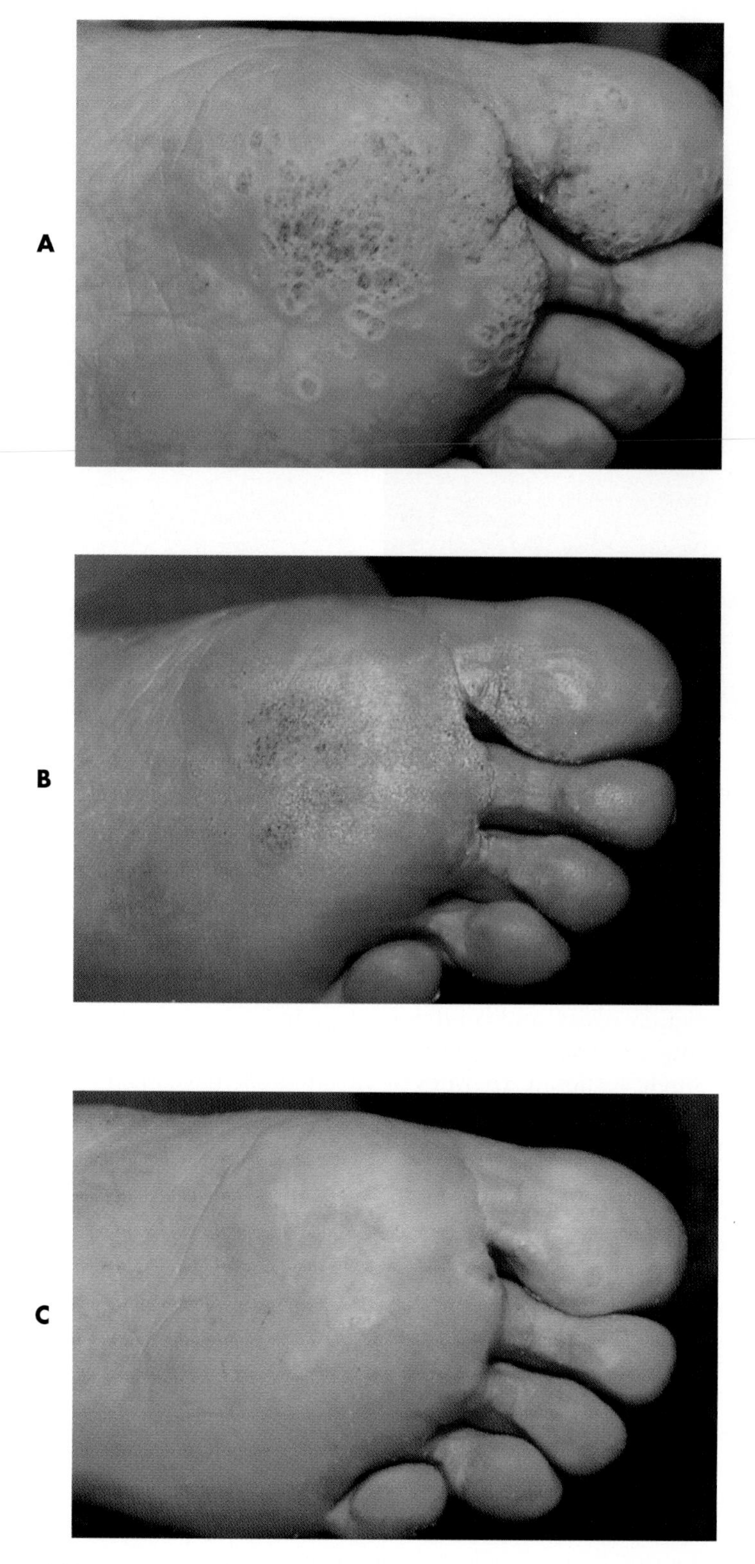

Figure 6-24 **A,** Extensive verruca vulgaris and plantaris in 14-year-old girl. **B,** One year after CO_2 laser vaporization with Coherent Ambulase laser used as continuous focused wave at 14 W with 2.5-mm spot size. Note only partial resolution. **C,** Three months after treatment with $UPCO_2$ laser at fluence of 250 mJ between 5 and 8 W using continuous mode with 2-mm spot size. Note complete resolution of verruca vulgaris and plantaris.

The most difficult group of patients are those who have failed multiple prior therapies using one or more modalities, particularly when the lesions are periungual in location. Reports of use of the CO_2 laser on these most difficult patients show cure rates of 32%,[169] 81%,[177] and 71%.[167] Because of the need for aggressive therapy, scarring occurred in 50% of one group,[174] and changes in the nail were noted in 29% of a second group.[167] This cure rate is far superior to that reported with the use of any other modality at present.

Several points should be emphasized concerning treatment of verrucae with the CO_2 laser. The use of magnification during the procedure to observe tissue characteristics is strongly recommended.[171,174,178] Wart tissue typically bubbles on laser impact, whereas normal tissue has fingerprint lines, or dermatoglyphs, and appears to contract with laser impact (Figure 6-25). Attention to these details will aid in identifying the endpoint of treatment.

Before using the laser, it is best to remove the dry, hyperkeratotic surface tissue. This proteinaceous debris requires much higher energy to vaporize because of its low water content and has a greater tendency to act as a heat sink, with resultant thermal diffusion. This tissue is easily removed by paring to a bleeding point. After one sweeps the CO_2 beam across the surface of the wart one to three times, a cleavage plane will appear at the dermal-epidermal junction.[167,177] As mentioned previously, this is a result of this junction's greater propensity to react to thermal injury. The tissue can then be removed with scissors or a scalpel by gently lifting and trimming its peripheral connections. At this point the laser is used for focal vaporization of persistent wart tissue (Figure 6-26). In addition to these techniques, it should also be noted that periungual warts often extend beneath and around the nail plate. The CO_2 laser is used to vaporize the overlying nail, thus avoiding nail avulsion. The underlying verrucae are then treated as described (Figure 6-27).

We examined the results of treatment of 46 patients having 300 warts, using the CW CO_2 laser, the superpulsed CO_2 laser, and the ultrapulsed CO_2 laser. Eighty-five percent of these patients had been treated with other modalities and had recurrences of their lesions. As the control of thermal damage was progressively increased by use of lasers with more appropriate parameters, we were capable of more precise

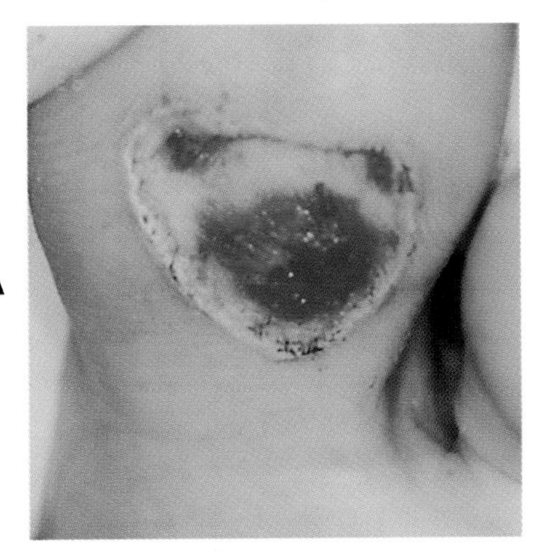

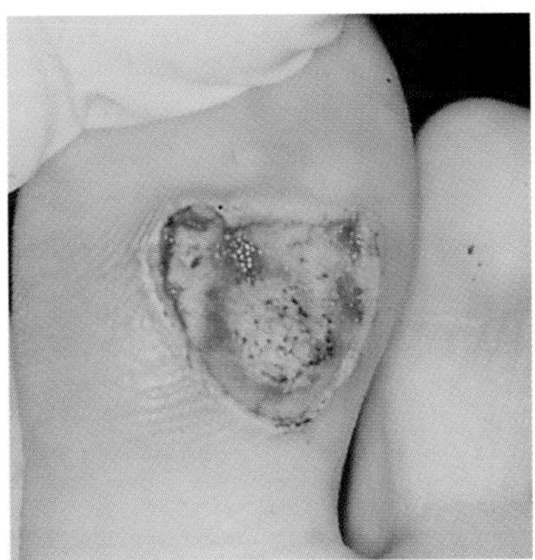

Figure 6-25 **A,** Large wart on plantar surface of great toe immediately after wart has been stripped off at dermal-epidermal juncture. In center of lesion is remaining wart tissue, surrounded by healthy, normal dermis. **B,** After second pass with $UPCO_2$ laser (8 W, 40 Hz, 693 μsec), dermis is seen to contract inward with a yellow color and texture similar to chamois cloth, while central wart tissue bubbles and vaporizes. This tissue should now be wiped clean with saline and any residual wart vaporized until entire base of lesion has a uniform appearance.

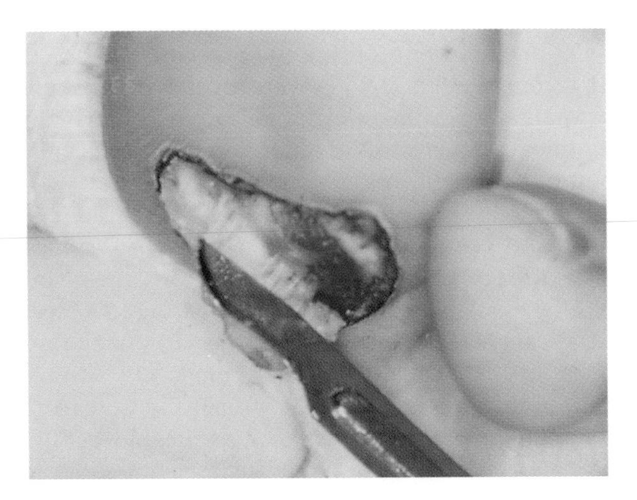

Figure 6-26 After sweeping CO_2 beam across surface of wart, vaporizing outer portion, a cleavage plane will appear at dermal-epidermal juncture. This tissue can then be removed by trimming the peripheral connections and gently lifting away wart tissue. After this has been accomplished, any remaining wart tissue can then be vaporized, as in Figure 6-24.

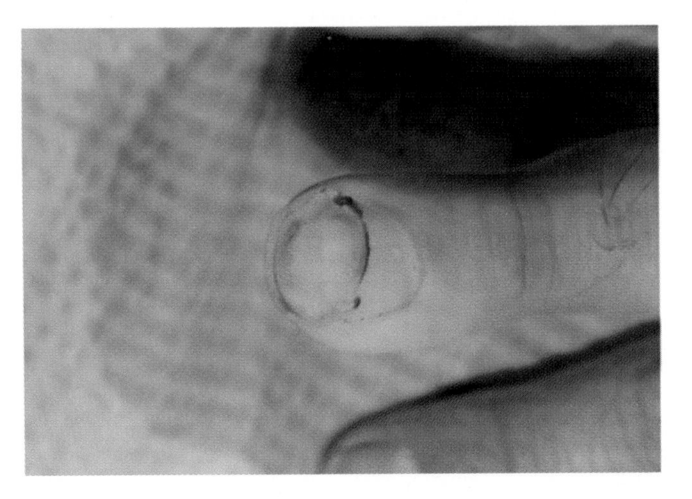

Figure 6-27 Verruca vulgaris of right third finger of 40-year-old man after treatment with $UPCO_2$ laser at 250 mJ and 5 W in continuous mode. After three passes, entire wart has been vaporized. Note preservation of remaining nail.

lesional vaporization with decreased residual thermal damage. This is reflected in the increasing cure rate and decreasing scar rate as we moved from CW to superpulsed to ultrapulsed lasers. The CW mode had a 68% success rate and a 54% incidence of scarring; the superpulse group had a 68% success rate and 33% incidence of scarring; and the ultrapulse group had a 90% success rate and 7% incidence of scarring (Table 6-2).

Removal of periungual warts without causing onychodystrophy and removal of plantar warts and condylomata in a single procedure are definite clinical advantages. The Candela flashlamp-pumped pulsed dye laser (FLPDL) laser may be appropriate for some of these lesions (see Chapter 2). However, multiple treatments are usually necessary, and thick lesions may be difficult to treat.

When a wart or any other tissue is vaporized by the CO_2 laser, a plume of smoke develops, consisting of steam and particulate matter from the vaporized tissue. These particles are usually minuscule, having mean diameters of 0.1 to 0.3 μm.[179] Viability of infectious organisms in the plume was demonstrated in 1986, when it was found that bacterial spores could survive in the plume at irradiances below 500 W/cm^2.[180] However, this same study and another[181] have shown that, in general, particularly with high irradiances, the CO_2 laser sterilizes and devitalizes exposed tissue. Although intact cells are rendered nonviable in the laser plume, the potential still exists for intact virions or viral DNA, both of which may be infectious, in the laser plume.[182] Although naked viral DNA can be infectious,[183-185] *virions* represent a much greater theoretic hazard because their specific infectivity is several orders of magnitude higher.[186]

Concern has arisen from reports detecting both viral DNA[182,186,187] and virions[186] of *papillomavirus* in laser plumes of vaporized warts from patients and animal models using both pulsed and CW CO_2 laser irradiation at both high and low irradiances. These reports and others[188-190] are consistent with the probability of finding viral DNA in laser plumes being related to both the concentration of virus in the lesion and the effects of subsurface tissue explosions forcefully ejecting nonaerosolized particles into the plume.[188] Whether these particles are potentially infectious cannot be answered definitively, because the current lack of a reproducible in vitro infectivity assay for human papillomavirus (HPV) particles makes this assessment virtually impossible to perform. However, a sensitive assay does exist for bovine papillomavirus, and infectious papillomavirus has been cultured from the CO_2 laser plume after vaporization of bovine warts.[186] A study of tissue specimen of condylomata acuminata charred with a CO_2 laser revealed that in 10 of 12 specimens (83%), **HPV DNA** was found.[191] Natural transmission of HPV during a laser procedure has not been demonstrated to date. However, the risks do exist and can be minimized with attention to the following facts:

1. Of all clinical wart types containing HPV type 1, *plantar warts* appear to be the richest in viral particles.[189-196]
2. The major risk of development of HPV infection from inhalation occurs with treatment of *genital warts* because types 6 and 11 are found in both genital warts and respiratory papillomatosis.[194,196-199] Warts generally are not highly contagious, and adults are usually fairly resistant to infection, except for genital warts that are sexually transmitted. In contrast to warts on the extremities, genital warts typically have low numbers of viral particles.[186]
3. The most important precaution is the diligent use of a *smoke evacuation system.* It has been shown that smoke evacuators with a volume capacity of 40 cubic feet per minute (CFM) and the capacity to filter particles greater than 0.1 μm will remove 99% of plume particulate matter if the nozzle is held within 1 cm of the treatment site.[199,200] However, this efficiency rapidly falls to 50% when the nozzle orifice is moved to just 2 cm from the treatment site.[201]

4. *Surgical masks* have been shown to filter aerosolized viral particles effectively.[186] The masks used effectively filtered 99.7% of particles 0.5 to 5 μm in diameter. Because papillomavirus virions are only 55 nm in diameter, one would not expect them to be filtered. Because these very small particles were filtered as well, however, it is thought that the charged microfiber web of the mask used (3M Company) may serve as an electrostatic filter to entrap the smallest particles. The mask must fit tightly to minimize airflow around the mask edges.

The presence of HPV viral particles in the laser plume raises the question of the potential for exposure to aerosolized, potentially infectious particles from patients infected with hepatitis virus or human immunodeficiency virus (HIV).

One study has shown the presence of HIV viral DNA in the laser plume from vaporization of concentrated tissue culture pellets infected with HIV.[179] However, the experimental tissue pellets used contained viral concentrations about 1 million times higher than that normally encountered in infected human blood, and the aerosolized virus did not survive longer than 2 weeks.[201] A separate study demonstrated that the plume from vaporization of concentrated simian immunodeficiency virus–infected cells yielded negative cultures for an 8-week incubation period.[202]

It would be wise to consider the plume of smoke from CO_2 laser vaporization to be infectious for viral diseases and to exercise the appropriate precautionary techniques mentioned to minimize the risk of contact with potentially infectious particles.

Squamous cell carcinoma (SCC) in situ. Vaporization of SCC in situ by use of the CO_2 laser may be particularly advantageous when the lesions are large, multifocal, or poorly defined and gradually blending in with a field of sun-damaged skin and actinic keratoses. This is basically a resurfacing procedure in which the sun-damaged surface of actinic keratoses and SCC in situ is vaporized to the papillary dermis and then allowed to heal by secondary intention (Figure 6-28). Vaporized sites should be examined closely with magnification to determine that all abnormal tissue is removed. Treatment may be combined with trichloroacetic acid (TCA) to peel the surrounding field of actinic keratoses at the same time. This combined approach

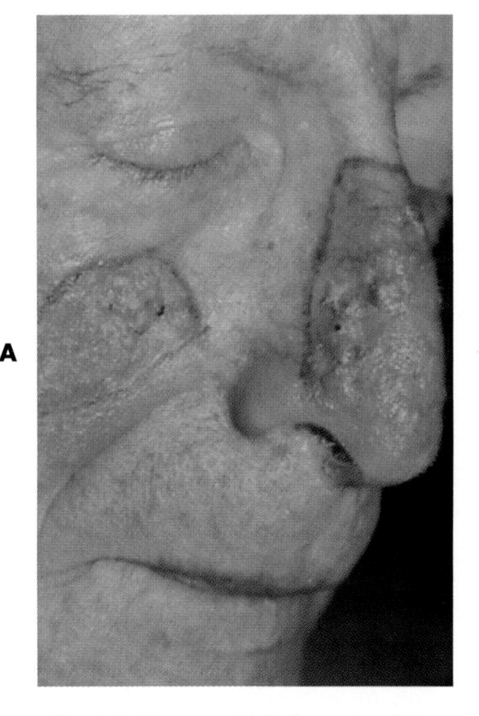

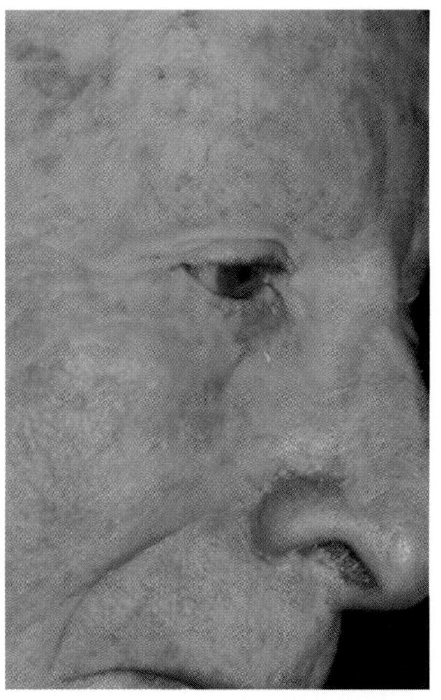

Figure 6-28 **A,** Multiple hypertrophic actinic keratoses and squamous cell carcinoma in situ (per biopsy evaluation) involving right cheek and nose of 83-year-old man. **B,** Six months after vaporization with superpulsed CO_2 laser (12 W, 250 Hz, 200 μsec), complete resolution of lesions without recurrence.

(CO_2 laser plus TCA peel) is especially beneficial in treatment of multiple, large, and recurrent actinic keratoses of the bald scalp when the entire scalp and forehead are involved. Alternatively, the entire scalp may be resurfaced with the pulsed CO_2 laser (see Chapter 7).

The CO_2 laser is particularly useful when the lesion is located in a difficult surgical area, such as the tip of the nose or the upper lip (Figure 6-29). This same surgical

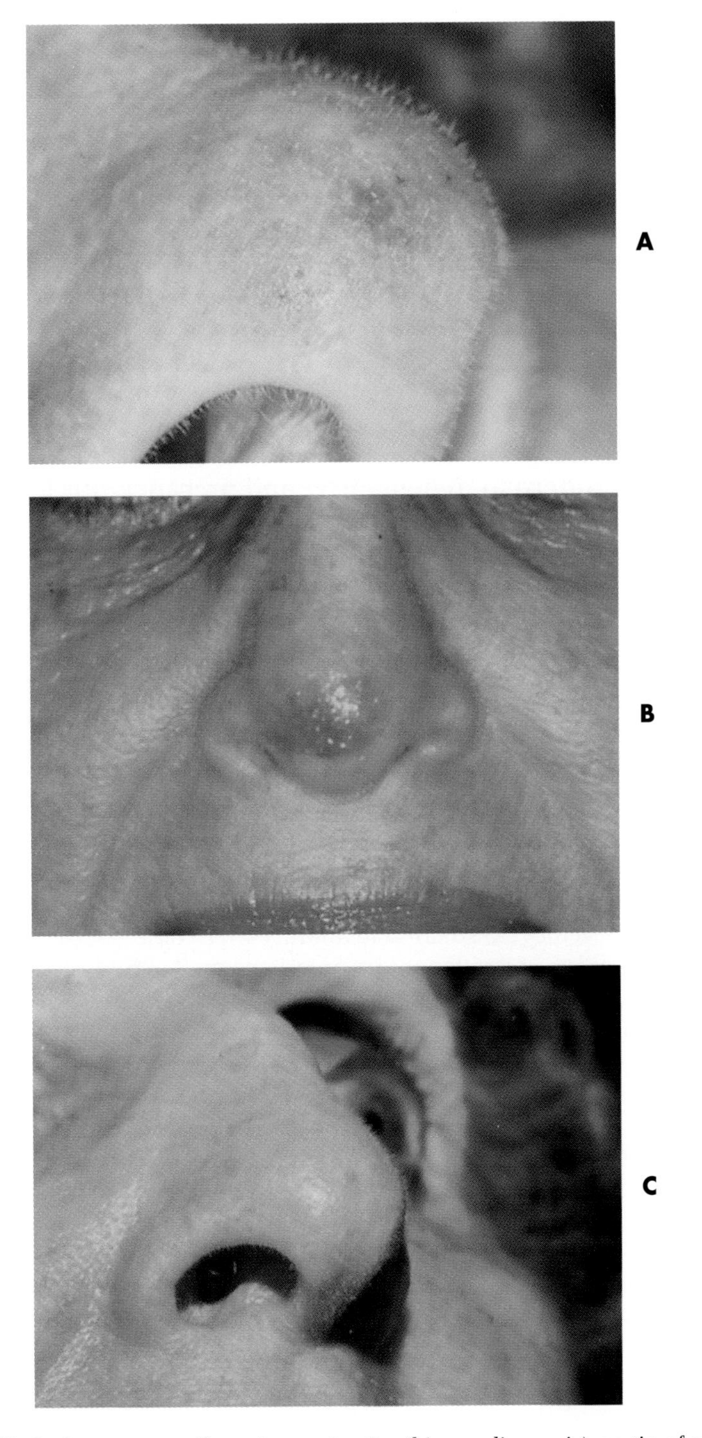

Figure 6-29 **A,** Squamous cell carcinoma in situ (biopsy diagnosis) on tip of nose of 67-year-old woman. **B,** One week after vaporization with UPCO_2 laser (250 mJ, 4 W, 702 μsec, 20 Hz, 2-mm-diameter spot size), superficial crust has developed over healing wound. **C,** Four months later, no sign of lesion and no scarring or pigment changes.

technique has been used to great advantage in the management of premalignant and noninvasive malignant lesions of SCC of the penis.[203] Three reports describe treatment of erythroplasia of Queyrat using the CO_2 laser.[204-206] The CO_2 laser has been combined with the neodymium:yttrium-aluminum-garnet (Nd:YAG) laser for more invasive penile lesions.[207-211] Recurrence rates have been equally as good (16% versus 17.6%) as those obtained by partial penectomy but have avoided the surgical mutilation.[212] Malek[203] found no recurrences of 22 superficial lesions treated with lasers after 2 years' follow-up.

Intraepithelial carcinoma of the vulva has been treated with the CO_2 laser as well. Two large series reported eradication rates of 91%[213] and 94%.[214] In both trials, however, repeated treatment sessions were used to eliminate untreated foci of recurrence at the borders of the lesion. Using a pulsed CO_2 laser would allow safe treatment of a wider margin around the visible lesion and eliminate the need for multiple treatment sessions.

Successful CO_2 laser treatment of *Bowen disease* of the vulva[215] and of the finger[216] has been reported. Effective treatment of precancerous lesions, such as porokeratosis of Mirbelli, has been reported with the CO_2 laser as well.[217-220]

The use of the CO_2 laser has also been advocated for cancerous and precancerous lesions of the oral cavity.[221-225] No significant advantage appears to exist with CO_2 laser treatment of cancerous lesions of the oral cavity, but obliteration of precancerous lesions may result in a lower recurrence rate.[221,222]

Other intraepidermal malignancies and precancerous lesions. The treatment of choice of *lentigo maligna* (melanoma in situ) is complete but conservative excision. However, some lesions may not be easily excised because of their large size and difficult surgical location, potentially resulting in considerable deformity. In these situations, topical treatment with 15% acetic acid or 5% fluorouracil,[226,227] radiation treatment,[228] electrodesiccation and curettage, dermabrasion, cryosurgery,[226] and argon laser treatment[229] have all been reported with variable success. Recurrences with these methods are attributed to atypical melanocytes along the adnexal epithelium not being destroyed. A recent series of four patients treated with the CO_2 laser showed them all to be free of recurrences with a mean follow-up of 15 months.[230]

Treatment of extramammary *Paget disease* has been reported with CO_2 laser vaporization of tissue fluorescing with δ-aminolevulinic acid (ALA) and Wood's light illumination.[231] Extramammary Paget disease typically occurs in the genital, axillary, or perianal areas. When lesions are widespread in these locations, surgical excision may not be easily achieved, so laser ablation is a welcome alternative.

Treatment of other premalignant or superficial malignant lesions in difficult surgical sites (e.g., penis, nose and upper lip, oral mucosa) can be accomplished with the same benefits using the CO_2 laser. These lesions include balanitis xerotica obliterans, lichen sclerosus,[232-236] bowenoid papulosis, oral florid papillomatosis, and sublingual keratosis. Lupus pernio of the face has also been treated by CO_2 laser ablation in order to avoid complex surgical repairs of the involved areas.[237]

Superficial basal cell carcinoma (BCC). CO_2 laser vaporization of large-circumference, superficial, multifocal BCC of the torso, scalp, and extremities may be very useful as well, particularly when the patient has multiple lesions or is elderly. We often obtain a superficial shave biopsy at the base of any skin cancer that has been treated if there is any question of surgical clearance of the lesion. It is important to assess the depth and aggressiveness of the lesion by biopsy before treatment. This technique may be combined with curettage in the same manner that electrodesiccation is used with curettage to remove BCC. Wheeland et al[238] reported the results of treatment of 370 superficial BCCs in 52 patients. No recurrence was seen after a mean follow-up of 20 months. A 5% incidence of hypertrophic scarring was noted.

Superficial multifocal BCC and BCCs on the extremities are rarely associated with aggressive growth characteristics[238-240] or tumor recurrence.[241] Because of the large size and multiple numbers of these lesions, a variety of nonexcisional surgical approaches to treatment have been used, including curettage and electrodesiccation,[242-245] cryosurgery,[246,247] and nonsurgical treatments of radiation therapy,[248] topical 5-fluorouracil,[249] and oral retinoids.[250] A previous report of vaporization of BCCs without attention to assessing the wound for complete tumor removal revealed a recurrence rate (or residual tumor rate) of 50% and emphasizes the need to use proper technique in treatment of BCC.[251]

The UltraPulse CO_2 laser is preferable for this procedure with a power of 5 to 10 W and beam size of 2 to 3 mm. It should be swept across the lesion's surface. This layer is then wiped clean with saline-soaked gauze, and the tissue is closely examined for residual BCC, which is visible as translucent whitish tissue that can be very friable and bleeds easily. A curet may be used at this point if desired. The residual BCC is then vaporized until normal dermis is encountered. Most of these lesions are very superficial.

We have reported the results of treatment of 15 patients having SCC in situ of the nose, upper lip, and cheeks, as well as 12 patients having large, multifocal BCC.[252] All lesions were clinically clear after follow-up periods of 6 to 18 months, and scarring was minimal, particularly with facial lesions of SCC in situ. All patients were treated with the UltraPulse CO_2 laser.

The advantages of using the CO_2 laser in such cases are the rapid operative time and avoidance of scarring and extensive and complex excisional surgery. The CO_2 laser allows excellent visualization of the wound because of the bloodless field and minimizes nonspecific thermal injury to adjacent tissue, which results in minimal scarring and rapid wound healing.

Débridement of necrotic or infected tissue

The second area where the CO_2 laser offers a distinct advantage is in the vaporization of necrotic or infected tissue. This may prove most valuable in the *débridement of burns.* Although the CO_2 laser has been demonstrated to be capable of performing burn débridement without interfering with graft survival and with significant hemostasis and preservation of blood volume,[253-255] hemostasis has proved to be the only benefit of the CW CO_2 laser because the investigators have shown that 700-μm layer of residual thermal damage impedes graft survival.[79,100,256,257] The use of the CO_2 laser for this application has never gained clinical support for three reasons: (1) it is a cumbersome procedure; (2) the CW CO_2 lasers have generated conflicting data regarding wound healing and graft survival; and (3) it is a slow and tedious procedure if a large area is involved.

Work on burn débridement has been performed at Massachusetts General Hospital using a pulsed, transversally excited atmospheric pressure (TEA) CO_2 laser,[59,75,101] which is a very-high-power laser with a very short pulse (100 nsec) that controls thermal damage and allows use of a large spot size. This laser has been shown to be capable of removing necrotic burn tissue rapidly and with less than 100 μm of thermal damage. Such a small layer of damage heals in the same time as a dermatome wound and does not interfere with graft survival. The ability to vaporize necrotic burn tissue and immediately graft the areas would avoid many of the fluid loss, transfusion, and infection complications that are so frequently seen in patients with extensive burns. The CO_2 laser has been shown to be bactericidal at high fluences (50 J/cm^2).[255] Although the TEA CO_2 system is not clinically available at this time, the work in this area has been very encouraging. Work is also in progress to develop an intelligent scanning mechanism that would be able to differentiate necrotic skin from viable tissue in débridement of burns.

Treatment of *hidradenitis suppurativa* by abalation of the involved areas and healing by secondary intention has been reported as an effective and efficient treatment of this difficult disease.[259-261] Sterilization of the surgical field by CO_2 abalation is thought to be advantageous in this situation.

Control of bleeding

Another area of definite clinical advantage is the CO_2 laser's use as an *incisional instrument* in surgical procedures involving two specific circumstances. The first is related to *patient peculiarities:* those patients having pacemakers or monitoring devices in whom the use of electrical spark coagulation of bleeding vessels may interfere with pacemaker or monitoring function, those having intrinsic bleeding disorders or taking clinical anticoagulants or other medications having a side effect of prolonged bleeding, those in whom blood loss may be life threatening, and those in whom the use of epinephrine to control cutaneous bleeding is contraindicated. The second circumstance is related to *site peculiarities:* a tissue site that is particularly prone to bleeding because of the preponderance of vessels, such as the scalp and vascular tissues.

Angiomatous tumors. A definite clinical advantage with the CO_2 laser is in the vaporization of various angiolymphoid and angiofibromatous conditions. These lesions are characterized generally as being exophytic and having either a significant fibrous component that must be removed with the vascular component or such vascular bulk that treatment with the vascular-specific lasers may be difficult. This group includes adenoma sebaceum of tuberous sclerosis, angiokeratomas, pyogenic granulomas, lymphangioma circumscriptum,[262-264] and some venous lakes. These lesions generally respond to the use of the argon laser as well, but the CO_2 laser offers greater precision and more thorough therapy. The use of the CO_2 laser in treatment of *lymphangioma circumscriptum* has been particularly beneficial because of its ability to seal lymphatics and stop the persistent lymphatic drainage often associated with these lesions. It also allows the use of a more benign and controlled surgical procedure for treatment of superficial lesions, avoiding the need for surgical excision and the resultant cosmetic deformity from scarring (Figure 6-30).

Control of thermal damage

In this situation, tissue must be ablated, and avoiding thermal damage to the tissue is critical to surgical success. Electrocoagulation devices for control of bleeding are contraindicated because the surgery must be as atraumatic as possible. Primary examples are the excisional debulking of keloids and the excision of acne keloid. Although the initial articles on treatment of keloids alleged a therapeutic advantage in vaporization or excision of keloids by use of the CO_2 laser,[125,255] this has not withstood the test of time.[265] Keloids exhibit a proliferative capability that may be extremely aggressive and requires secondary treatment with an agent that will suppress that proliferative activity, that is, intralesional cortisone[266] or interferon[267,268] or intralesional fluorouracil. However, the capability of excising bulky lesions before use of these agents and without significant risk of aggravating the lesion is a significant benefit.

The extreme heat generated by the CO_2 laser sterilizes the operative field[258] and prevents further infectious processes. This latter point also justifies the use of the CO_2 laser in surgical excisions performed on infected tissue in general. Débridement of decubitus ulcers, exuberant granulation tissue, and various cutaneous infections (botryomycosis, leishmaniasis) and ablation of nails infected with dermatophytes has been successfully accomplished with the CO_2 laser.[43] In treatment of acne keloid or perifolliculitis capitis abscedens et suffodiens (both diseases of the occipital scalp of black males characterized by nodules, abscesses, sinus tracts, and scarring alopecia), the CO_2 laser is used to excise the involved area, which is left to heal by secondary intention.[269,270] Excellent healing without lesion recurrence has been reported. This is also true in the treatment of acne keloid[269] and perifolliculitis capitis abscedens et suffodiens.[270]

Treatment of axillary osmidrosis (bromhidrosis) by careful ablation of subcutaneous and deep dermal apocrine glands through an axillary incision has also been reported.[271]

Another situation in which this precise control of residual thermal damage may be significant clinically is the preparation of a site for epithelial sheet grafting in

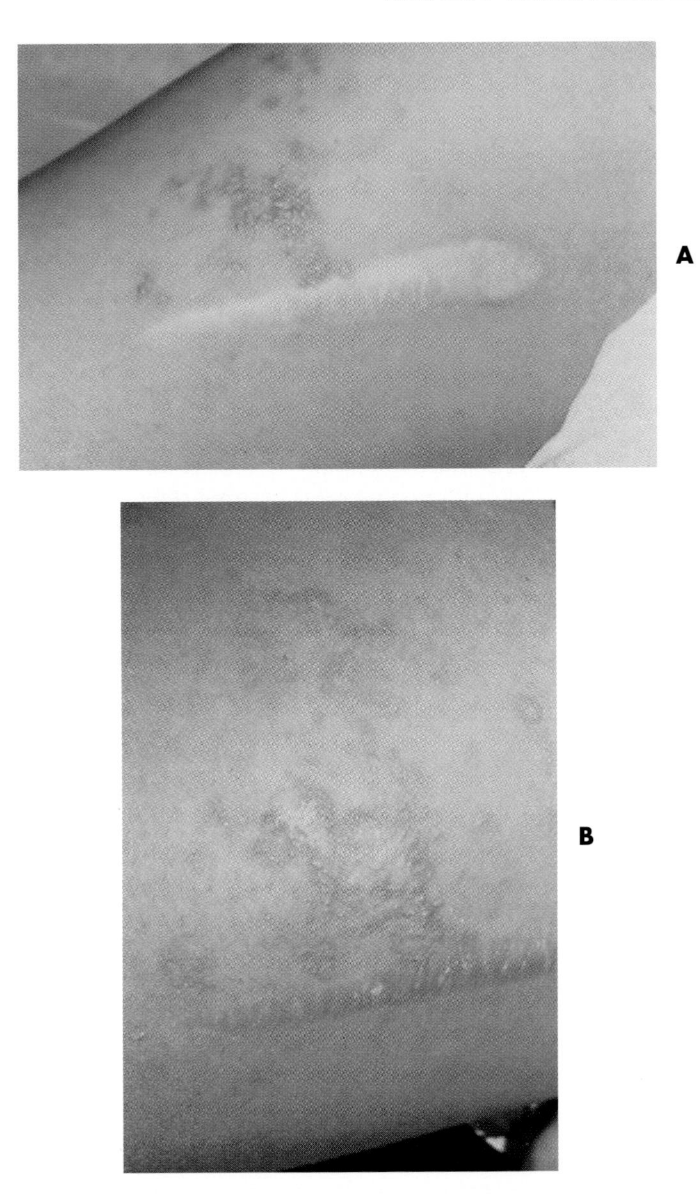

Figure 6-30 **A,** Patches of lymphangioma circumscriptum on thigh of 15-year-old girl. Adjacent scar is from excision of vascular hamartoma. **B,** Six months after vaporization of lesions with ultrapulsed CO_2 laser, some scarring has resulted from multiple treatment sessions.

treatment of vitiligo or depigmented scars.[272-274] Removal of the epithelium of the recipient site was performed with a short-pulsed (90-μsec) CO_2 laser, and a 90 μm ultrathin graft was placed over the recipient site. The thin layer of thermal necrosis (10-24 μm) did not interfere with graft survival.[272] This would be anticipated from Green et al's work[275] showing that laser-induced thermal necrosis greater than 160 μm $\pm$ 60 μm interferes with the skin graft take.

Lesions for which CO_2 Laser Is Potentially Treatment of Choice

Although lesions in this group may be treated with other therapeutic modalities, the CO_2 laser offers such significant benefit that it should always be the first consideration. Most of these lesions are best treated with the CO_2 laser because of the difficult surgical sites, the need for precision, and the control of bleeding and swelling. The CO_2 laser allows more aggressive local therapy and the ability to avoid excisional surgery.

Actinic cheilitis

The best example in this group is the treatment of actinic cheilitis. Although this condition has also been treated with excisional vermilionectomy,[276-280] liquid nitrogen cryosurgery,[280,281] and 5-fluorouracil,[282,283] the CO_2 laser offers the benefits of less scarring, shorter healing time, and less pain with a procedure that is both simpler and more effective. Again, however, the avoidance of thermal damage beneath the vaporized lesion is critical in achieving these goals.

Actinic cheilitis is a premalignant condition usually of the lower lip resembling chapping, but it is caused by chronic sun exposure associated with SCC. It is characterized by a variegated red and white, blotchy, and generally atrophic appearance with focal thickenings, flaking, crusting, and fissures (Figure 6-31). The vermilion border may be indistinct. SCC may be subtle in its development: three of six patient biopsy specimens with a diagnosis of actinic cheilitis showed histologic evidence of SCC in one series.[284] In addition, five of ten patients diagnosed clinically as having benign hyperkeratosis had histologic evidence of well-differentiated SCC. Thirteen patients having a clinical diagnosis of actinic cheilitis were studied with serial sections taken at 1-mm intervals. The investigators found 42 separate regions of dysplasia and 12 regions of carcinoma.[285]

Investigators estimate that SCC may result from actinic cheilitis after a latent period of 20 to 30 years, but this interval may vary.[286] In addition, a second SCC in a different site will develop in 5% to 14% of patients having SCC of the lip.[287-289] These studies and those of Slaughter et al[290] note the multicentric origin of actinic cheilitis and SCC of the lip and that the time of transition to malignancy may not be clinically apparent or predictable. This is a strong argument for removal of the entire surface of the vermilion of the lower lip to achieve effective therapy, not only to treat symptoms, but also to prevent the development of SCC. This is particularly important when considering that SCC of the lip metastasizes in approximately 11% of patients[290-292] in contrast to the rare occurrence of metastases from SCC of the skin arising in a previous actinic keratosis. All these facts underscore the importance of performing a biopsy on ulcerated or indurated lesions of actinic cheilitis.[293]

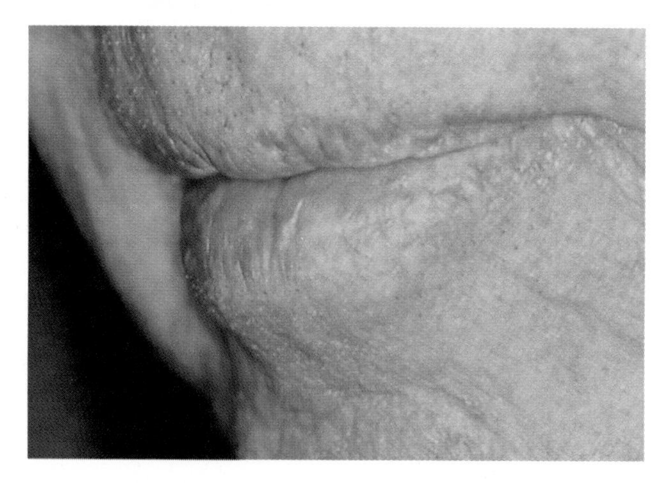

Figure 6-31 Severe actinic cheilitis involving both lower and upper lip of 57-year-old professional fisherman. Variegated red, brown, and white colors, generalized atrophic appearance with blurring of vermilion border, and focal thickenings are visible. This is a premalignant condition that may progress to squamous cell carcinoma.

Vermilionectomy with mucosal advancement was once considered the treatment of choice[294] because of its effectiveness combined with acceptable cosmetic results. However, the procedure causes considerable morbidity: 15.4% of patients experienced labial scar tension, 25% had paresthesias, 71.7% noted a prickling sensation caused by misaligned beard hairs, and 7.7% had visible scars.[278] Cryosurgery has produced unpredictable results,[295] and 5-fluorouracil treatment is difficult because of the prolonged therapeutic and healing time as well as the pain and discomfort involved.

A single case of CO_2 laser ablation vermilionectomy was reported in 1968,[296] but the procedure was not well accepted until after David's report[297] of successful treatment of eight cases with an average follow-up of 34 months in 1985. Since then, the results of treatment of 123 patients having average follow-up of 11 to 36 months have been reported.[295,298-301] Only two of these patients were found to have focal recurrences.

Healing time was reported to range from 3 to 8 weeks in these various studies but was more closely followed in one group with a reported mean of 98.5% reepithelialized at 4 weeks.[301] Scarring was not described in detail except in two studies. One reported one hypertrophic scar and two linear scars among 13 patients (23%),[294] and the second reported one hypertrophic scar (that gradually resolved) among 12 patients (8%).[301]

Minimal scarring is related to both proper wound care with avoidance of infection[294] and avoidance of thermal damage to the healing vermilion surface. As has been discussed, this can be achieved with proper pulse parameters and attention to details of laser-tissue interaction. A third factor is the depth of vaporization. Because of the variegated appearance of the vermilion surface and the potential for undiagnosed occult SCC, surgeons tend to vaporize the surface to a deeper level than necessary. Because actinic cheilitis is a purely epidermal process in an area devoid of hair follicles, superficial treatment that completely removes the epidermis should be adequate.[301]

The epidermis is vaporized by moving the laser spot (2-3-mm diameter) at 4 to 5 W across the skin surface at a speed of approximately 1 cm per second, resulting in whitening, bubbling, and vesiculation of the epidermis, which can then be wiped away with saline-soaked gauze. After this initial pass, two distinctive tissue qualities are visible. The majority of the tissue usually appears pink and pliable, whereas other areas are spotty gray, gray-white, or yellowish and appear fibrotic. It is usually recommended that these spots be vaporized to an endpoint of a cotton-white color, based on the presumption that they represent deeper actinic damage.[295,297,299] However, the significance of these tissue differences remains unknown. A recent study has provided evidence that these areas do not represent deeper involvement of actinic cheilitis and that vaporization at most to the papillary dermis should be adequate therapy for actinic cheilitis[301] and also should allow faster healing with avoidance of scarring.

Our patients having actinic cheilitis of the lower lip who were treated with a CW CO_2 laser required an average of 5.5 weeks to heal, and 44% healed with some degree of scarring visible. Those patients treated with a CW, rapid-pulse, low-fluence superpulsed laser required 4.5 weeks to heal and had a 33% incidence of scarring. Patients who were treated with the same superpulsed laser but with a secondary 50-msec shuttered pulse required only 2.5 weeks to heal and had a 6% incidence of scarring.[49] A final group was treated with the UltraPulse laser, which has more ideal pulse parameters. This group required an average of 13 days to heal, and none had scarring (Table 6-3). Those patients treated with the CW CO_2 laser and the CW rapid-pulse superpulsed CO_2 laser were treated without attention being focused on the avoidance of tissue charring (Figure 6-32). The focus of attention on this aspect of CO_2 laser surgery would be expected to improve overall results with the use of any type of CO_2 laser. The comparison of these four groups of patients offers a

Table 6-3
CO_2 laser treatment of actinic cheilitis

Laser	Pulse Width (μsec)	Repetition Rate (Hz)	Pulse Energy (mJ)	Power (W)	Beam Size (mm)	No. Patients	Healing Time (days)	Scar (%)
Continuous	N/A	N/A	N/A	5-10	2.5	17	37	44
Superpulse	200	250	32	4	2.5	18	30	33
Gated superpulse*	50	4	384	4	2.5	15	17	6
UltraPulse	600	20	250	5	2.5	20	13	0

N/A, Not available.
*Same superpulse laser as line above, used with 50-msec shuttered pulse.

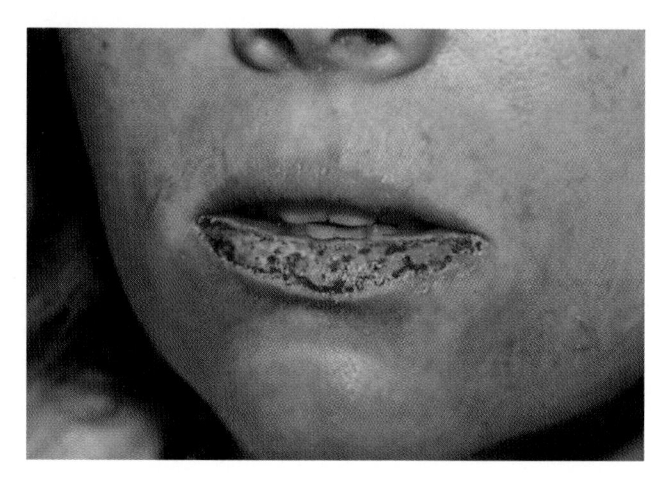

Figure 6-32 Charring of lower lip is apparent after treatment of actinic cheilitis using a continuous-wave (CW) CO_2 laser at 10 W.

valuable demonstration of the dramatic improvement in results that can be achieved by selection of proper pulse parameters and by attention to the details of clinical technique[49] (Figure 6-33).

Combinations of wedge excision simultaneously with CO_2 laser vermilionectomy have been reported as well.[302]

Eyeliner tattoo

Excision of unwanted eyeliner tattoo is a complex procedure because of the need to avoid damage to the eyelash follicles and prevent ectropion scarring. The use of the Q-switched lasers for removal of this tattoo can be accomplished in some cases, but it is awkward because the location is so near the eyelashes and lid margin, and multiple treatments are required. The extreme precision afforded by the use of the CO_2 laser allows vaporization of the aberrant tattoo without damage to the follicles or lid margin.[303] Healing is by secondary intention but results in a scar line that is clinically inapparent (see Chapter 4).

Rhinophyma

Treatment of rhinophyma has been accomplished by dermabrasion,[304-309] sculpting with a scalpel or razor blade[310-313] or a dermatome,[305,311,314,315] cryosurgery destruction,[315-319] and electrosurgical destruction,[305,306,316,317,320-322] as well as by the CO_2 laser.[320-333] Dermabrasion is generally a difficult procedure because of technical factors involved and often leaves incomplete results. The use of cryosurgery to obtain an even

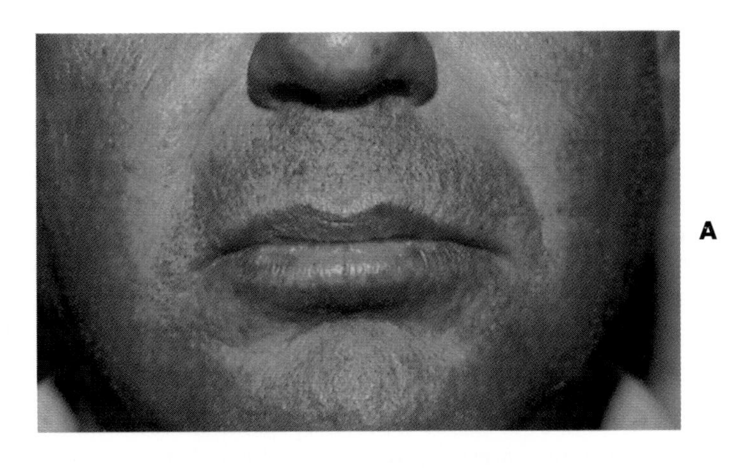

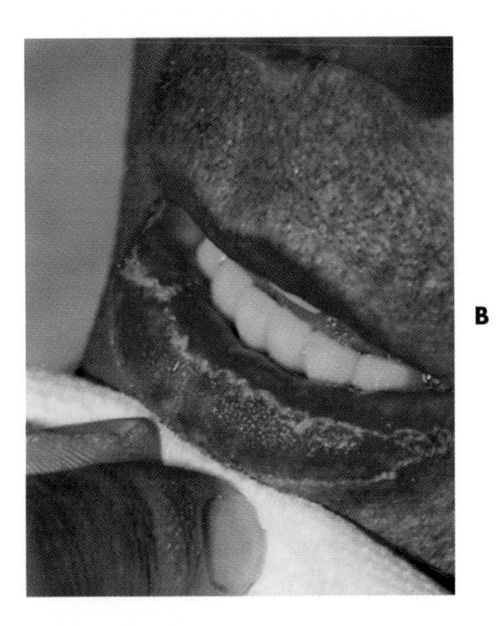

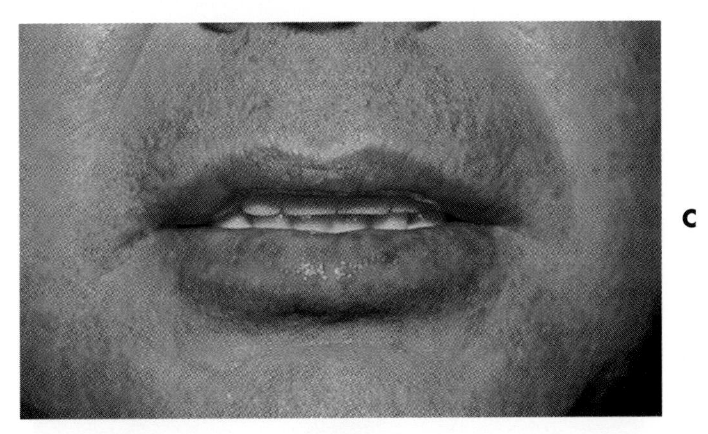

Figure 6-33 **A,** In 47-year-old man with 3-year history of chronic chapped lips, treatment over two 6-week periods with 5% 5-fluorouracil resulted in only limited improvement despite severe inflammatory reaction. **B,** Immediately after treatment with UPCO_2 laser at 250 mJ averaging 3 W. Vermilion surface was vaporized with overlapping 2.5-mm-diameter pulses and then wiped clear with saline, revealing a pink papillary dermis. **C,** Fourteen days after treatment; complete healing occurred within 10 days.

depth of tissue destruction is very difficult and often results in incomplete destruction and scarring or hypopigmentation. Use of a thermal scalpel and thermal destruction results in easier tissue removal but has a significant risk of scarring from heat conduction to deeper tissues. Sculpting with scalpels, razors, and dermatomes is fraught with significant bleeding, which requires excessive coagulation for hemostasis and compounds the difficulty of achieving a smooth tissue plane as an endpoint because of poor visualization and uneven tissue contouring and focal tissue destruction from electrocautery.

Use of the CO_2 laser is advantageous because of the greater precision and ease of tissue removal and the ability to sculpt the nasal contours hemostatically and precisely.[334] However, a definite risk of scarring exists from heat conduction when a CW CO_2 laser is used and tissue removal is taken to a deep level[328] (Figure 6-34). The UltraPulse CO_2 laser allows greater freedom in removal of bulky tissue with a decreased risk of scarring but does not completely eliminate this risk, and the surgeon must pay close attention to presentation of the oil gland structures (Figure 6-35).

The CO_2 laser is used with power settings of 5 to 20 W and can be used initially with a small spot size to excise excessive tissue before vaporization with use of a large spot size.* If the rhinophyma is mild to moderate, it is best to use vaporization only, but with a major rhinophyma, laser excision of excessive tissue before vaporization is helpful.[140,330] Tissue is vaporized methodically layer by layer until the desired level of recontouring is achieved. During vaporization the dermis contracts and causes expression of sebum from the sebaceous glands. This, as well as squeezing the nose and producing sebum extrusion, is a sign that intact sebaceous glands remain and that vaporization has not extended to a depth below these glands and will not result in healing with scarring.[333] Reepithelialization requires 2 to 4 weeks. In a study of 30 patients treated with a CW CO_2 laser, leukoderma, hypertrophic scarring, and alar retraction were each seen in one patient.[329] The most common complication was the presence of large dilated pores, representing exposure of the larger-diameter infundibulum and gland of the sebaceous follicle.

Epidermal nevi

Removal of linear epidermal nevi can be very difficult, and these lesions were virtually untreatable before the advent of the CO_2 laser.[335,336] Treatment by dermabrasion is almost invariably followed by lesion recurrence if the treatment is superficial

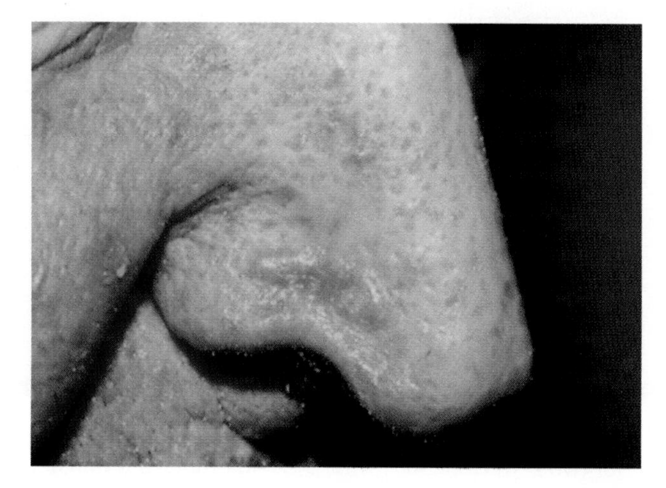

Figure 6-34 One year after treatment of rhinophyma with superpulsed CO_2 laser, retraction of nasal ala is visible. This has occurred because of thermal diffusion under vaporized tissue, resulting in damage to cartilage. Other than this location, results are excellent.

*References 25, 322, 326, 329, 331, 333.

or by scarring if the lesion is treated more aggressively. Excision of the lesions is usually not an option because of their size and location. Vaporization of these lesions with use of the CO_2 laser has been much more successful in prevention of both scarring and lesion recurrence. However, to avoid recurrence, it is necessary to ablate the lesion below the inferior tips of the rete pegs. This requires the use of magnification during surgery to visualize the depth of vaporization and extreme attention to detail to avoid scarring from deep ablation.

The degree of precision achievable with the CO_2 laser is not possible with other modalities, but a fine line exists between excellent results without lesion recurrence and ablating too deeply, resulting in healing with some degree of scarring. At times we have combined the use of the CO_2 laser with a pigment-targeted laser (e.g., the pigment lesion laser) in an effort to reduce further the risk of scarring. The CO_2 laser

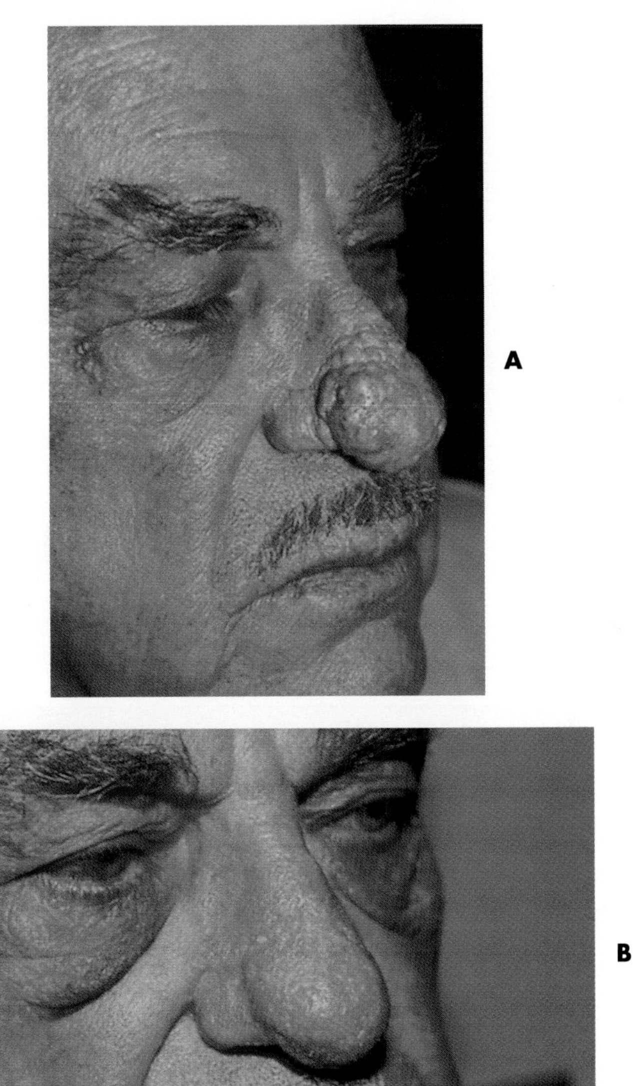

Figure 6-35 **A,** Long history of acne rosacea and multicystic rhinophyma in 67-year-old man. **B,** Three weeks after treatment with UltraPulse CO_2 laser using 10 to 20 W, 250 mJ/pulse, and 2.5-mm spot. Entire rhinophyma was sculpted to a smooth surface.

is used first to ablate all visual components of the lesion in a superficial manner. During the same operative session the area that has been treated with the CO_2 laser is again treated with high fluences (3.5-4.0 J/cm^2) of the pigment laser in hopes of selectively destroying any remaining epidermal cells without causing damage to the surrounding dermis. Our early results are encouraging, but long-term follow-up is necessary to evaluate the incidence of lesion recurrence (Figure 6-36).

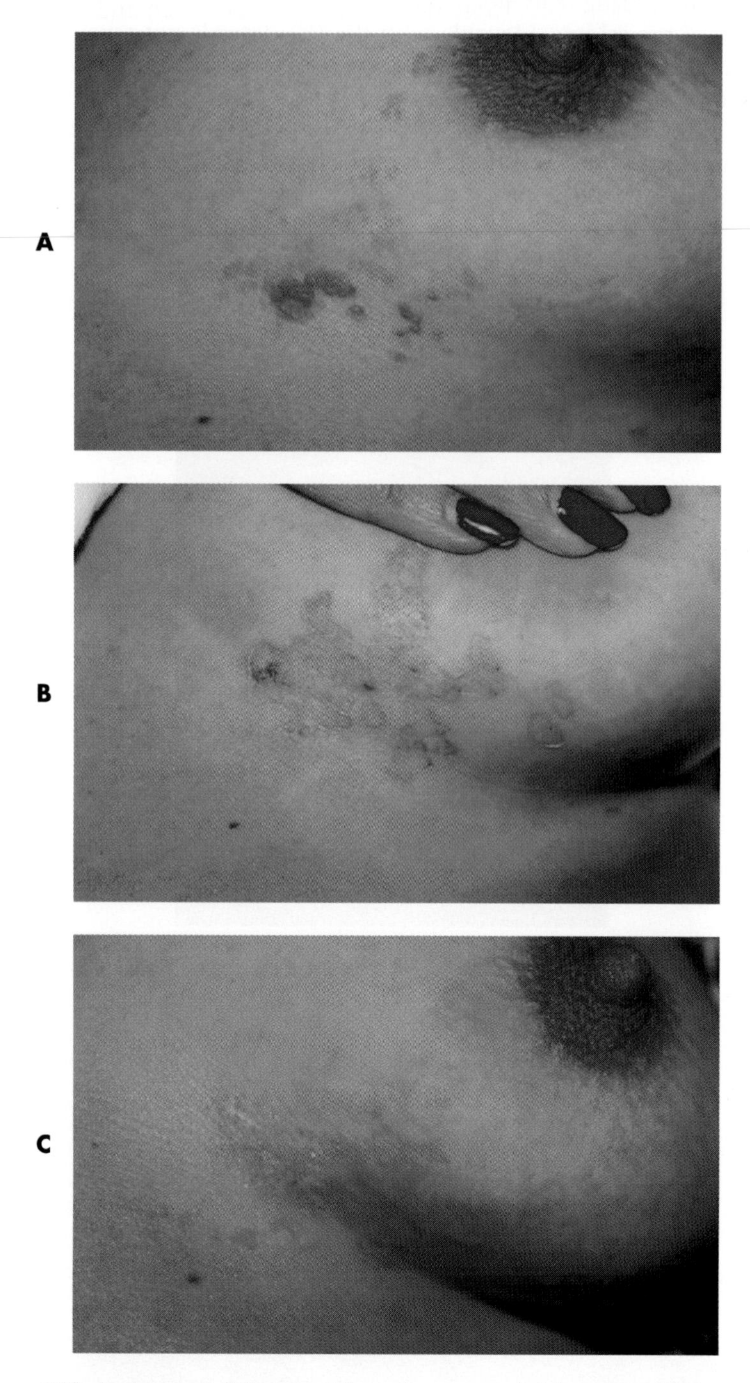

Figure 6-36 **A,** Congenital linear epidermal nevus on left breast and chest wall of 38-year-old woman. **B,** Immediately after treatment with UPCO_2 laser at fluence of 250 mJ and energy of 7 W. A 2-mm spot size was used in a continuous mode in multiple passes over lesion until clearance was obtained. DuoDerm dressing (Convatec, Princeton, NJ) was applied, with complete healing in 7 days. **C,** Ten weeks after treatment, complete resolution of nevus.

Benign dermal tumors

Another area where the CO_2 laser offers definite advantage is in vaporization of selected benign dermal tumors. These include neurofibromas,[337] granuloma faciale,[338] trichoepitheliomas, apocrine hydrocystomas, myxoid cysts, tricholemmomas of Cowden disease,[44] syringomas,[45,162] sebaceous hyperplasia, adenoma sebaceum of tuberous sclerosis,[46,163] syringocystadenoma papilliferum,[339] and chondrodermatitis nodularis chronica helicis.[340,341] These dermal tumors have been and still are treated by a variety of other surgical techniques, including excision and repair, shave excision, dermabrasion, cryosurgery, electrocautery, and argon, potassium titanyl phosphate, and Nd:YAG lasers, and with various acids and tretinoin (Retin-A). However, all these techniques have had one or more of the following disadvantages: scarring or surface textural change, cumbersome or slow surgical technique, lesion recurrence, and incomplete lesion removal.

The primary advantage of the CO_2 laser for removal of these lesions are the extreme precision afforded by the pulsed CO_2 laser, leaving minimal damage to adjacent normal tissue, and the ability to achieve microscopic control by magnified intraoperative visualization of the vaporized site. In addition, the speed of the treatment of multiple lesions, the bloodless field, and the diminished postoperative pain and swelling are definite advantages. As noted by Wheeland et al[46] and Apfelberg et al,[47] the use of the superpulsed CO_2 laser maximizes these benefits. In fact, with ultrapulsed CO_2 lasers, this is probably the treatment of choice for many of these conditions.

Cutaneous resurfacing procedures

The capability of the CO_2 laser to vaporize discrete cutaneous tumors precisely, as well as treat larger cutaneous surface areas of diseases such as psoriasis[342] and Hailey-Hailey disease[343] (Figure 6-37), with excellent cosmetic results has led to its use for various resurfacing procedures for cosmetic benefit.[344] The CO_2 laser may be used alone or in combination with TCA as a chemical peeling agent.

Focal and discrete irregularities such as punch grafts for acne scars,[345-347] chickenpox scars,[346] hypertrophic scars,[346,348] and full-thickness grafts[348] have been reported to respond with excellent cosmetic results to CO_2 laser vaporization, particularly with the superpulse mode.[347] The limited ability to obtain a uniform and smooth depth of vaporization over large areas has discouraged the use of the CW CO_2 laser alone as a facial resurfacing method for cosmetic purposes. The use of a computer-assisted scanning device with a CW CO_2 laser to achieve this goal has been reported[349] but was not regarded as generally useful[347,348] because of its tendency to create an unnatural, well-circumscribed depression. The development of the pulsed CO_2 lasers has revolutionized this procedure and has resulted in laser resurfacing to be the treatment of choice for resurfacing photodamaged skin for medical and cosmetic benefit (see Chapter 7).

Other superficial lesions

Another area where the pulsed CO_2 laser may offer distinctive clinical advantage is in treatment of various diseases limited to the superficial dermis and epidermis in difficult surgical locations. Hailey-Hailey disease,[343,350] lichen sclerosus et atrophicus, xanthelasma,[47,351,352] Zoon balanitis (erythroplasia),[353] balanitis xerotica obliterans,[233,234] lichen planus of the penis,[354] and oral florid papillomatosis[178] and psoriasis[342] have all been reported to be successfully treated with the CO_2 laser. These conditions are primarily on the genitalia, eyelids, and intertriginous surfaces, and the advantages of the CO_2 laser are related to the surgical difficulties imposed by the anatomic location, with the exception of psoriasis. *Psoriasis* is not generally treated by surgical means, but the vaporization of chronic plaques of psoriasis has been reported to achieve long-lasting results.[342,355] This may be secondary to obliteration of the abnormal epidermis and papillary dermis. Use of the CO_2 laser for

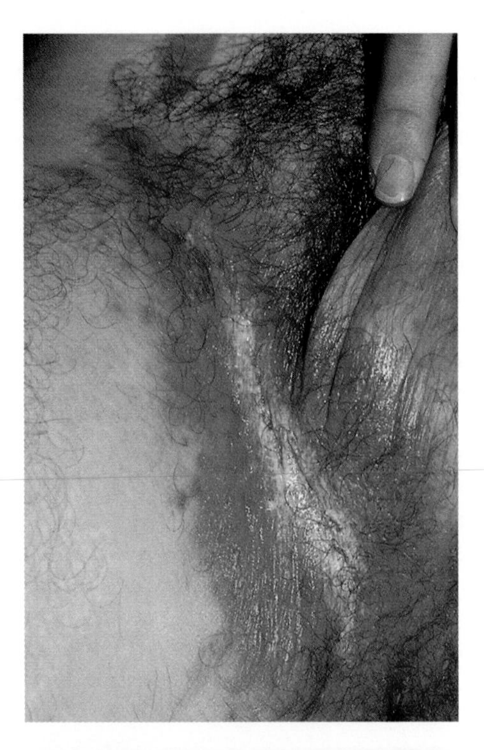

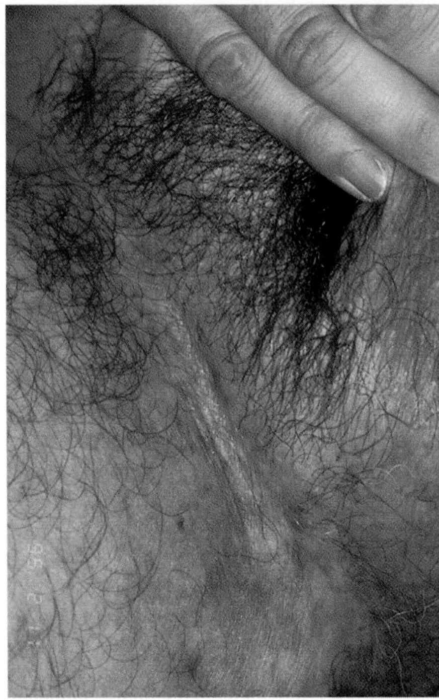

Figure 6-37 Hailey-Hailey disease in 50-year-old-male recalcitrant to topical therapy with corticosteroids and retinoids. **A,** Appearance before treatment. **B,** Five years after one treatment with UltraPulse CO_2 laser, which vaporized entire lesion to papillary dermis (Figure 6-14). Lesion has maintained remission in all treated areas.

psoriasis is limited, however, and does present the possibility of healing with scarring, so it should be approached cautiously until further data are generated.

Use of the CO_2 laser for the other conditions just listed has been reported to be extremely efficacious, and for the most part, other treatments have not been successful enough to be considered a treatment of choice. In each of these conditions the CO_2

laser therapy has been shown to result in long-term, possibly permanent control of a condition that has had no generally satisfactory treatment. Further use of the CO_2 laser in treatment of these diseases has resulted in the recommendation that this treatment modality be the treatment of choice, particularly with ultrapulsed CO_2 lasers.

REFERENCES

1. Goldman L: Laser treatment of melanoma. In Goldman L, editor: *Laser cancer research,* New York, 1966, Springer-Verlag.
2. Goldman L, Rockwell RJ Jr: *Lasers in medicine,* New York, 1971, Gordon & Breach.
3. Goldman L: The laser in the current cancer program, *Ann NY Acad Sci* 267:324, 1976.
4. Goldman L: Laser surgery in skin cancer, *NY State J Med* 77:1897, 1977.
5. Goldman L: Surgery by laser for malignant melanoma, *J Dermatol Surg Oncol* 5:141, 1979.
6. Stellar S, Polanyi TG: Lasers in neurosurgery: a historical overview, *J Clin Laser Med Surg* 10:399, 1992.
7. Polanyi TG, Bredemeier HC, Davis TJ Jr: *CO_2 laser for surgical research and medical and biological engineering,* New York, 1970, Pergamon.
8. Polanyi TG: Laser physics, *Otolaryngol Clin North Am* 16:753, 1983.
9. Aschler P, Ingolitsch E, Walter G et al: Ultrastructural findings in CNS tissue with CO_2 laser. In Kaplan I, editor: *Laser surgery II,* Jerusalem, 1976, Academic Press.
10. Ben-Bassat M, Ben-Bassat J, Kaplan I: An ultrastructural study of the cut edges of skin and mucous membrane specimens excised by carbon dioxide laser. In Kaplan I, editor: *Laser surgery,* Jerusalem, 1976, Academic Press.
11. Hall RR: Haemostatic incisions of the liver: CO_2 laser compared with surgical diathermy, *Br J Surg* 58:538, 1971.
12. Fidler JP, Hoefer RW, Polanri TG et al: Laser surgery in exsanguinating liver injury, *Surg Forum* 23:350, 1972.
13. Kirschner RA: Cutaneous plastic surgery with the CO_2 laser, *Surg Clin North Am* 64:871, 1984.
14. Slutzki S, Shafir R, Bornstein LA: Use of the carbon dioxide laser for large excisions with minimal blood loss, *Plast Reconstr Surg* 60:250, 1977.
15. Lyons GD, Lousteau RJ, Mouney DF: CO_2 laser as a clinical tool in otolaryngology, *Laryngology* 87:689, 1977.
16. Bellina JH: Gynecology and the laser, *Contemp Obstet Gynecol* 4:24, 1974.
17. Kaplan I, Goldman J, Ger R: The treatment of erosions of the uterine cervix by means of the CO_2 laser, *Obstet Gynecol* 41:795, 1973.
18. Goldman L et al: CO_2 laser surgery for cancer of man, *Laser J* 3:21, 1971.
19. Kaplan I, Sharon U, Ger R: The carbon dioxide laser in clinical surgery. In Wolbarsht M, editor: *Laser applications in medicine and biology,* vol 2, New York, 1974, Plenum.
20. Gamaleja NF, Polischuk EI: The experience of skin tumour treatment with laser radiation, *Panminerva Med* 17:238, 1975.
21. Kaplan I, Sharon V: Current laser surgery, *Ann NY Acad Sci* 267:249, 1976.
22. Stellar S, Ger R, Levine M et al: CO_2 laser for excision of burn eschars, *Lancet* 1:945, 1971.
23. Stellar S, Levine N, Ger R et al: Laser excision of acute third-degree burns followed by immediate autograft replacement: an experimental study in the pig, *J Trauma* 13:45, 1973.
24. Stellar S, Meijer R, Walia et al: Carbon dioxide laser débridement of decubitus ulcers followed by immediate rotation flap or skin graft closure, *Ann Surg* 79:230, 1974.
25. Goldman L, Perry E, Stefanovsky D: A flexible sealed tube transverse radio frequency excited carbon dioxide laser for dermatologic surgery, *Lasers Surg Med* 2:317, 1983.
26. Labandter H, Kaplan I: Experience with a “continuous” laser in the treatment of suitable cutaneous conditions: preliminary report, *J Dermatol Surg Oncol* 3:527, 1977.
27. Kaplan I, Peled I: The CO_2 laser in the treatment of superficial telangiectases, *Br J Plast Surg* 28:214, 1975.
28. Kaplan I, Labandter H: Onychogryphosis treated with the CO_2 surgical laser, *Br J Plast Surg* 29:102, 1976.
29. Friedman M, Gal D: Keloid scars as a result of CO_2 laser for molluscum contagiosum, *Obstet Gynecol* 70:394, 1987.
30. Shapshay SM, Rebeiz EE, Bohigian RK et al: Benign lesions of the larynx: should the laser be used? *Laryngoscope* 100:953, 1990.

31. Lanzafame RJ, Naim JO, Rogers DW et al: Comparison of continuous-wave, chop-wave, and super-pulse laser wounds, *Lasers Surg Med* 8:119, 1988.
32. Hobbs ER, Bailin PL, Wheeland RG et al: Superpulsed lasers: minimizing thermal damage with short duration, high irradiance pulses, *J Dermatol Surg Oncol* 13:955, 1987.
33. Kamat BR, Carney JM, Arndt KA et al: Cutaneous tissue repair following CO_2 laser irradiation, *J Invest Dermatol* 87:268, 1986.
34. Walsh JT, Hruza GJ, Flotte TF et al: Comparison of tissue ablation using TEA CO_2 and Er:YAG laser. In *Technical Digest Conference on Lasers and Electro-Optics,* Washington, DC, 1987, Optical Society of America.
35. Wright VC, Riopelle MA: *Laser physics for surgeons: the carbon dioxide laser,* Houston, 1982, Biomedical Communications.
36. Ben-Barucg G, Fidler JP, Wessler T et al: Comparison of wound healing between chopped mode-superpulse mode CO_2 laser and steel knife incision, *Lasers Surg Med* 8:596, 1988.
37. Baggish MS, Mohamed ME: Comparison of electronically superpulsed and continuous-wave CO_2 laser on the rate of uterine horn, *Fertil Steril* 45:120, 1986.
38. Rattner NH, Rosenberg SK, Fuller T: Difference between cutaneous wave and superpulse CO_2 laser in bladder surgery, *Urology* 13:264, 1979.
39. Rosenberg SK, Fuller T, Jacobs H: Rapid superpulse carbon dioxide laser treatment of urethral condylomata, *Urology* 2:149, 1981.
40. Fitzpatrick RE, Ruiz-Esparza J, Goldman MP: The depth of thermal necrosis using the CO_2 laser: a comparison of the superpulsed mode and conventional mode, *J Dermatol Surg Oncol* 17:340, 1991.
41. Fitzpatrick RE, Ruiz-Esparza J, Goldman MP: The clinical advantage of the superpulse carbon dioxide laser, *Lasers Surg Med Suppl* 2:52, 1990.
42. Fitzpatrick RE, Goldman MP, Ruiz-Esparza J: Clinical advantage of the CO_2 laser superpulsed mode: treatment of verruca vulgaris, seborrheic keratoses, lentigines and actinic cheilitis, *J Dermatol Surg Oncol* 20:449, 1994.
43. Olbricht SM: Use of the carbon dioxide laser in dermatologic surgery: a clinically relevant update for 1993, *J Dermatol Surg Oncol* 19:364, 1993.
44. Wheeland RG, McGillis ST: Cowden's disease—treatment of cutaneous lesions using carbon dioxide laser vaporization: a comparison of conventional and superpulsed techniques, *J Dermatol Surg Oncol* 15:1055, 1989.
45. Apfelberg DB, Maser MR, Lash H et al: Superpulse CO_2 laser treatment of facial syringomata, *Lasers Surg Med* 7:533, 1987.
46. Wheeland RG, Bailin PL, Kantor GR et al: Treatment of adenoma sebaceum with carbon dioxide laser vaporization, *J Dermatol Surg Oncol* 11:861, 1985.
47. Apfelberg DB, Maser MR, Lash H et al: Treatment of xanthelasma palpebrarum with the carbon dioxide laser, *J Dermatol Surg Oncol* 13:149, 1987.
48. Fitzpatrick RE: The ultrapulse CO_2 laser: selective photothermolysis of epidermal tumors, *Lasers Surg Med Suppl* 5:56, 1993.
49. Fitzpatrick RE, Ruiz-Esparza J: The superpulsed CO_2 laser. In Roenigk RK, Roenigk H, editors: *New trends in dermatologic surgery,* London, 1993, Martin Dunitz.
50. Hallock GG, Rice DC: In utero fetal surgery using a milliwatt carbon dioxide laser, *Lasers Surg Med* 9:482, 1989.
51. Dover JS, Smoller BR, Stern RS et al: Low-fluence carbon dioxide laser irradiation of lentigines, *Arch Dermatol* 124:1219, 1988.
52. Kamat BR, Tang SV, Arndt KA et al: Low-fluence CO_2 laser irradiation: selective epidermal damage to human skin, *J Invest Dermatol* 85:274, 1985.
53. Benedict LM, Cohen B: Treatment of Peutz-Jeghers lentigines with the carbon dioxide laser, *J Dermatol Surg Oncol* 17:954, 1991.
54. Dobry MM, Padilla RS, Pennino RP et al: Carbon dioxide laser vaporization: relationship of scar formation to power density, *J Invest Dermatol* 93:75, 1989.
55. Fisher JC: A short glossary of laser terminology for physicians and surgeons, *J Clin Laser Med Surg* 10:345, 1991.
56. Absten GT: Laser biophysics for the physician. In Ratz JL, editor: *Lasers in cutaneous medicine and surgery,* Chicago, 1986, Mosby.
57. Zweig AD, Meierhofer B, Muller OM et al: Lateral thermal damage along pulsed laser incisions, *Lasers Surg Med* 10:262, 1990.

58. Walsh JT, Flotte TJ, Anderson RR et al: Pulsed CO_2 laser tissue ablation: effect of tissue type and pulse duration on thermal damage, *Lasers Surg Med* 8:108, 1988.
59. Green HA, Domankevitz Y, Nishioka NS: Pulsed carbon dioxide laser ablation of burned skin: in vitro and in vivo analysis, *Lasers Surg Med* 10:476, 1990.
60. Reid R: Physical and surgical principles governing carbon dioxide laser surgery on the skin, *Dermatol Clin* 9:297, 1991.
61. Allwood MC, Russell AD: Thermally induced changes in the physical properties of *Staphylococcus aureus, J Appl Bacteriol* 32:68, 1969.
62. Wood TH, Roberts ER: Exchange of nitrogen between carboxypeptidase and labelled substrates, *Biochem Biophys Acta* 15:217, 1954.
63. Allwood MC, Russell AD: Mechanisms of thermal injury in nonsporulating bacteria, *Adv Appl Microbiol* 12:89, 1970.
64. Razin S, Arganon M: Lysis of microplasma, bacterial protoplasts, spheroplasts and L-forms by various agents, *J Gen Microbiol* 30:155, 1963.
65. Glover JL, Bendick PJ, Link WJ: The use of thermal knives in surgery: electrosurgery, lasers, plasma scalpel. In Ravitch M, editor: *Current problems in surgery,* Chicago, 1978, Mosby.
66. Trost MD, Zacherl RN, Smith MFW: Surgical laser properties and their tissue interaction. In Smith MFW, McElveen JT Jr, editors: *Neurological surgery of the ear,* St Louis, 1992, Mosby.
67. Henriques FC, Moritz AR: Studies of thermal injury. I. The conduction of heat to and through skin and the temperatures attained therein: a theoretical and experimental investigation, *Am J Pathol* 23:531, 1947.
68. Moritz AR, Henriques FC: Studies of thermal injury. II. The relative importance of time and surface temperatures in the causation of cutaneous burns, *Am J Pathol* 23:695, 1947.
69. Allwood MC, Russell AD: Thermally induced changes in the physical properties of *Staphylococcus aureus, J Appl Bacteriol* 32:68, 1969.
70. McKenzie AL: A three-zone model of soft-tissue damage by a CO_2 laser, *Phys Med Biol* 31:967, 1986.
71. Schomacker KT, Walsh JT, Flotte TJ et al: Thermal damage produced by high-irradiance continuous wave CO_2 laser cutting of tissue, *Lasers Surg Med* 10:74, 1990.
72. Fuller TA: Laser tissue interaction: the influence of power density. In Baggish MS, editor: *Basic and advanced laser surgery in gynecology,* East Norwalk, Conn, 1985, Century-Crofts.
73. Mage G, Pouly JL, Bruhat MA: Laser microsurgery of the oviducts. In Baggish MS, editor: *Basic and advanced laser surgery in gynecology,* Norwalk, Conn, 1985, Century-Crofts.
74. McKenzie AL: How far does thermal damage extend beneath the surface of CO_2 laser incisions? *Phys Med Biol* 28:905, 1983.
75. Green HA, Burd E, Nishioka NS et al: Middermal wound healing: a comparison between dermatomal excision and pulsed carbon dioxide laser ablation, *Arch Dermatol* 128:639, 1992.
76. Hall RR: The healing of tissues incised by a carbon-dioxide laser, *Br J Surg* 58:222, 1971.
77. Stellar S: The carbon dioxide surgical laser in neurological surgery, decubitus ulcers and burns, *Lasers Surg Med* 1:15, 1980.
78. Gillis TM, Strong MS: Surgical lasers and soft tissue interactions, *Otolaryngol Clin North Am* 16:775, 1983.
79. Willscher MK, Filoso AM, Jako GJ et al: Development of a carbon dioxide laser cystoscope, *Laser Surg Med* 1:183, 1980.
80. McKensie AL: How far does thermal damage extend beneath the surface of CO_2 laser incision? *Phys Med Biol* 28:905, 1983.
81. Beucker JW, Ratz JL, Richfield DF: Histology of port wine stain treated with carbon dioxide laser: a preliminary report, *J Am Acad Dermatol* 10:1014, 1984.
82. Tang SV, Kamat B, Ardnt KA et al: Low energy density CO_2 laser irradiation causes intraepidermal damage, *Lasers Surg Med* 3:329, 1984 (abstract).
83. Flemming AFS, Frame JD, Dhillon R: Skin-edge necrosis in irradiated tissue after carbon dioxide laser excision of tumor, *Laser Med Sci* 1:263, 1986.
84. Hambley R, Hebda PA, Abell E et al: Wound healing of skin incisions produced by ultrasonically vibrating knife, scalpel, electrosurgery, and carbon dioxide laser, *J Dermatol Surg Oncol* 14:1213, 1988.

85. Rainoldi R, Candiani P, Virgilis G et al: Connective tissue regeneration after laser CO_2 therapy, *Int Surg* 68:167, 1983.
86. Montgomery TC, Sharp JB, Bellina JH et al: Comparative gross and histological study of the effects of scalpel, electric knife, and carbon dioxide laser on skin and uterine incisions in dogs, *Lasers Surg Med* 3:9, 1983.
87. Gamaleya NF: Biomedical research in the USSR. In Wolbarsht ML, editor: *Laser applications in medicine and biology,* vol 3, New York, 1974, Plenum.
88. Mihashi S, Jako GJ, Incze J et al: Laser surgery in otolaryngology: interaction of CO_2 laser and soft tissue, *Ann NY Acad Sci* 267:263, 1976.
89. Hall RR, Hill DW, Beach AD: A carbon dioxide surgical laser, *Ann R Coll Surg Engl* 48:181, 1971.
90. Madden JE, Eslich RF, Custer JR et al: Studies in the management of the contaminated wound, *Am J Surg* 119:222, 1970.
91. Fisher SE, Grame JIW, Browne RM et al: A comparative histological study of wound healing following CO_2 laser and conventional surgical excision of canine buccal mucosa, *Arch Oral Biol* 28:287, 1983.
92. Kaplan L, Ger R: The carbon dioxide laser in clinical surgery, *Isr J Med Sci* 9:79, 1973.
93. Hishimoto K, Rockwell JR, Epstein RA et al: Laser wound healing compared with other surgical modalities, *Burns* 1:13, 1973.
94. Moreno RA, Hebda PA, Zitelli JA et al: Epidermal cell outgrowth from CO_2 laser- and scalpel-cut explants: implications for wound healing, *J Dermatol Surg Oncol* 10:863, 1984.
95. Rainoldi R, Candiani P, Virgilis G et al: Connective tissue regeneration after CO_2 laser therapy, *Int Surg* 68:167, 1983.
96. Fox JL: The use of laser radiation as a surgical "light knife" source, *J Surg Res* 9:199, 1969.
97. Buell BR, Schuller DE: Comparison of tensile strength in CO_2 laser and scalpel skin incisions, *Arch Otolaryngol* 109:465, 1983.
98. Cochrane JPS, Beacon JP, Creasey GH et al: Wound healing after laser surgery: an experimental study, *Br J Surg* 67:740, 1980.
99. Norris CW, Mullarky MB: Experimental skin incision made with the carbon dioxide laser, *Laryngoscope* 92:416, 1982.
100. Fry TL, Gerbe RW, Botros SB et al: Effects of laser, scalpel and electrosurgical excision on wound contracture and graft "take," *Plast Reconstr Surg* 65:729, 1980.
101. Green HA, Burd E, Nishioka NS et al: Skin graft take and healing after CO_2 laser and 193 nm excimer laser ablation of graft beds, *J Invest Dermatol* 92:436, 1989 (abstract).
102. Fidler JP, Bendick PJ, Glover JH et al: Effects of CO_2 laser on wound healing and infection, *Lasers Surg Med* 3:109, 1983 (abstract).
103. Badawy SZA, Mohamed EM, Baggish MS: Comparative study of continuous and pulsed CO_2 laser on tissue healing and fertility outcome in tubal anastomosis, *Fertil Steril* 47:843, 1987.
104. Chan P, Vincent JW, Wagemann RT: Accelerated healing of carbon dioxide laser burns in rats treated with composite polyurethane dressing, *Arch Dermatol* 123:1042, 1987.
105. Falanga V, Zitelli JA, Eaglstein WH: Wound healing, *J Am Acad Dermatol* 19:559, 1988.
106. Fidler JP: Techniques of laser burn surgery. In Goldman L, editor: *The biomedical laser: technology and clinical applications,* New York, 1981, Springer-Verlag.
107. Walsh JT, Deutsh TF: Pulsed CO_2 laser ablation: measurement of the ablation rate, *Lasers Surg Med* 8:264, 1988.
108. Van Gemert MJC, Welch AJ: Time constants in thermal laser medicine, *Lasers Surg Med* 9:405, 1989.
109. Brugmans MJP, Kemper J, Gijsbers GHM et al: Temperature response of biological materials to pulsed non-ablative CO_2 laser irradiation, *Lasers Surg Med* 11:587, 1991.
110. Schomacker KT, Walsh JT, Flotte TJ et al: Thermal damage produced by high-irradiance continuous wave CO_2 laser cutting of tissue, *Lasers Surg Med* 10:74, 1990.
111. Frenz H, Romano V, Zweig AD et al: Instabilities in laser cutting of soft media, *J Appl Phys* 66:4496, 1989.
112. Flemming MG, Brody N: A new technique for laser treatment of cutaneous tumors, *J Dermatol Surg Oncol* 12:1170, 1986.
113. Zweig AD, Frenz M, Romano V: A comparative study of laser tissue interaction at 294 μm and 10.6 μm, *J Appl Phys B* 47:259, 1988.

114. Herbich G: Epidermal changes limited to the epidermis of guinea pig skin by low-power carbon dioxide laser irradiation, *Arch Dermatol* 122:132, 1986.
115. Moritz AR: Studies of thermal injury. III. The pathology and pathogenesis of cutaneous burns: an experimental study, *Am J Pathol* 23:915, 1947.
116. Kamat BR, Tang SV, Arndt KA et al: Low-fluence CO_2 laser irradiation: selective epidermal damage to human skin, *J Invest Dermatol* 85:247, 1985.
117. Olbricht SM, Arndt K: Lasers in cutaneous surgery. In Fuller TA, editor: *Surgical lasers: a clinical guide,* New York, 1987, Macmillan.
118. Olbricht SO, Arndt KA: Carbon dioxide laser treatment of cutaneous disorders, *Mayo Clin Proc* 63:297, 1988.
119. Ratz JL, Bailin PL, Levine HL: CO_2 laser treatment of port-wine stains: a preliminary report, *J Dermatol Surg Oncol* 8:1039, 1982.
120. Apfelberg DB, Maser MR, Lash H: Argon laser treatment of cutaneous vascular abnormalities, *Ann Plast Surg* 1:14, 1978.
121. Noe JM, Barsky S, Gerr D et al: Port-wine stains and the response to argon laser therapy: successful treatment and the predictive role of color, age and biopsy, *Plast Reconstr Surg* 65:130, 1980.
122. Dixon JA: Lasers in surgery, *Curr Probl Surg* 21:11, 1984.
123. Cosman B: Experience in the argon laser therapy of port-wine stains, *Plast Reconstr Surg* 65:119, 1980.
124. Apfelberg DB, Maser MR, Lash H et al: The argon laser for cutaneous lesions, *JAMA* 245:2073, 1981.
125. Bailin PL, Ratz JL: Use of the carbon dioxide laser in dermatologic surgery. In Ratz JL, editor: *Lasers in cutaneous medicine and surgery,* Chicago, 1986, Mosby.
126. Levine H, Bailin P: Carbon dioxide treatment of cutaneous hemangiomas and tattoos, *Arch Otolaryngol* 108:236, 1982.
127. Ratz JL, Bailin PL: The case for use of the carbon dioxide laser in the treatment of port-wine stains, *Arch Dermatol* 123:72, 1987.
128. Bailin PL: Treatment of port wine stains with the CO_2 laser: early results. In Arndt KA, Noe JM, Rosen S, editors: *Cutaneous laser therapy: principles and methods,* New York, 1983, Wiley & Sons.
129. Van Gemert MJC, Welch AJ, Tan OT et al: Limitations of carbon dioxide lasers for treatment of port-wine stains, *Arch Dermatol* 123:71, 1987.
130. Van Gemert MJC, Welch AJ, Amin AP: Is there an optimal laser treatment for port-wine stains? *Lasers Surg Med* 6:76, 1986.
131. Buecker JW, Ratz JL, Richfield DF: Histology of port-wine stain treated with carbon dioxide laser, *J Am Acad Dermatol* 10:1014, 1984.
132. Apfelberg DB, Kosek J, Maser MR et al: Histology of port wine stains following argon laser treatment, *Br J Plast Surg* 32:232, 1979.
133. Finley JL, Barsky SH, Geer DE et al: Healing of port-wine stains after argon laser therapy, *Arch Dermatol* 117:486, 1981.
134. Solomon H, Goldman L, Henderson B et al: Histopathology of the laser treatment of port wine stains, *J Invest Dermatol* 50:141, 1968.
135. Campiglio GL, Candiani P, Maturri L: Port-wine stains: long-term histologic changes induced by argon and CO_2 laser treatment, *Acta Chir Plast* 37:25, 1995.
136. Tang SV, Arndt KA, Gilchrest BA et al: Clinical comparison of millisecond versus conventional argon laser treatment of in vivo vascular skin lesions, *Lasers Surg Med* 5:177, 1985.
137. Welch AJ, Motamedi M, Gonzalez A: Evaluation of cooling techniques for the protection of the epidermis during neodymium-YAG laser irradiation of the skin. In Joffe SN, editor: *Neodymium-YAG laser in medicine and surgery,* New York, 1983, Elsevier.
138. Lanigan SW, Cotterill JA: The treatment of port wine stains with the carbon dioxide laser, *Br J Dermatol* 123:229, 1990.
139. Apfelberg DB, Maser MR, Lash H et al: Benefits of the CO_2 laser in oral hemangioma excision, *Plast Reconstr Surg* 75:46, 1984.
140. Marsili M, Cockerell CJ, Lyde CB: Hemangioma-associated rhinophyma, *J Dermatol Surg Oncol* 19:206, 1993.
141. Shafir R, Slutzki S, Bornstein LA: Excision of buccal hemangioma by carbon dioxide laser beam, *Oral Surg* 44:347, 1977.

142. Ohshiro T: The CO_2 laser in the treatment of cavernous hemangioma of the lower lip: a case report, *Lasers Surg Med* 1:337, 1981.
143. Aronoff BL: The use of lasers in hemangiomas, *Lasers Surg Med* 1:323, 1981.
144. Bailin PL: Use of the CO_2 laser for non-PWS cutaneous lesions. In Arndt KA, Noe JM, Rosen S, editors: *Cutaneous laser therapy: principles and methods,* New York, 1983, Wiley & Sons.
145. McBurney EI: CO_2 laser treatment of dermatologic lesions, *South Med J* 71:795, 1978.
146. Brady SC, Blokmanis A, Jewett L: Tattoo removal with the carbon dioxide laser, *Ann Plast Surg* 2:482, 1978.
147. Beacon JP, Ellis H: Surgical removal of tattoos by carbon dioxide laser, *J R Soc Med* 73:298, 1980.
148. Bailin PL, Ratz JL, Levine HL: Removal of tattoos by CO_2 laser, *J Dermatol Surg Oncol* 6:997, 1980.
149. Reid R, Muller S: Tattoo removal by CO_2 laser dermabrasion, *Plast Reconstr Surg* 65:717, 1980.
150. Dixon J: Laser treatment of decorative tattoos. In Arndt KA, Noe JM, Rosen S, editors: *Cutaneous laser therapy: principles and methods,* New York, 1983, Wiley & Sons.
151. Morgan BDG: Tattoos, *Br Med J* 3:34, 1974.
152. Ruiz-Esparza J, Fitzpatrick RE, Goldman MP: Tattoo removal: selecting the right alternative, *Am J Cosmetic Surg* 9:171, 1992.
153. Ruiz-Esparza J, Goldman MP, Fitzpatrick RE: Tattoo removal with minimal scarring: the chemo-laser technique, *J Dermatol Surg Oncol* 14:1372, 1989.
154. Taylor CR, Gange RW, Dover JS et al: Treatment of tattoos by Q-switched ruby laser: a dose-response study, *Arch Dermatol* 126:893, 1990.
155. Kilmer SL, Lee MS, Grevelink JM et al: The Q-switched Nd:YAG laser (1064 nm) effectively treats tattoos: a controlled, dose-response study, *Arch Derm* 8:971, 1993.
156. Fitzpatrick RE, Goldman MP: Tattoo removal using the alexandrite laser (755 nm, 100 ns), *Arch Dermatol,* 130:1508, 1994.
157. Anderson RR, Geronemus R, Kilmer SL et al: Cosmetic tattoo ink darkening, *Arch Dermatol* 129:1010, 1993.
158. Herbich GJ: Ultrapulse carbon dioxide laser treatment of an iron oxide flesh-colored tattoo, *Dermatol Surg* 23:60, 1997.
159. Kaplan I: The CO_2 laser in plastic surgery, *Lasers Surg Med* 6:385, 1986.
160. Baker SS, Muenzler WS, Small RG et al: Carbon dioxide laser blepharoplasty, *Ophthalmology* 91:238, 1984.
161. David LM, Sanders G: CO_2 laser blepharoplasty: a comparison to cold steel and electrocautery, *J Dermatol Surg Oncol* 13:110, 1987.
162. David LM: The laser approach of blepharoplasty, *J Dermatol Surg Oncol* 14:741, 1988.
163. David LM, Abergel RP: Carbon dioxide laser blepharoplasty: conjunctival temperature during surgery, *J Dermatol Surg Oncol* 15:421, 1989.
164. Mittelman MD, Apfelberg DB: Carbon dioxide laser blepharoplasty: advantages and disadvantages, *Ann Plast Surg* 24:1, 1990.
165. Morrow DM, Morrow LB: CO_2 laser blepharoplasty: a comparison with cold steel surgery, *J Dermatol Surg Oncol* 18:307, 1992.
166. Lask G: Laser may be faster and better than scalpel for blepharoplasty, *Skin Allergy News,* May 1992.
167. Street ML, Roenigk RK: Recalcitrant periungual verrucae: the role of carbon dioxide laser vaporization, *J Am Acad Dermatol* 23:115, 1990.
168. Bar-Am A, Shilon M, Peyser MR et al: Treatment of male genital condylomatous lesions by carbon dioxide laser after failure of previous nonlaser methods, *J Am Acad Dermatol* 24:87, 1991.
169. Apfelberg DB, Druker D, Maser MR et al: Benefits of the CO_2 laser for verruca resistant to other modalities of treatment, *J Dermatol Surg Oncol* 15:371, 1989.
170. Mueller TJ, Carlson BA, Lindy MP: The use of the carbon dioxide surgical laser for the treatment of verrucae, *J Am Podiatr Med Assoc* 70:136, 1980.
171. Apfelberg DB, Rothermel E, Widtfeldt A et al: Preliminary report on use of the carbon dioxide laser in podiatry, *J Am Podiatr Med Assoc* 74:509, 1984.
172. McBurney EI: CO_2 laser treatment of dermatologic lesions, *South Med J* 71:795, 1978.
173. Wheeland RG, Walker NPJ: Lasers—25 years later, *Int J Dermatol* 25:209, 1986.

174. McBurney E, Rosen D: Carbon dioxide laser treatment of verrucae vulgaris, *J Dermatol Surg Oncol* 10:45, 1984.
175. Bunney M, Nolan MW, Williams DA: An assessment of the methods of treating viral warts by comparative treatment trials based on a standard design, *Br J Dermatol* 94:667, 1976.
176. Fereczy A, Mitao N, Nagai N et al: Latent papillomavirus and recurring genital warts, *N Engl J Med* 313:784, 1985.
177. Leavitt KM: CO_2 laser surgery for verrucae: a technique, *Laser Lett Int Soc Podiatr Laser Surg*, 23, 1991.
178. Persky MS: Carbon dioxide laser treatment of oral florid papillomatosis, *J Dermatol Surg Oncol* 10:64, 1984.
179. Baggish MS, Poiesz BJ, Joret D et al: Presence of human immunodeficiency virus DNA in laser smoke, *Lasers Surg Med* 11:197, 1991.
180. Walker NPJ, Matthews J, Newsom SWM: Possible hazards from irradiation with the carbon dioxide laser, *Lasers Surg Med* 6:84, 1986.
181. Mullarky MB, Norris CW, Goldberg ID: The efficacy of the CO_2 laser in the sterilization of skin seeded with bacteria: survival at the skin surface and in the plume emission, *Laryngoscope* 95:186, 1985.
182. Garden JM, O'Banion K, Shelnitz LS et al: Papillomavirus in the vapor of carbon dioxide laser-treated verrucae, *JAMA* 259:1199, 1988.
183. Ito Y: A tumor producing factor extracted by phenol from papillomatous tissue (Shope) of cottontail rabbits, *Virology* 12:596, 1960.
184. Ito Y, Evans CA: Induction of tumors in domestic rabbits with nucleic acid preparations from partially purified Shope papillomavirus and from extracts of the papillomas of domestic and cottontail rabbits, *J Exp Med* 114:485, 1961.
185. Lowy DR, Dvoretzky I, Shober R et al: In vitro tumorigenic transformation by a defined sub-genomic fragment of bovine papillomavirus DNA, *Nature* 287:72, 1980.
186. Sawchuk WS, Weber PJ, Lowy DR et al: Infectious papillomavirus in the vapor of warts treated with carbon dioxide laser or electrocoagulation: detection and protection, *J Am Acad Dermatol* 21:41, 1989.
187. Andre P, Orth G, Evenou P et al: Risk of papillomavirus infection in carbon dioxide laser treatment of genital lesions, *J Am Acad Dermatol* 1:131, 1990.
188. Matchette LS, Faaland RW, Royston DD et al: In vitro production of viable bacteriophage in carbon dioxide and argon laser plumes, *Lasers Surg Med* 11:380, 1991.
189. Abramson AL, DiLorenzo TP, Steinberg BM: Is papillomavirus detectable in the plume of laser-treated laryngeal papilloma? *Arch Otolaryngol Head Neck Surg* 116:604, 1990.
190. Ferenczy A, Bergeron C, Richart RM: Human papillomavirus DNA in CO_2 laser–generated plume of smoke and its consequences to the surgeon, *Obstet Gynecol* 75:114, 1990.
191. Hong-Xia LI, Wen-Yuen Z, Ming-Yu X: Detection with the polymerase chain reaction of human papillomavirus DNA in condylomata acuminata treated with CO_2 laser and microwave, *Int J Dermatol* 34:209, 1995.
192. Grussendorf-Cohen E, Gissman L, Holters J: Correlation between content of viral DNA and evidence of mature viral particles in HPV-1, HPV-4 and HPV-6-induced virus acanthomata, *J Invest Dermatol* 81:511, 1983.
193. zur Hausen H: Human pathogenic papilloma viruses, *Arzneimittelforschung* 27:212, 1977.
194. Laurent R, Agache P, Coume-Marquet S: Ultrastructure of clear cells in human warts, *J Cutan Pathol* 2:140, 1975.
195. Jenson AB, Sommer S, Payling-Wright C et al: Human papillomavirus frequency and distribution in plantar and common warts, *Lab Invest* 47:491, 1982.
196. Laurent R, Kienzler JL, Croissant O et al: Two anatomicoclinical types of warts with plantar locations: specific cytopathogenic effects of papillomavirus, *Arch Dermatol Res* 274:101, 1982.
197. Mounts P, Shah KV, Kashima H: Viral etiology of juvenile- and adult-onset squamous cell papilloma of the larynx, *Proc Natl Acad Sci USA* 79:5425, 1982.
198. Gissman L, Wolnik L, Ikenberg H et al: Human papillomavirus types 6 and 11 sequences in genital and laryngeal papillomas and in some cervical cancers, *Proc Natl Acad Sci USA* 80:560, 1983.
199. Smith JP, Topmiller JL, Shulman S: Factors affecting emission collection by surgical smoke evacuators, *Lasers Surg Med* 10:224, 1990.

200. Trevor M: Presence of virus in CO_2 laser plumes raise infection concern, *Hosp Infect Control* 166, 1987.
201. Mihashi S, Ueda S, Hirano M et al: Some problems about condensates induced by CO_2 laser irradiation. Paper presented at Fourth Annual Meeting of International Society for Laser Surgery, Tokyo, November 1981.
202. Starr JC, Kilmer SL, Wheeland RG: Analysis of the carbon dioxide laser plume for simian immunodeficiency virus, *J Dermatol Surg Oncol* 8:297, 1992.
203. Malek RS: Laser treatment of premalignant and malignant squamous cell lesions of the penis, *Laser Surg Med* 12:246, 1992.
204. Greenbaum S, Glogau R, Stegman S et al: Carbon dioxide laser treatment of erythroplasia of Queyrat, *J Dermatol Surg Oncol* 15:747, 1989.
205. Rosenberg S: Carbon dioxide laser treatment of external genital lesions, *Urology* 25:555, 1985.
206. Rosenberg S, Fuller T: Carbon dioxide rapid superpulse laser treatment of erythroplasia of Queyrat, *Urology* 16:181, 1980.
207. Blatstein LM, Finkelstein LH: Laser surgery for the treatment of squamous cell carcinoma of the penis, *J Am Osteopathol Assoc* 90:338, 1990.
208. Hofstetter A, Frank F: *The neodymium-YAG laser in urology,* Basel, 1980, Hoffman-LaRoche.
209. Rosenberg SK: Lasers and squamous cell carcinoma of external genitalia, *Urology* 27:430, 1986.
210. Boon TA: Sapphire probe laser surgery for localized carcinoma of the penis, *Eur J Surg Oncol* 14:193, 1988.
211. Malloy TR, Wein AJ, Carpiniello VL: Carcinoma of penis treated with neodymium YAG laser, *Urology* 31:26, 1988.
212. Gursel EO, Georgountzos C, Uson AC et al: Penile cancer: clinicopathologic study of 64 cases, *Urology* 1:569, 1973.
213. Baggish M, Dorsey J: CO_2 laser for the treatment of vulvar carcinoma in situ, *Obstet Gynecol* 57:371, 1981.
214. Townsend D, Levine R, Richast R: Management of vulvar intraepithelial neoplasia by carbon dioxide laser, *Obstet Gynecol* 60:49, 1982.
215. Landthaler M, Haina D, Brunner R et al: Laser therapy of bowenoid papulosis and Bowen's disease, *J Dermatol Surg Oncol* 12:1253, 1986.
216. Gorden KB, Robinson J: Carbon dioxide laser vaporization for Bowen's disease of the finger, *Arch Dermatol* 130:1250, 1994.
217. McCullough TL, Lesher JL: Porokeratosis of Mibelli: rapid recurrence of a large lesion after carbon dioxide laser treatment, *Pediatr Dermatol* 11:267, 1994.
218. Rabbin PE, Baldwin HE: Treatment of porokeratosis of Mibelli with CO_2 laser vaporization versus surgical excision with split-thickness skin graft, *J Dermatol Surg Oncol* 19:199, 1993.
219. Merkle T, Hohenleutner U, Braun-Falco O et al: Reticulate porokeratosis—successful treatment with CO_2 laser vaporization, *Cline Exp Dermatol* 17:178, 1992.
220. Groot DW, Johnston PA: Carbon dioxide laser treatment of porokeratoses of Mibelli, *Lasers Surg Med* 5:603, 1985.
221. Pinheiro ALB, Frame JW: Surgical management of premalignant lesions of the oral cavity with the CO_2 laser, *Braz Dent J* 7:103, 1996.
222. Cheisa F, Sala L, Costa L et al: Excision of oral leukoplakias by CO_2 laser on an outpatient basis: a useful procedure for prevention and early detection of oral carcinomas, *Tumori* 72:307, 1986.
223. Flynn MB, White M, Tabah RJ: The use of carbon dioxide laser for the treatment of premalignant lesions of the oral mucosa, *J Surg Oncol* 37:232, 1988.
224. Frame JW, Das Guptas AR, Dalton JA et al: Use of the carbon dioxide laser in the management of premalignant lesion of the oral mucosa, *J Laryngol Otol* 98:1251, 1984.
225. Horch HH, Gerlarch KL, Schaefer HE: CO_2 laser surgery of oral premalignant lesions, *Int J Oral Maxillofac Surg* 15:19, 1986.
226. Coleman WP, Davis RS, Reed RJ et al: Treatment of lentigo maligna and lentigo maligna melanoma, *J Dermatol Surg Oncol* 6:476, 1980.
227. Nazzarro-Porro M, Passi S, Balus L et al: Effect of dicarboxylic acids on lentigo maligna, *J Invent Dermatol* 72:296, 1979.
228. Goldschmidt H, Breneman JC, Breneman DL: Ionizing radiation therapy in dermatology, *J Am Acad Dermatol* 30:157, 1994.

229. Arndt KA: New pigmented macule 4 years after argon laser treatment of lentigo maligna, *J Am Acad Dermatol* 14:1092, 1986.
230. Kopera D: Treatment of lentigo maligna with the carbon dioxide laser, *Arch Dermatol* 131:735, 1995.
231. Becker-Wegerich PM, Fritsch C, Schulte KW et al: Carbon dioxide laser treatment of extramammary Paget's disease guided by photodynamic diagnosis, *Br J Dermatol* 138:169, 1998.
232. Kartamaa MK, Reitamo S: Treatment of lichen sclerosus with carbon dioxide laser vaporization, *Br J Dermatol* 136:356, 1997.
233. Ratz JL: Carbon dioxide laser treatment of balanitis xerotica obliterans, *J Am Acad Dermatol* 10:925, 1984.
234. Rosenberg SK, Jacobs H: Continuous wave carbon dioxide treatment of balanitis xerotica obliterans, *Urology* 19:539, 1982.
235. Rosenberg SK: Carbon dioxide laser treatment of external genital lesions, *Urology* 25:555, 1985.
236. Windahl T, Hellsten S: Carbon dioxide laser treatment of lichen sclerosus et atrophicus, *J Urol* 150:868, 1993.
237. Stack BC, Hall PJ, Goodman AL et al: CO_2 laser excision of lupus pernio of the face, 19:529, 1998.
238. Wheeland RG, Bailin PL, Ratz JL et al: Carbon dioxide laser vaporization and curettage in the treatment of large or multiple superficial basal cell carcinomas, *J Dermatol Surg Oncol,* 13:119, 1987.
239. Salasche SJ: Status of curettage and desiccation in the treatment of primary basal cell carcinoma, *J Am Acad Dermatol* 10:285, 1984.
240. Roenigk RK, Ratz JL, Bailin PL et al: Trends in the presentation and treatment of basal cell carcinomas, *J Dermatol Surg Oncol* 12:860, 1986.
241. Dubin N, Kopf AW: Multivariate risk score for recurrence of cutaneous basal cell carcinoma, *Arch Dermatol* 119:373, 1983.
242. Knox JM, Lyles TW, Shapiro EM et al: Curettage and electrodesiccation in the treatment of skin cancer, *Arch Dermatol* 82:197, 1960.
243. Edens BL, Bartlow GA, Haghighi P et al: Effectiveness of curettage and electrodesiccation in the removal of basal cell carcinoma, *J Am Acad Dermatol* 9:383, 1983.
244. d'Aubermont PCS, Bennett RG: Failure of curettage and electrodesiccation for removal of basal cell carcinoma, *Arch Dermatol* 120:1456, 1984.
245. Spiller WF, Spiller RF: Treatment of basal cell epithelioma by curettage and electrodesiccation, *J Am Acad Dermatol* 11:808, 1984.
246. Torre D, Lubritz RR, Graham GF: Cryosurgical treatment of basal cell carcinomas, *Prog Dermatol* 12:11, 1978.
247. Kuflik EG: Cryosurgical treatment for large malignancies on the upper extremities, *J Dermatol Surg Oncol* 12:575, 1986.
248. Belisario JC: An appraisal of therapeutic methods for skin carcinomas by scalpel or electrosurgery, ionizing radiations, electrochemosurgery and local chemotherapy, *Acta Derm Venereol* 44 (suppl 56):1, 1964.
249. Shelley WB, Wood MG: Nodular superficial pigmented basal cell epitheliomas, *Arch Dermatol* 118:928, 1982.
250. Peck GL, Gross EG, Butkus D et al: Chemoprevention of basal cell carcinoma with isotretinoin, *J Am Acad Dermatol* 6:815, 1982.
251. Adams EL, Price NM: Treatment of basal-cell carcinomas with a carbon-dioxide laser, *J Dermatol Surg Oncol* 5:803, 1979.
252. Fitzpatrick RE: The ultrapulse CO_2 laser: selective photothermolysis of epidermal tumors, *Lasers Surg Med Suppl* 5:56, 1993.
253. Levin NS, Salisbury RE, Peterson HD et al: Clinical evaluation of the carbon dioxide laser for burn wound excisions: a comparison of the laser, scalpel, and electrocautery, *J Trauma* 15:800, 1975.
254. Fidler JP, Law E, MacMillan BG et al: Comparison of carbon dioxide laser excision of burns with other thermal knives, *Ann NY Acad Sci* 267:254, 1976.
255. Stellar S, Levine N, Ger R et al: Laser excision of acute third-degree burns followed by immediate autograft replacement: an experimental study in the pig, *J Trauma* 13:45, 1973.
256. Fidler JP, Rockwell RJ, Siler VE et al: Early laser excision of thermal burns in the white rat and miniature pig, *Burns* 1:5, 1974.

257. Norris CW, Mullarky MB: Experimental skin incision made with the carbon dioxide laser, *Laryngoscope* 92:416, 1982.
258. Talebzadeh N, Morrison RP, Fried MP: Comparative cell targeting in vitro using the CO_2 laser, *Lasers Surg Med* 14:164, 1994.
259. Lapins J, Marcusson JA, Emstestam L: Surgical treatment of chronic hidradenitis suppurativa: CO_2 laser stripping–secondary intention technique, *Br J Dermatol* 131:551, 1994.
260. Finley EM, Rata JL: Treatment of hidradenitis suppurative with carbon dioxide laser excision and second-intention healing, *J Am Acad Dermatol* 34:465, 1996.
261. Dalrymple JC, Monaghan JM: Treatment of hidradenitis suppurativa with the carbon dioxide laser, *Br J Surg* 74:420, 1987.
262. Eliezri YD, Sklar JA: Lymphangioma circumscriptum: review and evaluation of carbon dioxide laser vaporization, *J Dermatol Surg Oncol* 14:357, 1988.
263. Bailin PL et al: Carbon dioxide laser vaporization in lymphangioma circumscriptum, *J Am Acad Dermatol* 14:257, 1986.
264. Arndt KA, Noe JM, Rosen S, editors: *Cutaneous laser therapy: principles and methods,* New York, 1983, John Wiley & Sons.
265. Apfelberg DB, Maser M, White D et al: Failure of carbon dioxide laser excision of keloids, *Lasers Surg Med* 9:382, 1989.
266. Murray JC, Pollack SV, Pinnell SR: Keloids: a review, *J Am Acad Dermatol* 4:461, 1981.
267. Berman B, Duncan MR: Short-term keloid treatment in vivo with human interferon alpha-2B: results in a selective and persistent normalization of keloidal fibroblast collagen, glycosaminoglycan, and collagenase production in vitro, *J Am Acad Dermatol* 21:694, 1989.
268. Granstein RD, Rook A, Flotte TJ et al: A controlled trial of intralesional recombinant interferon-J in the treatment of keloidal scarring, *Arch Dermatol* 126:1295, 1990.
269. Kantor GR, Ratz JL, Wheeland RG: Treatment of acne keloidalis nuchae with carbon dioxide laser, *J Am Acad Dermatol* 14:263, 1986.
270. Glass LF, Berman B, Laub D: Treatment of perifolliculitis capitis abscedens et suffodiens with the carbon dioxide laser, *J Dermatol Surg Oncol* 15:673, 1989.
271. Park JH, Cha SH, Park SD: Carbon dioxide laser treatment vs. subcutaneous resection of axillary osmidrosis, *Dermatol Surg* 23:247, 1997.
272. Kahn AM, Ostad A, Moy RL: Grafting following short-pulse carbon dioxide laser deepithelialization, *Dermatol Surg* 22:965, 1996.
273. Khan AM, Cohen MJ: Treatment of depigmentation following burn injuries, *Burns* 22:552, 1996.
274. Khan AM, Cohen MJ: Vitiligo: treatment by dermabrasion and epithelial sheet grafting, *J Am Acad Dermatol* 33:646, 1995.
275. Green HA, Burd EE, Nishioka NS et al: Skin graft take and healing following 193-nm excimer, continuous-wave carbon dioxide (CO_2), pulsed CO_2 or pulsed holmium:YAG laser ablation of the graft bed, *Arch Dermatol* 129:979, 1993.
276. Grotting JK: Chronic lower lip lesions: treatment by the "lip-shave" operation, *Minn Med* 39:527, 1956.
277. Spira M, Hardy SB: Vermilionectomy: review of cases with variation in technique, *Plast Reconstr Surg* 33:39, 1964.
278. Sanchez-Conejo-Mir J, Perez-Bernal AM, Moreno-Gimenez JC et al: Follow-up of vermilionectomies: evaluation of the technique, *J Dermatol Surg Oncol* 12:180, 1986.
279. Birt BD: The "lip shave" operation for pre-malignant conditions and micro-invasive carcinoma of the lower lip, *J Otolaryngol* 6:407, 1977.
280. Cataldo E, Doku HC: Solar cheilitis, *J Dermatol Surg Oncol* 7:989, 1981.
281. Lubritz RR, Smolewski SA: Cryosurgery cure rate of premalignant leukoplakia of the lower lip, *J Dermatol Surg Oncol* 9:235, 1983.
282. Epstein E: Treatment of lip keratoses (actinic cheilitis) with topical fluorouracil, *Arch Dermatol* 113:906, 1977.
283. Robinson JK: Actinic cheilitis: a prospective study comparing four treatment methods, *Arch Otolaryngol Head Neck Surg* 115:848, 1989.
284. LaRiviere W, Pickett AB: Clinical criteria in diagnosis of early squamous cell carcinoma of the lower lip, *J Am Dent Assoc* 99:972, 1979.
285. Schmitt CK, Folsom TC: Histologic evaluation of degenerative changes of the lower lip, *J Oral Surg* 26:51, 1968.

286. Nicolau SG, Balus L: Chronic actinic cheilitis and cancer of the lower lip, *Br J Dermatol* 76:278, 1964.
287. Wurman LH, Adams GL, Meyerhoff WL: Carcinoma of the lip, *Am J Surg* 130:470, 1975.
288. Paletta FX, Coldwater L, Booth F: The treatment of leukoplakia and carcinoma in situ of the lower lip, *Ann Surg* 145:74, 1957.
289. Moller R, Reymann F, Hou-Jensen K: Metastases in dermatological patients with squamous cell carcinoma, *Arch Dermatol* 115:703, 1979.
290. Slaughter DP, Southwick HW, Smejkal W: "Field cancerization" in oral stratified squamous epithelium: clinical implications of multicentric origin, *Cancer* 6:963, 1953.
291. Lund HZ: How often does squamous cell carcinoma of the skin metastasize? *Arch Dermatol* 92:635, 1965.
292. LaRiviere W, Pickett AB: Clinical criteria in diagnosis of early squamous cell carcinoma of the lower lip, *J Am Dent Assoc* 99:972, 1979.
293. Epstein JH: Carbon dioxide laser treatment of actinic cheilitis, *West J Med* 156:192, 1992.
294. Knabel MR, Koranda FC, Olejko TD: Surgical management of primary carcinoma of the lower lip, *J Dermatol Surg Oncol* 8:979, 1982.
295. Defresne RG, Garrett AB, Bailin PL et al: Carbon dioxide laser treatment of chronic actinic cheilitis, *J Am Acad Dermatol* 19:876, 1988.
296. Goldman L, Shumrick DA, Rockwell J: The laser in maxillofacial surgery: preliminary investigative surgery, *Arch Surg* 96:397, 1968.
297. David LM: Laser vermilion ablation for actinic cheilitis, *J Dermatol Surg Oncol* 11:605, 1985.
298. Whitaker DC: Microscopically proven cure of actinic cheilitis by CO_2 laser, *Lasers Surg Med* 7:520, 1987.
299. Stanley RJ, Roenigk RK: Actinic cheilitis: treatment with the carbon dioxide laser, *Mayo Clin Proc* 63:230, 1988.
300. Zelvekson BD, Roenigk RK: Actinic cheilitis: treatment with the carbon dioxide laser, *Cancer* 65:1307, 1990.
301. Johnson TM, Sebastien TS, Lowe L et al: Carbon dioxide laser treatment of actinic cheilitis: clinicohistopathologic correlation to determine the optimal depth of destruction, *J Am Acad Dermatol* 27:737, 1992.
302. Vinciullo C: Combination carbon dioxide laser vermilionectomy and wedge excision of the lip, *Aus J Dermatol* 57:111, 1996.
303. Fitzpatrick RE, Goldman MP, Dierickx C: Laser ablation of facial cosmetic tattoos, *Aesthetic Plast Surg*, 18:91, 1994.
304. Albom M: Electrosurgical treatment of rhinophyma, *J Dermatol Surg Oncol* 2:189, 1976.
305. Staindl O: Surgical management of rhinophyma, *Acta Otolaryngol* 92:137, 1981.
306. Cheney ML, Graves TA, Blair PA: Rhinophyma: a surgical management, *J La State Med Soc* 139:13, 1987.
307. Kemble JVH: Correction of deformities of the nose, *Practitioner* 224:399, 1980.
308. Fulton JE: Modern dermabrasion techniques: a personal appraisal, *J Dermatol Surg Oncol* 13:780, 1987.
309. Fisher WJ: Rhinophyma: its surgical treatment, *Plast Reconstr Surg* 45:466, 1970.
310. Anderson R, Dykes ER: Surgical treatment of rhinophyma, *Plast Reconstr Surg* 30:397, 1962.
311. Freeman BS: Reconstructive rhinoplasty for rhinophyma, *Plast Reconstr Surg* 46:265, 1970.
312. Karge HK, Konz B: Surgical methods in the treatment of rhinophyma, *J Dermatol Surg* 1:31, 1975.
313. Gursel B, Yalciner G: Rhinophyma: treatment by excision and silver impregnated amniotic membrane, *Rhinology* 26:63, 1988.
314. Matton G, Pickrell K, Huger W et al: The surgical treatment of rhinophyma, *Plast Reconstr Surg* 30:403, 1962.
315. Strempel H: A new dermatome for surgical treatment of rhinophyma, *J Dermatol Surg Oncol* 7:153, 1981.
316. Linehan JW, Goode RL, Fajardo LF: Surgery vs electrosurgery for rhinophyma, *Arch Otolaryngol* 91:444, 1970.
317. Verde SF, Oliveira ADS, Picoto ADS et al: How we treat rhinophyma, *J Dermatol Surg Oncol* 6:560, 1980.
318. Nolan JO: Cryosurgical treatment of rhinophyma, *Plast Reconstr Surg* 52:437, 1973.

319. Sonnex TS, Dawber RPR: Rhinophyma: treatment by liquid nitrogen spray surgery, *Br J Dermatol* 109(suppl 24):18, 1983.
320. Greenbaum SS, Krull EA, Watnick K: Comparison of CO_2 laser and electrosurgery in the treatment of rhinophyma, *J Am Acad Dermatol* 18:363, 1988.
321. Eisen RF, Katz AE, Bohigian RK et al: Surgical treatment of rhinophyma with the Shaw scalpel, *Arch Dermatol* 122:307, 1986.
322. Farina R: Rhinophyma: plastic correction, *Plast Reconstr Surg* 6:461, 1950.
323. Ali KM, Callari RH, Mobley DL: Resection of rhinophyma with CO_2 laser, *Laryngoscope* 99:453, 1989.
324. Bohigian RK, Shapshay SM, Hybels RL: Management of rhinophyma with carbon dioxide laser: Lahey Clinic experience, *Lasers Surg Med* 8:397, 1988.
325. Roenigk RK: CO_2 laser vaporization for treatment of rhinophyma, *Mayo Clin Proc* 62:676, 1987.
326. Wheeland RG, Bailin PL, Ratz JL: Combined carbon dioxide laser excision and vaporization in the treatment of rhinophyma, *J Dermatol Surg Oncol* 13:172, 1987.
327. Shapshay SM, Strong MS, Anastasi GW et al: Removal of rhinophyma with the carbon dioxide laser, *Arch Otolaryngol* 106:257, 1980.
328. Amedee RG, Routman MH: Methods and complications of rhinophyma excision, *Laryngoscope* 97:1316, 1987.
329. Hassard AD: Carbon dioxide laser treatment of acne rosacea and rhinophyma: how I do it, *J Otolaryngol* 17:336, 1988.
330. Hallock GG: Laser treatment of rhinophyma, *Aesth Plast Surg* 12:171, 1988.
331. Haas A, Wheeland RG: Treatment of massive rhinophyma with the carbon dioxide laser, *J Dermatol Surg Oncol* 16:645, 1990.
332. Greenbaum SS, Krull EA, Watnick K: Comparison of CO_2 laser and electrosurgery in the treatment of rhinophyma, *J Am Acad Dermatol* 18:363, 1988.
333. el-Azhary R, Roenigk RK, Wang TD: Spectrum of results after treatment of rhinophyma with the carbon dioxide laser, *Mayo Clin Proc* 66:899, 1991.
334. Simo R, Shama VL: Treatment of rhinophyma with carbon dioxide laser, *J Laryngol Otol* 110:841, 1996.
335. Ratz JL, Bailin PL, Lakeland RF: Carbon dioxide laser treatment of epidermal nevi, *J Dermatol Surg Oncol* 12:567, 1986.
336. Garden JM, Geronemus RG: Dermatologic laser surgery, *J Dermatol Surg Oncol* 16:156, 1990.
337. Roenigk RK, Ratz JL: CO_2 laser treatment of cutaneous neurofibromas, *J Dermatol Surg Oncol* 13:187, 1987.
338. Wheeland RG, Ashley JR, Smith DA et al: Carbon dioxide laser treatment of granuloma faciale, *J Dermatol Surg Oncol* 10:730, 1984.
339. Jordan JA, Brown OE, Biavati MU et al: Congenital syringocystadenoma papilliferum of the ear and neck treated with CO_2 laser, *Int J Pediatr Otorhinolaryngol* 38:81, 1996.
340. Karam F, Bauman T: Carbon dioxide treatment of chondrodermatitis nodularis helicis, *Ear Nose Throat J* 67:757, 1988.
341. Taylor MB: Chrondrodermatitis nodularis chronica helicis: successful treatment with the carbon dioxide laser, *J Dermatol Surg Oncol* 17:862, 1991.
342. Morselli M, Anselmi C, Farinelli F et al: CO_2 laser peeling for psoriasis, *Lasers Surg Med* 7:97, 1987.
343. Don PC, Carney PS, Lynch WS et al: Carbon dioxide laserabrasion: a new approach to management of familial benign chronic pemphigus (Hailey-Hailey disease), *J Dermatol Surg Oncol* 13:1187, 1987.
344. Spandoni D, Cain CL: Facial resurfacing using the carbon dioxide laser, *AORN J* 50:1007, 1989.
345. Solotoff S: Treatment for pitted acne scarring: postauricular punch grafts followed by dermabrasion, *J Dermatol Surg Oncol* 12:10, 1986.
346. Henahan JF: CO_2 laser used to correct facial defects, *Dermatol Times*, April 1992.
347. Garrett AG, Dufresne RG, Ratz JL et al: Carbon dioxide laser treatment of pitted acne scarring, *J Dermatol Surg Oncol* 16:737, 1990.
348. Wheeland RG: Revision of full-thickness skin grafts using the carbon dioxide laser, *J Dermatol Surg Oncol* 14:130, 1988.
349. Brauner G, Schliftman A: Laser surgery in children, *J Dermatol Surg Oncol* 13:178, 1987.

350. McElroy JA, Mehregan DA, Roenigk RK: Carbon dioxide laser vaporization of recalcitrant symptomatic plaques of Hailey-Hailey disease and Darier's disease, *J Am Acad Dermatol* 23:893, 1990.
351. Giler S, Kaplan I: The use of the CO_2 laser for the treatment of cutaneous lesions in an outpatient clinic. In Atsumi K, Minsakal N, editors: *Laser Tokyo '81, Proceedings of the 4th Congress of the International Society for Laser Surgery,* Tokyo, 1983, Intergroup.
352. Alster TS, West TB: Ultrapulse CO_2 laser ablation of xanthelasma, *J Am Acad Dermatol* 34:848, 1996.
353. Baldwin H, Geronemus R: Carbon dioxide laser vaporization of Zoon's balanitis: a case report, *J Dermatol Surg Oncol* 15:491, 1989.
354. Bain L, Geronemus R: The association of lichen planus of the penis with squamous cell carcinoma in situ and verrucous squamous cell carcinoma, *J Dermatol Surg Oncol* 15:413, 1989.
355. Bekassy Z, Astedt B: Carbon dioxide laser vaporization of plaque psoriasis, *Br J Dermatol* 114:489, 1986.

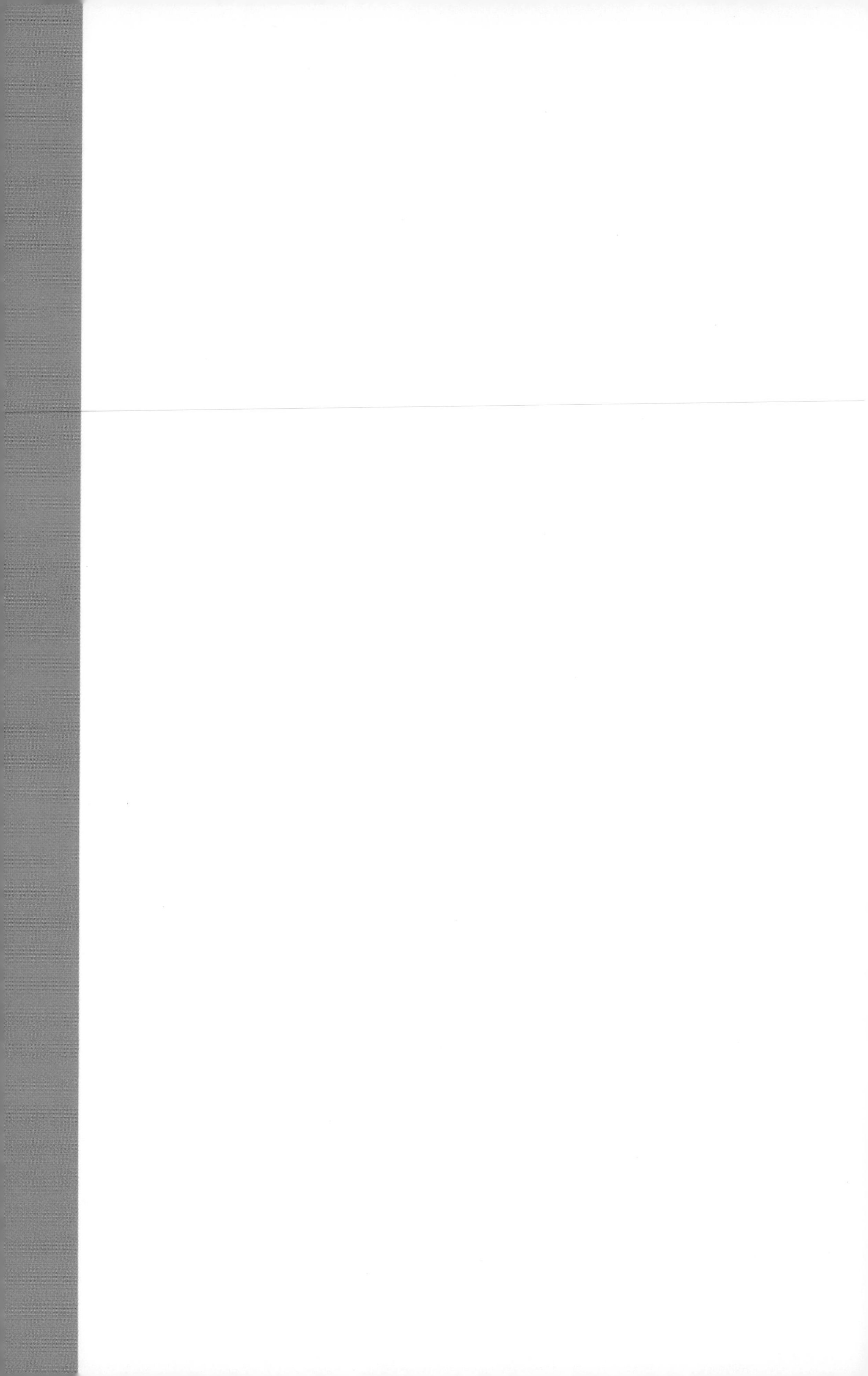

CHAPTER seven

Skin Resurfacing with Carbon Dioxide and Erbium Lasers

Richard E. Fitzpatrick and Mitchel P. Goldman

Pulsed carbon dioxide (CO_2) laser resurfacing of photodamaged skin has rapidly become the treatment of choice for rejuvenation of photoaging facial skin, and along with pulsed erbium:yttrium-aluminum-garnet (Er:YAG) laser resurfacing, is currently being explored for similar treatment of the skin of the neck and hands. To achieve the excellent results possible with this treatment modality, one must understand the pathophysiology of photodamaged skin, details of laser-tissue interaction, factors in the proper choice of patients, and optimal laser treatment parameters. In addition, knowledge of photoaging of skin and its modulation with topical agents and assessment of fundamentals of cutaneous wound healing allow intelligent choices to be made in the determination of preoperative and postoperative regimens.

Interest has surrounded facial rejuvenation for centuries. The use of topical agents such as soured milk, vegetable extracts, and mud packs has been documented in ancient civilizations. However, only in the last decade has rejuvenation been approached from a scientific basis. With the aging of the American population, particularly those 76 million individuals referred to as the "baby boomers" turning age 50, much attention has been focused on "antiaging" therapies. In particular, the use of retinoic acid, alpha-hydroxy acids, and antioxidants in conjunction with sunscreens and sunblocks has been investigated to prevent or reverse the photoaging process. Although these agents may have significant benefit, they generally fall short of the clinical expectations of those using them as a primary rejuvenation treatment.

To achieve a more dramatic clinical endpoint, a variety of chemical agents have been used to induce a layer of necrosis of variable depths, effectively peeling away the outermost layer of sun-damaged skin, with subsequent dermal healing and reepithelialization resulting in a more youthful appearance. Similar results have been achieved by mechanically removing these outer layers with dermabrasion. This chapter details the use of the CO_2 and Er:YAG lasers to rejuvenate the skin.

PHOTOAGING OF THE SKIN

Free Radicals and Antioxidants

Skin is constantly exposed to noxious environmental stimuli, including pollutants, pesticides, and herbicides; extremes of heat and cold; and chemicals that act as irritants and allergens. By far the most significant and damaging stimulus is sun exposure. All these stimuli, however, share one characteristic: the ability to generate and propagate the formation of reactive oxygen species, or *free radicals*. The biologic relevance of these free radicals has been studied extensively. Both the epidermis and the dermis are at risk from the adverse effects of these very reactive species.[1-7] Much, if not most, of the damage to the skin that results from sun exposure occurs through the action of free radicals.

The primary target of these free radicals is the lipid bilayer making up the cell membrane. Unsaturated lipids within the cell membrane react very readily with free radicals. A single free radical can initiate a chain reaction whereby many lipid molecules are disrupted and the integrity of the entire cell membrane is compromised. In addition, both deoxyribonucleic acid (DNA) and ribonucleic acid (RNA) are degraded by free radicals, which may result in mutations. Proteins are adversely affected as well. Enzyme inhibitors may be rendered nonfunctional and proteolytic balances deregulated, resulting in unwanted tissue destruction. All the components of connective tissue have been shown to be altered or degraded by free radicals.

If these processes continued unchecked, death would be the endpoint. Fortunately, various defense mechanisms function to contain these reactions. Cellular and extracellular free-radical "quenchers" include superoxide dismutase, catalase, glutathione, vitamin E (α-tocopherol), vitamin C (ascorbic acid), ubiquinone, and heme oxygenase.[8-15] These antioxidant systems act as primary intracellular defenses against reactive oxygen species before their interaction with macromolecules. Nonenzymatic antioxidants (ascorbate, tocopherol, β-carotene, reduced coenzyme Q, or ubiquinol and reduced glutathione) are small molecues that act in both intracellular and extracellular spaces, although predominantly extracellularly in connective tissue spaces.[16] *Tocopherol* and *β-carotene* are the main lipid-soluble nonenzymatic antioxidants and are primarily localized to cell membranes. Because of its

Table 7-1
Cellular and extracellular antioxidants and ultraviolet (UV) radiation

Antioxidant	Studies Conducted to Show Blockage of UV Damage with Topical Application	Small Molecule, Primarily Extracellular	Known Effects of UV Radiation	Comments
Catalase			Inactivated	
Glutathione		X	Reduced	Spares α-tocopherol; substrate for enzymatic antioxidant functions
α-Tocopherol	+	X	Depleted	Most abundant antioxidant; located in cell membranes; lipid soluble
Ascorbic acid	+	X	Depleted	Main water-soluble free-radical quencher; reduces tocopherol radical to α-tocopherol
Ubiquinone		X	Depleted	Reduces tocopherol radical
Heme oxygenase			—	
β-Carotene	+	X	Reduced	Efficient quencher of singlet O_2; lipid soluble; protects cell membranes
Lycopene	+	X	Reduced	Twice as active as β-carotene
Coenzyme Q			—	
Superoxide dismutase	+		Reduced	Large molecule
Pyruvate			—	Readily enters cells and promotes cell survival

location on cell membranes, tocopherol inhibits already-initiated lipid peroxidation. Beta-carotene interacts primarily with singlet oxygen (Table 7-1).

Ascorbate is the main water-soluble nonenzymatic antioxidant. It is an ideal free-radical scavenger, being available in most tissues in adequate supply and capable of accumulating within cells. It is also versatile in its reactions and capable of being recycled. Vitamin C is necessary for hydroxylation of procollagen, resulting in collagen production. Ascorbate may also stimulate collagen synthesis by directly and specifically activating collagen gene regulation, both by increasing the transcription rate and stabilizing RNA procollagen.[17,18]

Although these antioxidant systems are up-regulated after ultraviolet (UV) light exposure, they are easily overwhelmed. Catalase is directly inactivated, and vitamins E and C, as well as ubiquinones, are shown to be depleted, while superoxide dismutase, glutathione peroxidase, and glutathione are reduced. Thus the net effect of UV irradiation of the skin is a cascade of damaging free radicals.[19-29] In addition, because a major chromophore for UV-B radiation is DNA, much of the cellular damage done by the UV-B wavelengths of sunlight occurs independent of free-radical formation. However, UV-A radiation imparts its damage in a manner that appears to be mediated primarily through free-radical formation.

Aging Processes

Aging effects of the skin are generally characterized as resulting from both an intrinsic and an extrinsic process. *Intrinsic aging* refers to those processes that result purely from the passage of time. These effects are thought to be secondary to cell membrane damage from free-radical formation as well. These effects generally start to become visible around age 30 to 35 and generally are subtle until more advanced years (generally over age 60). They are most easily visualized in non-sun-exposed areas of the skin. These effects include thinning of the epidermis, hypocellularity of the dermis, and a gradual decrease in numbers of dermal blood vessels, collagen, and elastic tissue. This results in pallor and fine wrinkling with loss of elasticity and sagging of the skin.[30-34]

Extrinsic aging is caused primarily by the effects of environmental UV radiation, thus the terms *photoaging* and *photodamage.* For the average person the vast majority of this sun exposure occurs during multiple brief exposures to the sun during daily normal activities, not in the pursuit of a tan or as a consequence of a sunburn. Photodamage is thought to account for more than 90% of the unwanted changes in skin appearance in sun-exposed areas. These changes include fine to coarse wrinkling, laxity, leathery and coarse skin texture progressing to atrophy in severe photodamage, irregular pigmentation, dry scaling and roughness of the skin surface, telangiectasia, sallowness, and easy bruisibility.[30,35-37]

Solar elastosis represents the deposition of an abnormal, yellow, amorphous elastotic material in the upper dermis that replaces normal collagen and elastin and does not have the resiliency or structure of normal elastic tissue.[30,31,38-40] The walls of the reduced numbers of blood vessels become thin and fragile, resulting in clinical purpura from mild trauma. The compromised maturation of keratinocytes and abnormal melanization of the epidermis result in irregular pigmentation as well as precancerous and cancerous epidermal cells (Figure 7-1).

The extracellular matrix of the dermis provides the bulk of skin tissue and its supporting framework. It is composed primarily of type I collagen, with lesser amounts of type III collagen, elastin, proteoglycans, and fibronectin.[41]

Collagen, a protein fiber, accounts for approximately 80% of the dry weight of the dermis. Its architectural organization of fine, interlacing fibers parallel to the epidermis provides the basic structure and strength of the skin. *Elastin,* another protein fiber, composes 2% to 4% of the dry weight of the dermis. Elastin is arranged in a delicate meshwork of individual fibers perpendicular to the epidermis that provides the skin with

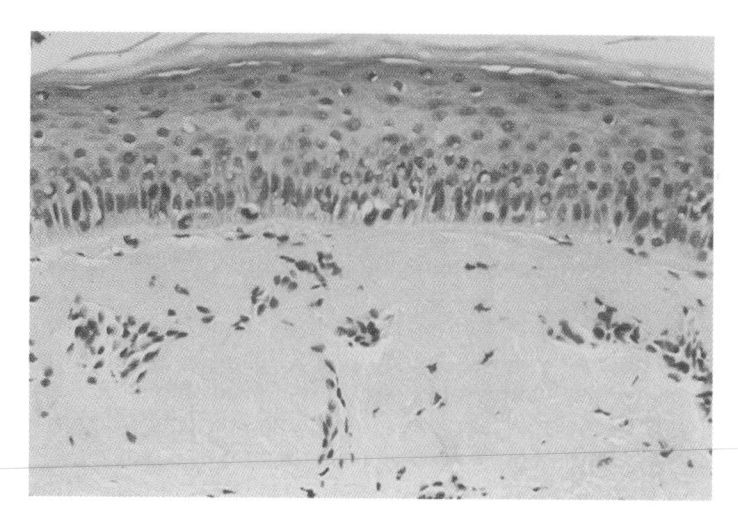

Figure 7-1 Ultraviolet (UV) light damage to skin results in epidermal atrophy and flattening of rete ridges with development of precancerous and cancerous epidermal cells. Amorphous elastotic material (solar elastosis) replaces normal collagen and elastin. Capillaries become reduced in number with thin fragile walls.

elasticity (stretch) and resilience (recoil). Changes in this framework result in the most visible clinical alterations associated with aging skin: wrinkles, manifested histologically as the disorganization of collagen fibrils[42] and the accumulation of abnormal elastin-containing material.[43] The normal dense network of collagen fibers is replaced by thin, haphazardly arranged fibers. Between the epidermis and solar elastosis is a very thin layer of normal collagen, termed the *Grenz* or *border zone*. This thin layer appears to be secondary to growth factors secreted from the epidermis that stimulate fibroblasts to create a healthy layer of dermal tissue on which the epidermis can rest.

The visible and functional degree of textural abnormality (pebbly, uneven, or crepelike changes), wrinkling and furrowing, and sagging skin laxity correlates with the density and depth of solar elastosis in the dermis.

Immunochemistry studies have demonstrated fragmentation of collagen fibers in areas of solar elastosis.[44,45] In addition, a statistically significant decrease (20%) in total collagen content of sun-damaged skin versus sun-protected skin has been demonstrated[45] and confirmed in other studies.[46,47] Further investigation has shown collagen production to remain unchanged, but increased collagen degradation in sun-damaged skin results in a net decrease in steady-state collagen levels, predominantly within the paillary dermis.[42] In vitro studies have suggested a role for fibroblast-derived collagenase in this process of photoaging. UV exposure has been shown to stimulate collagenase production directly by human fibroblasts[48] and to up-regulate collagenase gene expression.[49]

Additional biochemical evidence of connective tissue alterations in photoaged skin includes reduced levels of types I and III collagen precursors[50] and cross-links,[51] an increased ratio of type III to type I collagen,[52] and an increased level of elastin.[53]

Collagenase is one of the matrix-degrading *metalloproteinases* (MPs), proteolytic enzymes that specifically degrade collagen, elastin, and other proteins in connective tissue and bone.[54,55] These enzymes are critical for matrix remodeling during wound healing.[56] Their activities are regulated by specific inhibitors[57] to prevent excessive matrix degradation.[58,59] Collagenases are the only proteases capable of hydrolyzing fibrillar collagen within its triple-helix structure and are required for normal collagen turnover in adult mammals.[60] Once cleaved, collagen is further broken down by gelatinases and stromelysins.

In a study using a dose of UV light equivalent to 5 to 15 minutes of midday sun exposure, both single exposure and four exposures at 48-hour intervals were shown to induce the same maximal elevation of three matrix MPs.[61] Degradation of endogenous type I collagen fibrils was increased by 58% in UV-irradiated skin compared with nonexposed skin. From a practical view, this means that brief sun exposures on an every-other-day basis should maintain elevation of these matrix-degrading enzymes and cause breakdown of skin connective tissue and premature skin aging without the induced erythema associated with a clinical "sunburn."

Glycosaminoglycans (GAGs) are complex sugars that make up the majority of the remaining extracellular matrix supporting living skin. These sugars have the ability to bind up to 1000 times their weight in water. GAGs are composed primarily of hyaluronic acid and dermatan sulfate, with smaller amounts of chondroitin sulfate and heparan sulfate. The water-holding properties of *hyaluronic acid* swell the extracellular matrix and allow the rapid diffusion of water-soluble molecules. Hyaluronic acid increases with rapid tissue proliferation, regeneration, and tissue repair.[62,63] It is involved in the structure and organization of the extracellular matrix and preserves tissue hydration.[64-69] It has been proposed that decreased turgidity of the skin, decreased support of microvessels, wrinkling, and altered elasticity associated with aging may be the result of variations in the levels of hyaluronic acid in the dermis[68] and that disappearance of wrinkles may result from increased levels of GAGs.[70] A steady decline of hyaluronic acid in the epidermis has been shown to occur with aging[65] and higher levels of bound hyaluronic acid versus free hyaluronic acid, and an overall decrease with aging has been postulated.[71-76]

Almost all these extracellular components of the dermis are synthesized by dermal fibroblasts, which are influenced by cytokines, inflammatory cells, and the extracellular matrix components themselves.

The effects of intrinsic aging on the dermis represents a diminished ability to remodel collagen and maintain a functional elastic fiber network. This results from decreasing responsiveness of dermal fibroblasts and cytokines and decreasing levels of collagenase, the enzyme that helps degrade and remodel collagen.

Chronic cumulative UV exposure also is medically significant, because it results in the development of actinic keratoses, squamous cell carcinoma (SCC), basal cell carcinoma (BCC), and melanoma. UV light is considered a "complete carcinogen"; that is, it not only initiates cancers through DNA mutations but also promotes their growth through the inflammatory processes associated with cumulative UV exposure.[77] This cutaneous photodamage has resulted in the annual appearance of greater than 1 million new cases of BCC and SCC as well as more than 38,000 new cases of melanoma annually in the U.S. population.[77,78] The additional effect of ozone depletion in the atmosphere has been predicted to increase these skin cancers.

REVERSAL OF PHOTOAGING

Effective topical therapies to reverse photoaging have included the use of retinoids, alpha-hydroxy acids, and antioxidants in addition to sunscreens.

Retinoids

Retinoids have been shown to play a role in modulating cellular differentiation and proliferation, possibly through nuclear retinoid receptors.[79] In the area of topical agents, more information is available regarding *tretinoin* or its metabolic precursor *retinoic acid* (Retin-A, Renova), and its effects on photoaging than any other compound now used.[79-97] Improvement in the appearance of photoaged skin after treatment with tretinoin is associated with the restoration of type I procollagen to levels approaching those seen in non-sun-exposed skin.[87] Studies in mice and humans have demonstrated that topical retinoic acid reduces the wrinkled appearance of UV radiation–damaged skin.[88-90] This results at least in part from an increase in new dermal collagen formation[91] and occurs in a dose-dependent manner.

Retinoic acid has also been shown to stimulate the synthesis of hyaluronic acid.[97-102] A recent study has shown that treatment of photoaged skin with topical retinoic acid resulted in a 23% increase in the thickness of the vital epidermis related to increasing hyaluronic acid.[97]

Tretinoin has been shown to stimulate proliferation of keratinocytes and fibroblasts, resulting in normalization of the epidermis and stimulation of new collagen in the upper dermis, and to inhibit UV-B-induced collagen degeneration.[88,92-94] In addition, new blood vessel formation, elastin formation, and redistribution of epidermal melanin pigment have been demonstrated. In recent 6-month clinical trials, approximately 65% of patients were found to have improvement in fine wrinkling and irregular pigmentation, whereas 80% noted some overall improvement.[84-86,88]

Long-term studies of topical retinoic acid for photodamage have shown that the maximal efficacy is obtained after at least 10 months of treatment. Long-term treatment is needed to maintain clinical benefit.[95] Recently, hypertrophic scars and keloids,[103] acne scars,[104] and striae distensae (atrophicae)[105] have been shown to improve with prolonged treatment with topical retinoic acid. These improvements would be explained by new collagen formation and remodeling.

Pretreatment of skin with tretinoin inhibits by 70% to 80% the induction of the three MPs that are necessary to degrade skin collagen fully.[54,58,96] It is thought that the ability to block the induction of matrix MPs by UV light through agents such as tretinoin or retinol[106,107] may prevent dermal damage that leads to photoaging.

As previously mentioned, a study using UV radiation doses equivalent to 5 to 15 minutes of midday sun in single and multiple exposures in vivo demonstrated induction of matrix MPs that was sustained with multiple exposures. Pretreatment of skin with tretinoin substantially inhibited the induction of collagenase, 92-kilodalton gelatinase, and stromelysin-1, but not the tissue inhibitor of matrix MPs-1.[61] These studies provide a rationale for treating photodamaged skin with tretinoin.

Alpha-hydroxy Acids

Alpha-hydroxy acids (AHAs), particularly *glycolic acid,* have been enthusiastically received by the public and by physicians involved in rejuvenative medicine. These topical preparations are widely available from many manufacturers and have been shown to have some benefit in treating abnormal distributions of epidermal pigmentation as well as acne.[108] Although antiaging benefits for treatment of extrinsic aging are alleged by anecdotal reports, no significant peer-reviewed controlled studies demonstrate beneficial dermal effects. However, AHAs can increase epidermal and dermal GAGs and skin thickness. This is secondary to the increased GAGs content with its associated water binding.[109,110] A recent study has also reported increased collagen production.[110] Thickening of the dermis as well as increased collagen content was observed, even though no inflammation was seen.

If AHAs do have a dermal effect, it probably results from chemical irritant effects, which may be related to deeper penetration of formulations with a pH of 3 or lower. A stinging or burning sensation is indicative of dermal penetration. Large molecules attached to AHAs (polyhydroxy acids) may limit penetration and result in a more superficial effect.

Antioxidants

The use of antioxidants to protect against damage incurred from free-radical formation is logical. Dietary supplementation of vitamin C and a mixture of antioxidants have been shown to reduce UV-B-induced neoplasms in mice.[111,112] High levels of dietary vitamin E in mice have resulted in increased skin levels adequate to inhibit solar induced lipid hydroperoxides.[113]

The use of antioxidants topically to protect the skin from the harmful effects of UV radiation has become an area of intense investigation. The first antioxidant studied was vitamin E, and in 1979 it was shown to prevent UV-B erythema, even when applied several minutes after UV exposure.[114] Other studies confirmed the photoprotective effects of topically applied vitamin E when used in concentrations of 2%.[115-117] These studies demonstrated the effectiveness of α-tocopherol, but not its acetate derivative. For the acetate to be effective, it must be converted to α-tocopherol. This conversion does occur in skin[118] but is limited and requires days.[116,119] In addition, vitamin E absorbs at 297 nm and therefore contributes partially as a sunscreen as well.

Tocopherols are the most abundant and efficient free-radical scavengers in biologic membranes. Primary water-soluble antioxidants include ascorbate and cellular thiols. Glutathione is an important substrate for enzymatic antioxidant functions. Carotenoids are lipid soluble and important in protecting cell membranes.

Vitamin E is the most important inhibitor of lipid membrane damage, acting by intercepting reactive, lipid-derived radical intermediates before they can propagate the damage.[10] Vitamin E has been shown to be capable of breaking a chain reaction of oxidation in the cellular membrane and is important in scavenging lipophilic radicals, which are formed either within the membrane or by an attack of aqueous radicals on the membranes. Although water-soluble antioxidants, especially vitamin C, act as a first defense against free radicals generated in plasma and extracellular fluids, they cannot scavenge lipophilic radicals within the membranes.[120] However, only a few vitamin E molecules exist for every thousand lipid molecules in membranes. To react catalytically, there must be a mechanism to regenerate the parent vitamin E molecule, α-tocopherol. One of the main functions of vitamin C, which is much more plentiful, is to reduce the tocopherol radical back to α-tocopherol, thereby making it available to inhibit yet another chain reaction in cell membranes.[10,121-123] Ubiquinone and lipoic acid also have this capability.[13,14]

Dihydrolipoate[124-126] and other thiols[122] can also protect membranes and prevent lipid peroxidation and spare tocopherol. The thiols associated with membrane proteins may have an antioxidant role and the protection of protein thiols by glutathione may be considered as sparing tocopherol as well.[127-129]

Vitamin C is water soluble and is one of the most effective antioxidants in quenching reactive oxygen species such as singlet oxygen and superoxide.[11] In plasma it is the predominant inhibitor of low-density lipoprotein (LDL) oxidation.[12] However, it is an extremely unstable molecule that begins to degrade in minutes when near neutral pH, which makes it very difficult to be used effectively in topical preparations. Fortunately, an acidic pH helps stabilize vitamin C significantly, with an increase in percutaneous absorption without significant skin irritation.[130]

A patented formulation using vitamin C in 10% concentration and in combination with zinc and tyrosine in an acidic pH (Cellex-C), has been shown to result in tissue levels of vitamin C 20 times normal with penetration up to 500 μm into the dermis.[23] Vitamin C has been shown to act as an antioxidant at these tissue concentrations and to block UV-A and UV-B tissue damage.[10,131-133] In addition, it is thought to be a cytokine that directly stimulates fibroblasts to produce collagen.[134-138] One study using a neutral-pH ascorbic acid formulation showed no significant effect in protection against UV-A-induced wrinkling in mouse skin.[139] It is thought that the ascorbic acid would be 100% ionized at this pH and therefore unable to be absorbed into the skin. The pH of the vitamin C formulation therefore may be a critical variable.

As with vitamin E, stabilized derivatives of ascorbic acid must be converted metabolically to vitamin C to be effective. This conversion has been reported with ascorbic acid-2-phosphate,[140] Ester-C,[141] and ascorbic acid-2-glucoside.[142]

Lipid solubility would seem to be an advantage for a compound to penetrate the stratum corneum. *Ascorbyl palmitate* has a polar ascorbate head and lipophilic tail. It is stable for at least 6 months and is hydrolyzed to L-ascorbate by phosphatases present in skin. Ascorbic acid–palmitate has great lipophilicity, enhancing its ability to penetrate into the skin, and has been reported to be moderately protective against UV-B sunburn, even when applied after UV-B irradiation.[143] Cutaneous levels of ascorbyl palmitate have not been measured, and adequate topical concentrations for the desired biologic effects are not known. Some researchers allege that the optimal concentration would be greater than 20% ascorbyl palmitate. However, one study did show that penetration of L-ascorbate in human skin was 15% that of ascorbyl palmitate and 29% that of α-tocopherol, but these levels did not correlate with antioxidant activity.[16]

Because vitamins C and E interact naturally, it was thought that a combination of both would be superior to either alone as a photoprotectant, and this combined effect has been demonstrated.[144] In this study, vitamin E was superior to vitamin C in protecting against UV-B light, whereas vitamin C was superior regarding UV-A protection.

Beta carotene, a carotenoid and a natural antioxidant, has also been used as a photoprotectant. It is an efficient quencher of singlet oxygen. It has been shown to inhibit UV-B-induced tumor formation in mice when given orally[145] and UV-B-mediated lipid damage[146] as well as 8-methoxypsoralen & UVA-induced erythema[147] when used topically in animal models. The carotenoids include lycophene in addition to β-carotene. *Lycophene* has the greatest quenching ability, twice that of β-carotene.[129] The carotenoids have also been shown to have anticancer activity.[148-150]

Superoxide dismutase is a large molecule and thus unlikely to penetrate the stratum corneum, but one study showed it can inhibit PUVA-induced erythema.[147] Encapsulation into liposomes has been used to enhance its absorption, but the penetration depth in this type of formulation is unknown. However, studies using liposomal superoxide dismutase have shown that it inhibits UV-induced lipid peroxidation[151] and prevents UV-induced loss of intrinsic superoxide dismutase activity.[152]

Pyruvate and other α-ketoacids react rapidly with H_2O_2 to protect cells from cytolytic effects.[153] *Pyruvate* is one of the few antioxidants that readily enters cells[154] and promotes cellular survival. It was recently reported that mammalian cells secrete pyruvate as an antioxidative defense against oxygen radicals.[154] Sodium pyruvate was shown to increase the proliferative rate of epidermal keratinocytes and to protect against lipid peroxidation[129,153,155,156]

Selenomethionine[157] and extracts of green tea (high in polyphenoic cathechol-like compounds)[158] are other antioxidants that have been shown to have photoprotective benefits when applied topically.

Photoprotective Effects

Antioxidants clearly add biologic protection to help prevent the damage that both UV-A and UV-B may do to the skin. Their addition to a topical preparation containing sunscreens provides more than additive protection and allows the skin to repair more readily the damage that does occur. However, their specific formulation and concentrations are critical parameters that affect their effectiveness in topical preparations.

Fibroblasts play a pivotal role in maintaining the dermal architecture. These cells are quiescent until they respond to stimuli. Inflammation and wounding stimulate collagenase proteolytic activity. Growth factors induce cellular proliferation through procollagen production and collagenase inhibition. Fibroblasts become increasingly proteolytic with age. They underexpress procollagen and collagenase inhibitory factor and overexpress collagenase. The net result is a diminishing ability to maintain the structural integrity of the dermis. Thus medical treatment of cellular aging involves down-regulating proteolytic activity and up-regulating structural protein synthesis.[159,160]

Most of the clinical improvement seen with the use of topical tretinoin has been shown to correlate with new type I collagen formation.[87] This effect is both time and dose related and may be significant in treatment of both sun-exposed and non-sun-exposed skin.[90,161]

Whether these topical preparations are capable of reversing photodamage to the degree that is clinically desirable by patients seeking a more youthful appearance is somewhat controversial, and most physicians believe that they are adjuncts to surgical resurfacing procedures. Retinoic acid has been shown to enhance wound healing when used preoperatively for dermabrasion and chemical peels[162-167] and recently in a porcine study of laser resurfacing with and without retinoic acid before treatment.[168] Most physicians recommend its use preoperatively and postoperatively for laser resurfacing.[169] Topical vitamin C has had the same type of support for enhancing wound healing from anecdotal reports, although no published reports to date have established its value objectively.

• • •

In summary, photoaging results in alterations in the epidermis that have the potential of developing into skin cancers and precancers as well as pigment abnormalities. Dermal alterations result in structural changes that manifest as wrinkling and loss of normal skin texture and elasticity. To repair this damage, sunscreens are essential, but a variety of topical medications and agents may be beneficial as well. Retinoids may be useful in stimulating both epidermal and dermal repair. AHAs have been shown to assist at least with epidermal normalization. Topical antioxidants, especially vitamins C and E, not only may be protective against photodamage,

Table 7-2
Topical agents to reverse photodamage

Agent	Demonstrated Benefit
Tretinoin (Retin-A)	Normalization of epidermis; elimination of precancers
	Elastin formation
	Normalization of pigment
	New capillary formation
	New collagen formation; inhibition of collagen degeneration; may modulate collagen remodeling
	Increases glycosaminoglycans (GAGs); stimulation of synthesis of hyaluronic acid
	May modulate collagen remodeling
Retinol	Converted to retinoic acid in skin
	Less irritation topically than retinoic acid
Alpha-hydroxy acids	Normalization of epidermis
	Normalization of pigment
	Increase GAGs
	Possible increase in collagen through direct irritant effect
Vitamin C	Biologically blocks ultraviolet (UV) damage to skin (UV-A more than UV-B)
	Direct stimulant to fibroblasts for new collagen
Ascorbyl palmitate	Lipid soluble
	Converted to ascorbic acid in skin
Vitamin E	Biologically blocks UV damage to skin (UV-B more than UV-A); easily absorbed in skin
Hyaluronic acid	Enhances water content of both epidermis and dermis
	May modulate wound healing

but also may allow better regenerative capabilities by not exhausting normal defenses, as well as through potentiation of collagen production by vitamin C. Hyaluronic acid enhances the water content of both the epidermis and the dermis.

All these agents should be part of a pretreatment regimen to prepare the skin for laser resurfacing by making the skin as healthy as possible (Table 7-2). Studies of topical application of these agents have shown their effects to be both time and dose dependent. Therefore longer periods of application preoperatively are preferable to shorter periods. For optimal results, periods of 3 to 6 months are advisable. However, even the use of these agents for only 2 weeks preoperatively may be beneficial, because it may stimulate fibroblasts to an active phase, enhance epidermal proliferation, and provide stores of vitamin C in tissue. Resumption of this regimen postoperatively as early as possible (generally 2 to 3 weeks) and continuation for at least 6 months, but preferably indefinitely, as an ongoing maintenance regimen are advantageous and advisable.

NONLASER TREATMENT OF PHOTOAGING

Because photoaging results in skin changes that are most pronounced at the skin surface, physically removing these layers, with subsequent regeneration of healthy new epidermis and papillary dermis, has always been a more aggressive alternative approach to reversal of photodamage.

Traditionally, surgical treatments for photoaging have involved the removal of this outer layer of the most severely photodamaged tissue (epidermis and upper dermis) using various acids or dermabrasion[170] and then allowing the healing process to replace this tissue with healthy, non-solar-damaged dermal and epidermal tissue. Alternatively, lifting procedures such as rhytidectomy and blepharoplasty may be performed to remove redundant loose tissue or excessive or bulging subcutaneous tissue.

The difficulty in achieving a specific and repeatedly predictable depth of tissue removal with chemicals and dermabrasion has led to variable results, although dramatic improvement may be achieved with either modality in some patients. To avoid the risks of hypopigmentation, prolonged erythema, and scarring that may be associated with deep levels of resurfacing, the practice has been to treat more superficially, resulting frequently in insufficient cosmetic improvement. The depth of chemical peeling may be variable, depending on cutaneous characteristics, time of application, skin preparation, amounts and types of acid applied, and other factors affecting penetration, resulting in uneven clinical effects with patches of hypopigmentation or scarring and persistence of photodamage and wrinkles in other areas in the same patient.[171-176] In addition, phenol preparations are cardiotoxic and in high doses can be nephrotoxic and hepatotoxic.[174] Superficial peels (AHAs, Jessner's solution, 10%-15% trichloroacetic acid [TCA]) produce injury to the epidermis primarily and only minimal upper papillary dermal injury. These peels produce a wound depth of 60 to 100 μm. Medium-depth and deep chemical peels (35%-50% TCA, 50%-100% phenol, 50%-55% phenol mixed with croton oil, salicylic or lactic acid) produce more extensive papillary dermal and reticular dermal damage. Medium-depth peels induce a wound depth of 200 to 450 μm. Deep peels penetrate to the midreticular dermis, 500 to 800 μm deep.[175,176]

Dermabrasion is a technique-dependent procedure that must be used with caution on thin skin, such as the delicate tissue of the eyelid. It typically produces variable results in the same patient because of subtle technique differences, sometimes related to difficulties in visualizing intraoperative depths of resurfacing. In addition, dermabrasion continues to lose favor because of the potential for exposure to bloodborne pathogens.[176-178]

CARBON DIOXIDE LASER

Although physicians showed considerable interest in development of resurfacing parameters with the CO_2 laser in the early to middle 1980s, the safety profile for use of the continuous-wave (CW) CO_2 laser prohibited its use in this manner. Successful low-fluence CW CO_2 laser removal of the epidermis was reported[179,180] as well as revision of skin grafts[181] and treatment of acne scars[182] in 1985 through 1991. However, this technique was found to be too risky to use over large surface areas because it has too high a risk of scarring. These treatment techniques can be traced back to Leon Goldman's report of treatment of actinic cheilitis with the CO_2 laser in 1968.[183] This treatment technique, however, was not widely used for this condition until popularized by David's report of a series of patients in 1985.[184]

The more limited use of the CO_2 laser in combination with TCA peeling was reported first by Brauner and Schliftman[185] in 1987 and by David et al [186] in 1989 for the treatment of wrinkling.

Laser Development

The development of superpulsed CO_2 lasers, in conjunction with Anderson and Parrish's development of the theory of selective photothermolysis[187] and work being done on burn débridement, allowed the potential for defining the necessary laser parameters for skin resurfacing. Work done by our group[188-193] plus critical information obtained by Green et al[194-196] led to the realization that cutaneous resurfacing could be accomplished with a high-energy, pulsed CO_2 laser. From 1988 to 1991, however, no laser manufacturer showed interest in developing such a CO_2 laser for this purpose. Fortunately, however, Coherent had developed such a laser for ear-nose-throat and gynecologic use. This laser was poorly received in these fields and was about to be withdrawn from production when I was told of its existence and that it might be just the laser I was seeking.[197]

Working with Dale Koop of Coherent, we modified this laser for resurfacing by developing a collimated handpiece, increasing the pulse energy to 500 mJ, enlarging the spot size to 3 mm, and developing a computer pattern generator (CPG) to standardize the placement of laser impacts on the skin surface. Protocol involving treatment with single-pulse vaporization was developed and involved single-impact passes with approximately 10% to 20% spot overlap of a gaussian beam and wiping away desiccated tissue debris between passes.

Initially the laser was used in treatment of various cutaneous lesions, as traditionally performed with CW or superpulsed CO_2 lasers, to understand the potential limitations or complications of the laser. At the same time, a histologic study was performed on a porcine model to explore the wound depths and healing characteristics in comparison to commonly used resurfacing modalities.[198] Relatively predictable depths of injury, ranging from intraepidermal to 350 μm, could be produced by varying the pulse energy and the number of laser passes (Figure 7-2).

Weinstein[199] reported the first series of patients treated with the high-energy, pulsed CO_2 laser for cosmetic benefit. She reported 36 patients who had upper and lower lid laser blepharoplasty in conjunction with periorbital resurfacing. Excellent results (complete eradication of static periocular lines) was seen in 81%; reepithelialization required 8.4 days on average and erythema 4.7 weeks to fade. One patient had transient scarring, one had transient ectropion, and three had mild hypopigmentation. Lowe et al[200] reported that 100 patients had been successfully treated and that gradual improvement was seen over the first 6 months postoperatively, with average improvement being 4.17 on a scale of 6.0 (maximum). The initial use of the laser was confined to the perioral and periorbital regions, because

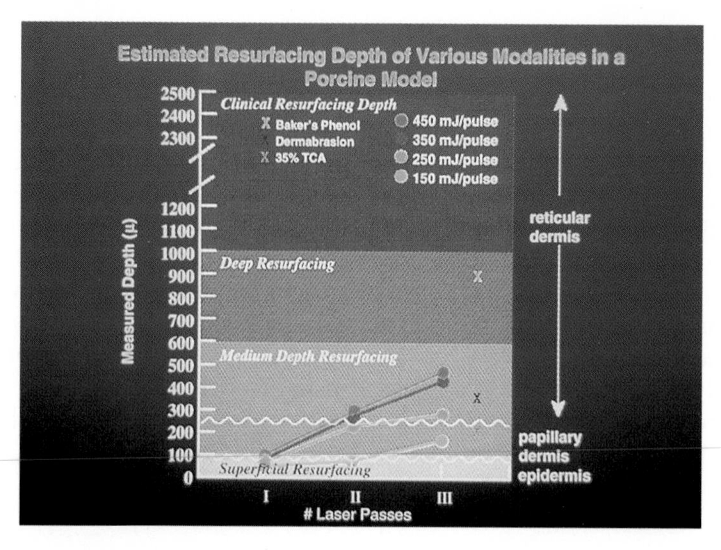

Figure 7-2 Varying pulse energies and passes of UltraPulse CO_2 laser resulted in resurfacing depths comparable to those of trichloroacetic acid (TCA) peels or dermabrasion, but not those of phenol peels.

these areas were most difficult to treat by traditional methods. Improvement in pretreatment photodamage by approximately 50% or more was reported by our group[202] (Figure 7-3). It became apparent that full-face resurfacing was possible and resulted in even better cosmetic improvement.

Simultaneously, the SilkTouch scanning system (Sharplan Laser Corp., Allendale, NJ) was being developed and used for ablative rectal surgery,[202] laser uvuloplasty[203] in the management of obstructive sleep apnea, and hair transplantation.[204] This laser system was also being evaluated in a single pass for laser cutaneous resurfacing.[205] Our protocol of multiple single passes with wiping between passes was adapted for this system as well. The first clinical series reports appeared in 1995.[206, 207]

The first reports of 47 patients and 40 patients showed an average improvement of greater than 50% and 3.5 on a scale of 6.0.[206,207] Erythema was seen to last 1 to 4 months[206] or averaged 6 weeks.[207] Persistent erythema was seen to correlate with depth of ablation. Postinflammatory hyperpigmentation was the most common complication, occurring in 17%, exclusively in patients with skin types III or IV. Bacterial infections occurred in 6%, with herpes simplex disseminating in one patient.[206]

A third laser, the SurgiPulse XJ150 (Sharplan) uses two paried 200-mJ energy peaks rather than a single 500-mJ peak as seen with the Coherent UltraPulse CO_2 laser. With a peak energy of 200 mJ, very little energy actually exceeds the critical irradiance required for tissue vaporization. Because of this, an increased number of laser passes was found to be necessary for treatment, and a 63% mean average improvement was seen, compared with 82% mean improvement after UltraPulse laser treatment.[208]

These recent advances in high-energy, pulsed CO_2 lasers, combined with the development of safe and effective treatment protocols, have resulted in an explosion of interest, promotion, and use of these lasers for rejuvenation of facial photodamage.[199-201,205-218]

Advantages

The potential advantages of pulsed-laser cutaneous resurfacing relate to the precise control of tissue vaporization, minimization of residual thermal damage, and achievement of hemostasis. These advantages are achieved by single-pulse vaporization of

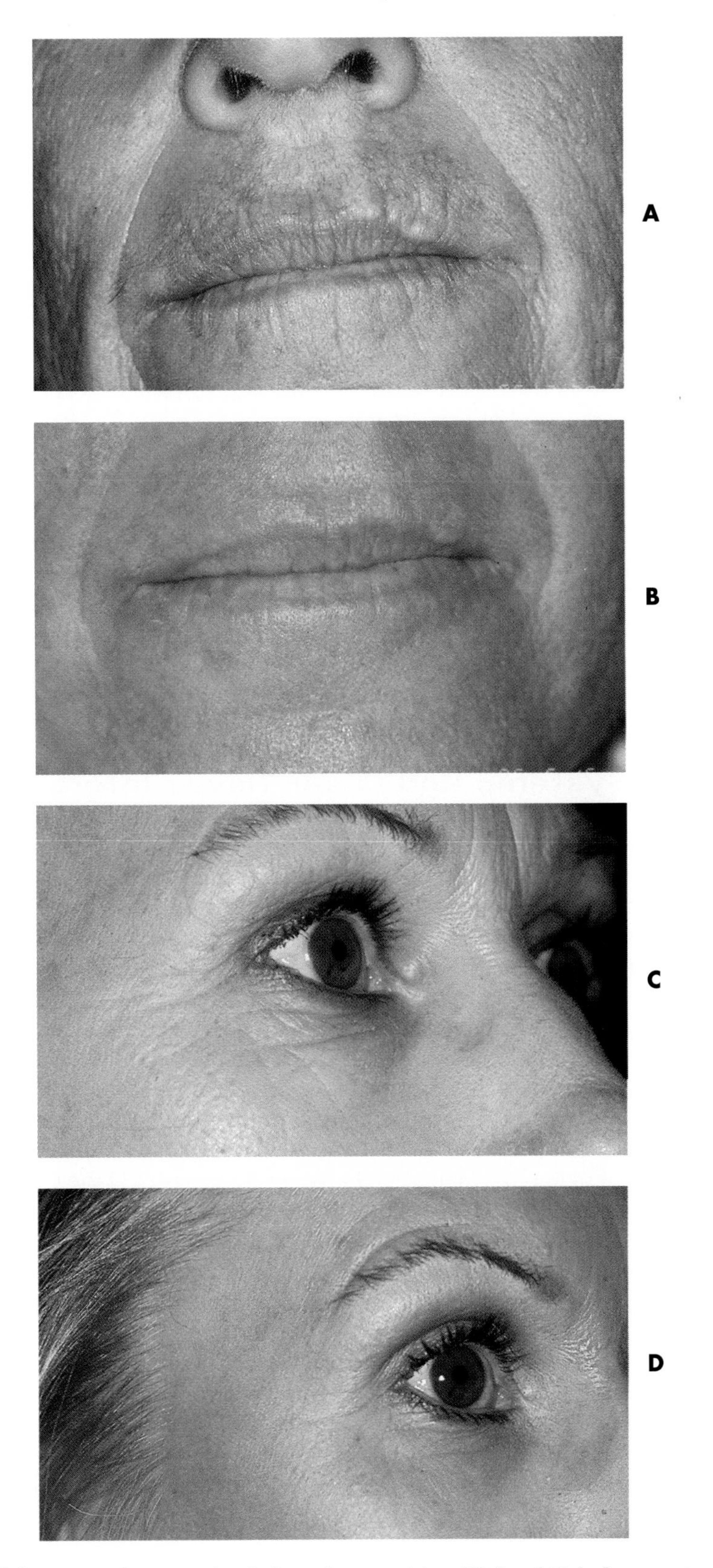

Figure 7-3 **A,** Significant perioral photodamage (class III, level 7) before treatment. **B,** Six months postoperatively, dramatic improvement, with photodamage now rated class I, level 2. **C,** Periorbital photodamage (class II, level 6) before treatment. **D,** Nine months postoperatively, significant improvement, with photodamage now rated class I, level 3.

tissue using a high-energy, submillisecond, pulsed CO_2 laser. The CO_2 wavelength (10,600 nm) is efficiently absorbed in water, resulting in an optical penetration depth of 20 to 30 μm.[195,196,219] The absoprtion coefficient (μa) of water at 10.6 μm is approximately 790 cm^{-1} and in tissue 553 cm^{-1} (790 cm^{-1} × 70%, assuming water content of tissue to be 70%).[219] Each pulse exposure should remove about one optical penetration depth (20-30 μm) of tissue and leave two to four times that (40-120 μm) of residual thermal damage. In cutaneous applications, intracellular water is the laser's target, and on absorption, heat transfer results in instantaneous tissue heating to greater than 100° C boiling of water and its vaporization and cellular ablation. If this energy is delivered with a continuous beam, the tissue becomes progressively desiccated, and because of loss of its water target, heat accumulates in tissue, reaching temperatures of up to 600° C. This results in diffusion of heat to several hundred micrometers below the level of vaporization.

A layer of thermal necrosis greater than 100 μm interferes with wound healing and may result in significant scarring when it extends deeper into the dermis.[192,220,221] To avoid this scenario, the laser energy must be delivered rapidly, in less time than it takes the tissue to cool (estimated to be 1 msec or less).* If the individual pulses do not deliver adequate energy to vaporize tissue, multiple pulses become necessary and complicate the situation because of heat diffusion between pulses.[192] Ideally the tissue should be vaporized in a single pulse, because this dissipates heat away from the treated tissue and does not allow significant heat diffusion to occur below the level of vaporization.

Delivery Systems and Laser-Tissue Interactions

A study regarding the effects of pulse duration on the ablation threshold and residual thermal damage[226] revealed a number of significant findings regarding the laser-tissue interaction. These findings included that (1) when tissue ablation occurs, the pulse duration is not critical because a rapid temperature drop occurs just below the ablation front,[227,230] (2) residual thermal damage in this situation approaches a theoretic minimum of 50 μm,[227,229-232] and (3) increases in pulse width cause increased thermal damage at the edges of craters resulting from a gaussian beam. Also, an increase in the ablation threshold at longer pulse durations is related to thermal diffusion during the pulse. To confine thermal damage, the velocity of ablation is critical and requires a value of 0.65 cm/sec or greater to achieve minimal thermal damage.

The ablation depth per pulse at 7.5 J/cm^2 was found to be 35 μm, too small to account for the clinical improvement seen in two or three passes of the CO_2 laser in treating wrinkles measuring 300 μm in depth. This aspect is discussed in greater detail later.

As an alternative to pulsed delivery, a CW CO_2 laser may be used with a scanning system that sweeps the beam across tissue rapidly enough that the tissue dwell time is less than the thermal relaxation time of the tissue, simulating the tissue effects of a pulsed delivery system.[200,206]

The laser beam may be delivered using a *focused* system, in which the beam is focused with lenses to a point having maximal fluence or irradiance. The distance from that focal point is a major determinant of tissue reaction, resulting in decreasing energies with increased handpiece-to-tissue distances. Alternatively, the beam may be delivered in a *collimated* manner, in which the beam is parallel and nondivergent, having the same fluence or irradiance independent of handpiece-to-tissue distances.

Although several new pulsed lasers were introduced in the mid-1990s, two laser systems have been used to pioneer this field and have generated virtually all the published data available: the UltraPulse laser (Coherent) and the SilkTouch scanner

*References 187, 192, 195, 196, 198, 222-238.

(Sharplan). The UltraPulse laser can deliver up to 500 mJ in a single pulse with a duration of less than 1 msec. This energy is delivered with a 3-mm collimated beam, generally used with 3 to 5 W resulting in a repetition rate of 6 to 10 Hz. Rapid, precise placement of these high-energy pulses ensuring single-pulse tissue interaction is achieved with a CPG,[233-236] using a 2.25-mm beam, 300 mJ per pulse, and a power of 60 W resulting in a placement of 81 pulses in one of six patterns at a rate of 220 Hz and with pulse densities varying from no overlap to 60% overlap (Figure 7-4).

The Sharplan system uses a standard CW CO_2 beam focused to a 200-μm spot that is manipulated through rotating mirrors to scan tissue rapidly, resulting in a tissue dwell time of less than 1 msec. Scanning patterns of 4, 6, or 9 mm may be chosen.

In clinical use, two passes with the Sharplan SilkTouch systems appear to be approximately equal to three passes with the UltraPulse laser in terms of the amount of tissue removed and the depth of residual thermal necrosis.[237]

Experimental data and theoretic calculations reveal the necessary pulse fluence to vaporize epidermal tissue to be approximately 5 J/cm^2.[219] To utilize a large spot size and deliver a pulse less than 1 msec in achieving this threshold fluence, a very high irradiance is necessary. When a spot size of 2.5 mm is used, 250 mJ must be delivered in less than 1 msec.[192] This is generally delivered with a gaussian beam, so a peripheral ring of about 10% may exist in which this threshold may not be reached. This suprathreshold energy will immediately vaporize intracellular water, leaving behind cellular proteinaceous debris. The depth of vaporization is proportional to the pulse energy. However, when the laser is interacting with the dermis, a new situation exists. Water is now primarily extracellular, in the dermal matrix, which is dominated by the structural proteins collagen and elastin. Type I collagen will melt at temperatures greater than 60° C but requires fluences much greater than 5 J/cm^2 for vaporization. Nonvaporization heating of the dermis will have little adverse effect as long as the pulse width is less than 1 msec and pulses are delivered to the same tissue spot at rates less than 5 Hz. If the delivery rate is greater than this, heat will accumulate between pulses, and thermal damage by diffusion may occur. This can result in poor wound healing or scarring.

Histologic studies have revealed a relationship between depth of ablation and pulse energy as well as the number of passes.[198,219,222-228,238] A comparision between the CO_2 laser used with various pulse energies and numbers of passes and TCA peeling, dermabrasion, and Baker's phenol peel on a porcine model showed that typical

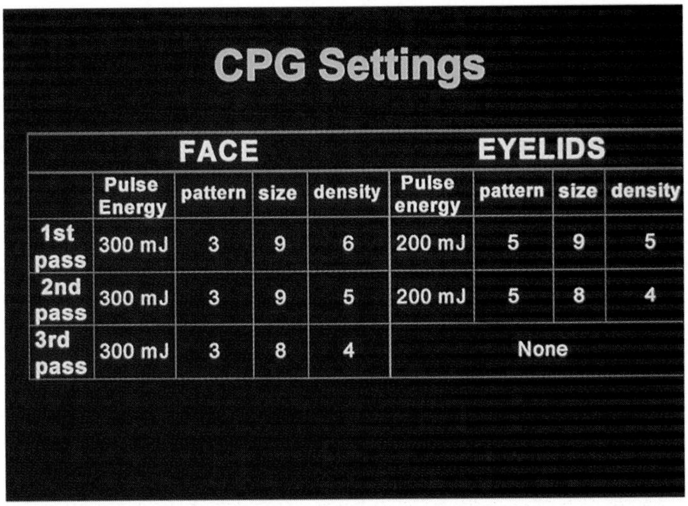

CPG Settings

	FACE				EYELIDS			
	Pulse Energy	pattern	size	density	Pulse energy	pattern	size	density
1st pass	300 mJ	3	9	6	200 mJ	5	9	5
2nd pass	300 mJ	3	9	5	200 mJ	5	8	4
3rd pass	300 mJ	3	8	4	None			

Figure 7-4 Computer pattern generator (CPG) settings should not use densities greater than 6 if cumulative thermal damage from excessive pulse overlap is to be avoided.

pulse energies at one to three passes produced a wound depth intermediate between a 35% TCA peel and dermabrasion, but much more superficial than a phenol peel.[198] Most histologic studies have shown the first CO_2 laser pass to result in epidermal ablation and subsequent passes to result in variable depths of dermal ablation and necrosis. The amount of residual thermal necrosis has also been shown to correlate with both pulse energy and number of passes, with each pass delivering the same amount of energy with less vaporization and more extensive heat absorption because of the layer of desiccated tissue at the treatment surface[198,222-225,228] (Table 7-3 and Figure 7-5).

Pubished reports have correlated clinical signs with anatomic depths of ablation.[239] A pink color of tissue was found to correlate with superficial papillary dermis, chamois-cloth appearance for deeper papillary dermis, and waterlogged cotton-thread appearance for reticular dermis. We have found this to be true, but only in deep ablation, such as with treatment of plantar warts or BCC of the back. When thinner layers of ablation are used, as in resurfacing, these subtle clinical signs are not seen. Unfortunately, a second report has received a tremendous amount of attention in which color changes were stated to be an indication of depth of ablation: pink indicating epidermis, gray indicating papillary dermis, and chamois yellow indicating reticular dermis.[212] These color changes are actually a misinterpretation of anatomic changes and not a reliable indicator of tissue depth. If little residual thermal necrosis (less than 30 μm) exists, thermal reaction will not be sufficient to coagulate fine papillary vessels, and the tissue will be pink because of the visible capillary blood flow. This is typical of the appearance of the tissue after a single laser pass removing the epidermis. After a second or third laser pass, the laser is reacting with the dermis and leaves 70 to 100 μm of thermal necrosis, adequate for hemostasis and resulting in whitish gray tissue. Further laser passes tend to leave more thermal injury, resulting in progressive yellow-brown discoloration, which is a sign of thermal injury, not an indication of penetration into the reticular dermis.

These color changes probably do correlate to some degree with depth of injury, but many inexperienced physicians have interpreted this report too literally and spend much wasted time attempting to recognize subtle color changes, when attention to the laser-tissue interaction with better comprehension would be much more informative.

One study used posttreatment biopsies to compare three pulsed CO_2 lasers with a CW CO_2 laser. After one, two, and three passes, the depth of residual thermal damage measured 30, 80, and 150 μm, respectively, with the SilkTouch laser; 30, 100, and 150 μm with the SurgiPulse laser; and 20, 50, and 70 μm with the UltraPulse laser.[222] The CW CO_2 laser left a 400-μm layer of thermal necrosis.

Although early studies appeared to show a relatively constant amount of tissue to be ablated per pass[198] (approximately 75 μm), it became clear in clinical use that a decreasing amount of tissue was ablated per pass. To investigate this hypothesis, as well as the effects of single-pulse vaporization versus multipulse vaporization, or

Table 7-3
Residual thermal necrosis with CO_2 laser treatment*

Laser Passes	Area of Necrosis (μm)
One	15.5 ± 7.0
Two	53.0 ± 21.2
Three	40.0 ± 21.7
Four	50.2 ± 26.4

Data from E. Bernstein, UltraPulse CO_2 Multicenter Clinical Trial.
*Pulse width less than 1 msec, fluence 7.1 J/cm^2.

"pulse stacking," and its possible relationship to scarring, a study on excised tissue was done.[240] Skin excised for "face-lift" surgery was treated with one through ten passes, wiping with saline between passes and using single-pulse, double-pulse, and triple-pulse impacts at 10 Hz on the same impact site. Biopsies were done to study the depth of ablation as well as residual thermal necrosis. Whether single, double, or triple pulses were used at either 250 mJ or 500 mJ per pulse, a similar curve was generated showing that an ablation plateau was reached after three or four passes at 225 to 250 μm in the dermis (Figure 7-6).

Residual thermal necrosis showed a linear relationship to both pulse energy and number of passes, with single-pulse vaporization gradually increasing to a maximum of 100 μm at pass number seven. However, pulse stacking had a marked impact on residual thermal necrosis, because double pulses added significantly more thermal injury per pass and triple pulses even more per pass, about 30 μm (Figure 7-7). This additional thermal injury may significantly affect wound healing and result in a much deeper wound than intended. Pulse stacking may occur intentionally by concentrating repeated laser impacts on the same tissue site or unintentionally

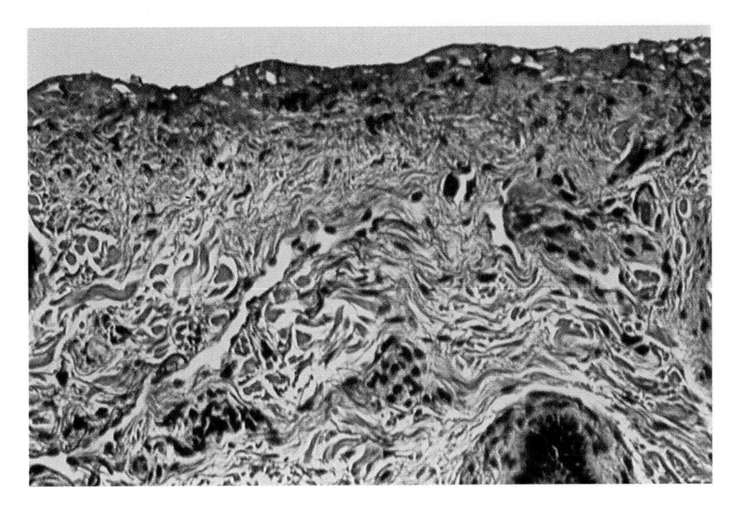

Figure 7-5 Residual thermal damage after two or three passes of UltraPulse CO_2 laser averages approximately 70 μm.

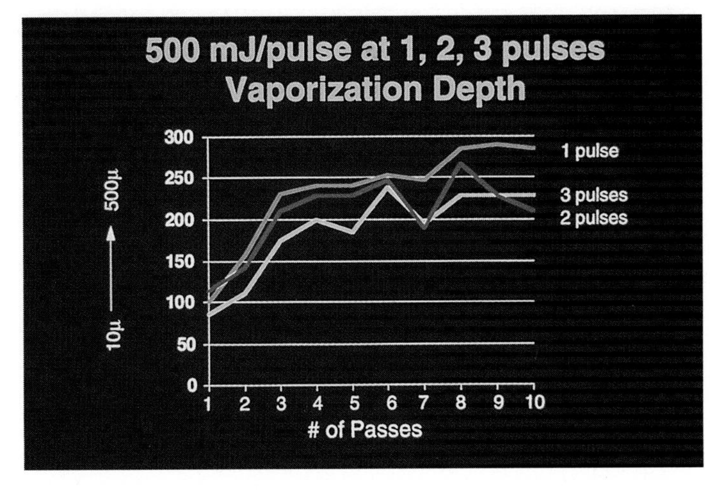

Figure 7-6 With pulsed CO_2 laser ablation, using one, two, or three pulses per impact site at 10 Hz, ablation plateau is reached in three to four passes, limiting ablation depth to approximately 250 μm.

by moving the handpiece at too slow a pace or by using a CPG density that results in too much pulse overlap (densities 7, 8, and 9) corresponding to 40%, 50%, and 60% overlap. This may be a significant factor in causing scarring, hypopigmentation, or poor wound healing (Figure 7-8).

Another finding from this study is that in using single-pulse vaporization with a fluence of 3 to 7 J/cm^2 and a pulse width of less than 1 msec, CO_2 laser resurfacing is a self-limiting procedure, plateauing at a depth of 250 to 300 μm in the dermis, too superficial a wound to result in scarring because of depth alone. Therefore adherence to proper treatment techniques is critical in avoiding excessive thermal injury.

Previous histologic studies of dermabraded skin[170,178] revealed a new, orderly epidermis overlying an upper papillary dermal band of new collagen or "scar." Similar results (increased collagen I formation in the papillary dermis) have been reported after 10 months of treatment with topical tretinoin for photoaged skin.[86] Biopsy specimens obtained at baseline and 3 and 12 weeks after dermabrasion were

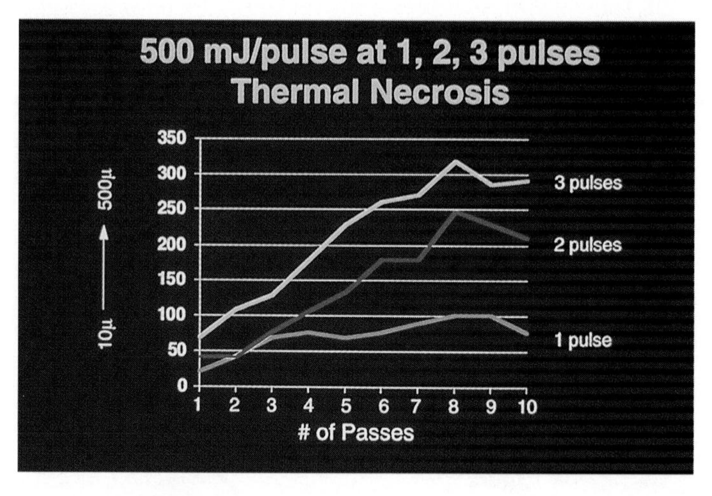

Figure 7-7 When multiple pulses impact same site at 10 Hz (double or triple sets), a cumulative thermal effect occurs resulting in increasing loss of control of residual thermal necrosis. Single tissue impacts, however, result in excellent control of residual thermal damage, even after 10 laser passes.

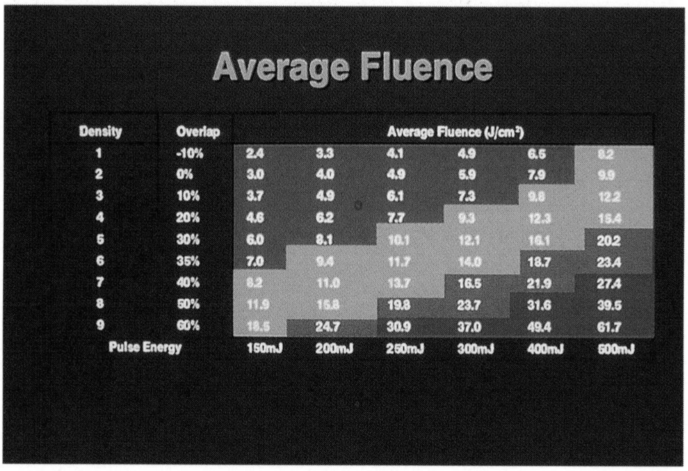

Average Fluence

Density	Overlap	Average Fluence (J/cm^2)					
1	-10%	2.4	3.3	4.1	4.9	6.5	8.2
2	0%	3.0	4.0	4.9	5.9	7.9	9.9
3	10%	3.7	4.9	6.1	7.3	9.8	12.2
4	20%	4.6	6.2	7.7	9.3	12.3	15.4
5	30%	6.0	8.1	10.1	12.1	16.1	20.2
6	35%	7.0	9.4	11.7	14.0	18.7	23.4
7	40%	8.2	11.0	13.7	16.5	21.9	27.4
8	50%	11.9	15.8	19.8	23.7	31.6	39.5
9	60%	18.5	24.7	30.9	37.0	49.4	61.7
Pulse Energy		150mJ	200mJ	250mJ	300mJ	400mJ	500mJ

Figure 7-8 Most effective fluences for treatment are 5 to 18 J/cm^2, corresponding to green and yellow zones of this chart. CPG settings of 9 can result in a fluence as high as 60 J/cm^2.

analyzed and correlated with clinical assessment.[241] Clinical reduction in wrinkling correlated significantly with an increase in fibroblast procollagen-1 in RNA and an increase in procollagen-1 protein, suggesting that clinical improvement may be a result of increased collagen synthesis. Similar increases in Grenz zone collagen have been reported after laser resurfacing,[223,224,228] which we have found as well.[242] This new collagen production and remodeling may be a significant factor in achieving rejuvenation of facial photodamage, as well as in improvement in atrophic acne scars (Figure 7-9). Continued improvement in facial wrinkling has been noted to occur for as long as 6 months postoperatively and in acne scars for 12 months or more. Long-term biopsies (up to 4 years postoperatively) have shown reversal of epidermal dysplasia, maintenance and continued thickening of the Grenz zone, and marked improvement in the layer of solar elastosis underlying the Grenz zone, with reduction in overall depth and development of a more fibrillar character (Figure 7-1 and Figure 7-10).

A further consideration is that consecutive passes with the laser result in the laser encountering desiccated, thermally denatured collagen with little water to act as a target for the laser. This results in a progressively decreased depth of vaporization per pulse. When less of the pulse energy goes into vaporization, progressively more energy is deposited into the tissue, potentially causing thermal necrosis by diffusion. In this situation the pulse width and repetition rate become critical.

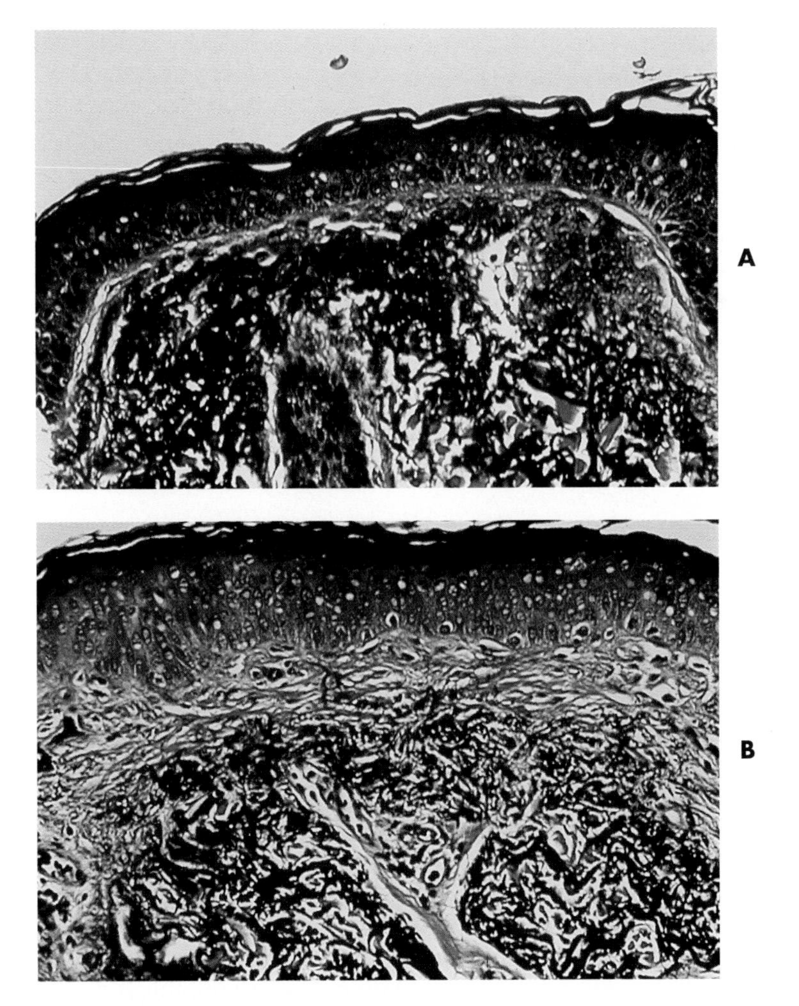

Figure 7-9 **A,** Before treatment. **B,** Using elastic tissue stains, a 600% increase in Grenz zone is noted 90 days after resurfacing, indicating new collagen formation. In addition, layer of solar elastosis is reduced.

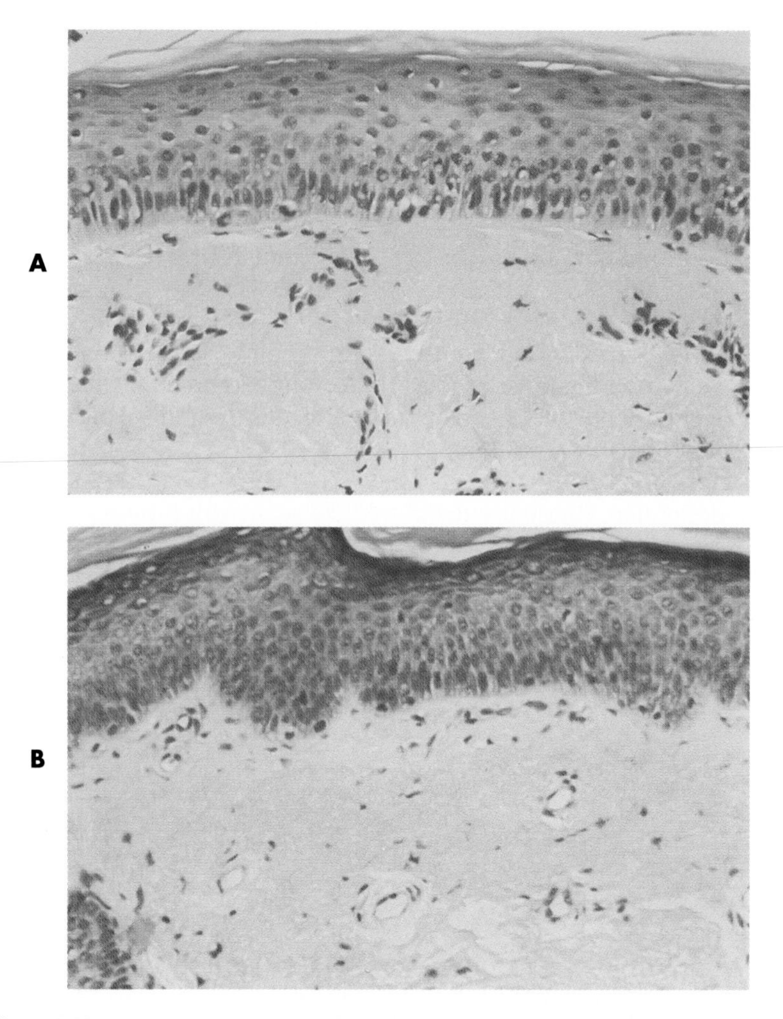

Figure 7-10 Long-term biopsies (2 years or more postoperatively) have demonstrated normalization of epidermis, continued gradual thickening of Grenz zone, and reduction of solar elastosis. In addition, solar elastosis was found to become progressively less homogenous and amorphous with much greater fibrillar content. See also Figure 7-1.

In addition to the vaporization and coagulation effects of these lasers removing up to 250 to 300 μm of tissue in the dermis, with decreasing tissue ablation with each sequential pass, a second mechanism of laser-tissue interaction appears to be important in achieving the desired clinical results. A discernible shrinkage of the skin is visible as the laser reacts with the dermis, tightening loose folds of skin. This is thought to be a result of heat-induced collagen shrinkage.[201]

When the CO_2 laser interacts with tissue, three distinct zones of tissue alteration correlate to the degree of tissue heating. The *zone of direct impact* results in vaporization of intracellular water and tissue ablation. Underlying this is a *zone of irreversible thermal damage and denaturation* resulting in tissue necrosis. Below this layer is a *zone of reversible, nonlethal thermal damage* (see Figure 7-11), in which collagen shrinkage is thought to occur, accounting for the visible tissue tightening observable as the CO_2 laser interacts with the dermis.

COLLAGEN SHRINKAGE

Collagen fibers provide the framework and mechanical strength of skin. The microscopically visible fiber is composed of a bundle of fibrils that are readily distinguishable by electron microscopy. These fibrils are made up of a unit filament, the *protofibril,* which has the same chemical and configurational structure as the collagen molecule.

The collagen molecule is a highly unique and unusual protein containing three polypeptide chains in a helical conformation with the presence of hydroxyproline and hydroxylysine. The repetitive positioning of glycine at every third amino acid locus accounts for its unique helical conformation.

Intermolecular cross-links provide collagen connective tissue with unique physical properties of high tensile strength and substantial elasticity. This cross-linking is mediated by the copper-dependent enzyme lysyl oxidase and can be chemically inhibited by β-aminopropionitrile. This cross-linking reaction is also inhibited by heat and photonic energy.

Thermal Effects

The knowledge regarding collagen shrinkage and tightening comes from a variety of sources, including biochemistry and thermokinetics,[243-263] tissue studies,[264-276] thermokeratoplasty,[277-319] orthopedics,[320-325] and tissue-welding studies.[251,326-359] The group having the closest clinical correlation to tissue shrinkage during resurfacing is found in tissue-welding studies, but clinical studies in orthopedics and ophthalmology have involved the thermal effects of type I collagen and are directly translatable to cutaneous work. The changes in collagen that occur in resurfacing mirror the collagen changes seen in all these areas of collagen research.

The response of collagen to heat is different than that of other body tissues. The hydrothermal shrinkage of collagen fibers has long been recognized as a characteristic of collagen.[280] The mechanism of this thermal contraction is proposed to be a molecular structure transition between the triple helix and a random coil.[243-246] Temperature elevation ruptures the ultrastructural cross-links that stabilize the collagen helix and results in immediate contraction in the fibers to about one-third their original length, with a corresponding increase in the caliber of individual fibers without alteration in the structural integrity of the tissue. Although the application of heat dissociates the interpeptide bonds, the cross-linkage between tropocollagen molecules remains intact, and the contraction of these linked molecules leads to shortening of the collagen fiber.[284]

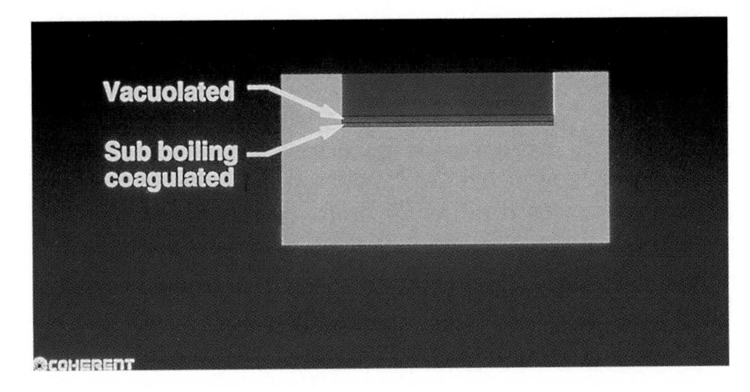

Figure 7-11 Zones of thermal damage in tissue instantaneously heated above 70° C but below 100° C. Normal tissue has a temperature of 37° C. Between this 70°-C layer and normal 37°-C tissue is a gradient of temperature in which collagen shinkage occurs, ideally at 63° C.

The thermal stability of collagen is also species dependent as well as related to its hydroxylation. As new collagen is formed, it becomes progressively more cross-linked with time, so younger, newer collagen is less heat stabile than mature collagen and contracts at a lower temperature. The shrinkage temperature for collagen lies within a very narrow range within which collagen fibers will shrink without destroying collagen fibrils. The higher the amino acid content, the more stable is the helix. The temperature at which half the helical structure of molecular strands is lost is called the *melting temperature* (Tm). For intact collagen fibers, the comparable index is the *shrinkage temperature* (Ts). For calf skin, the Tm of tropocollagen has been shown to be 39° C (only 2° C above body temperature), whereas the collagen Ts is 65° C.[246] The relationship between denaturation of collagen in the solid state and in the dissolved state has possible physiologic significance. It has been proposed that denaturation of extractable collagen in vivo at physiologic temperatures is a necessary state in the catabolism of collagen, preparing it for proteolytic digestion.[247,248]

The viscosity of a tropocollagen solution drops sharply at 39° C as the helical structure is disrupted to random coils and a disrupted structure called *gelatin* results. This same type of reaction with intact collagen results in visible shrinkage along the long axis of collagen fibers and occurs at a very specific temperature. Rabbit cornea has been shown to shrink 40% to 50% at 65° C.[280] Mammalian collagen, including human scleral and skin tissue, shrinks at 61° to 63° C, whereas human cornea shrinks at a lower temperature, 55° to 58° C.[282] However, the thermal properties of collagen vary with both the age of the animal and the environmental conditions.[249,264,265] Hyalinization of collagen, a characteristic microscopic finding of thermal injury, indicates merger of unraveled, swollen collagen fibers and has been reported to occur at temperatures greater than 58° C. Changes in birefringence (double refraction), indicating thermally coagulated collagen with unraveling of collagen fibrils and loss of unique striations, reportedly occurs at 70° to 75° C.[266]

In a well-organized discussion of photothermal effects induced by laser irradiation of tissue, Thomsen[266] separates these biologic thermal effects into three different thermodynamic processes based on observations by Pearce,[267] as follows:

1. Lower-temperature (about 43°-150° C) damage by heat accumulation processes, which may be lethal or nonlethal depending on times of heat exposure
2. Higher-temperature (100° C+) effects, dominated by water vaporization and effects of water vapor release
3. High-temperature ablation (about 300°-1000° C), resulting in tissue vaporization, combustion, molecular dissociation, and plasma formation

Thermal Coagulation

The visible thermal changes seen in collagen on light microscopy represent thermally induced, irreversible alterations of proteins and other biologic molecules, organelles, membranes, and cells, referred to as *thermal coagulation*. These alterations are caused primarily by thermal denaturation of structural proteins, are seen immediately after heating, and are always lethal. This differs from the low-temperature tissue injury that occurs, which may be demonstrable with electron microscopy or enzyme histochemistry in the first 24 hours or through light microscopy 48 to 72 hours after cellular death. Nonlethal changes may be more difficult to document because staining artifacts can mimic the pathologic alterations.

Thermally induced partial loss and complete loss of native birefringence and hyalinization of thermally coagulated collagen are easily recognizable. The normally seen birefringence is related to the regular arrangement of molecules forming the collagen fibrils. Thermally coagulated collagen examined by electron microscopy reveals unraveling of collagen fibrils with loss of the unique striations of collagen and an increase in fibrillar diameters.[265] The unraveled strands merge, and the individual fibers become less distinct, forming the swollen, hyalinized (glassy) collagen fibers seen with light microscopy. Birefringence changes induced by thermal reaction in collagen include a gradual loss of bright image intensity as well as color shifts of histologic stains. The loss of bright image intensity in thermally coagulated collagen may result from thermal disruption of the intramolecular and intermolecular bonds of collagen, leading to destruction of the regular arrangement among collagen molecules. The unraveling of collagen fibrils may expose new dye-binding sites and thus result in the color shifts seen. Normal fibers have been found to be intermixed with altered fibers in examination of tissue-welding sites induced by thermal changes from laser irradiation.[250,326,327]

The easily recognizable changes of thermal necrosis of collagen reflect the effects of higher temperatures (70°-75° C) that result in cellular death and therefore are not necessarily desirable in resurfacing procedures, at least not greater than 200 to 300 μm in depth. Whether more subtle alterations in birefringence and color shifts can be definitively correlated with corresponding electron microscopy changes and shown to represent a layer of nonlethal thermal injury, but irreversible structure change, has not been demonstrated. Our hypothesis is that such a layer exists just below the layer of visibly altered thermal changes. However, the only, or *primary,* collagen shrinkage may occur in the area of tissue necrosis. If this is true, maintenance of tissue shrinkage seen would depend on efficient collagen replacement of this necrotic layer while maintaining this shortened tissue matrix. This would be difficult to achieve, because this layer sloughs within 1 week in normal wound healing, much faster than the synthesis and cross-linking of new collagen occur.

In general, however, researchers agree that the thermal profile of laser-tissue interaction must be controlled to prevent excessive tissue heating and thermal necrosis when performing laser resurfacing. If, in addition, a tissue layer of collagen can be heated in the range of 60° to 70° C to achieve the desired shrinkage without completely denaturing collagen or changing the skin's structural integrity, and if this thermally altered collagen persists in this state, then maintenance of this shortened, tightened condition would be achieved. Replacement of this altered collagen in the healing process might cause regression of the collagen contraction achieved.[316] Indeed, in the absence of trauma, the half-life of type I collagen has been shown to be consistent with the life span of the experimental animal.[268] Some authors assume this to be true of human collagen as well, but the stability and longevity of collagen and its normal homeostatic replacement are for the most part unknown. It is known to be an ongoing process controlled by fibroblasts and dependent on collagenase secretion. The half-life of corneal collagen is reported to be 10 years or more; however, this is a unique location because it has no direct vascular supply.[269]

Collagen Structure

Collagen is a protein that undergoes self-assembly into macromolecular structures. Collagen solutions will readily polymerize into collagen fibrils that are indistinguishable from those found in vivo. Reactive carbonyl moieties generate intermolecular cross-links (collagen aldehydes reacting with other collagen amino acids), uniting the collagen molecules into a continuous polymeric network.[251] Thus collagen molecules, which contain carbonyl groups, self-assemble into fibers, which then become cross-linked because of reactions between the carbonyl groups and other amino acids of adjoining molecules. This structure is maintained by hydrogen bonds.[252]

Collagen protofibrils are composed of laterally aggregated, staggered molecules, which when cross-linked, form a strong, macroscopic three-dimensional network. The molecular stagger results from interactions between the amino acid side chains and consequently has the requisite precision to bring the lysyl side chains into proximity to form intermolecular cross-links.[254] This occurs in a spontaneous, progressive manner. As previously mentioned, this precise intermolecular cross-linking is species specific, because the relative abundance of different cross-links varies greatly depending on the tissue of origin of the collagen.[251]

Flexibility in side-chain interactions suggest that rather than a unique reaction being involved, a myriad of conformations occur at the molecular surfaces.[254] The fluidity of the surface domains would allow collagen molecules in soft tissues to slip relative to one another when stress is applied.[255]

Denaturation

The loss of the specific structure of a macromolecule without chemical degradation is considered to be denaturation. Collagen in solution undergoes denaturation at about of 30° C. Reconstitution of collagen fibrils from these heated solutions is no longer possible, so its biologic function is destroyed as well. However, this process tends to be reversible. The polypeptide strands making up the original collagen molecule have a considerable but incomplete capacity to resume the intrachain characteristics of the native state.[255] Therefore the denaturation temperature involves a considerable range that is both time and temperature dependent. The shrinkage process also has been described as a *rate phenomenon;* in general a 2°-C rise in temperature reduces the time for shrinkage by half.[256]

A similarity exists between the denaturation of soluble collagen and the thermal shrinkage of collagen. A study of the shrinkage temperature of normal human skin versus that of various pathologic states revealed a range of 57° to 65° C, with normal skin having an average shrinkage temperature of 62.9° C and abnormal skin averaging 61.9° C.[270] A transient lengthening was observed just before the instantaneous shrinkage. An energy of activation near 140 kcal is found for tendon collagen. From thermodynamic considerations, it is concluded that the only bonds involved in thermal shrinkage are the hydrogen bonds between chains. The cooperative nature of the "melting" of hydrogen bonds remains as the common feature of both the denaturation of soluble collagen and the hydrothermal contraction of collagenous tissue.[252]

Mammalian collagen, either skin or tendon, contracts sharply at 60° to 70° C (Ts) to about one-third to one-quarter its initial length. The tensile strength of the fiber is greatly lowered and shows "rubber-like elasticity."[256] Completely shrunken collagen loses its orderly structure. This structural alteration is an irreversible process once it is completed. The disoriented collagen formed is in a low state of entropy and consequently tends to fold into a more random configuration, thereby gaining in entropy.

The change from an oriented structure to a random state of configuration of the protein units is a natural consequence of the structure's tendency to increase its entropy. Instantaneous shrinkage of collagen takes place at temperatures at which the free energy of activation is about 25 kcal per mole, and the heat of the activation process has been determined to be 25 cal per gram.[256]

At about 60° C the process is initiated in tendon collagen by the appearance of tiny nodules. As the temperature is raised, more energy is available to rupture additional cross-links, which increases the thermal movement of the chains. A point will be reached at which the structure is weakened to the extent that it will assume a more stable configuration by chain folding. The nodules visibly enlarge and coalesce, and shrinkage of the tendon takes place. Further heating results in loss of structure and relaxation of collagen strands. This threshold for relaxation was found to be 78° C, but it rises with increasing age because of an increase in the number of thermally stable bonds.[264] In one study, human tendons were shown to contract sharply to 70% of their original length at about 70° C but to fall apart physically at temperatures higher than 80° C.[271]

Studies of *thermokeratoplasty,* in which corneal flattening is achieved through application of heat, have shown that in the corneal stroma the highest temperatures do not achieve additional shrinkage, but rather result in thermal injury and necrosis.[280,314] White et al[341,356] and Kopchok et al[357] have shown in tissue-welding studies that collagen bonding occurs if tissue apposition is precise and the temperature is controlled to prevent denaturation of the tissue elements. Higher energies and higher temperatures have also been shown to disrupt the laser seal when tissue-welding vessels.[355-358] Furthermore, kinetic modeling of the laser-tissue fusion process was done with guidelines such that excessive heating desiccates collagen fibers to a brittle state unsuitable for fusion.[257] Clearly, overheating collagen is counterproductive.

On the other hand, a number of studies have demonstrated that the percent shrinkage of collagen is directly proportional to the heat applied to tissue while remaining within a narrow range and without exceeding the excessive heating threshold.[228,271-273,316,336] However, when evaluating percent shrinkage of various tissues, the clinician must keep in mind that the degree of shrinkage of tissue will depend not only on the collagen contraction, but also on the mechanical properties of the surrounding tissue.

Tissue Welding

Numerous studies have demonstrated that nonablative laser energies can alter the ultrastructural and biochemical properties of tissue containing collagen.* Many of these studies have focused on tissue fusion occurring with laser tissue welding. Tissue welding occurs at temperatures that do not cause charring or gross desiccation. Early desiccation of tissue is noted as immediate whitening and then tanning of tissue occur, followed rapidly by tissue shrinkage and welding. In an early study,[280] collagen fibrils were found to lose their periodicity, greatly increase their caliber, and split into fine-fiber substructures with a roughly concentric arrangement on cross section. Although not separated because they were in control specimens, these fibrils were closely interdigitated. It was thought that covalent cross-links formed as the tissue cooled, resulting in tissue welding. Other authors have speculated that collagen fibrils uncoil above a certain temperature threshold and then randomly re-form interstrand and intrastrand cross-links as the tissue cools.[251,330-332] As the temperature increases, the molecular dynamics of the collagen are changed, and increasingly flexible side chains exist.[254,332] A variety of covalent collagen cross-links can occur spontaneously as the tissue cools.[251,332]

Laser welding of tissue is thought to occur either by formation of cross-links or by denaturation and reannealment of structural proteins. Supporting the latter theory is a study by Bass et al[328] showing absence of the helical structure in the collagen of laser-treated tendon with no evidence of covalent bonding. Noncovalent interactions between denatured collagen molecules were theorized to be responsible for the weld. Overexposure of full-thickness incisions to THC:YAG energy resulted in separation of fused tissue edges.[332] Adequate welding of tissue can occur without covalent bonds because the necessary conditions exist for the production of strong noncovalent bonds. The denatured, randomly oriented collagen has the opportunity to aggregate noncovalently in a variety of disordered forms.

Others have postulated the production of strong hydrophobic interstrand bonds in nonhelical domains of collagen.[259] A kinetic model for tissue fusion proposes that laser fusion depends on thermal denaturation of tissue collagen.[257] The authors suggest that collagen fibrils unravel with heating and then reentwine during the cooling phase. In addition, Serure et al[355] proposed that tissue adhesion in CO_2 laser

*References 258, 280, 283, 314, 315, 330, 331.

welds of microvascular anastomoses resulted from collagen denaturation in the media and adventitia of the vessel, as well as from fibrin polymerization. Epstein and Cooley[359] demonstrated that seals in CO_2 laser–welded microvessels consist of denatured cells and collagen, which reorganize over the first 2 to 4 weeks of healing.

Reports supporting the formation of cross-links include biochemical studies,[251,258,330-332] electron microscopy studies,[326,331,337,341,356] and tissue studies,[340,358] all of which agree with the hypotheses of Anderson et al[334] and others.[335,336] Electron microscopy reveals collagen fibers fusing with interdigitation of bundles across the cut, reflecting end-to-end as well as parallel cross-linking.[326,341] In addition, normal fibers were found to be intermixed with modified fibers (fused, swollen, dissolved), indicating collagen fibers with different reactions to the same temperature. This was also found to be true in previous studies,[250,326,327] showing that collagen fibers do not completely denature with laser welding. This may reflect the presence of more than one type of collagen having different proportions of hydroxyproline present and may be related to a mixture of young collagen in with mature collagen. This may indicate an ongoing process of tissue remodeling, absorption of damaged collagen, and its replacement with new collagen fiber by fiber rather than en bloc.[250]

White et al[337] reported loss of striation and swelling of collagen fibrils to 100 to 400 μm (normal 70 μm). These ultrastructural changes could be explained either by covalent cross-linking or by protein denaturation with noncovalent bonding in either a helical or an aggregate form. These studies suggest that covalent cross-linking occurs.

Clinical Developments

Thermally induced changes in collagen were first investigated in refractive surgery 100 years ago by Lans,[277] who applied electrocautery to the peripheral cornea of rabbit eyes and achieved correction of astigmatic changes of up to 6.00 diopters. However, he found variability in the predictability of the curvature changes induced. In 1914 Wray[278] successfully used cautery clinically to treat a patient with hyperopic astigmatism, and O'Connor[279] confirmed its benefit in selected cases in 1933 and reported persistence of refractive correction for 10 years postoperatively.

The determination of corneal collagen shrinkage temperatures in 1964[282] resulted in greater interest in thermokeratoplasty, and in the mid-1970s several investigators explored this as a treatment option for keratoconus.[280,281,285-287] Because of reports of a high incidence of regression[287] and various complications,[288-290] this procedure was never widely used, although Itoi[291] advocated its use because only 7% of his 750 patients treated subsequently required corneal transplantation.

In the 1980s, radiofrequency devices[292,293] and a retractable thermal probe (Michrome wire)[294-296] were used in an attempt to deliver heat in a more controlled manner but were abandoned because of poor predictability and regression of effects.[297,298]

Since then lasers have been investigated as devices to deliver heat more precisely with selective targeting,[299] based primarily on a theoretic model developed by Mainstern.[300] At least five different lasers have been studied: CO_2[301-304] yttrium-erbium-glass (Y-Er-glass),[305] cobalt:magnesium fluoride,[283] hydrogen fluoride,[303-306] and holmium:YAG (Ho:YAG).[299,307-319] Only the Ho:YAG has been evaluated in clinical trials. In general, long-term follow-up (up to 2 years) has shown treatment with the Ho:YAG laser to induce moderate curvature changes with no significant complications. However, a small percentage (27% in one study)[312] of patients had continuous regression of the retractive changes throughout the first year. Some of this regression may be related to the treatment parameters used, and many unanswered questions remain at this time. Evidence indicates that persistent local contraction of collagen is present in treated rabbit eyes and that new collagen formation occurs as well. The significance of this new collagen formation and its effects on regression of the refractive benefits is controversial. Inhibition of new collagen formation by corticosteroids has been suggested as a potential method of preserving postoperative refractive stability.[314]

Collagen remodeling and new collagen formation are thought to be possibly counterproductive, because the brisk stromal wound healing may result in replacement of the thermally altered collagen by newly synthesized molecules not maintaining the new, shortened profile. In addition, the new collagen may adversely affect the refraction by having a different ultrastructure, as would a scar, or by altering curvature through filling in interstices, thickening the stroma, or counteracting the curvature changes.

Mechanical tissue factors such as the elasticity (or loss of it) of adjacent tissues may contribute to regression even though the collagen contraction is maintained. Epithelial hyperplasia resulting from laser injury also is thought to be a secondary event that may alter refraction.

Studies have shown that keratocyte injury occurs when stromal collagen is heated to 79° C.[304,319] Avoiding injury to the epithelium and keratocytes by development of a better delivery system and maintaining corneal temperature in the narrow range of 60° to 75° C would be optimum: above the shrinkage temperature of corneal collagen and below that lethal to keratocytes.

A natural transition from the use of collagen shrinkage as a therapeutic modality in ophthalmology to its use in orthopedics was reported by Fing et al,[320] who used heat not on the eye itself, but on extraocular muscle tendon. They reported the successful treatment of strabismus by shrinking the muscle tendon. Indeed, much of the basic knowledge regarding collagen shrinkage secondary to heating has been obtained through laboratory studies using excised tendons as the collagen source, so these clinical results are not surprising.

An in vitro study using a rabbit model was performed to investigate the potential of using laser energy (Ho:YAG laser) to the joint capsule of the shoulder to decrease capsular redundancy in patients with shoulder instability.[321] This study showed a significant and strong correlation between energy density applied and percent shrinkage of capsular tissue. Up to 40% shrinkage was seen without loss of normal relaxation properties of the tissue, indicating normal stability in response to stress. However, the higher energies resulted in a decrease in stiffness, indicating more compliant tissue. Once again, as seen in other tissue studies, this indicates that overheating may cause adverse tissue effects and disruption of collagen bonds.

In a multicenter clinical trial, patients with glenohumeral instability were shown to have dramatic improvement 6 months postoperatively after nonablative reduction of their joint capsule using the Ho:YAG laser.[324]

A further study using tissue baths heated to a designated temperature was performed on cadaver shoulders to determine the specific tissue effects of a range of temperatures.[325] This study revealed significant tissue shrinkage to occur at temperatures at or above 65° C. The percent shrinkage correlated with the temperature applied and ranged from 11% ± 15% at 65° C to 59% ± 5.4% at 80° C. Histologic and electron microscopy (EM) studies revealed progressive alterations in collagen, with hyalinization on light microscopy and loss of distinct edges of fibers visible with EM at 65° C, but complete homogenization with light microscopy and loss of fibrillar structure with EM seen at 80° C. This study revealed that distinct fibrillar structure was lost at or above 70° C, indicating transition of fibrillar collagen to an amorphous state. A previous EM study using the Ho:YAG laser to shrink the joint capsule, however, revealed that fibril diameters increased dramatically with less distinct edges, but with preservation of individual fibers. The difference may be secondary to the methods of heating or other factors. The authors point out, however, that wound healing factors must be considered and postulate that after adequate healing, the tissue may have normal architectural properties with maintenance of its shortened length.

After laser resurfacing, EM studies have revealed three distinct zones of collagen morphology.[274] In the most superficial tissue at the base of tissue vaporization is a *zone of homogenous, completely denatured collagen* without discrete fibrillar components. This corresponds with the layer of thermal necrosis visible on light microscopy. An intact tertiary structure is necessary for diffraction of polarized light (birefringence). Loss of this structural integrity is associated with loss of birefringence and with tinctorial changes resulting from exposure of stain-binding sites within the unraveled collagen fiber.[274] These changes result in the area of thermal necrosis that is visible on light microscopy. The exact correlation of the EM zones to this visible zone is not known at this time. However, below the first homogenous zone is a *zone of significant population of less structurally defined collagen fibers of increased diameter* interspersed among normal collagen fibers. Below this is a *zone of normal collagen fibers.*

Skin Rejuvenation

Clinical observations have confirmed the value of collagen shrinkage in rejuvenation of photodamaged skin. This is a significant component of the clinical improvement seen in laser resurfacing. Its exact mechanism and relative importance have been debated. We have hypothesized that the shortened collagen fibers result in a shrunken matrix on which collagen remodeling occurs, resulting in preservation of this tightened skin. That the tightened skin does persist to variable degrees is confirmed by study of photographs over time, as well as by the occurrence of laser-induced *ectropion,* a condition of excessive tissue tightening.

Tissue contraction is grossly visible on impact of the pulsed CO_2 laser with skin during resurfacing, being most profound on the first and second dermal passes after removal of the epidermis. Although some component of this tissue contraction is undoubtedly secondary to tissue volume loss as a consequence of vaporization of tissue water, a large portion is thought to be from collagen contraction. Gardner et al[228] found a positive linear correlation between the number of passes and the degree of skin shrinkage. A linear regression model showed a 6% size reduction per pass with the SilkTouch laser and a 5% reduction per pass with the UltraPulse laser. Rehydrating the tissue between passes resulted in only slight correction of the shrinkage (Figure 7-12). Analysis of a single specimen treated with the SilkTouch laser for five consecutive passes with rehydration between passes revealed about 15% reduction on the first pass and a plateau at about 31% reduction after three to five passes. Temperature

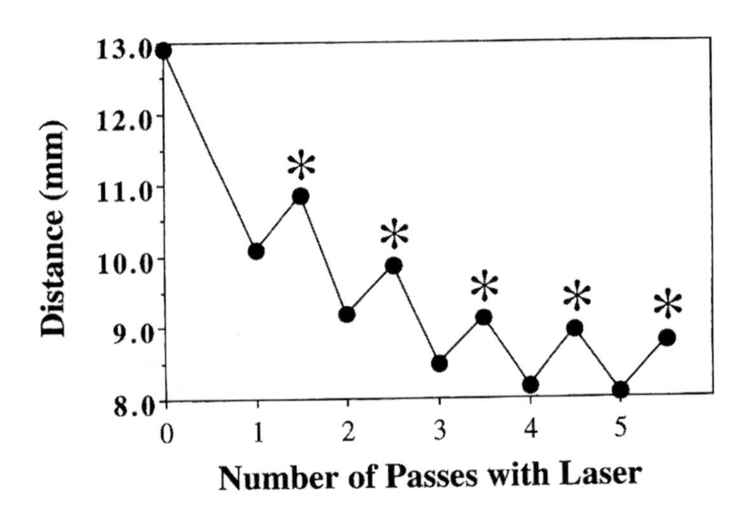

Figure 7-12 Collagen shrinkage as seen per pass with UltraPulse CO_2 laser. Asterisks represent rehydation between passes. (From Gardner ES, Reinisch L, Stricklin GP et al: *Lasers Surg Med* 19:379, 1996.)

elevation in the tissue was approximately 20° C and unchanged with each pass. Ross et al[273] observed a positive correlation between contraction of the treated area and both fluence and the number of laser passes in their studies on pig skin.

RESURFACING TECHNIQUE

The most important factor in performing CO_2 laser resurfacing is *single-pulse laser-tissue interaction.* If vaporization is accomplished in a single pulse, the heat of the laser-tissue interaction is released in the vapor created, and thermal diffusion deep into the treated tissue will not occur. If the tissue cannot be vaporized (i.e., the threshold for vaporization is not reached), it is critical that the pulse duration be less than the thermal diffusion time. In this situation the laser-tissue interaction site will cool off before there is time for thermal diffusion to occur. If laser pulses are stacked one on top of another, additive thermal effects will occur because of heat retention. For the CO_2 laser, the pulse repetition rate must be less than an estimated 5 Hz to allow tissue cooling between pulses and to avoid cumulative thermal effects.[275]

The technique used with the Coherent UltraPulse 5000 is described here. Similar techniques with appropriate modifications specific to individual systems to achieve the same laser-tissue interaction may be used for other systems as well.

UltraPulse Technique

When performing resurfacing procedures by hand with a 3-mm collimated beam, it is critical to move the handpiece at a rate that allows single-pulse laser-tissue interaction, with minimal overlapping (generally a rate of 4 to 10 Hz). When using the CPG, the patterns should not be overlapped, and the individual laser impacts within the pattern should have minimal overlap (generally densities of 3 to 6).

The surface is covered with a single pass of laser impacts, resulting in white, desiccated debris composed of proteinaceous epidermal tissue remaining after intracellular tissue water vaporization (Figure 7-13). This tissue debris should be wiped away with saline-moistened gauze to remove the remaining epidermis. The first pass

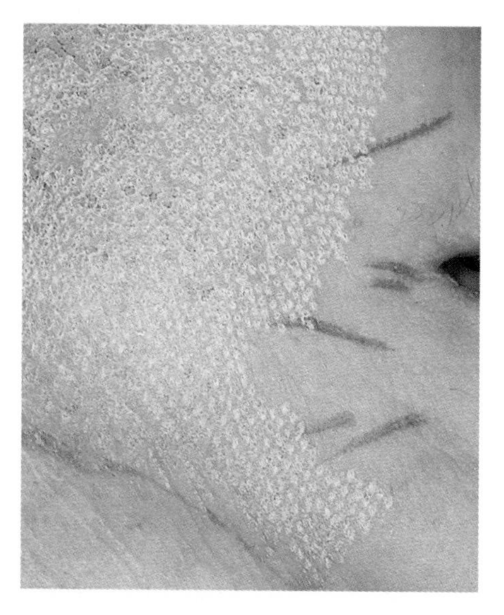

Figure 7-13 Initial CO_2 laser pass effectively removes epidermis by vaporizing a 40- to 50-μm layer and causing a subepidermal vesicle to form. Surface is covered with white, desiccated, proteinaceous debris from epidermis immediately after first pass. This needs to be wiped away with saline-soaked gauze.

generally removes the epidermis and leaves only minimal residual thermal damage (10-30 μm) depending on epidermal thickness, with more thermal damage in thin epidermis, such as eyelid or neck skin. This same procedure is repeated over the entire surface to be treated for the second pass. The only difference is that during this pass, the CPG is oriented at 90 degrees to the direction used for the first pass. The reason for this is to avoid the appearance of linear pigment streaks that may be associated with the pattern of the CPG (Figure 7-14).

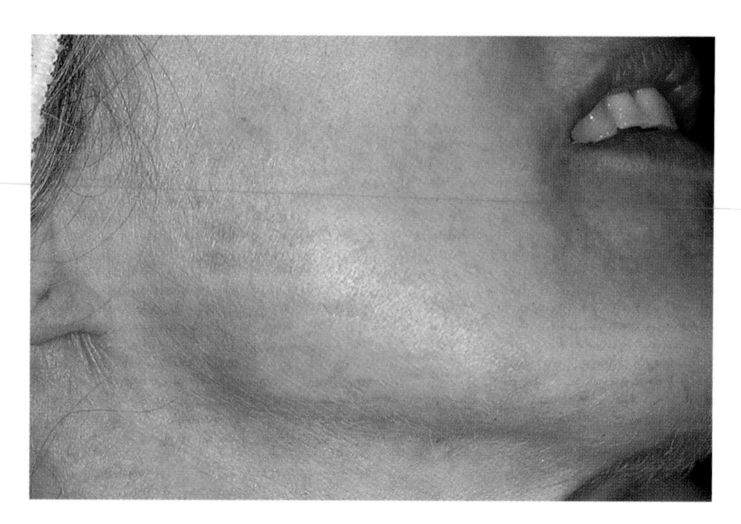

Figure 7-14 Single pass of CPG may result in linear streaks of hyperpigmentation, resulting from differential thermal effects leaving a mixture of non-sun-damaged cells and sun-damaged cells. To prevent this, a second pass is performed at 90 degrees to first pass.

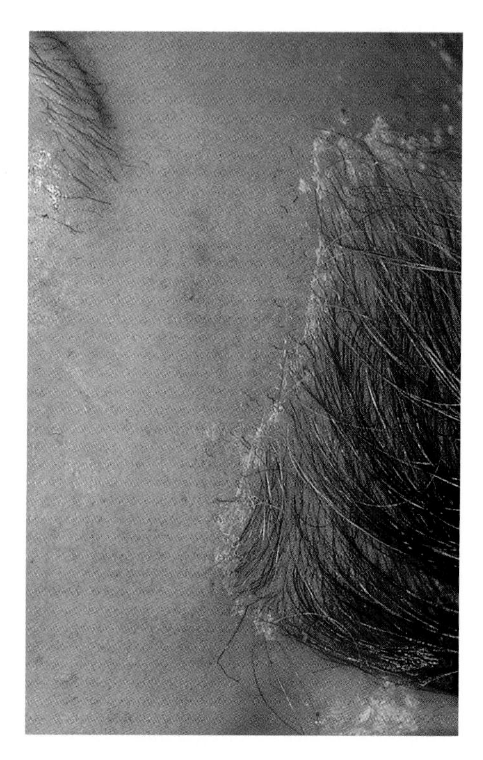

Figure 7-15 "Feathering" into hairline 5 to 15 mm to avoid leaving a line of contrast anterior to hairline. Hair will regrow normally in this feathered zone, but it is not possible to treat inside scalp without coagulating shaft of hairs.

Generally, the third pass is applied more selectively to areas of more significant photodamage and wrinkling. If photodamage remains visible over the entire treatment area, the entire area is treated again. In general, however, the third pass is confined to the glabellar area, upper lip, nasolabial folds, and lateral cheeks. A fourth pass with the Coherent CPG is only rarely needed except in cases of advanced, severe photodamage and is therefore not recommended (Figure 7-4).

Generally after the third pass with the Coherent CPG, treatment with the 3-mm beam is used in selective areas to flatten high tissue points by vaporization and to tighten loose skin or ablate wrinkles by pulling the base of wrinkle lines up and achieving as smooth a surface as possible to act as a base for new collagen formation.

In performing resurfacing, clinicians should keep in mind the following:

1. Always "feather" the peripheral areas by decreasing the density of pulse application as well as the pulse energy (decrease to 200-250 mJ), or angle the beam at 45 degrees to spread the fluence over a larger surface area.
2. Feather into the hairline a distance of 5 to 15 mm and well under the jawline (3-5 cm) (Figure 7-15).
3. Use feathering parameters to treat the eyelid surfaces, and use no more than two passes in the immediate periorbital area, except isolated spot application to persisting folds of tissue.
4. Carefully observe the laser-tissue interaction of the eyelids to avoid excessive tightening of tissue and possible scleral show or ectropion, especially in patients with a prior blepharoplasty.
5. Use the 3-mm beam to make a single pass along the vermilion borders of the upper and lower lips, because this is the most common area of persistence of wrinkle lines. This also helps to emphasize the vermilion border.
6. Do not routinely cross the vermilion border. Treat up to the border, because this will make the lips appear fuller and emphasize the vermilion border as a result of the collagen tightening of the lip.
7. Treat lines that cross the vermilion border individually by tracing over the line with the laser once all the other areas have been treated, rather than treating the entire vermilion surface.
8. After completion of treatment with the CPG, carefully search the treatment surface for signs of residual seborrheic keratoses, actinic keratoses, or SCC in situ and for thickened scars, and vaporize these to a flat surface using the 3-mm beam with pulse-stacking treatment technique or with the Er:YAG laser.
9. Always carefully observe the immediate tissue response regarding contraction or yellow-brown discoloration. If this discoloration persists after wiping with saline, this is a sign of thermal necrosis (Figure 7-16).

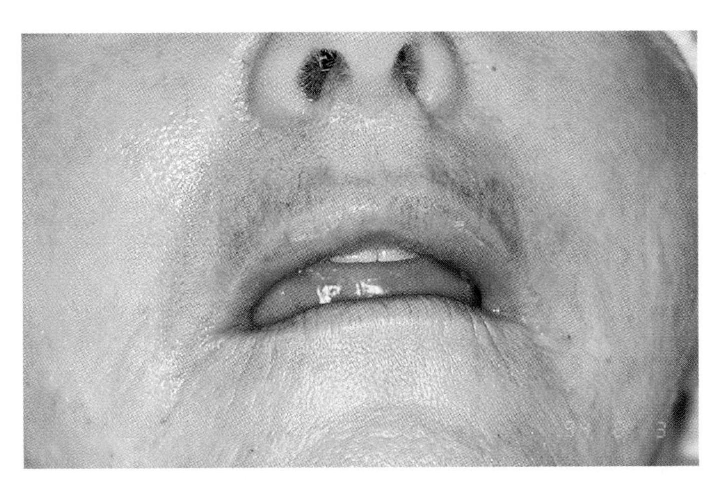

Figure 7-16 Persistent yellow-brown discoloration of dermis after wiping with saline is a sign of thermal injury that may be extending deeper into dermis.

10. Use the 3-mm spot in placing impact sites at 3- to 5-mm intervals to achieve tightening of the skin without significant thermal risk (concentric lines of these treatment spots moving away from a site to be tightened is effective). This is particularly useful on the eyelids and midcheeks.

The endpoint of treatment is when one of the following conditions is seen:

1. The wrinkle or scar is removed.
2. A yellow-brown discoloration indicating thermal damage is seen.
3. No further skin tightening is observed.

No reason exists to continue treating an area when any of these signs is observed. Leave that area untreated from that point on and concentrate on other tissue sites.

SilkTouch Technique

The treatment technique using the Sharplan SilkTouch embodies the same basic principles, but with modifications specific to the system. Because the beam is not collimated, one must be careful to hold the handpiece at the proper distance from the skin at all times and to avoid movement during the scan of each "pulse." Also, the beam is not gaussian in its energy distribution, so no built-in compensation exists for overlap of patterns. However, the scan pattern is a circle, which necessitates either having skip spaces with nonoverlapping pattern placement or overlapping each pattern on four sides to create a square. Caution must be observed in monitoring these pattern overlaps for signs of excessive thermal injury to the treated tissue. A square-pattern scan has recently been added to the capabilities of the scanner, as well as "light-touch" capabilities, with a scanning system similar to Coherent's CPG, using a small spot size but a true pulse of laser energy with less than 1-msec duration.

Either a 3.7-mm scan using 5 to 8 W or a 6.5- or 9.0-mm scan with 15 to 20 watts is chosen. With the Sharplan system, increasing the power results in an increased depth of vaporization: 18 W vaporizes deeper than 16 W. Typical settings are 18 W for the 6.5- and 9.0-mm scan and 7 W for the 3.7-mm scan. Scan duration is 0.2 sec *on* and 0.3 to 0.4 sec *off* in the repetitive mode.

Generally, two passes of one of the larger patterns are used, then the 3.7-mm scan and spot is used in the same manner as with the Coherent 3-mm collimated beam at the vermilion border and along "shoulders" of persistent lines. Feathering is accomplished by decreasing the power and angling the handpiece to less than 90 degrees. The eyelids are treated with decreased wattage as well and generally only a single pass.

With the newer FeatherTouch-SilkTouch system, it is easier to obtain superficial resurfacing using the FeatherTouch mode, scanning circles or squares 3 to 15 mm in diameter.

Weinstein[360] reports the histologic findings using a 10-mm square at 36 W, corresponding to a fluence of 10 J/cm^2, as follows:

1. Single pass: epidermal vaporization with dermal coagulation necrosis of 10 μm
2. Two passes: epidermal vaporization with dermal coagulation necrosis of 30 μm
3. Three passes: epidermal vaporization with dermal coagulation of 50 μm

The depth of vaporization into the dermis is not given.

When the same settings are used on the SilkTouch mode, the pattern is scanned twice: once inward, then outward. The total time on tissue is longer, the fluence is higher (28 J/cm^2), and the thermal injury is greater, as follows:

1. Single pass: epidermal vaporization with dermal coagulation necrosis of 70 μm
2. Two passes: epidermal vaporization with dermal coagulation necrosis of 100 μm

The depth of vaporization into the dermis is not reported.

• • •

To accomplish excellent results, it is necessary to have an understanding of the basic mechanisms of action of laser resurfacing. Basically, four mechanisms are involved:

(1) single-pulse vaporization, (2) collagen shrinkage and skin tightening, (3) new collagen formation and remodeling of collagen, and (4) multipulse coagulation of collagen.

Single-pulse Vaporization

Single-pulse vaporization uses the concepts of selective photothermolysis. The pulse width of the laser should be less than 1 msec to have interaction of tissue and delivery of heat in less than the thermal relaxation time of the tissue to be removed. It is also important that the pulse energy be high enough to accomplish complete vaporization of the tissue in a single pulse. For a beam size of 2.5 mm or greater, pulse energies greater than 250 mJ are necessary. These pulses should be delivered with minimal overlap. The gaussian distribution of energy across the beam will allow overlap of pulses without significantly changing the energy delivered at the periphery of the pulse. Using this type of mechanism, superficial layers of the dermis can be removed. First the epidermis is removed, then the superficial layers of the papillary dermis, but in general, vaporizing deeper than 250 to 300 μm is not done. Using this mechanism alone, removal of superficial wrinkle lines can be achieved. These include fine wrinkles anywhere on the face (Figure 7-17).

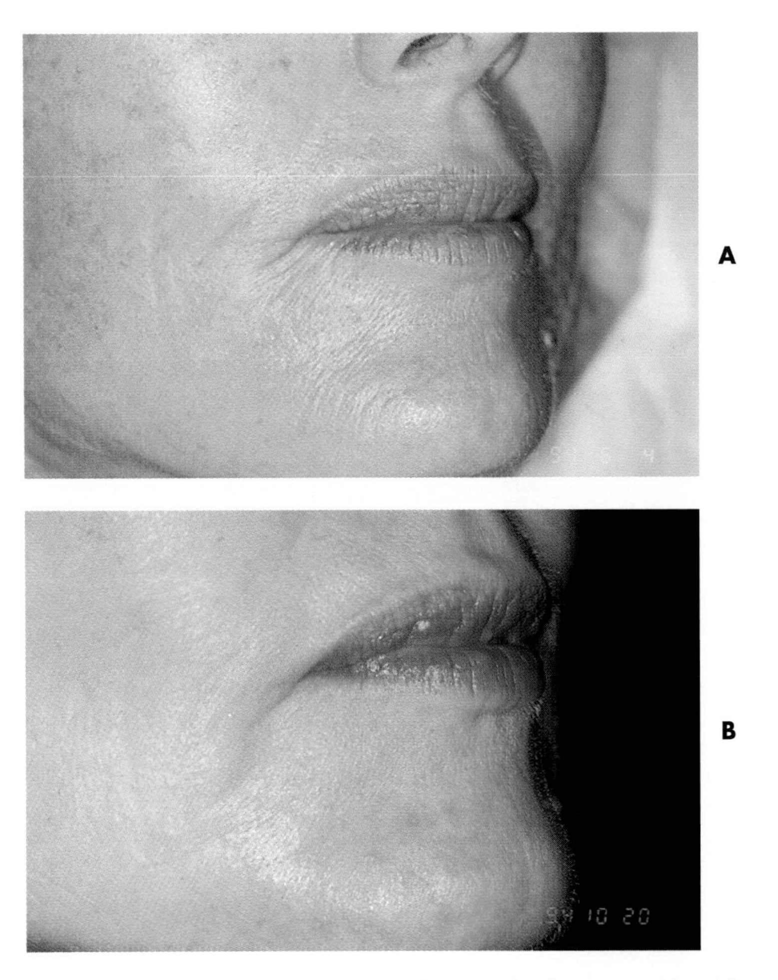

Figure 7-17 **A,** Relatively superficial lines may be completely removed by ablating to depth of wrinkle line. **B,** Improvement depends on ablation of solar elastosis and wound healing. Collagen shrinkage and new collagen formation are not necessary for this improvement to occur.

Collagen Shrinkage and Skin Tightening

It was not initially anticipated that collagen shrinkage would be a component of the laser-tissue interaction. However, unexpected improvement in redundant folds of the eyelids, loose skin of the cheeks, nasolabial folds, and the other deep wrinkle lines, coupled with the visible skin tightening observable with the laser-tissue interaction, has led to use of heat-induced collagen shrinkage for clinical benefit (Box 7-1).

This skin-tightening effect allows achievement of comparable clinical results at a more superficial level of tissue removal than is necessary with other resurfacing modalities, such as dermabrasion and chemical peels. The amount of tightening observed depends on the number of passes delivered, unknown specific tissue factors (possibly the numbers and health of intact collagen fibers), tissue thickness, and anatomic location. Thin tissue such as eyelid and neck skin tightens very readily and often profoundly, even to the point of causing ectropion in eyelid skin. Temporal skin is generally thinner compared with other facial skin and also tightens more significantly. Tightening of cheek skin may be important in reducing nasolabial fold prominence and "jowls" under the jaw line. Tightening may be used very selectively to achieve desired clinical effects (Figure 7-18). Precise tightening of folds of loose eyelid tissue (Figure 7-19) or atrophic scars (Figure 7-20) can dramatically improve clinical results without significant risk if careful clinical observation is used.

By targeting high points of glabellar and forehead lines, better smoothing of these areas may be achieved. This type of tissue change has been shown to persist 4 years or more and is thought to be a permanent structural change in the skin once the new collagen formation has occurred.

Box 7-1 Collagen shrinkage with CO_2 laser

Collagen molecule

- Three polypeptide chains in helical conformation result from repetitive positioning of glycine at every third amino acid locus.
- Intermolecular cross-links provide tensile strength and are inhibited by heat.
- Heat dissociates interpeptide bond; molecules remain intact.
- Hydrothermal shrinkage occurs through molecular structure transition from a triple helix to a random coil.
- Immediate contraction of fibers occurs to about one-third their original length.
- Collagen is progressively more cross-linked with time, so new collagen is less stable and contracts at lower temperature.

Collagen-heat reaction

- Polypeptide strands of heated tissue have capacity to resume the original intrachain characteristics.
- Collagen readily self-assembles into fibrils, which cross-link in a spontaneous, progressive manner.
- A myriad of molecular conformations are possible.
- Denaturation process is both time and temperature dependent; in general a 2°-C rise in temperature reduces shrinkage time by 50%.
- Very narrow temperature range exists for shrinkage without destroying fibrils.
- Instantaneous shrinkage temperature of human collagen was found to be 62.9° C, with range of 57° to 65° C.
- As temperature rises, more and more cross-link bonds are broken until loss of structure and denaturation occur.
- Percent shrinkage is directly proportional to heat applied, while not exceeding threshold for denaturation.

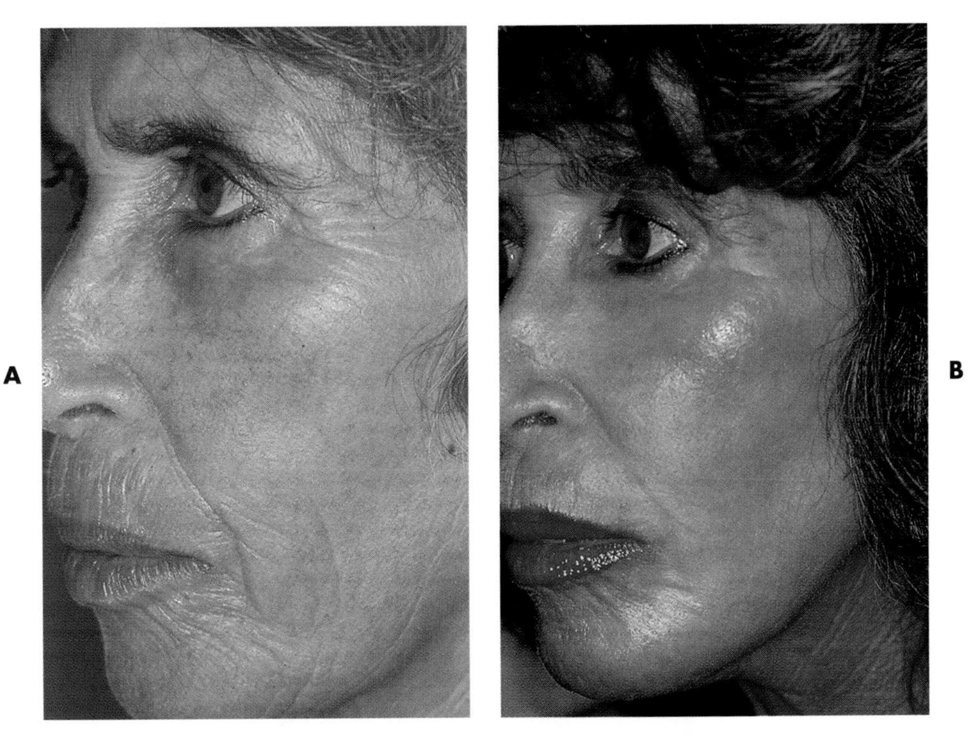

Figure 7-18 Skin tightening and collagen shrinkage result in clinical improvement in nasolabial folds and cheeks. **A,** Before treatment. **B,** One year after full-face CO_2 laser resurfacing.

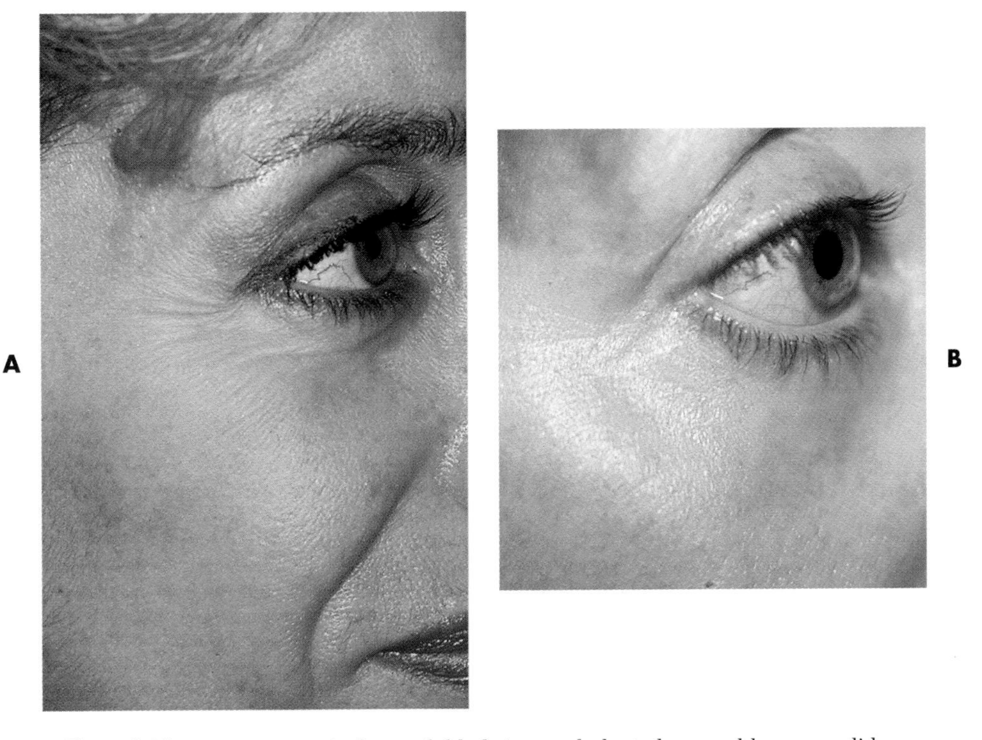

Figure 7-19 Improvement in loose, folded tissue of photodamaged lower-eyelid skin usually occurs primarily from collagen tightening. **A,** Before therapy. **B,** Four months after CO_2 laser resurfacing.

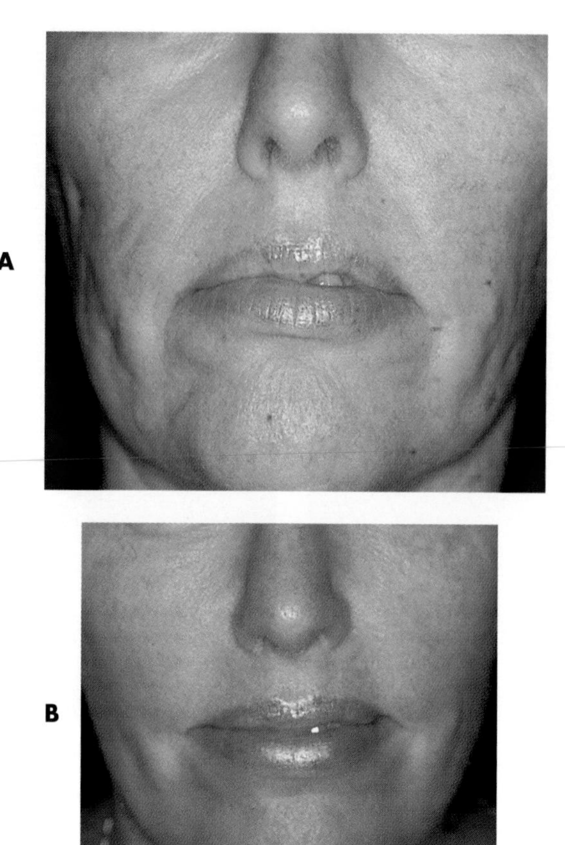

Figure 7-20 Atrophic acne scars may respond dramatically to a single treatment with CO_2 laser by using collagen tightening selectively and artfully to elevate scars. **A,** Before treatment. **B,** Four months after CO_2 laser resurfacing.

New Collagen Formation and Collagen Remodeling

To avoid excessive thermal injury, it is recommended that the laser resurfacing procedure be discontinued when signs of thermal injury are seen, that is, yellow-brown discoloration of the skin. Often, when treatment is discontinued because of visible thermal effects, visible wrinkle lines are still present, particularly on the glabella and forehead and upper lip (Figure 7-21, *A* and *B*). These lines may gradually improve during the healing process and may gradually subside over 6 to 12 weeks (Figure 7-21, *C* and *D*). This occurs as a consequence of new collagen formation and collagen remodeling.

A multicenter study demonstrated that UltraPulse laser resurfacing results in up to a 600% increase in the Grenz zone layer. A new layer of healthy, fine collagen fibrils is laid down parallel to the epidermis and measures 100 to 400 μm in depth, replacing the layer of solar elastosis vaporized by the laser.

Multipulse Coagulation

The most efficient fluences for vaporizing the epidermis have been shown to be in the range of 5 to 19 J/cm^2. Single-pulse vaporization generally uses fluences of about 7 J/cm^2. However, when one pulse is stacked on top of another without sufficient tissue cooling time, additive thermal effects occur. When using the CPG with

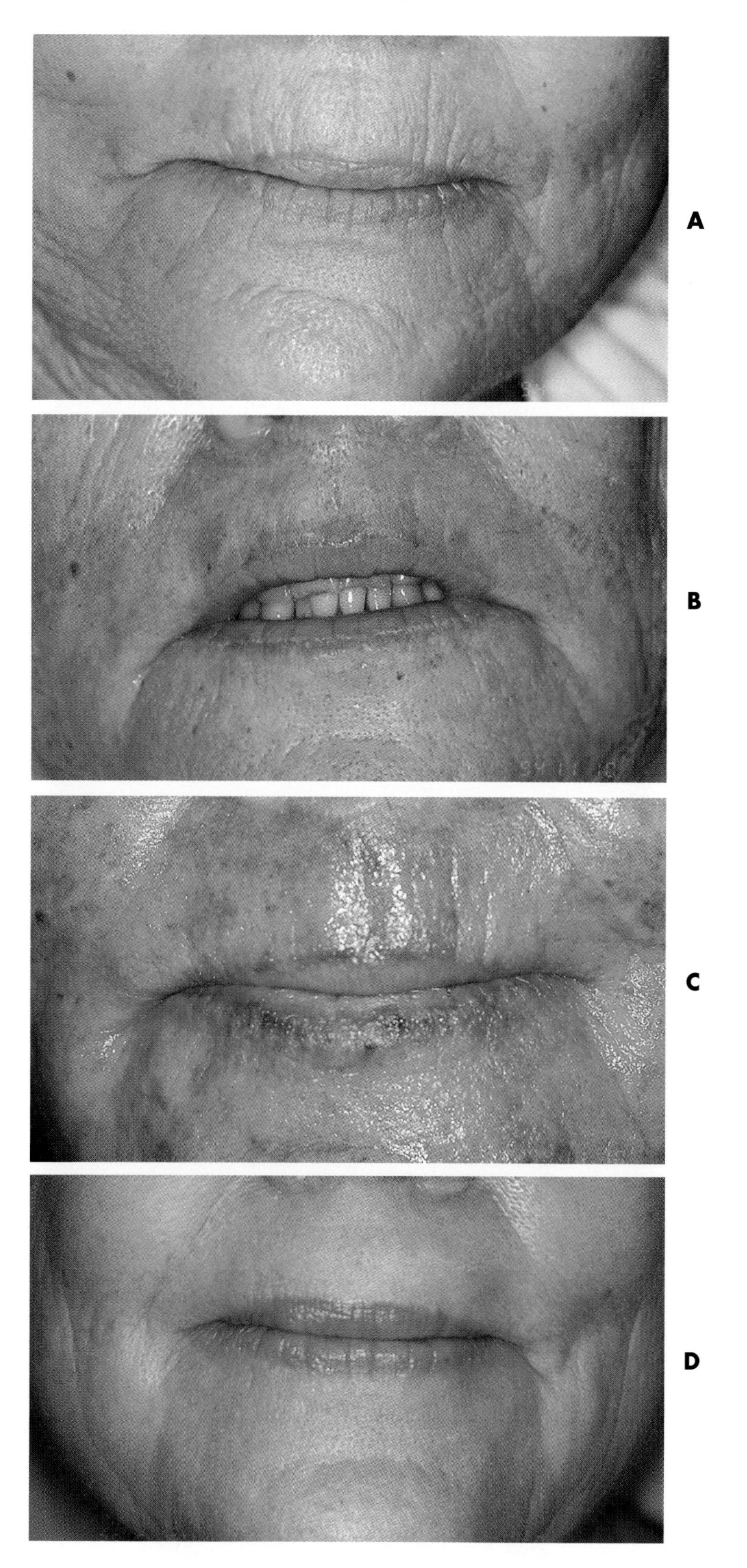

Figure 7-21 Clinical improvement often occurs in a delayed manner secondary to new collagen formation and collagen remodeling. **A,** Deep upper-lip lines before treatment. **B,** Immediately after treatment, these lines remain very visible. **C,** Three days after treatment, swelling intensifies visibility of some lines. **D,** Six months later, lines are gone.

the UltraPulse laser, a density of 9 results in as high an energy density as 60 J/cm^2 to be delivered to the tissue. It has been clinically observed that after making three or four passes with the UltraPulse laser using CPG densities of 4 to 6, nothing visible appears to occur to the tissue. Neither the depth of vaporization nor the thermal injury appears to be increasing. Biopsy studies confirm this impression, as long as single-pulse vaporization is being used.[240]

However, these same tissue studies have shown that with stacking pulses on top of one another, the zone of thermal necrosis gradually increases and may increase to greater than 300 μm, even though the depth of vaporization remains basically unchanged. The procedure of vaporization appears to level off because the tissue target (i.e., water) changes as the procedure progresses. In the first pass the laser is interacting with intracellular water. Once the epidermis has been stripped away, however, the laser is acting primarily with extracellular water in the dermis. In addition, the water content of the epidermis is closer to 80%, whereas in the dermis the water content is closer to 60%. The dermis is made up primarily of protein fibrils of collagen and elastic tissue. These fibers have a much higher threshold of vaporization than water. Therefore the amount of tissue vaporized with each pass becomes less and less.

Complicating the situation even further, is the layer of thermal necrosis, which measures generally between 50 and 100 μm, is desiccated and has very little water. Therefore it is difficult to vaporize deeper than 200 to 300 μm using single-pulse vaporization with a collimated beam. However, stacking pulses results in cumulative thermal effects and may allow deeper vaporization because of the higher fluence that results from rapid pulse succession.

This is a hazardous procedure because the residual thermal damage is greater with pulse stacking and may progress to the point of interfering with wound healing, which may cause scarring. This occurs without obvious clinical signs of potential problems, but subtle signs may be distinguished by experienced observation. When stacking pulses on top of each another, a yellow-brown discoloration of the tissue is observed clinically. This is initially subtle and clears with saline wiping. As

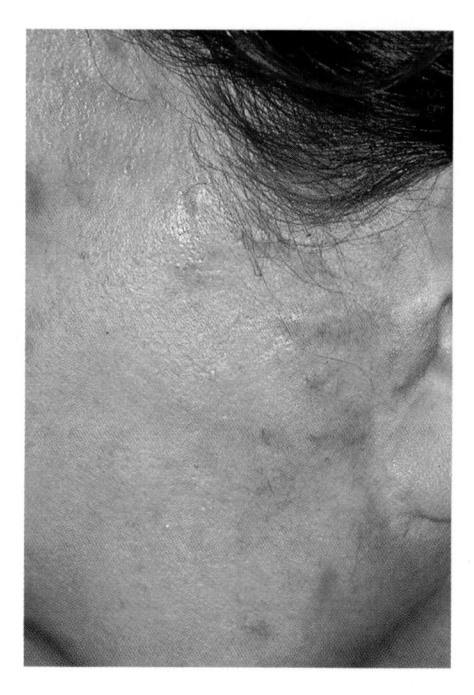

Figure 7-22 Failure to adhere carefully to single-pulse vaporization may result in inadvertently stacking pulses and extending thermal necrosis deeply into dermis. This may result in delayed wound healing and scarring.

further passes are performed, the yellow color gradually deepens to brown and will not wipe away. When this yellow-brown discoloration is seen, the physician can be certain that this area will be the last to heal and that this tissue will slough. Although this pulse-stacking technique can be used to resurface deeper because of the resultant tissue slough, it is a potentially dangerous technique that can result in poor wound healing and scarring (Figure 7-22).

If a decision is made to use this technique clinically, it is imperative to learn the signs of depth of injury by observation of tissue healing with variable levels of treatment on repeated occasions. As mentioned earlier, the three endpoints of treatment are elimination of the wrinkle or scar, a yellow-brown discoloration indicating thermal damage, and no further collagen shrinkage or tightening. When any one of these is reached, the laser procedure should be terminated in that area of the face. It is much safer to re-treat residual lines after an adequate healing time of 6 months or longer.

FACIAL WRINKLING

To evaluate the severity of wrinkling and photodamage present and therefore achieve some degree of predictability of response to resurfacing, a clinical classification and numeric scoring system has been adapted from other photodamage assessment systems. Although other wrinkling and photodamage assessment scales exist, the need for a system related purely to visible wrinkling and visible textural changes secondary to solar elastosis was thought to be more relevant to the topic of wrinkle eradication.[201]

Use of this scoring system allows broad classification into mild, moderate, and severe categories as well as a subjective numeric severity score (Table 7-4). Assessing patients both before and after treatment in a study with an average follow-up of about 90 days revealed that the average patient's preoperative score decreased approximately 50% as a consequence of resurfacing.[208] This means that mild wrinkles generally resolve completely, moderate wrinkles become mild, and severe wrinkles become moderate. Other studies[199,200,206] using different assessment systems have come to basically the same conclusion: wrinkles generally improve 50% to 70%, with superficial lines eliminated, deeper lines softened, skin texture normalized, precancerous lesions eliminated, and lentigines and seborrheic keratoses eliminated. These are realistic expectations for the patient, although occasionally even severe wrinkles may completely resolve. The treated area may continue to improve for several months after laser resurfacing as collagen remodeling takes place. Studies of long-term benefit are now being conducted by various investigators.

Table 7-4
Facial wrinkling: Clinical classifications

Class	Wrinkling	Score	Degree of Elastosis
I	Fine wrinkles	1-3	Mild: fine textural changes with subtly accentuated skin lines
II	Fine to moderate-depth wrinkles; moderate number of lines	4-6	Moderate: distinct papular elastosis (individual papules with yellow translucency under direct lighting) and dyschromia
III	Fine to deep wrinkles; numerous lines; with or without redundant skin folds	7-9	Severe: multipapular and confluent elastosis (thickened, yellow, and pallid) approaching or consistent with cutis rhomboidalis

Our studies of patients with an average follow-up of 2 years postoperatively (range 1-4 years) have revealed an excellent preservation of these results. Generally, as anticipated, the lines first to recur are those caused by muscle motion ("crow's feet," glabellar, forehead). Excellent preservation of results was seen, however, because 3-month versus 25-month scores revealed an average improvement in preoperative photodamage scores periorally of 49% versus 38%, respectively, while periorbital scores were 46% versus 31% improved (Figure 7-23). Interestingly, patient

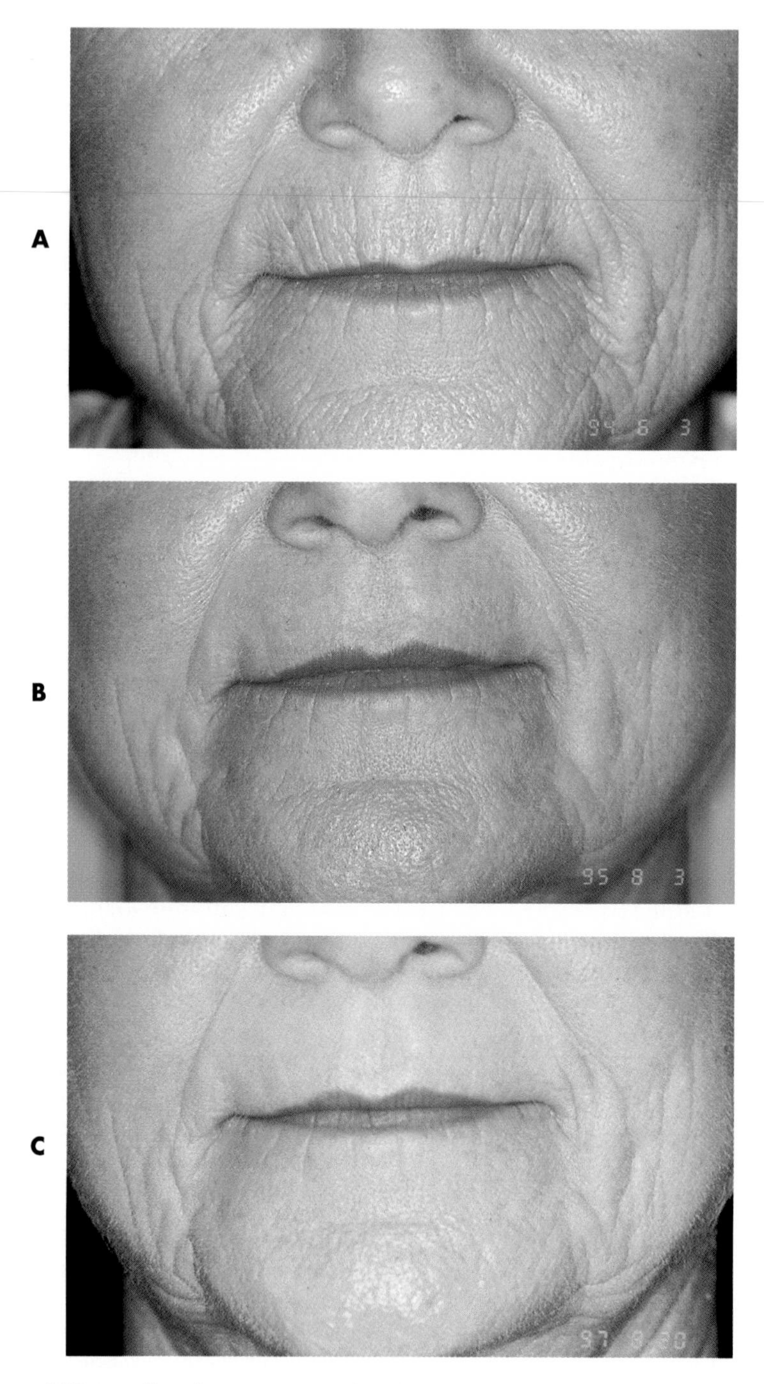

Figure 7-23 Excellent long-term results after CO_2 laser resurfacing of facial wrinkles. **A,** Before surgery: class III, level 8. **B,** Fourteen months postoperatively: class II, level 4. **C,** Thirty-nine months postoperatively: class II, level 4. Note progression of photoaging of medial cheeks, which were not treated.

satisfaction for these two areas was 55% for the perioral area and 80% for the periorbital area. Overall, 94 of 104 patients (90%) considered laser resurfacing to be a beneficial procedure that they would recommend to others.[361] This may be true because the laser removes the textural and pigmentary abnormalities (the "weathered" look) even though the muscles may still be able to fold the skin into wrinkles.

Other investigators have found similar results. Burns[362] had independent observers grade 95 consecutive full-face resurfacing procedures at 90 days and 1 year postoperatively using a scale of 1 to 8 and found an average decrease in photodamage scores as follows:

Area	90 days	1 year
Perioral	69%	64%
Cheeks	89%	72%
Forehead	80%	48%
Periorbital	79%	52%

No difference was seen in outcome whether patients were treated with the Coherent system or the Sharplan system.

Ross et al[363] reported the long-term results of 28 patients treated with either the SilkTouch or the UltraPulse laser and found that their pretreatment photodamage scores continued to improve from 60 days to the reassessment point at 1 year. Scores improved 43% in the SilkTouch group and 34% in the UltraPulse group, but no statistical difference was seen between the two groups. The immediate thermal damage was found to be about 30% greater in the SilkTouch group, with a wider zone of fibroplasia (220 μm vs. 150 μm in the UltraPulse group) at 1 year postoperatively. No statistical difference was seen in adverse effects for the two groups, although focal hypopigmentation was noted in two patients treated with the SilkTouch laser and one patient treated with both. Weinstein[360] reports that follow-up of her patients for as long as 5 years after resurfacing has shown that improvement visible at 6 months was still present at 5 years and that the overall results are indeed long-lasting.

In addition, 24 subjects were treated with the SilkTouch laser on one side of the face and 35% TCA on the opposite, for correction of periorbital wrinkling. Using a scoring system of 1 to 5, pretreatment scores were found to diminish 56% with laser treatment versus 20% with chemical peeling at 6 months. The outcome difference was statistically significant. Posttreatment erythema, however, lasted 4.5 months versus 2.5 months for the respective groups.[364]

Long-term follow-up of 12 patients having photodamage treated with dermabrasion and followed for 6 months to 8 years showed that not only did cosmetic improvement persist over these time periods, but the need for continued treatment of premalignant and malignant lesions was virtually eliminated.[178] All patients were noted to have maintenance of smooth, supple skin with pigmentation slightly lighter than adjacent nondermabraded skin.

OTHER INDICATIONS

Acne

Laser resurfacing can achieve significant improvement in acne scarring. The procedure can be made very precise by sculpting the edges of the scars and vaporizing more tissue away only in the areas of scar tissue while doing only superficial resurfacing in the rest of the cosmetic unit being treated. The tissue-tightening effects can achieve dramatic improvement in soft atrophic scars with sloping walls (Figure 7-20). Some "ice pick" and bound-down scars should first be removed with punch

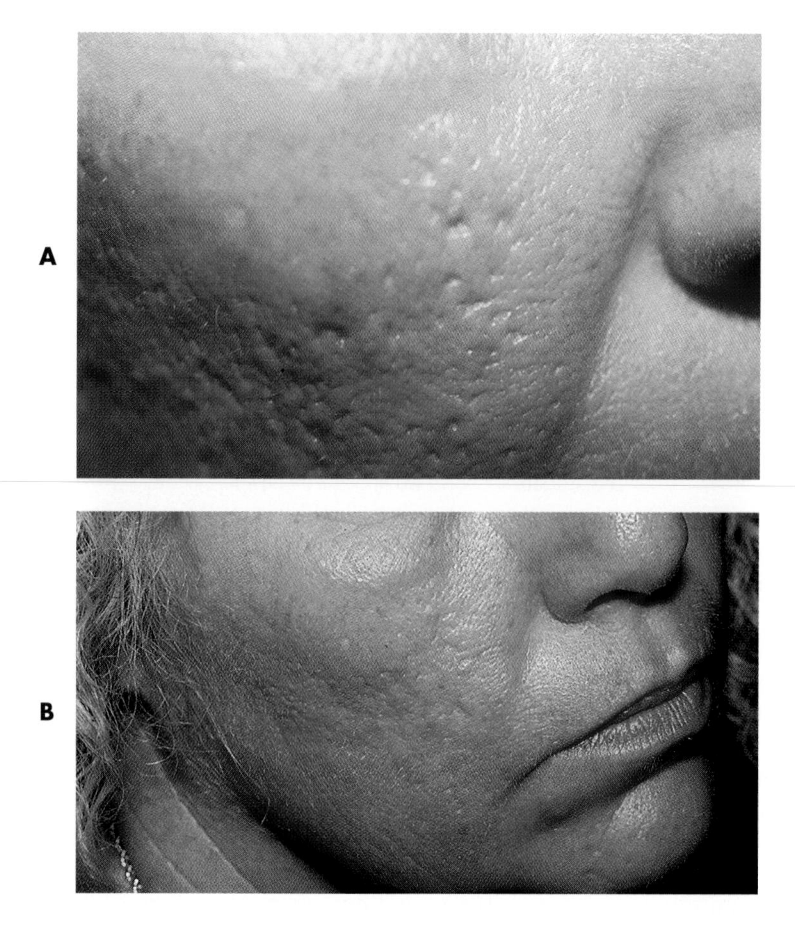

Figure 7-24 "Ice pick" or bound-down scars will improve greatly if scar excisions are performed before CO_2 laser resurfacing. **A,** Before excision. **B,** One year after laser resurfacing.

excision, punch elevation, or punch grafting, with laser resurfacing performed 6 to 12 weeks later if maximum improvement is desired[365] (Figure 7-24). Those not treated first with excision will improve, but the degree of improvement achieved will depend on the scar's depth and the operator's skill. In general, a 30% to 50% improvement is the treatment goal. However, a study using the Coherent UltraPulse CO_2 laser to treat moderate to severe atrophic acne scars in 50 patients revealed an average clinical improvement of 81% at 6 months after treatment, with progressive improvement occurring during that period.[366]

Patients should be advised that acne scars are always difficult to treat by any method, and the patient rarely reaches the level of satisfaction desired in a single surgical procedure. The same is true for laser resurfacing, but additional laser procedures add significant degrees of improvement.

Scars

Crateriform varicella scars and isolated acne scars can be improved with spot laser resurfacing. The area around and over the scar is vaporized with one laser pass. Additional passes are concentrated along the edge of the scar crater until it has been completely effaced.

Postsurgical (Figure 7-25) and traumatic scars and skin grafts (Figure 7-26) can be dramatically improved if resurfaced.[181,182,367] It is best to wait until the scar has completely healed (3 to 6 months) (Figure 7-27). This is an artistic endeavor and involves the vaporization of elevated tissue high points as well as skin tightening to elevate loose atrophic tissue. This is often a process of trial and error, attempting various maneuvers in small selective areas with observation of tissue effects before deciding to use an approach in a larger surface area.

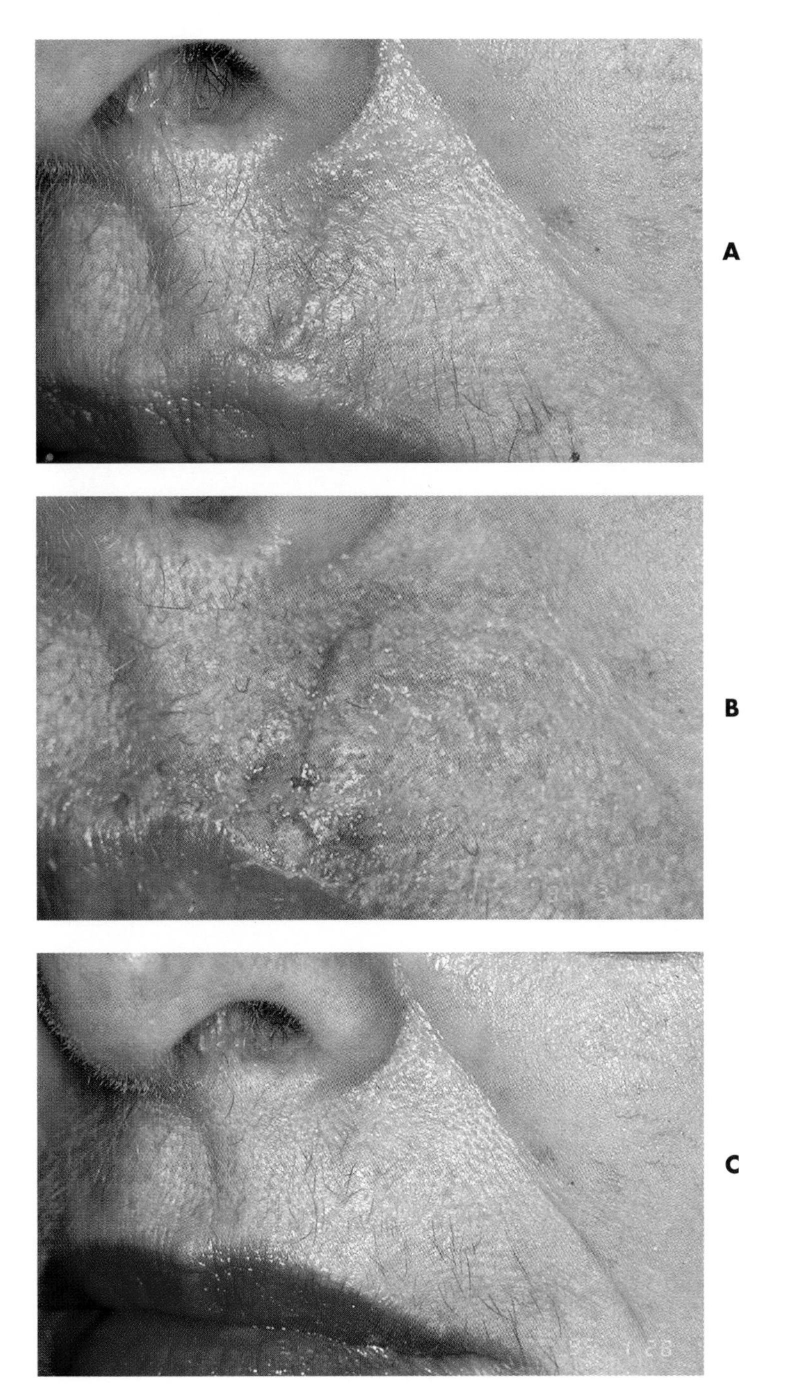

Figure 7-25 **A,** Linear scar 6 weeks after repair of Mohs surgical defect. **B,** Immediately after resurfacing with UltraPulse CO_2 laser at 500 mJ, 3-mm-diameter spot size, with three passes given to vaporize scar. **C,** Nine months after resurfacing, virtual disappearance of scar.

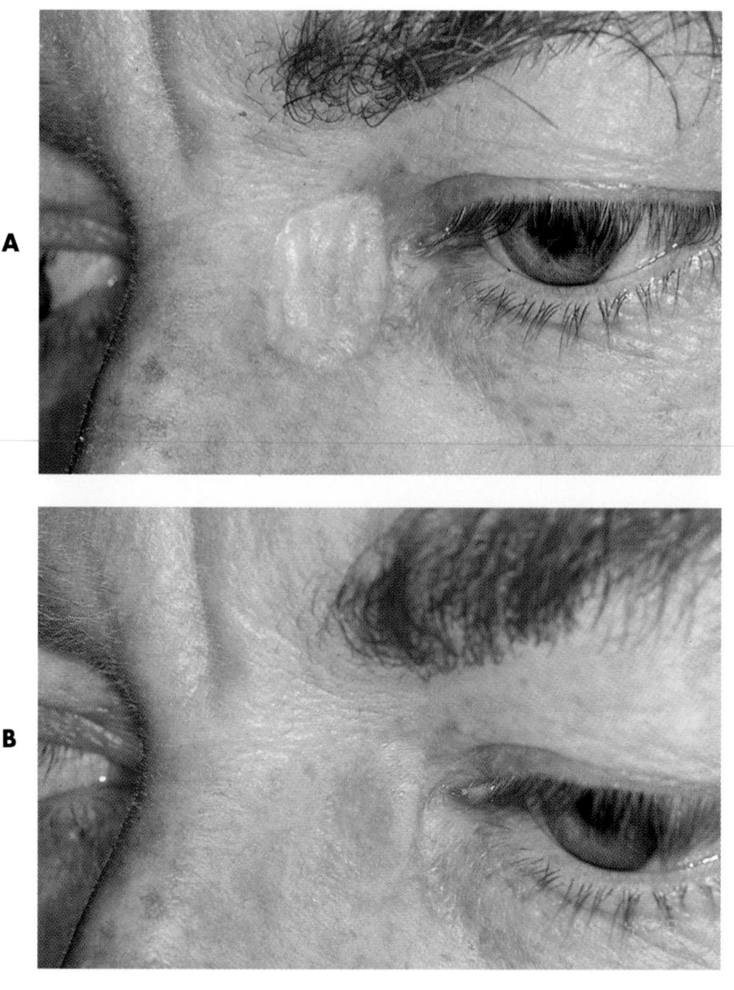

Figure 7-26 **A,** Six weeks after full-thickness skin graft repair of Mohs surgical defect. **B,** Four months after laser resurfacing of skin graft with laser parameters identical to those in Figure 7-27.

Actinic Cheilitis

Actinic cheilitis has proved to be a condition for which CO_2 laser therapy is considered the treatment of choice.[184,368-377] It can be successfully treated by performing a laser *vermilionectomy* using any of the resurfacing lasers.[365] This procedure usually requires only one pass with the laser over the vermilion surface and then spot treatment of persistently visible actinic damage. This has significantly reduced postoperative healing to approximately 10 days, in contrast to the 4 weeks required when the conventional CO_2 laser was used in the past.[184,368-377] Also, the risk of scarring is greatly reduced because the extent of thermal damage is much less.

Actinic keratoses unresponsive to conventional treatment with liquid nitrogen and topical 5-fluorouracil can be treated by removing the epidermis with one pass and then concentrating treatment on visible dermal extensions using one of the resurfacing lasers. This is especially useful on the dorsal hands and scalp but may be a primary or sole indication for laser resurfacing.

In our experience, treatment of these lesions in large surface areas results in much greater efficacy of treatment, with significantly decreased numbers of lesions occurring and their interval of recurrence greatly lengthened (see Chapter 6).

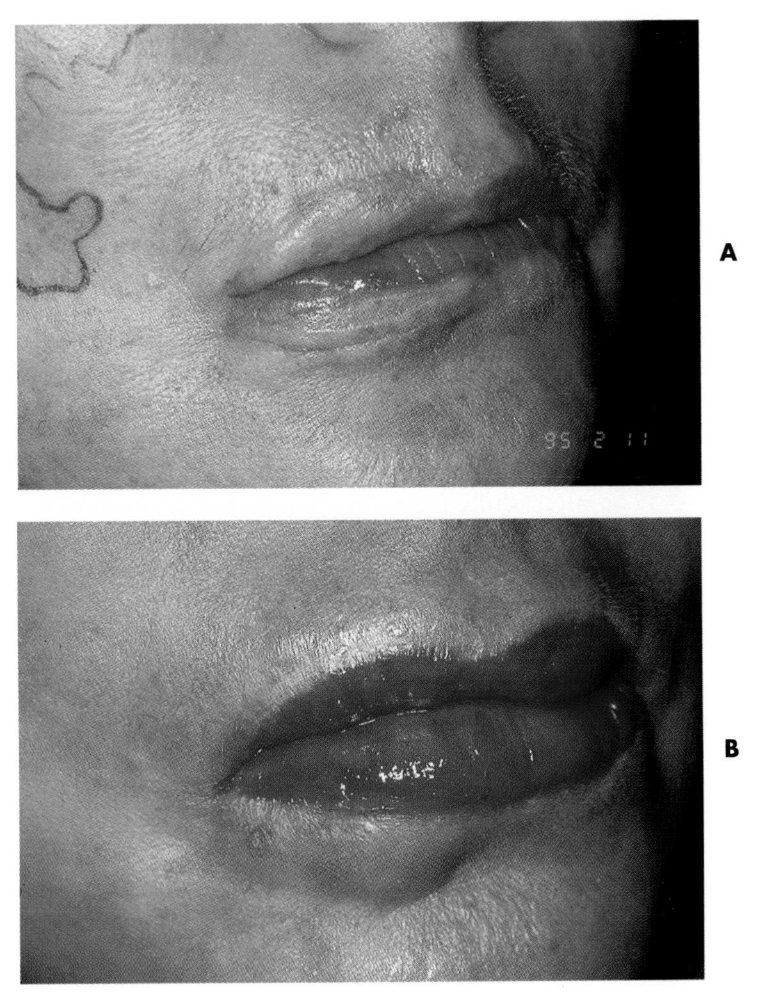

Figure 7-27 **A,** Obvious deformity of scarred lips after full-thickness tissue loss and reconstructive surgery. **B,** UltraPulse CO_2 laser was used to sculpt scar tissue and normalize lip contours.

Pigmentation

Pigmentation irregularities such as postinflammatory *hyperpigmentation* or *melasma* can sometimes be improved with laser resurfacing. It is very important to use tretinoin (Retin-A) and hydroquinones for an extended period before and after the procedure.[378,379] Other lasers more specific for melanin or medium-depth chemical peels are often preferable because they do not require anesthesia and recovery time is much shorter.[380-384] Melasma responds variably, in a similar manner to its response to other modalities.[385] Usually these pigment abnormalities are a secondary component of treatment and not the primary treatment objective. If they are the primary reason for treatment, care must be taken to ensure that other, more pigment-specific therapies are not desirable for whatever reason.

Rhinophyma and Benign Growths

Rhinophyma[386,387] and various small benign growths such as syringoma,[388] trichoepithelioma,[389] dermatosis papulosa nigra, xanthelasma,[390] adenoma sebaceum,[391] sebaceous hyperplasia, and epidermal nevi[392,393] have traditionally been treated with the conventional CO_2 laser and respond in an even more excellent manner to the resurfacing CO_2 lasers (see Chapter 6).

SURGICAL CONSIDERATIONS

Regional Versus Full-Face Resurfacing

The two areas of photodamage and wrinkling that have been shown to respond dramatically well to laser resurfacing are the *perioral and periorbital regions.*[201] These areas are not improved by face-lifting procedures, and although blepharoplasty may improve the skin laxity, it does not smooth away the wrinkle lines and textural changes of the periorbital region. Chemical peels and dermabrasion have given disappointing results in both these regions after treatment by the average practitioner. Treatment success in these regions has given laser resurfacing its popularity. Either of these areas may be successfully treated as an isolated region, but if both areas are to be treated, it is far better to treat the entire face.

In general, *full-face resurfacing* will give a better clinical result in all patients, because treatment of the full cheeks results in better tightening of the nasolabial lines, lateral "crow's feet," and midcheek creases. The same is true of treating the entire forehead and its effects on glabellar lines, lateral temporal lines, and upper aspects of crow's feet. In addition, the even pigmentation and smoothing of the skin results in a much more pleasant cosmetic appearance than blending new, smooth skin to photodamaged skin and creating a patchwork pattern. From a practical standpoint, it is also much easier for the patient to deal with postoperative erythema that is uniform over the full face rather than patchy erythema with multiple borders to blend. We rarely treat only a single anatomic unit, almost never treat an isolated wrinkle or scar, and never treat two isolated anatomic units simultaneously without treating the intervening skin. In our office, 90% to 95% of patients receive full-face treatment.

Timing of Treatment

Whether to treat early or later is an issue that frequently arises. The potential advantages of treating early, rather fine, subtle wrinkle lines is that the procedure can be done more superficially and with less risk of prolonged erythema, pigment changes, or scarring. Also, greater potential exists for removing all the photodamaged tissue, achieving a more long-lasting result, and providing a preventive benefit regarding future wrinkling. However, these early changes are usually relatively subtle clinically and, even when fully removed, result in only modest cosmetic benefits. The primary benefit may be in halting progression of photodamage.

The pros and cons of performing a relatively aggressive procedure for a relatively minor cosmetic problem need to be discussed in detail with the patient and a decision made with realistic expectations (Table 7-5). The alternative is to place the patient on a topical therapeutic program for reversal of photodamage and to use mild topical peels such as salicylic acid, AHA, or Jessner's solution. In addition, the use of pigment-specific lasers and vascular-specific lasers can be offered for the removal of individual pigmented and vascular lesions.

Degree of Photodamage and Pigmentation

When dealing with more advanced photodamage, full-face resurfacing is almost always necessary. Complete removal of deep lines in a single procedure may not be possible, as previously discussed. The anticipated improvement is 50% to

Table 7-5
Early versus later CO_2 laser treatment of wrinkles*

Pros	Cons
Treatment of Early Wrinkling	
More superficial resurfacing necessary	Improvement may be subtle
Less risks of scarring, prolonged erythema, and pigment loss	Use of relatively aggressive treatment for relatively minor cosmetic problem
Complete elimination of wrinkles typically achieved	Must weigh risk/benefit ratio
Long-lasting results achieved with good maintenance program	Patients often very demanding and critical of less-than-perfect results
Treatment of Late Wrinkling	
Dramatic improvement often achieved	Deeper resurfacing procedure and more aggressive therapy necessary
Medical benefit (e.g., removal of actinic keratoses, squamous cell carcinoma in situ) common	Greater risks of scarring, prolonged erythema, and pigment loss
Significant psychologic benefit	More than one procedure necessary for complete elimination of wrinkles
Patient satisfied with improvement, with no expectation of complete eradication of wrinkles	Persistence of benefits variable, depending on depth of preexisting damage as well as maintenance program

*Both are successful. Both patient and physician must have realistic expectations. In general, earlier treatment preferable to later treatment because of decreased risks and enhanced ability to achieve excellent results.

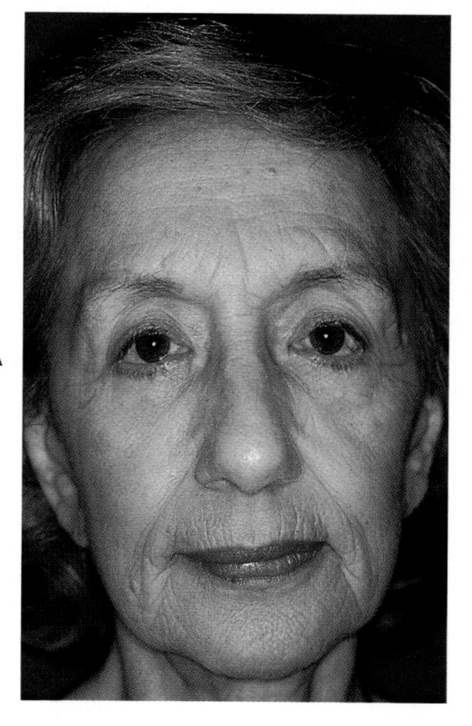

A

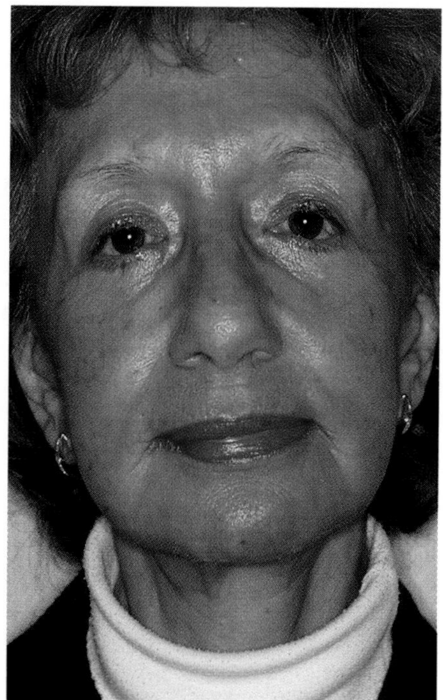

B

Figure 7-28 Anticipated improvement results for full-face resurfacing are 50% to 70%. Complete elimination of some wrinkle lines definitely will occur, but other lines may only soften. **A,** Before surgery. **B,** Three months postoperatively.

70%[199-201,206-208] (Figure 7-28). If further improvement is desired, a second treatment may be done after 6 to 12 months to allow new collagen formation and collagen remodeling. Patients with more advanced photodamage are usually very pleased with their clinical improvement even though it may not be complete eradication of wrinkle lines. Complete elimination of wrinkle lines usually is not the patient's goal, and overaggressive treatments may result in prolonged healing or hypopigmentation from deep levels of tissue ablation and deep resurfacing. The physician must effectively communicate to the patient that some degree of decreased pigmentation is a consequence of treatment.

Sun-damaged skin, with a history of decades of sun exposure, has a different pigmentation than non-sun-damaged skin that is related to the depth of resurfacing. Removal of the epidermis alone may result in healing with a population of melanocytes derived from the most superficial aspect of the follicular epithelium. These melanocytes have a significant history of prior sun damage and may produce persistent dyspigmentation. Deeper resurfacing results in progressive elimination of this sun-exposed subset of follicular epithelial melanocytes, yielding a more uniform pigmentation. An effective means of communicating this to patients is to have them compare the pigment of a non-sun-exposed area, such as the skin of the medial upper arms, to that of their face. This is likely to be the color of their newly healed skin, with non-sun-exposed epithelium and papillary dermis having developed during the healing process. If a strong color contrast is seen, a decision must be made regarding (1) selection of epidermal resurfacing only, which can be accomplished with a 20% TCA peel or careful CO_2 or Er:YAG laser resurfacing, and (2) consideration of forming the transition zone from treated to nontreated skin.

The natural shadowing under the jaw line makes this area a good transition area. For some patients the contrast will be too great if they do not wear makeup. It may be preferable, however, to have this contrast occur at the jaw line rather than at midneck (chosen by some physicians because the upper neck heals better than the lower neck and can be treated more aggressively), the clavicular level, or the V of the neck or upper chest. Resurfacing of the neck to the clavicles or down to the middle anterior chest has not been recommended with the CO_2 laser because the risk of side effects is too high. The erbium laser may be used successfully in this regard with proper technique. Some physicians use 20% to 25% TCA applied in a light coat, with only spotty frosting occurring. The latter two choices may be appropriate for a woman who always wears a collared shirt and rarely or never has her entire upper chest and shoulder area visually exposed. When these areas are more visible from the clothing worn, especially in those frequently involved in athletics, women may prefer more superficial resurfacing and a transition zone at the jaw line.

To preserve normal pigmentation, even though it may be reduced in contrast to sun-damaged skin, it is necessary to avoid deep, midreticular dermal tissue removal. This type of pigment loss is considered a complication and is usually associated with prolonged erythema (Figure 7-29). It should be avoidable by adhering to our recommended techniques.

Lines of Expression

Lines of expression—forehead lines, glabellar lines, and particularly "crow's feet" lateral canthal lines—are caused by muscle contraction and will always recur, even if completely erased after the procedure. As long as the muscles involved continue to fold the skin, a crease is formed. Several surgical procedures may be used to denervate or demuscle some of these areas. However, a very useful adjunctive procedure is the injection of botulin toxin type A (Botox) to block nerve transmission to these muscle groups.[394-397] These injections may be performed 1 to 2 weeks preoperatively or postoperatively to block these muscle groups and prevent motion in

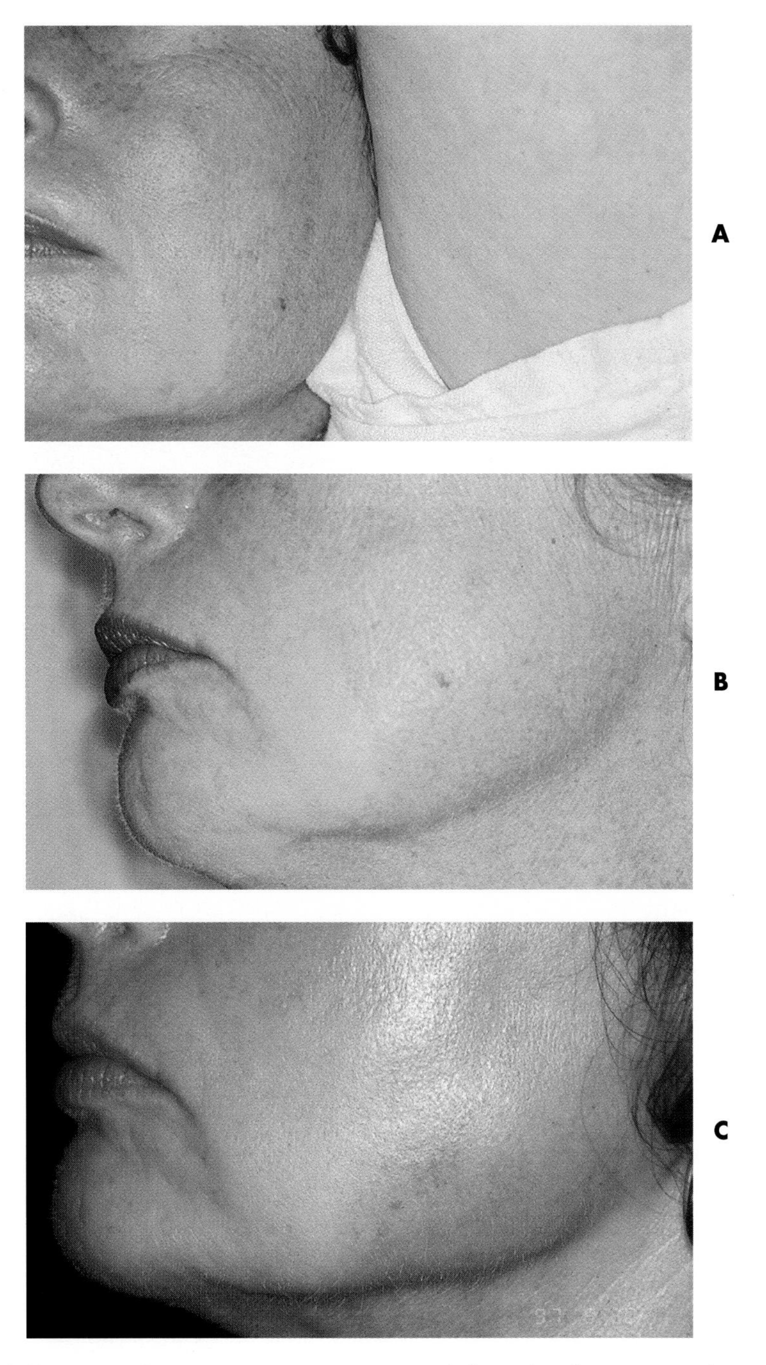

Figure 7-29 **A,** True hypopigmentation occurs with loss of melanocytes and results in pigment loss that is usually more significant than that of non-sun-exposed skin. **B,** This type of pigment loss contrasts sharply with photodamaged skin. **C,** Treatment of this condition is oriented toward removal of contrasting photodamaged skin.

these areas for 4 to 6 months during the time of new collagen formation and remodeling. Enhanced results are seen and should give a more lasting clinical improvement (Figure 7-30). If desired, the Botox injections may be done repeatedly, with longer-lasting results seen with each subsequent injection as the muscles atrophy. This generally requires four to five treatments before this longer-lasting effect is seen.

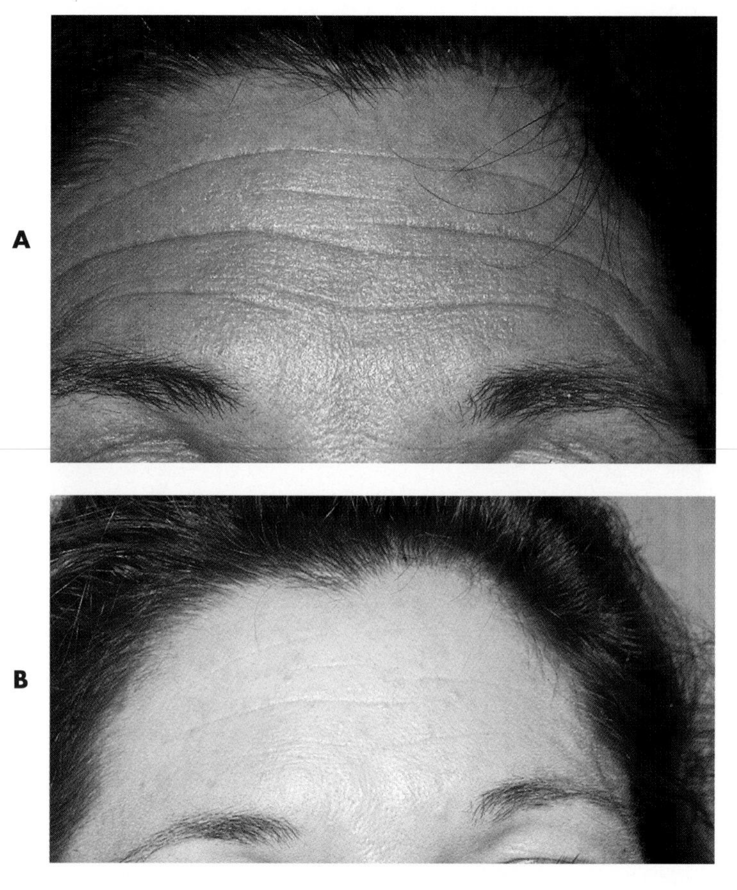

Figure 7-30 **A,** Deep lines of forehead, glabella, and lateral canthi caused by muscle movement frequently recur after laser resurfacing. **B,** Pretreatment with Botox results in more significant, longer-lasting improvement.

Contraindications

Box 7-2 lists possible contraindications to resurfacing.

PREOPERATIVE REGIMENS

Carefully selected preoperative and postoperative treatment regimens are necessary to achieve optimum results with skin resurfacing.[378,379,398] All patients apply topical retinoic acid (Retin-A, Renova) each night and topical vitamin C (Cellex-C) each morning, as well as a full-spectrum sunscreen such as TI-SILC (HumaTech) or a sunscreen containing Parsol 1789. As mentioned previously, these topical agents are thought to enhance the overall cosmetic benefit and promote quicker healing and reepithelialization. Although an arbitrary minimum preoperative treatment time of 2 weeks is often used, achieving maximum benefit requires months of use, and a minimum of 2 months is suggested (Figure 7-31).

Postinflammatory hyperpigmentation occurs frequently after laser resurfacing, although it is transient in nature and treatable, if not preventable. In general, the risk parallels the depth of the patient's natural color or pigment: the darker the color, the greater the potential. To reduce the incidence of postinflammatory hyperpigmentation, in addition to the topical agents already mentioned, patients with Fitzpatrick

Box 7-2 Contraindications to skin resurfacing

Possible abnormal wound healing
- Prior isotretinoin (Accutane) treatment within 1 to 2 years
- Keloids/hypertrophic scars
- Scleroderma/collagen vascular diseases
- Immunosuppressive drugs

Decreased adnexal structures of skin
- Prior radiation therapy
- Prior deep phenol peel
- Burn scars

Infectious diseases
- Human immunodeficiency virus/acquired immunodeficiency syndrome

Infectious diseases—cont'd
- Hepatitis C
- Active herpes simplex
- History of recurrent infections/anergy

Koebnerizing (isomorphic) diseases
- Labile psoriasis
- Severe eczema
- Vitiligo

Medical conditions
- Significant diabetes
- Problematic hypertension
- Significant cardiovascular/pulmonary disease

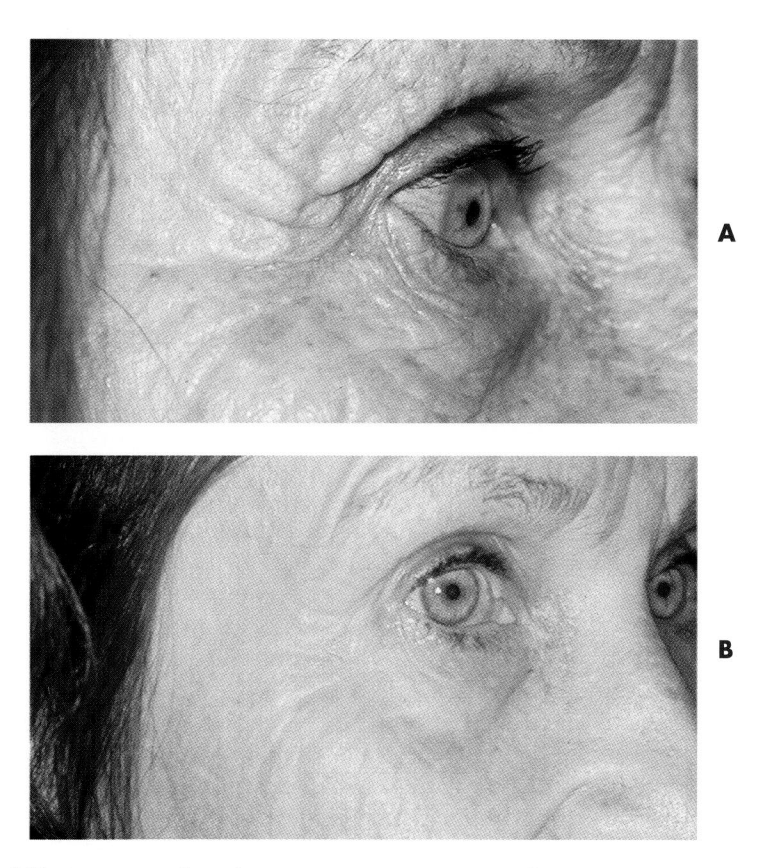

Figure 7-31 **A,** Severe photodamage. **B,** Pretreatment with tretinoin (Retin-A) and vitamin C for at least 6 months significantly enhances response to laser resurfacing.

types III to VI pigment are given topical preparations of hydroquinone, kojic acid, or azelaic acid to be used for 1 to 2 months preoperatively. Hydroquinone is cytotoxic to melanocytes and is the mainstay of treatment. Azelaic acid, kojic acid, and glucosamine inhibit tyrosinase and pigment synthesis. In addition, tretinoin promotes melanosome transfer and keratinocyte turnover. These agents are then started as soon as possible postoperatively (2-4 weeks). Care must be taken to limit inflammation from starting these products too early (Table 7-6).

Table 7-6
Agents to treat hyperpigmentation

Agent	Mechanism of Action
Hydroquinone	Cytotoxic to melanocytes
Azelaic acid	Inhibits tyrosinase and pigment synthesis
Kojic acid	Inhibits tyrosinase and pigment synthesis
Glucosamine	Inhibits tyrosinase and pigment synthesis
Tretinoin	Promotes melanosome transfer and keratinocyte turnover
Alpha-hydroxy acids	Promotes keratinocyte turnover

Prevention of Infections

To guard against *herpes simplex* infection triggered by surgical stress and to prevent its dissemination over the deepithelialized skin surface, patients are given an antiviral agent such as valacyclovir (Valtrex) or famcyclovir (Famvir) starting 3 days preoperatively if they have a prior history of herpes simplex infection or starting on the day of the procedure if no prior history. This treatment should be continued at least through the reepithelialization phase of wound healing (an additional 7-10 days). All patients should be treated with this regimen, because patients with no known prior history of herpes simplex infection have been noted to develop an acute episode in the immediate postoperative period.[201] Dissemination over the treatment area with resultant scarring has been observed to occur in these patients (Figure 7-32). An acute treatment dose rather than a suppressive dose should be used. Valtrex (500 mg twice daily) and Famvir (250 mg twice daily) provide higher and longer-lasting blood drug levels than does acyclovir (Zovirax, 400 mg four times daily). In patients with a known history of herpes simplex infection, the dosage is increased 50% (three times instead of twice daily), because the response of herpes simplex may be dose dependent, and use of significantly higher doses in treatment of herpes zoster has not been associated with an increased incidence of adverse effects.

Staphylococcal infection has been prevented by the prophylactic use of systemic antibiotics such as dicloxacillin, azithromycin, or ciprofloxacin. The use of intranasal mupirocin (Bactroban),[399] however, has not proved to be advantageous and may even worsen the situation. All staphylococcal infections occurred in the group of patients using intranasal Bactroban in a study of patients randomly assigned to use or not to use Bactroban for 3 days preoperatively and 7 days postoperatively.[240]

The layer of thermally necrotic tissue that results from CO_2 laser resurfacing requires several days to slough. This layer is treated with frequent to continuous soaking in order to promote débridement and enhance reepithelialization. Al-though moist wound care has been shown to enhance wound healing and reepithelialization, it also provides an environment that is ideal for bacterial growth, particularly the ubiquitous gram-negative organisms such as *Pseudomonas aeruginosa* and gram-positive *Staphylococcus aureus*. This is especially true when prophylactic antibiotics have diminished normal cutaneous flora. However, even normal cutaneous flora may proliferate on the wound surface in this situation and result in disruption of wound healing and reepithelialization. To help prevent this infection, meticulous attention to washing the hands with Techni-Care (Care-Tech Laboratories, Inc., St. Louis) daily during the postoperative phase should be done. Prophylactic treatment with ciprofloxacin (500 mg twice daily) has been advocated because of its anti-*Pseudomonas* coverage combined with its reasonable anti-*Staphylococcus* coverage.[400] Further study of this recommendation has revealed that only one infection occurred while patients were still taking ciprofloxacin.[401] All other infections occurred after

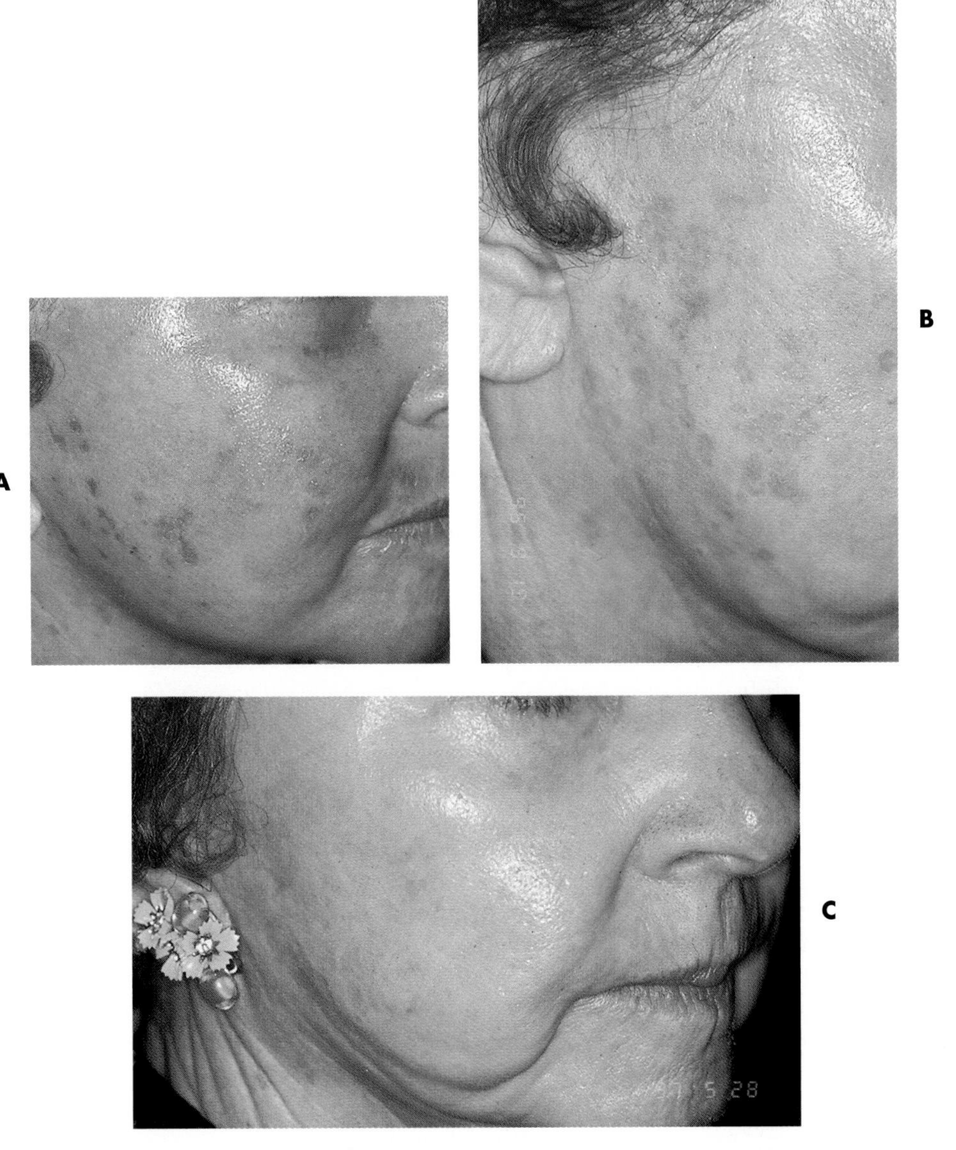

Figure 7-32 **A,** Dissemination of herpes simplex occurred on day 4 postoperatively in patient with no prior history of herpes simplex infection, despite pretreatment with acyclovir (Zovirax). Valacyclovir (Valtrex) has been found to be superior as a preventive medication because much higher drug blood levels are achieved. **B,** Ten months postoperatively, scarring from infection is apparent. **C,** Eight months later, marked improvement has been achieved with pulsed dye laser treatment of scars.

ciprofloxacin had been discontinued. We currently recommend that ciprofloxacin be continued for at least 10 days and possibly as long as 2 weeks.

The prevention of bacterial infections should not be taken lightly, because toxic shock syndrome (TSS) has been reported after a benign cutaneous infection with *S. aureus* after laser resurfacing in three patients to date. Also, scarring secondary to disruption of wound healing has resulted from *S. aureus, Pseudomonas,* and normal cutaneous overgrowth or infection.

Another postoperative infection that may result from the moist wound environment is *cutaneous candidiasis.* This has been found to correlate with a prior history of vaginal yeast infection.[400] Prophylaxis with a single dose of fluconazole (400 mg) on the day of surgery is recommended in these patients. To date, we have not seen a yeast infection occur in a patient who received this prophylactic treatment preoperatively. The presentation of this infection postoperatively may include typical signs and symptoms of cutaneous candidiasis, but also may be atypical and present only as slow wound healing, itching, and erythema. It should always be suspected in a patient with unexplained poor wound healing. A potassium hydroxide preparation from a scraping of a suspicious area or a culture usually confirms the diagnosis. (See Chapter 6.)

IMMEDIATE PREOPERATIVE MEASURES

The skin should be prepped with Techni-Care, a broad-spectrum, nontoxic microbicide that is antiviral, antifungal, and effective against both gram-positive and gram-negative bacteria. Thirty-second contact use has been shown to result in 99.99% bacterial reduction. Flammable agents such as chlorhexidine gluconate (Hibiclens) and isopropyl alcohol should not be used in the immediate preoperative stage unless thoroughly washed off with water preoperatively. Hibiclens and alcohol also have ocular toxicities, especially in a sedated patient (Table 7-7).

Metal eye shields should be inserted to protect the eyes.[402] Tetracaine (Tetcaine HCL Ophthalmic 0.5%) or a similar ophthalmic anesthetic solution is first placed in the eyes. Metallic eye shields with an external etching coated with sterile ophthalmic petrolatum should be used. Cox laser eye shields (Delasco, Council Bluffs, Iowa), which are available in three sizes, are inserted with a rubber vacuum plunger and have proved to be the most effective of those available because of ease of insertion and the ability to close the lids over them without distorting the overlying skin. When the eye shields are removed at the end of the procedure, the eyes should be flushed with sterile saline to wash out the petrolatum remaining on the conjunctival surface. This minimizes blurry vision postoperatively. If the periorbital area is not to be treated, the eyes may be protected with moistened gauze pads rather than eye shields.

The periphery of the patient's face should be draped with wet cloths before the procedure so that errant laser impacts do not contact a flammable surface or skin unintended for treatment. Some physicians advocate the use of aluminum foil, but

Table 7-7
Antimicrobials and microbicides as prophylaxis before skin resurfacing

	Chlorhexidine Gluconate (Hibiclens)	Providone-iodine (Betadine)	Linear Alcohol	Techni-Care
Substantivity (hours)	>6	3	None	>6
Occular irritation	Yes	Yes	Yes	Minimal
Scrub time (minutes)	8	3.5	11	0.5
Dermatitis potential	30%	30%	High	<1%
Formulation dependent	Yes	Yes	Variable	Yes
Amount needed (ml)	10	10	—	2.5
Tissue contraindications	Yes	Yes	Yes	None
Toxicity/chemical burns	Eyes, ears	Skin, genitalia	Eyes	Nontoxic*
Denatured by organic material	Minimal	Yes	No data	Minimal
Transdermal penetration/absorption	No	Yes	No	Yes
pH measurement	5.86	4.0	6.8	7.2

Data from a variety of sources.
*Safe for mucous membranes.

we find this to be impractable. If the glossy surface is the outer surface, reflection of an errant beam can occur; if the duller surface is exterior, reflection may still occur. Perhaps even more significantly, it is difficult to keep these foil sheets in place during the movement that necessarily occurs during the procedure. They are constantly falling off the surgical field, requiring replacement. A moist towel is easy to apply, is pliable, stays in place, and absorbs any errant laser beam that happens to hit it. The teeth may be protected by placement of wet gauze under the lips and over the teeth, but we have not found this to be necessary, except in patients with extensive porcelain crowns.

ANESTHESIA

For CO_2 laser resurfacing of the face, as for any surgical procedure, the goals of anesthesia are to provide optimal conditions for the surgeon while ensuring the patient's safety and comfort. Facial resurfacing is a highly stimulating and painful procedure requiring significant analgesia and alteration of consciousness level for optimal results. Muscle relaxation and loss of all reflexes are unnecessary and may be undesirable.

The sensory innervation of the face is complex and in some areas overlapping, making it difficult to attain adequate anesthesia using only nerve blocks. For complete and bilateral anesthesia, one must block the forehead; periocular, nasal, medial, and lateral face and cheeks; anterior areas of the ears; perioral region; and jaw lines. The medial forehead is blocked through the supraorbital and supratrochlear nerves. Sensory blockage of the entire face is difficult to achieve because a variety of nerves innervate this area and some of the blocks are very difficult to perform. The upper half of the ear is innervated through the mandibular nerve. The medial cheek, upper lip, and part of the skin overlying the nose are innervated through the infraorbital nerve. The lower lip and chin are innervated via the mental nerve. The upper outer cheek and lateral forehead are innervated through the maxillary nerve and the far lateral cheek and jaw line through the cervical plexus on each side.

Even with perfect technique, the 14 separate nerve blocks required for facial anesthesia may leave areas around the ear and lateral temporal region without adequate anesthesia.[403] Supplementation of the nerve blocks that are easily performed (infraorbital, mental, supraorbital, and supratrochlear) with local infiltration is painful and only partially effective.

Some physicians treat with only the use of topical anesthetic creams, such as lidocaine-prilocaine (EMLA Cream). We have found this to be very ineffective, because achievement of anesthesia results in maceration of tissue from the occlusive process, which then alters the laser-tissue interaction because of the excessive tissue water content. When this is not done, anesthesia is generally not achieved, and the procedure may be too painful to complete.

Another alternative now being popularized is *tumescent anesthesia:* using very dilute infiltration of 0.1% to 0.2% lidocaine (Xylocaine) in saline to distend the tissue subcutaneously, as is done with liposuction. This undoubtedly may produce adequate anesthesia but also may cause tissue distortion and alterations of the skin's mechanical properties. This interferes with identification of tissue laxity and its elimination through collagen shrinkage and skin tightening. Skin tightening depends not only on the pliability and ease of movement of the collagen, but also that of immediately adjacent tissue.

Some compromise in results would be anticipated with use of these local anesthetic techniques, either from inability to treat adequately because of incomplete anesthesia or alterations in the laser-tissue interaction. Local anesthesia techniques are generally supplemented with sedatives such as diazepam (Valium), midazolam (Versed), or lorazepam (Ativan) and analgesics such as meperidine (Demerol) or hydromorphine (Dilaudid), generally given orally or intrmuscularly (IM). Possible side effects from these drugs must be considered as well in the choice of anesthesia. We prefer intravenous (IV) propofol sedation as our anesthesia, if feasible.

General anesthesia with *endotracheal (ET) intubation* for full-face laser resurfacing is an acceptable technique and has certain advantages. It ensures airway control, is safe and quickly administered, and allows the administration of adequate narcotic analgesia without concern for respiratory depression. However, not all facilities are equipped to provide general anesthesia. Also, patients or physicians may be reluctant to use general anesthesia for this procedure. A method of deep IV sedation combined with the use of the *laryngeal mask airway* (LMA) allows the procedure to be accomplished without ET intubation or an anesthesia machine.

Propofol is the primary agent used and provides rapidly induced, easily maintained, and quickly terminated loss of consciousness. IV midazolam is used to provide initial sedation and amnesia, while analgesia is provided by fentanyl (Sublimaze) supplemented intermittently with ketamine (Ketalar). To counteract potentially troublesome side effects of ketamine, all patients receive glycopyrrolate (Robinul) as a drying agent and midazolam and propofol before receiving ketamine. By using this regimen and limiting the total ketamine dose to about 1 mg/kg, patients have had no problems with "bad dreams" or adverse psychic experiences.[403]

The requisite equipment for this technique consists of an electrocardiogram (ECG), blood pressure monitor, pulse oximeter, supplemental oxygen source, LMA, and an IV infusion pump, as well as an anesthesiologist to administer the anesthesia. Capnohepatography, while optional, is desirable to monitor adequacy of ventilation. Prudence dictates that any facility administering narcotics or sedatives have appropriately trained medical personnel, a fully stocked resuscitation cart, intubation equipment (laryngoscope, blades, ET tubes), a method for delivering positive-pressure ventilation (Ambu bag or Jackson-Rees circuit), and a charged and functional defibrillator. A recovery area staffed with qualified nursing personnel should have the capacity to monitor ECG, blood pressure, and pulse oximetry.

Concern over the safety of laser energy in proximity to oxygen and the patient's face is understandable. All modern inhaled anesthetics are nonflammable, and although oxygen and nitrous oxide support combustion, neither is itself flammable. It is imperative that flammable liquids not be used in the facial preparation. The patient must be instructed not to use hairspray or other topical skin and hair products before surgery to avoid the introduction of unknown chemicals into the surgical field.

The oxygen delivery system consists of the LMA and the tubing from a green oxygen mask connecting the oxygen cylinder and the LMA, which includes a small pilot tube used to inflate the pharyngeal cuff. The LMA is very resistant to damage from the laser. An informal study performed in our facility revealed it to be resistant to penetration or inflammation despite 60 consecutive laser impacts while oxygen was flowing to enrich the immediate open-air vicinity. The pilot tube also is very resistant to laser damage, requiring 22 impacts before it was cut through, but never ignited. The green oxygen tubing, on the other hand, is easily damaged, and a few pulses will melt it. However, the oxygen flowing through the tube will not ignite, although any flammable object present in the field (e.g., dry gauze, dry hair) will ignite. ET tubes and LMA tubes can be fully protected by wrapping them with saline-soaked gauze or towels. With proper procedures and caution that no combustible liquids or other products are used near surgical areas, laser resurfacing in the presence of oxygen and an anesthetic delivery system such as an ET tube or LMA is safe.

WOUND HEALING

Observations in animal models and clinical studies suggest a general sequence of events that occur in wound healing, largely controlled by fibroblasts.[404-410] This has been divided into three phases: inflammatory, proliferation, and maturation.

Inflammatory Phase

The inflammatory phase lasts 3 to 10 days.[407,410] After dermal trauma, blood vessels constrict, and leakage of plasma proteins (fibrinogen, fibronectin, plasminogen) and platelets occurs. Plasma and blood clot when exposed to tissue factors[411] and form a gel-like fibrin-fibronectin matrix. Inflammatory cells, new capillaries, and fibroblasts derived from the wound edges migrate into this matrix. Activated macrophages are probably the most important cells in this phase of healing, particularly for wound débridement.[412-415]

The fibrin-fibronectin matrix is degraded by inflammatory cells. Fibroblasts synthesize fibronectin, interstitial collagens, and GAGs to form a new fibrovascular connective tissue, or granulation tissue, within 2 to 4 days after injury.[404,416,417] Fetal wound healing has been found to proceed without scar formation, and unlike adult wounds, in which hyaluronic acid is present transiently, high levels of hyaluronic acid persist in fetal wounds until repair is completed. The fetal extracellular matrix contains abundant hyaluronic acid rather than collagen.[418,419] This may be the result of decreased degradation,[420] and other studies suggest that hyaluronic acid may have a regulatory effect on scarless fetal wound healing.[421,422] Topical treatment of wounds with hyaluronic acid was found to reduce scarring of tympanic membrane perforations.[423] Normal mature scars, hypertrophic scars, and keloids were found with distinctively different distributions of hyaluronic acid, possibly contributing to their different clinical appearances.[424]

Beneficial effects of topical hyaluronic acid have been demonstrated both clinically and histologically in cutaneous ulcer healing studies,[425-430] animal wound studies,[431-433] and in vitro and in vivo studies.[434-437]

Proliferation Phase

The prominent collagen formed during the inflammatory phase is type III collagen, which has a gel-like consistency.[438] Its synthesis is maximal between 5 and 7 days. The proliferation phase occurs over the next 10 to 14 days and is dominated by the proliferation of fibroblasts and synthesis of collagen as well as regeneration of the epidermis and neoangiogenesis. Reepithelialization is heralded by mitoses at wound edges and at appendages within 24 hours.[408] Epidermal proliferation is maximal at 24 to 72 hours.[409] Direct contact with fibronectin and type I collagen guides and stimulates epithelial cell migration in culture.[410] Soluble substances such as growth factors derived from platelets, macrophages, dermal parenchymal cells, and keratinocytes stimulate reepithelialization in animal models.[417] Continued collagen synthesis proceeds, stimulated by macrophage-derived and platelet-derived factors,[439] followed by capillary resorption and disappearance of fibroblasts.[440]

Lymphokines, complement, native collagens of types I to V, fibronectin, and platelet-derived growth factor may be potent mitogens and chemotactants for fibroblasts.[404,441] In addition, macrophages may be activated by blood and may play a key role in inducing a fibroproliferative response when there is significant blood within the healing wound.[404,413,442]

In the biosynthesis of collagen, *procollagen* is formed intracellularly by fibroblasts and secreted into the extracellular space.[440] It is then biochemically transformed into *tropocollagen* by proteases.[443-446] The tropocollagen molecules aggregate into immature soluble collagen fibrils, which are then cross-linked by the action of lysyl oxidase to form mature, stronger collagen fibers.[447]

Maturation Phase

The total amount of collagen in a wound reaches a maximum at 2 to 3 weeks, but collagen remodeling continues over months to years.[448] This characterizes the third phase of wound healing, the maturation phase. The earliest collagen fibers are thin and unorganized, becoming thicker, cross-linked, and parallel to skin tension lines with time. As new collagen is formed, abnormal or damaged collagen is broken down by collagenases and proteases produced by fibroblasts, macrophages, and inflammatory cells. *Proteoglycans,* responsible for water storage in the healing wound, decrease, and water is reabsorbed as the wound heals.[449,450]

Remodeling of the collagen matrix results in gradual shrinkage, thinning, and paling of the scar. Once the collagen bed is established as a stable matrix, collagen production and resorption continue in a steady, balanced state in a normally healed scar. Tensile strength increases from 5% of original strength at 2 weeks to 80% in a mature scar.[451] Contraction of a scar, which begins 1 week after wounding, is not caused by excessive deposition of collagen, but rather by the effects of transformation of fibroblasts to myofibroblasts.[452,453] These cells produce contractile proteins with characteristics of smooth muscle cells. Granulation tissue has been shown to contain as much actomyosin as an equivalent weight of smooth muscle.[454] Furthermore, it has been demonstrated that contraction of myofibroblasts can be inhibited by smooth muscle relaxants.[407,452] It has been proposed that migrating fibroblasts interact with their surrounding matrix components to reorganize connective tissue fibers to induce shrinkage.[455] These factors can result in as much as a 45% reduction in wound surface area.[407]

Effects of Treatment

The magnitude and timing of each phase of wound healing may vary significantly depending on the wounding procedures and modalities. A study was designed to characterize differential responses to cutaneous injuries of equal depth created by a dermatome, laser ablation, or standard thermal metal template.[456] When skin is wounded with a dermatome, the wound bed is immediately flooded with growth-factor-laden platelets and blood constituents. By contrast, the other thermal wounds are deficient in immediate blood-borne cytokines. At day 5, dermatome wounds showed an average reepithelialization of 54%, almost two times higher than that of laser injuries and four times higher than standard thermal burns. This difference had disappeared by day 10. At day 5, laser wounds contained the highest number of proliferating fibroblasts, which were significantly depressed in thermal burns. At day 10, this order was reversed, with thermal burns having the highest proliferative profile and laser wounds the lowest. Laser wounds showed the earliest peak in matrix metalloproteinase (MMP) expression, whereas burns showed the least expression at day 5. An assessment of angiogenesis showed peak values at day 5 in both excisional and laser wounds, with burns not peaking until day 10. Laser injuries appeared to mature the earliest. The amount of new granulation tissue in laser injuries was modest compared with excisional or burn injuries. Standard burns exhibited the highest degree of disorganization, a feature of immature wounds.

In summary, laser injuries showed early accelerated levels of angiogenesis, dermal fibroblast proliferation, and MMP expression but were dramatically slower to resurface. This delay in reepithelialization may be related to damage to keratinocytes that reside in the upper aspects of hair follicles and sweat ducts. More likely, the difference in laser wounds relate to the layer of necrotic tissue that needs to be digested before reepithelialization can proceed in non-laser-induced wounds. The differences in the MMP expression patterns of the three types of wounds raise questions regarding proteolytic enzymes within the wound clearing and activating precursor of cytokines beneficial to wound healing. The data suggest that the function of MMPs within these wounds is not the proteolysis of devitalized tissues but rather the active remodeling of the wound environment.

POSTOPERATIVE WOUND CARE

If the patient develops noticeable intraoperative swelling, usually detected in the periorbital area, dexamethasone (Decadron, 10-12 mg by IV push) and betamethasone (Celestone, 6 mg IM) are adminstered. Although some physicians routinely use a Decadron Dos-pak, oral prednisone (20 mg every day for 7 days), or triamcinolone (Kenalog, 40 mg IM) postoperatively, the effects on suppression of fibroblast activity and infection surveillance must be considered. Single-dose IV Decadron and IM Celestone are rapidly cleared and thus should not interfere with wound healing. Because postoperative swelling generally clears rapidly (2 to 5 days), the choice of the shorter-acting corticosteroids is preferable.

The patient is told to expect a mild burning sensation for the first 1 to 3 days and significant swelling for the first 2 to 5 days. During the first 3 to 5 days, significant serous exudate is present as well, related to the swelling and absence of an epithelial barrier. Use of topical antibiotics and other topical drugs should be particularly avoided during this phase, because the incidence of contact irritant and allergic dermatitis is enhanced by the absence of epithelium.[248] We have found the incidence to increase from about 3% to 4% when topical agents are used in non-laser-treated skin to 20% or higher when they are used in laser resurfacing. Bacitracin is a frequent sensitizer, with a fivefold increase in dermatitis reported from 1990 to 1994.[457] In addition, a compound such as petrolatum, which usually does not cause contact sensitivity, has a greater potential to sensitize in this situation.[240,458]

Open-wound care generally consists of frequent soaking with cool distilled water containing a small amount of white vinegar. One teaspoon per cup is generally the starting concentration (0.25% acetic acid). The mildly acidic pH has an antibacterial effect, which is especially important in suppressing *Pseudomonas* species. The skin should be soaked copiously every 1 to 2 hours. The objective is to soak away the serous exudate and any necrotic tissue on the skin surface. Just patting the skin with a moist gauze pad is not adequate. Between soakings, the skin should be liberally and continuously coated with petrolatum (Vaseline) or Theraplex. This coating may be gently removed with gauze or facial tissue before the next soaking. Ice packs or frozen peas may be applied during this period for symptomatic pain relief.

The application of petrolatum to the wound surface results in a semiocclusive, moist environment. Recent studies have shown that wounds treated with petrolatum compared with those treated with a topical antibiotic have no increased incidence of infection and heal at the same rate.[459] In contrast, in an earlier study of accidental burns treated with either petrolatum mesh gauze or nitrofurazone, 75% of the petrolatum group had bacteria reported as "too numerous to count" compared with only 10% of the nitrofurazone group.[460]

The composition of a bland emollient apparently may have an effect on wound healing. A U.S.P. petrolatum ointment decreased wound healing by 17%, a white petrolatum cream increased wound healing by 24%, and a lotion with propylene glycol without petrolatum increased wound healing by 15%.[461]

Wound-healing studies have shown that vehicles with the proper combination of fatty acids result in faster healing than do petrolatum or Aquaphor.[153] Fatty acids that reflect the composition of fatty acids in human membranes are required for the proliferation of epithelial cells.[154,155] This mixture of fatty acids also significantly enhances the ability of pyruvate and vitamin E to inhibit reactive oxygen production and improve membrane function and cellular viability. These three components—vitamin E, pyruvate, and essential fatty acids—have been shown to be synergistic in reducing oxidative stress to keratinocytes and enhancing wound healing.[153]

The benefit of occlusive dressings in accelerating wound healing was first demonstrated in 1962[462] and confirmed in numerous studies.[463-474] reepithelialization was shown to occur 30% to 45% more quickly, with decreased pain and inflammation and more cosmetically acceptable scar formation. In addition, new collagen formation has been shown to begin 3 days earlier than in open wounds,[475] with an increased rate of collagen synthesis.[476]

The increased rate of reepithelialization produced by occlusive dressings is generally attributed to the moist wound environment and the absence of a crust that may impede cellular movement. In addition, occlusive dressings provide an environment that maximizes exposure to various endogenous growth factors. Continued exposure to epidermal growth factor has been shown to quicken epidermal resurfacing.[477]

The semiocclusive dressings are a diverse and complex group of wound dressings produced by many different manufacturers and involving many dressings with unique features that are often poorly understood by clinicians (Table 7-8). The most frequently used dressings are the polyurethane films, the hydrocolloids, and the hydrogels. The *polyurethane films* are simple dressings made from a single sheet of polyurethane, often bonded to an adhesive. The dressing is permeable to water vapor and gases but impermeable to wound fluids. Silon II, however, has multiple puncture slits to allow passage of fluids, and Omniderm is bonded to acrylamide, a hydrophilic monomer, rather than to an adhesive. On contact with a moist surface, Omniderm immediately absorbs water and conforms to the skin surface. It must be wet to be removed.[478]

Table 7-8
Biosynthetic dressings

Classification	Composition	Examples	Transmits Oxygen
Polyurethane films	Polyurethane *or* co-polyester with adhesive backing	Op-Site Bioclusive, Opraflex, Uniflex, Blisterfilm, Visulin, Ensure, Clingfilm, Viofilm, Acuderm, Omniderm, Dermafilm, Silon II, Tegaderm	+
Hydrocolloids	Hydrophilic colloidal particles bound to polyurethane foam	DuoDerm, Actiderm, Tegasorb, Cutinova Hydro, Ultec, Comfeel Ulcus, Restore, Hydrapad, Granulfex E, Intrasite, Intact, Flexzan	–
Hydrogels	60%-99% water cross-linked polymer, such as polyethylene or polyvinyl	Vigilon, Second Skin, Biofilm, Geliperm, Cutinova Gel, Elasto-Gel, Intrasite Gel, Span Gel, ClearSite	?
Calcium alginate	Composite of fibers from calcium alginate	Sorbsan Kaltostat	?
Foams	Hydrophillic or hydrophobic polyurethane or gel film	Cutinova Plus Ulcer Care, Lyofoam, Sythaderm Allevin, Epigard	+
Others			
Biobrane	Silicone rubber with nylon and porcine collagen bilaminate		?
N-Terface	Monofilament plastic		+
Cellophane wrap (contains 65% glycerin)	Cellulose with glycerin	Saran Wrap	+

Hydrocolloid dressings use a water-impermeable polyurethane outer covering that is separated from the wound by a hydrocolloid material, usually carboxymethyl cellulose. This hydrocolloid interacts with the wound exudate to form a gel that does not adhere to the wound surface; however, these dressings do adhere to normal skin. Within the gel are endogenous enzymes that autolytically débride the wound.[474,479,480]

Hydrogel dressings consist of two layers of polyethylene or polyvinyl alcohol with water suspended between the layers, or in the case of Elasto-Gel (Southwest Technologies, Inc., North Kansas City, Mo), a 65% glycerin suspension. These dressings are hydrophilic and capable of marked fluid absorption, so they are well suited for exudative wounds. Their primary disadvantage is that the lack of adhesion requires a secondary dressing for immobilization.

The *foam dressings* are completely nonadherent and very absorptive of wound exudate. As with the hydrogels, they require a secondary dressing.

The *alginate dressings* are also similar because they are very absorptive of exudate and require a secondary dressing. The dressing is easily removed with saline irrigation because it is soluble in solutions containing sodium ions.[481] Alginates have been used in the food and pharmaceutical industries since 1881 and are salts of alginic acid, derived from brown seaweeds. They are unique as dressings because of their action as hemostatic agents[482,483] and have not been shown to induce adverse tissue

	Transmits Moisture Vapor	Absorbs Fluids	Transparent	Adhesive Dressing Required	Secondary Dressing Required	Comments
	+	–	+	+	–	Fluid retention may be problem Difficult to handle Omniderm or Silon II better suited for exudative wounds
	–	±	–	+	–	Gel formed by dressing often purulent in appearance and acrid in odor If wound very exudative, gel will leak beyond dressing
	+	+	±	–	+	Capable of significant fluid absorption Require frequent dressing change
	?	++	–	–	+	Significant hemostatic properties Very high absorbency
	+	±	–	–	+	Similar to hydrogels Can become incorporated in wound if wound dries
	?	–	–	–	–	May delay reepithelialization Excessive fluid accumulation occurs
	+	±	–	–	+	Wick effect transfers fluids to outer membrane
	+	–	+	–	–	Oxygen transmission increases 1000-fold when material is wet

changes.[484] They may be ideal dressings for resurfacing, especially erbium laser therapy, in regard to the capillary oozing that occurs postoperatively.

Biobrane, N-Terface, and cellophane wrap have not been used as often in resurfacing procedures, although each has its advocates as well as its critics.

Studies of varying the time of application or removal of an occlusive dressing have shown that for optimal healing, dressings need to be applied within 2 hours after wounding and should be left in place for at least 24 hours.[485] Waiting 24 hours before application almost precludes the occlusive dressing's effect on wound healing, but it still may have benefit in pain reduction. Early removal of the dressing greatly reduces the occlusive effects, but not if 24 or 48 hours has passed.

Biooclusive dressings are beneficial during the first 3 to 5 days because they keep the skin cleaner of exudate and allow faster reepithelialization. Popular dressings include Vigilon (Bard Patient Care Division, Murray Hill, NJ), Second Skin (Spenco Medical Corp., Waco, Texas), Flexzan (Dow-Hickman Pharmaceuticals, Sugar Land, Texas), and Silon II (BioMed Sciences, Inc., Bethlehem, Pa) (Figure 7-33).

These dressings have the disadvantage of being difficult to keep in place and time-consuming to apply (except for Silon II, which is applied in seconds). They also may encourage the development of infection because of the combination of moisture, necrotic tissue, and occlusion. When used, they must be changed daily. Only those dressings such as Silon II that have slits or punctures allowing fluid to soak through the dressing should be left in place for more than 1 or 2 days without changing. In addition, Flexzan hides the wound surface and makes it difficult to diagnose a wound infection at its earliest manifestation without removing the bandage. Despite these factors, patients appear to progress to a more cosmetically acceptable point faster if one of these dressings is used for the initial 3 to 5 days.

Long-term healing does not appear to be influenced by these dressings, but an increased incidence of postoperative wound infections from the occlusive dressing seems to occur if oral antibiotics are not used.[240] The question of potentially increasing the risk of infection by the use of occlusive dressings is not easy to answer,

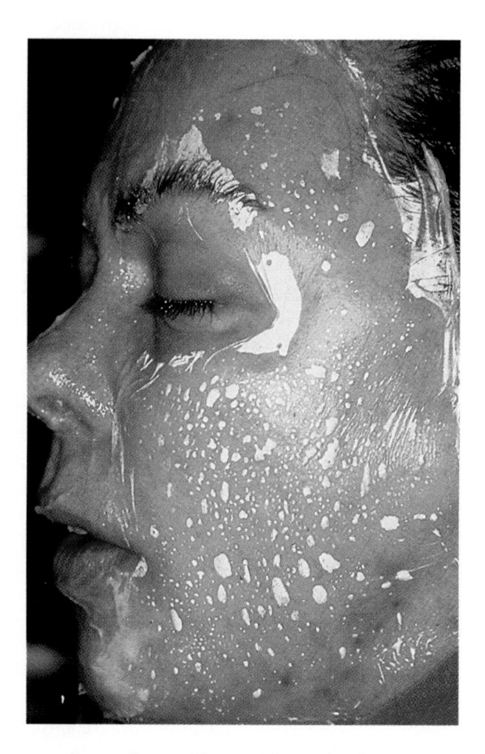

Figure 7-33 Silon II, a polyurethane film with multiple small slits, allows soaking directly through film and enhances wound healing during first 72 hours.

because petrolatum itself is occlusive, and the literature on the effects of an occlusive dressing on the bacterial population is contradictory. Application of an occlusive dressing to a contaminated wound clearly will worsen the situation. Some studies have shown that bacterial colonization under occlusion does not impair wound healing,[486-489] that wound fluid and exudate collecting under an occlusive dressing have bactericidal activity,[490,491] and that infection rates with occlusion are usually less than those with nonocclusive dressings.[474,491-494] However, a study comparing semiocclusive dressings exposed to open air showed not only an increased number of microorganisms, but also a shift toward gram-negative organisms.[486] Other investigators have shown a similar pattern on normal skin occluded with a plastic film.[489,495]

Pseudomonas aeruginosa favors a moist environment and readily colonizes burn wounds. A wound dressing that would provide the benefits of occlusion without encouraging the growth of *P. aeruginosa* in burn wounds might result in a more favorable prognosis for burn patients. Such a dressing would be beneficial in facial resurfacing as well.

A recent study evaluated three dressings regarding their ability to suppress *P. aeruginosa* inoculated on burn wounds of specific pathogen–free (SPF) pigs.[496] The three dressings evaluated were (1) a hydrogel containing 22% polyvinyl pyrrolidone, 18% propylene glycol, and 60% water (ClearSite, Conmed Corp.); (2) a hydrogel containing 65% glycerin, 17.5% water, and 17.5% polymeric matrix of acrylamide (Elasto-Gel); and (3) a hydrocolloid made of pectin and sodium carboxymethylcellulose (DuoDerm, Conva Tec). All the wounds were clinically infected. However, wounds covered with the hydrogel containing glycerin had a significantly lower number of *P. aeruginosa* than the other wounds at all points in time. An in vitro study also showed that the hydrogel with glycerin caused a significant reduction in *P. aeruginosa,* as well as in *Escherichia coli* and *S. aureus.* Glycerin has been reported to have an antimicrobial effect that is attributed to dehydration,[497] and a 10% solution of glycerin and ichthammol showed particular activity against *P. aeruginosa.*[498]

These results suggest that the hydrogel with glycerin may be advantageous in promoting wound healing while providing an environment that does not support bacterial proliferation; however, this has not been tried clinically. K-Y Jelly, which has 17% glycerin content, has often been found to be too irritating to use on freshly resurfaced skin. Whether the glycerin hydrogel would be less irritating is unknown at this time.

An increased susceptibility to gram-negative infections in resurfacing patients would reflect our clinical experience as well. If semiocclusive dressings are to be used postoperatively, most physicians now would advise that (1) antibiotic coverage should include gram-negative organisms, (2) dressings should be changed frequently if not daily, and (3) occlusve dressing should be used no more than 72 hours.

The next phase of wound healing lasts another 7 to 10 days. During this phase, no further weeping occurs and swelling has usually resolved. Maturation of the epithelium still requires a moist environment. Petrolatum may be used during this phase, but a lighter preparation is usually more comfortable. Theraplex emollient, Cetaphil moisturizer (Galderma Laboratories, Inc., Fort Worth, Texas), Norwegian Formula emulsion (Neutrogenia), and Curel (Bausch and Lomb, Inc., Rochester, New York) have been used during this phase. Biologic agents such as vitamin C, essential fatty acids, hyaluronic acid, aloe vera, and antioxidants may be incorporated into the moisturizer and may be beneficial in this phase. After the second week a lighter, high-moisture cream containing these biologic agents can be used and continued. Preoperative topical agents are restarted at 2 to 3 weeks postoperatively.

Close surveillance of patients during the postoperative period is important to provide emotional support and to detect abnormalities in the healing process at the earliest manifestation. Patients are seen at 2 to 3 days, 1 week later, and at 3 weeks, 6 weeks, 3 months, 6 months, and 1 year postoperatively.

COMPLICATIONS

As with all resurfacing procedures, the incidence of complications is related to both the depth of resurfacing and the patient's preexisting skin pigment type. Complications include infection, pigmentary changes, acne and milia, scarring, and ectropion. Swelling, erythema, petechiae, and itching are normal postoperative sequelae that may be more prominent in some patients.[378]

Postoperative Swelling

Postoperative swelling is generally mild to moderate, peaking on day 2 to 3 and most often resolving by day 5 to 7. At times, however, dramatic swelling may occur that is frightening and uncomfortable for the patient. Although we do not routinely use steroids in the postoperative course, in this situation of excessive swelling, IM Celestone (6-9 mg) or oral prednisone (40-60 mg daily for 3-5 days) may be valuable. Patients are also advised to soak their face frequently and to use ice packs or frozen peas as frequently as needed.

Erythema

Erythema occurs to some degree in all patients and reflects the increased blood flow and angiogenesis associated with dermal healing. The degree and persistence of erythema relate to the depth of resurfacing performed and the amount of nonspecific thermal injury produced, as well as to unidentified individual variables and possibly to preoperative and postoperative regimens. The regimens outlined previously appear to enhance wound healing and decrease erythema. In addition, the inflammatory reaction related to slough of thermal necrotic tissue may be a factor in prolonging erythema. Removal of this layer with the Er:YAG laser has been shown to be effective both in reducing erythema and infection and in enhancing the healing process and speeding its conclusion.

Itching

Itching is a common postoperative complaint, particularly during the second postoperative week. It can indicate infection, particularly candidiasis, but is then often accompanied by other signs, such as poor wound healing, beefy erythema in patches, and exudate. Contact dermatitis must be considered as well when pruritus occurs, particularly if any topical medications are being used. If these conditions are excluded, generally the itching will respond well to an antihistamine such as diphenhydramine (Benadryl, 10 or 25 mg) or loratadine (Claritin, 10 mg) or a topical steroid such as alclometasone dipropionate (Aclovate).

Infection

The combined incidence of bacterial, viral, and candidal infection has been found to be 4.7% in a multicenter study[499] and 4.3% in a retrospective study,[400] 12% in Burns' study,[362] 7.6% in our most recent study,[401] and 8.4% in the study of Waldorf et al.[206] Multiple organisms are typically found, and the microorganisms identified (*Staphylococcus* and *Pseudomonas* species) are similar to those found in burn injuries.[500-502]

The moist wound care and the layer of thermal necrosis provide an environment conducive to bacterial and candidal growth. The absence of the protective epidermal barrier further invites infection and allows dissemination of the infection across the surface of the treatment area. Biocclusive dressings further complicate the situation by trapping bacteria and increasing the incidence of infection.[400]

Infection should be suspected in the following situations:

1. Patient complains of persistent or new onset of pain.
2. Burning or intense itching is reported after day 2 or 3.
3. Patient has patchy, intense erythema, yellow exudate or crust, papules, pustules, or erosions.
4. "Reversal of healing" is seen; that is, previously reepithelialized areas become eroded.

Eighty percent of infections become symptomatic within 7 days, and pain is the most common complaint, reported by 50% of patients. However, as previously mentioned, the use of antibiotics may alter this pattern, and antibiotics used for 10 to 14 days may eliminate postoperative bacterial infections. A sensation of burning and itching is the second most common symptom, reported by a third of patients.

When an infection is suspected, direct smears and cultures for bacteria, yeast, and herpesvirus should be taken, because the physical findings of infection may be atypical, with the absence of the epithelium and presence of a necrotic layer and edema. Correct diagnosis requires proper identification of the infectious agent.

All patients should be given appropriate antiviral medication at surgery, because the laser resurfacing procedure may be a potent factor in herpetic reactivation.[503] Should this occur despite antiherpetic prophylaxis, it is best to switch from valacyclovir to famciclovir, or vice versa, and to increase the dosage.

When candidal infections are encountered, a 400-mg dose of fluconazole should be given and occlusive topical regimens discontinued.

Bacterial infections should be treated according to culture and sensitivity results. Serious consideration should be given to prophylactic use of ciprofloxacin (500 mg twice daily) starting the evening before surgery and continuing for 10 to 14 days postoperatively.

Acne and Milia

Many physicians report an unusually high incidence of milia formation after laser resurfacing as well as increased of exacerbation of acne. Although the use of petrolatum-based ointments may be an exacerbating factor in many patients, particularly those with a prior history of acne, the incidence of this complication appears to parallel the degree of thermal injury to the tissue. Thermal injury may lead to a shock effect on sebaceous glands, causing their disruption and dedifferentiation of adnexal structures and producing an aberrant re-formation of the canal.[504] Dermabrasion, by contrast, generally results in improvement in acne; some physicians believe this is an invariable consequence of dermabrasion, although degree of improvement may vary.

Treatment of acne and milia is that traditionally used for acne: minimize occlusive ointments, reinstitute tretinoin and AHAs, and administer systemic tetracycline or minocycline. Gentle acne surgery performed at 2- to 4-week intervals may be beneficial as well. Isotretinoin (Accutane) may be started if the acne fails to respond to more conservative measures.

Hyperpigmentation

Hyperpigmentation is generally related to the degree of natural pigmentation and occurs in 20% to 30% of those with Fitzpatrick type III skin and nearly 100% of patients with type IV skin if treatment is performed without preoperative preparation.[208] Almost all episodes will resolve within 2 to 4 months if aggressively treated. Strict sun avoidance is a fundamental aspect of treatment and is enhanced by daily use of full-spectrum sunscreens containing titanium dioxide or Parsol 1789. Hydroquinone is cytotoxic to melanocytes and is the mainstay of treatment. Tretinoin promotes melanosome transfer and keratinocyte turnover and is almost always beneficial as well. Azelaic acid, kojic acid, and glucosamine inhibit tyrosinase and pigment synthesis and may be added to the regimen when patients are responding slowly. Topical vitamins C and E function as free-radical scavengers and help prevent further stimulation of melanocytes by UV radiation. Pretreatment with these agents will minimize the occurrence of hyperpigmentation, as well as its degree of severity and its favorable response to therapy.

Hypopigmentation

Hypopigmentation is a delayed phenomenon, generally not apparent for 6 to 12 months. True hypopigmentation must be differentiated from *pseudohypopigmentation,* a situation in which the resurfaced area has normal pigmentation reflective of non-sun-exposed skin, but contrasts distinctively with the more darkly pigmented sun-damaged skin. *True hypopigmentation* reflects a diminished melanocyte content of the skin and correlates with both the depth of resurfacing and the degree of thermal injury. These patients generally have long-lasting erythema, often have had problems with milia and acne as well, and may have areas of scarring. These patients typically have been treated with free-hand techniques allowing pulse stacking or with CPG patterns having greater than 50% overlap. These patients often have received more than three laser passes as well.

Treatment of hypopigmentation has been unrewarding, including the use of PUVA. When segmental hypopigmentation or pseudohypopigmentation is present, resurfacing the remainder of the face will blend the area and decrease its visibility (Figure 7-29). An incidence of about 20% has been reported for hypopigmentation, but this must be examined carefully and pseudohypopigmentation separated as a different phenomenon, because it may not be preventable. In a review of 104 patients 1 to 4 years postoperatively, we found hypopigmentation in 19.2% (20 of 104). Pseudohypopigmentation was present in 65% of these patients and true hypopigmentation in 35%. Hypopigmentation was classified as mild in 85% of these patients. When examined more closely, these 20 patients with hypopigmentation were also the patients having the worst photodamage preoperatively, those with the most significant clinical improvement, and those who were most pleased with their results. Pseudohypopigmentation should be viewed as a *consequence* of resurfacing in significantly photodamaged skin rather than a complication. However, patients should be forewarned of this aspect of the procedure.

Petechiae

Although of almost no long-term significance, the appearance of small petechiae is often a source of much concern to the patient. They appear just as reepithelialization is complete, conflicting with the patient's desire to return to public view. Small subepithelial hemorrhages from the immature basement membrane and undeveloped rete appear to be the cause. These factors render the skin more fragile and easily damaged with minor trauma from rubbing or scratching. Petechiae may continue for several weeks after the procedure but clear quickly without treatment.

Scarring

Erythematous and hypertrophic scars often result from excessive depth of tissue injury. This is usually caused by excess tissue heating and residual thermal damage well beyond the depth of tissue vaporized by the laser. Incorrect "off" times, high scanner densities (greater than 40%), and failure to keep the handpiece moving during resurfacing are some of the treatment methods that lead to inadvertent overlap or "stacking" of pulses, with the resultant accumulation of heat and residual thermal damage.

Scarring is also seen more frequently in patients who develop a postoperative infection, particularly in those who have had multiple prior surgical procedures, altering the anatomy of the region. In addition, patients treated more aggressively, resulting in a thicker layer of thermal necrosis, may be more prone to infection. Careful preoperative history taking to rule out predisposing factors and immediate treatment of postoperative infections are mandatory.

Scarring is much more frequently seen in treatment of nonfacial areas, such as the neck. Decreased adnexal structures, thinner dermis, and increased tissue tension and traction secondary to motion are predisposing factors. In a trial of 10 patients receiving a single laser pass of 300 mJ with CPG density of 6, we encountered scarring of the lower one third of the neck in three patients and patchy hypopigmentation in four patients (Figure 7-34).

The earliest evidence for the development of a scar is usually erythema and pruritus. At this point the affected area should be cultured to rule out infection, and

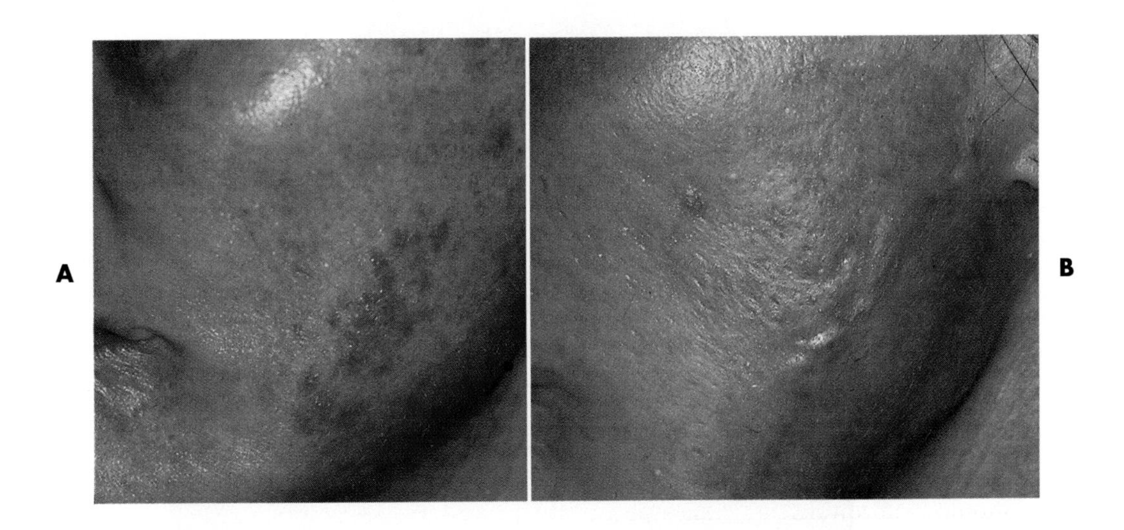

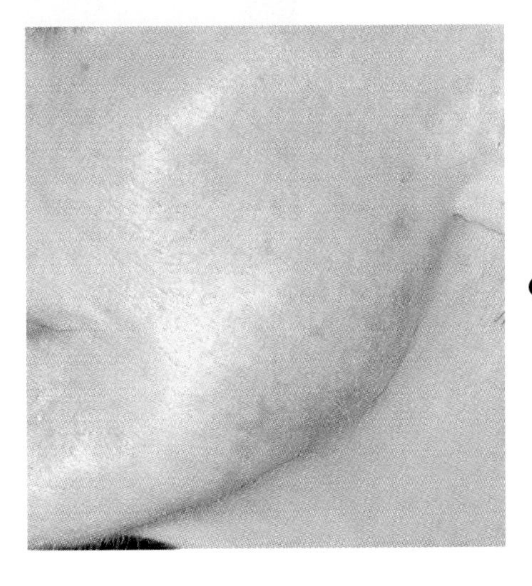

Figure 7-34 **A,** *Pseudomonas* infection developed on day 8 after single-pass laser resurfacing, resulting in nonhealing erosions on lower cheek. **B,** Although this area initially healed very well, at 4 months an obvious hypertrophic scar was developing, corresponding to site of infection. **C,** Intensive treatment with intralesional 5-fluorouracil (45 mg/ml) and triamcinolone (Kenalog, 1 mg/ml) followed by pulsed dye laser (6 J/cm^2) resulted in scar resolution after approximately 1 year.

A

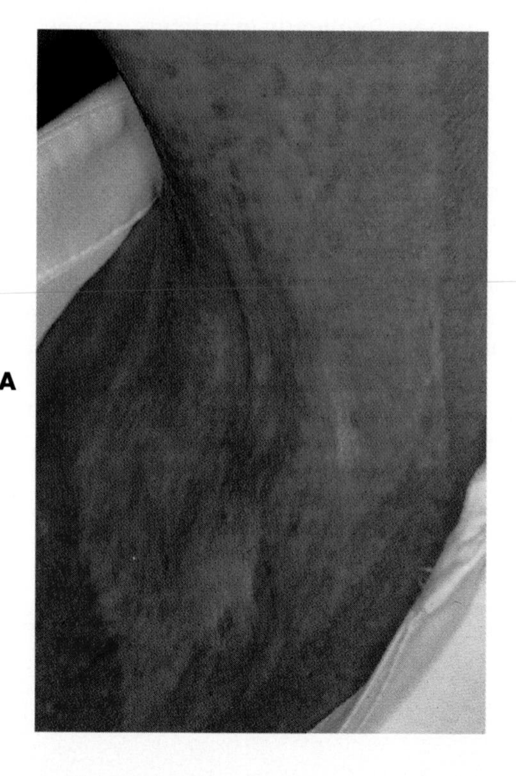

B

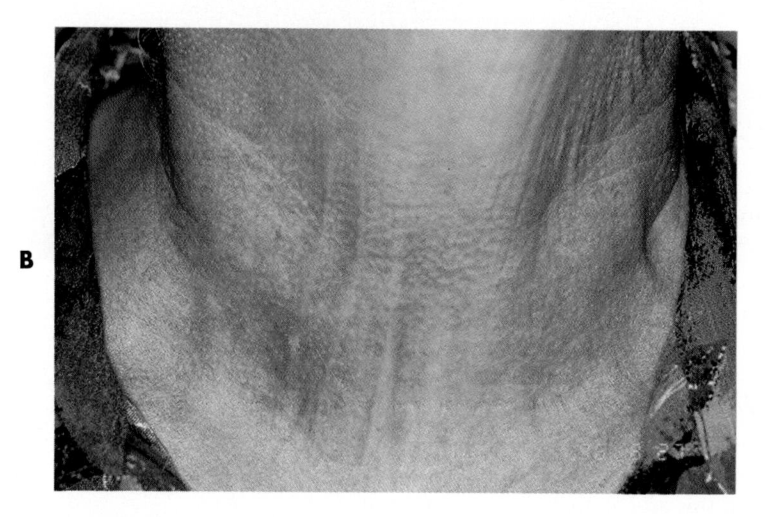

Figure 7-35 **A,** Treatment of the neck in same manner as the face may result in severe scarring. **B,** Treatment goals must be much more conservative, but even a single pass with the same laser parameters used for the face may result in scarring of the lower neck.

topical high-potency corticosteroids should be applied two or three times daily. If the affected area begins to thicken, intralesional injection of triamcinolone (10 mg/ml) with 5-fluorouracil (50 mg/ml) in a 1:9 dilution (1-mg triamcinolone with 45-mg 5-fluorouracil) should begin every 2 to 3 days. Topical silicone dressings should also be applied. If further progression occurs, we advise using the 585-nm flashlamp pumped pulse dye laser (FLPDL) or other vascular lasers or intense pulsed light (PhotoDerm VL) every 4 weeks. With these techniques, permanent scarring has been avoided (Figure 7-35).

Ectropion

Contraction of previously scarred tissue of the lower eyelid leads to excessive tightening and exposure of the conjunctiva. This avoidable complication usually occurs in patients who have undergone resurfacing after a lower-lid blepharoplasty without stabilizing the lateral canthal tendon. It may also occur if laser resurfacing is performed too aggressively in this region without attention to the laser-tissue interaction.

To minimize the occurrence of ectropion, we recommend that the patient's skin elastic recoil be tested, the so-called snap test, with close observation for loose tissue folds and the effect on the lid margin when tightened. If the lid margin moves easily, close observation during the procedure is essential to avoid excessive tightening of the lid. In addition, laser density should not exceed 20% to 30% in this region to limit nonspecific thermal damage of dermal tissue, and only one or two passes should be performed with careful attention to the tightening effect. The cheeks should be treated before the periorbital area so that the additive tightening effects of this area are known before periorbital resurfacing. Scleral show was found in 3% of patients less than 4 months postoperatively and in 2% more than 4 months postoperatively in a report of 1000 procedures.[505] Ectropion occurred in 0.3% of patients in this series.

Synechiae

Synechiae are adhesions that occur when two adjacent areas of deepithelialized skin are in contact with each other in a fold and a bridge of epithelium develops over the top of the fold. This occurs primarily on the lower eyelid and has the appearance of an unusual crease or faint white line 1 to 2 weeks postoperatively. Treatment consists of cutting the epidermal bridge with a fine-tipped scissors, lancet, or scalpel. The patient then must carefully roll a moist cotton-tipped applicator over the area frequently to avoid recurrence. Synechiae almost always resolve without problems.[505]

NEW RESURFACING LASERS

It is often stated that one of the main limitations of CO_2 laser resurfacing is the extensive erythema that persists for 1 to 3 months. Because of this perceived disadvantage, manufacturers have marketed lasers that may be capable of resurfacing with greater ease and more superficially and with delivery of less heat to the treated tissue.

TruPulse Laser

Based on technology developed at the Los Alamos National Physics Laboratory, a high-peak-power, short-pulse CO_2 laser has been developed by Tissue Technologies and approved by the U.S. Food and Drug Administration (FDA) for skin ablation.

This laser, called the TruPulse, produces high-peak-power pulses that can achieve fluences greater than 5 J/cm^2 (the ablation threshold of human skin) at variable pulse durations, from 30 μsec to 1 msec. By using shorter pulse durations than the UltraPulse CO_2 laser, in the range of 60 μsec per pulse, this device removes less tissue per pass (on the order of 30 μm). Therefore the TruPulse laser requires more passes to ablate significantly photodamaged skin effectively, but also leaves less residual thermal damage per pass (on the order of 15-30 μm). Early claims suggest that erythema after CO_2 laser resurfacing with the TruPulse is substantially less than with the other CO_2 lasers. However, evidence also suggests that collagen tightening is decreased as well, relative to the diminished heating of tissue, and that to achieve comparable clinical results, deeper resurfacing is necessary, resulting in prolonged erythema. In other words, equal results may require a similar period of erythema.

Erbium:YAG Laser

Other laser wavelengths have the capacity to resurface skin. The erbium:yttrium-aluminum-garnet (Er:YAG) laser produces light in the near-infrared (IR) portion of the electromagnetic spectrum at 2.94 μm. This wavelength was discovered by Soviet researchers in 1975,[506] and its clinical use developed in Europe.[507-512] The broad water-absorption band extends from just under 2 μm to beyond 10 μm, ensuring superficial absorption of near-IR light. The Q-switched Er:YAG laser ablates approximately 15 to 20 μm of skin and leaves such a thin layer of thermal damage (5 μm) that it is not hemostatic. The Er:YAG laser has been investigated using a Q-switched pulse of 90 μsec, but pulse-to-pulse instability and a low-intensity tail of a gaussian beam have made this beam profile undesirable. Instead, the laser is used in its normal-spiking mode, emitting a macropulse of approximately 250 μsec, made up by a train of 1-μsec micropulses with pulse-to-pulse stability of $\pm 2\%$.[513] The Er:YAG laser was first studied in this mode to determine whether it could be an effective resurfacing device.

Several companies now produce erbium lasers (Candela, Con-Bio, ESC, Coherent, and others). These lasers are purely ablative, causing minimal collagen tightening. Because of the high coefficient for absorption of water, very little tissue water is necessary for tissue reaction, allowing deep or very superficial vaporization, but both being done with minimal thermal injury. This may result in some unique clinical benefits, such as treatment of scars; treatment of the neck, chest, hands, and arms[514]; and removal of superficial photodamage and wrinkling with faster healing and decreased erythema.[515]

When the coefficient of absorption for water is compared directly, that for the CO_2 laser (10.6 μm) is approximately 790 μm^{-1}, whereas the erbium laser peak at 2.94 μm is approximately 13,000 μm^{-1}, more than 16 times greater than that of the CO_2 laser (Figure 7-36). This results in its energy being absorbed much more readily in a thinner layer of tissue than with the CO_2 laser. In fact, calculations of the absorption coefficient, assuming tissue to be 70% water, show this energy to be absorbed in about 1 μm of tissue.[507,509,513-519] This results in efficient tissue ablation with very little scattering of the beam and minimal residual thermal damage. However, actual clinical and experimental data reveal deeper tissue penetration than this calculated optical penetration.[519]

The ablation threshold for the Er:YAG laser is about 1.5 J/cm^2 [509,513,520] and the ablation efficiency about 2 to 3 μm/pulse/J/cm^2 up to about 10 J/cm^2.[509,513,516,518] However, ablation rates per pulse of 16 μm,[509] 30 μm,[517] and 400 μm (at 80 J/cm^2)[513] have been reported, which seem inconsistent with the reported penetration depth of the Er:YAG laser of about 1 μm.

This deeper ablation process occurs because ablation at 2.94 μm is an explosive process caused by rapid heating, vaporization, and consequent high-pressure expansion of irradiated tissue.[513,519] Explosive particle ejection occurs when a gradient exists

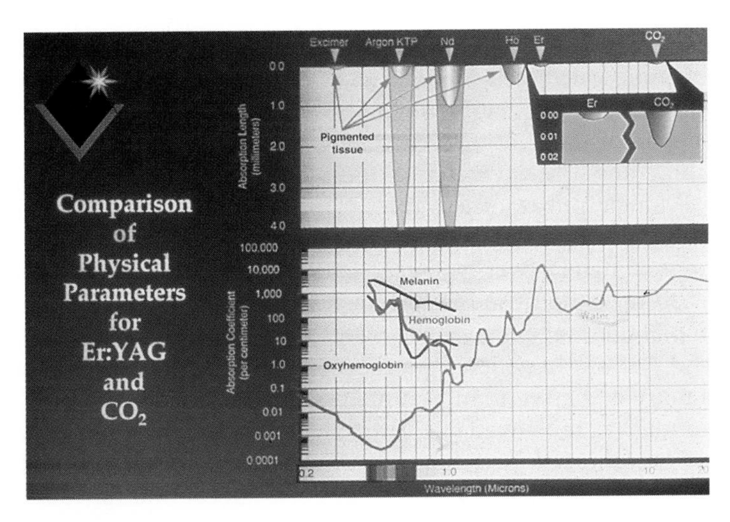

Figure 7-36 Erbium:YAG laser wavelength of 2.94 μm is absorbed 16 times more readily than that of CO_2 laser.

between the atmospheric pressure of the environment and pressure within tissue. When tissue water is evaporated and prevented from escaping from tissue fast enough, tissue pressures may exceed atmospheric pressures when temperatures exceed 100° C. Because the tissue surface is cooled by expansion of the vapor, temperature and pressure may then be higher in a subsurface layer. The steam pressure of water increases rapidly with increasing temperature. Indeed, these high-temperature, high-pressure gases forming at the absorption site are thought to result in explosive tissue removal.[513,519] High-speed photography has shown ablated material to leave the surface at supersonic velocities (10^3 m/sec).[521]

The ablation of tissue during the pulse of the Er:YAG laser is a dynamic process during which material heated at the beginning of the pulse is removed during the pulse, clearing a path for radiation to be deposited deeper in tissue during the same pulse.[513] High-speed photography has shown that tissue removal begins within 200 μsec after the beginning of the pulse.[522] The explosive ejection of this ablated material removes it from the beam pathway. Furthermore, water vaporized by the pulse has a much lower coefficient of absorption than does liquid water and therefore does not interfere with the beam, because it is essentially transparent.[513,519]

Interestingly, lower fluences (less than 10 J/cm^2) of a thermal energy analyzer (TEA) CO_2 laser using 2-μsec pulses result in the same ablation efficiency, supporting this instantaneous vaporization model.[513]

This in-depth absorption explains the tearing of tissue seen in vascular tissue, the large ablation depths per pulse, and the zones of residual thermal damage that increase greatly at high fluences.[513,519]

Increasing pulse numbers applied to one spot results in decreasing the ablation efficiency and increasing the zone of thermal necrosis. Using 14 J/cm^2 and a 1-Hz repetition rate resulted in a decrease of the ablation rate from 30 to 22 μm when the pulse numbers increased from 20 to 120.[518] These effects are avoided clinically by moving the beam over the ablation area, and in fact, tissue necrosis of less than 50 μm is seen even with high fluences.[509,519] Thermal necrosis zones not exceeding 30 to 50 μm have been confirmed both in vitro and in vivo.[509,510,517-520]

The absence of tissue coagulation, however, results in bleeding as the vessels of the superficial dermal plexus are severed. This may limit the depth of ablation that is achievable.[510,518,520]

Clinical use of high-fluence, small-diameter beams is undesirable, because it may result in an irregular surface because of the deep intantaneous ablation that results.

This energy is delivered with a pulse duration that is far below the 1-msec thermal relaxation time calculated for that layer of human skin heated by the pulsed CO_2 laser, with the pulse generally 250 to 350 μsec. However, because of the short penetration depth of the 2.94-μm wavelength, the laser-heated layer of tissue is only 1-μm thick and this layer has a thermal relaxation time of approximately 1 μsec.[231,519,522] Single pulses of less than 1-μsec duration are needed to minimize thermal diffusion during the laser pulse. In the normal-spiking mode, the Er:YAG laser emits approximately twenty 1-μsec micropulses in a macropulse burst of approximately 200 μsec. Because of efficient tissue vaporization and interpulse cooling time, minimal thermal damage occurs. Each micropulse can ablate tissue and act independently,[519,521] but in general the thermal damage from normal-spiking-mode irradiation is more extensive than that of Q-switched irradiation.

Most erbium lasers now available can deliver 1 to 2 J per pulse, so very high irradiances may be achieved, particularly with a focused beam. Although physicians and manufacturers typically report results as pulse energy and spot size, it would be much more meaningful and allow easier comparison if treatment parameters were discussed in fluence (J/cm^2) (Table 7-9). No shock-wave effect occurs in tissue, but clinically a pressure-wave effect seems to occur relative to the explosive vaporization that results when delivering such large amounts of energy to such a thin layer of tissue so rapidly. This is evidenced by significant intraoperative periorbital edema when treating the eyelids in virtually all patients and a high rate of recurrence of hypertrophic scars ablated by the erbium laser. These two observations are in contrast to what is seen with the CO_2 laser in the same circumstances.

The erbium laser therefore can be viewed as essentially a pure vaporizational or ablative laser, with insignificant thermal damage and minimal collagen shrinkage occurring in tandem.

The occurrence of prolonged healing, prolonged erythema, and even scarring secondary to the residual thermal damage seen with the CO_2 laser has resulted in many physicians looking for an alternative resurfacing modality that does not result in thermal injury to the tissue. This could potentially be more useful in treatment of early photodamage of the face and photodamage of the neck, chest, hands, and arms (Figure 7-37).

This has resulted in a new wave of enthusiasm for resurfacing, specifically with the Er:YAG laser. However, because of the newness of the technology and its promotion by eager physicians and laser manufacturers, a number of myths regarding the Er:YAG laser have been generated. These myths hold some element of truth but are based on generalization of those elements. These Er:YAG myths are as follows:

1. *The Er:YAG laser is painless and requires no anesthesia.* The Er:YAG laser can be used to remove the epidermis painlessly, because no nerve endings exist in the epidermis and

Table 7-9
Er:YAG laser fluences (J/cm^2)

Spot Size (mm)	Pulse Energy (J)					
	0.5	1.0	1.2	1.7	2.0	3.0
0.2	1592.4	3184.7	3821.7	5414.0	6369.4	9554.1
0.5	254.8	509.6	611.5	866.2	1019.1	1528.7
1	63.7	127.4	152.9	216.6	254.8	382.2
2	15.9	31.8	38.2	54.1	63.7	95.5
3	7.1	14.2	17.0	24.1	28.3	42.5
4	4.0	8.0	9.6	13.5	15.9	23.9
5	2.5	5.1	6.1	8.7	10.2	15.3
6	1.8	3.5	4.2	6.0	7.1	10.6

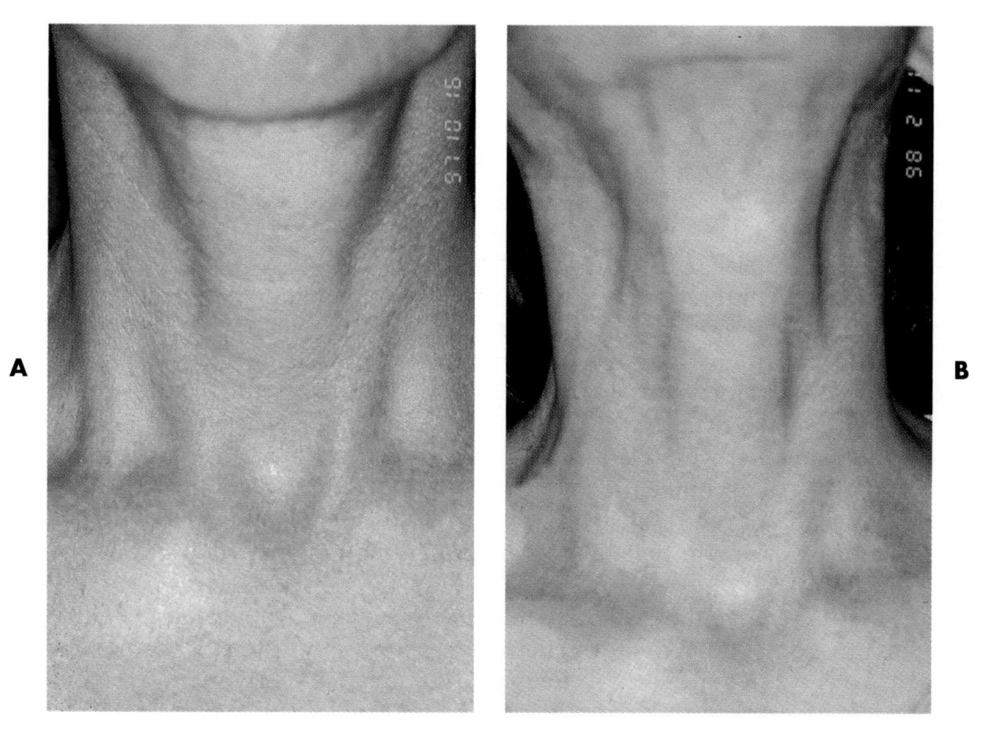

Figure 7-37 Treatment of neck using erbium laser allows removal of photodamaged epidermis without dermal injury. Improvement of skin texture and blending of color are reasonable goals. Improvement of 40% to 50% has been observed. **A,** Before treatment. **B,** Four months postoperatively.

insufficient heat is generated to stimulate the papillary dermal nerves. However, once the dermis is reached with a second pass of the laser, pain occurs just as readily as with any laser.

2. *Healing is faster with the Er:YAG laser, and redness (erythema) is minimal or less prolonged.* The Er:YAG laser does vaporize a thinner layer of tissue than the CO_2 laser and with less residual thermal injury to tissue, but the healing time correlates with the total depth of resurfacing, not the depth per pass. Equal results require equal depths of treatment. Ablation of deep lines with the Er:YAG laser still requires treatment into the dermis, with a consequently longer healing time. Rapid healing with minimal erythema can be achieved only with the most superficial treatment. When compared directly with CO_2 laser resurfacing, the total resurfacing depth of the CO_2 laser (ablation plus thermal necrosis and thermal injury) should be compared with that of the erbium laser, which is a difficult task to accomplish.
3. *Side effects are reduced with the Er:YAG laser, resulting in safer treatment.* Side effects such as hypopigmentation, scarring, erythema, and slow healing are generally depth related and therefore are reduced with more superficial treatment. Therefore, if the Er:YAG laser is used in a more superficial manner, the incidence of complications would be expected to be diminished as well. However, the same statement may be made regarding CO_2 laser resurfacing.

Surgical Technique

The depth of ablation is a function of the pulse energy and spot size or fluence. With the same pulse energy, a smaller spot size results in a higher fluence and therefore greater depth of vaporization. However, a smaller spot size also results in a tendency to create holes and an uneven texture. Also, the repetition rate and the pulse energy are inversely related, so a high pulse energy limits the repetition rate, at least within the limits of a 20-W laser. Virtually all systems that are currently available have an upper-limit repetition rate of 10 to 20 Hz, which limits the value of a pulse-scanning system, because these repetition rates can be manipulated by hand accurately by experienced laser surgeons.

Most often a spot size of 3 to 5 mm is used, with a pulse energy of 1 to 2 J (generally the maximum available). If a collimated beam is available, it is generally preferable at this stage. A repetition rate that can be easily handled is chosen (5-10 Hz), and spots are placed with 10% to 30% overlap.

Generally, two or three passes of the Er:YAG laser are required to remove the epidermis. It is much more difficult to ascertain when the epidermis is completely removed with the erbium laser compared with the CO_2 laser, because the epidermis does not separate with a subepidermal vesicle as it does with the CO_2 laser.

To determine the depth of vaporization into the skin, it is best to cover the skin in an orderly manner with relatively uniform passes rather than to treat with a random airbrush-type technique. This type of technique must be used cautiously because it leads to uneven results with much greater potential of inadvertent, deeper vaporization. Working in repetitive single passes allows better control and knowledge of depth.

It is best to remove the epidermis completely over the whole area to be treated and then to assess the dermal irregularities. Almost any patient being treated for photodamage will require some degree of dermal ablation, in addition to removal of the epidermis, because the textural irregularities and wrinkling originate in this layer. One to three passes are done in an even manner, just as was done with epidermal removal, with each pass ablating an additional 15 to 30 μm of tissue. At this point, dermal irregularities may be removed in a tissue-sculpting mode. This is most easily accomplished with a focused handpiece having a focal spot size of 1 to 2 mm. The distance between the tissue and the handpiece will then determine the fluence delivered, and the handpiece may be moved closer to or farther from the tissue depending on the amount of tissue ablation desired. This is best done holding the handpiece at an acute angle to tissue in a manner such that tissue elevations above the desired plane are preferentially irradiated, thereby decreasing the risk of cutting holes or troughs in the tissue (Figure 7-38).

Treatment using these techniques will result in maximal smoothing of tissue with minimal residual thermal damage. However, a second consequence of minimal thermal damage is that blood vessels are not cauterized, and therefore bleeding is encountered. Generally, the first dermal pass may result in scattered pinpoint bleeding at most

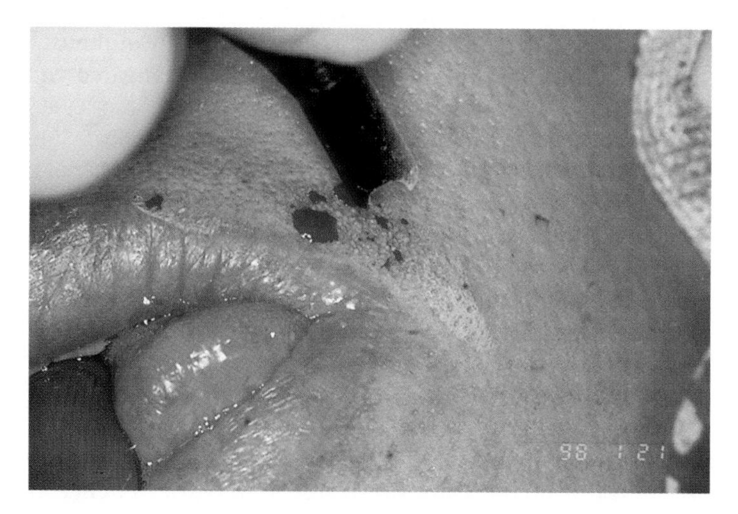

Figure 7-38 Tissue sculpting can be accomplished with the erbium laser, holding the beam at an acute angle to encounter higher tissue points selectively.

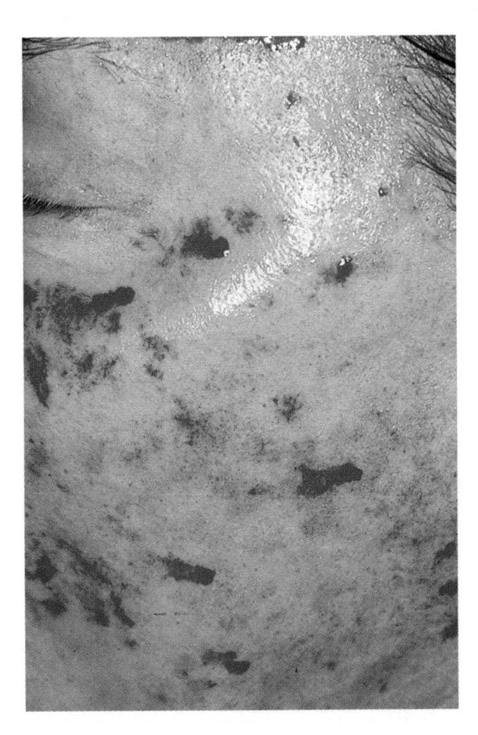

Figure 7-39 Because the erbium laser does not leave enough residual thermal necrosis to cauterize dermal vessels, bleeding will be encountered. Pinpoint bleeding is first seen in upper papillary dermis and becomes more significant as upper reticular dermis is reached.

as small dermal capillaries are encountered in the papillary dermis (Figure 7-39). After an additional one to three passes, larger vessels are reached, which results in more significant bleeding requiring application of pressure. Bleeding that is brisk enough to interfere with treatment is usually encountered only with rhinophyma.

Although many physicians using the Er:YAG laser do not wipe away the fine tissue debris on the surface of treated skin between passes, using dry to damp gauze for this purpose is beneficial. By wiping this fine layer away, the laser has direct access to tissue to be treated, and the physician can more easily and more accurately visualize the anatomic location of the plane being treated. Wiping is particularly useful when performing epidermal passes, because it allows better identification of epidermis and dermis. Fragments of residual epidermis or lesional tissue that remain on the surface may be wiped cleanly away, avoiding the need to ablate these spots of tissue and providing a more even plane of tissue to be treated on the next pass.

COMBINATION LASER TREATMENT

Both the CO_2 laser and the Er:YAG laser have unique qualities that can be exploited during resurfacing. The CO_2 laser is unique in the following ways:

1. Hemostasis is achieved.
2. A plateau of ablation is reached, limiting resurfacing depth if proper treatment protocols are followed.
3. Collagen (skin) tightening occurs as a heat-related phenomenon, resulting in correction of loose tissue and atrophic scars.
4. The first pass causes an epidermal/dermal split that allows easy and complete removal of the epidermis with a single pass.

The Er:YAG laser is unique in the following ways:

1. Minimal residual thermal damage or tissue heating occurs.
2. This pure-ablation laser continues to ablate with each pass and does not reach an ablation plateau with depth.
3. Only minimal tissue water is required for laser-tissue interaction.

The most successful use of lasers for resurfacing would utilize each laser to take advantage of its unique benefit and to eliminate the disadvantages of each as much as possible. Accordingly, the following protocols are followed for early photodamage and for moderate to advanced photodamage.

Early Photodamage and Superficial Scars

When treating early photodamage or when patients desire a more superficial treatment allowing early return to work and as little healing time as possible (Figure 7-40), the laser surgeon performs the following steps:

1. The epidermis is removed with a single pass of the CO_2 laser, usually with a density overlap of 20% to 30%. This can be accomplished very efficiently with the CO_2 laser, and biopsy studies have shown 0 to 10 μm of residual thermal necrosis with this single pass. If only epidermal removal is desirable, treatment is completed by using the Er:YAG laser to clean up any epidermal remnants and to feather the periphery. If dermal treatment of acne scars or photodamage is required, the areas of treatment are assessed with consideration of step 2.

2a. The CO_2 laser may be used with either the 3-mm spot or the CPG in small areas that will benefit from collagen tightening, such as the lower eyelids or medial cheeks and areas of atrophic acne scarring.

2b. The Er:YAG laser may be used uniformily in one or two passes to remove superficial photodamage and fine wrinkles and to feather the periphery.

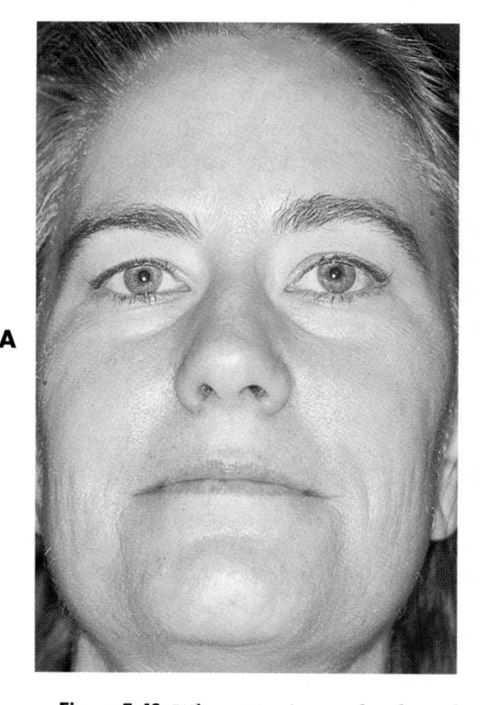

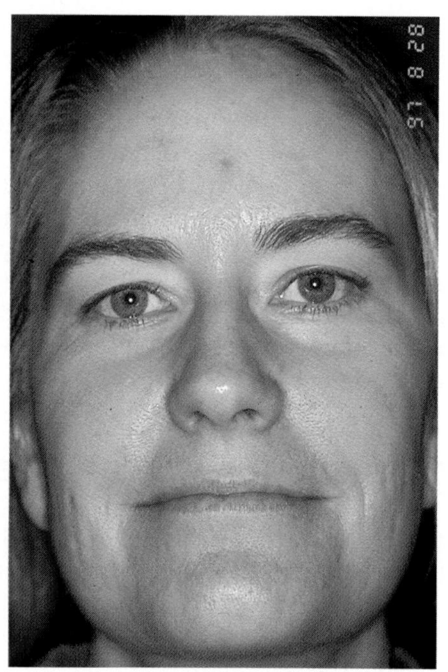

Figure 7-40 When treating early photodamage **(A)**, especially if patient desires to return to work with as little healing time as possible, epidermis is removed with CO_2 laser and superficial dermal resurfacing performed with erbium laser **(B)**. Although moderate improvement is seen, tissue tightening of cheeks and removal of deeper lines are not accomplished.

Significant Photodamage and Scars

When treating patients desiring the maximal improvement in a single treatment and having significant photodamage or acne scarring, the laser surgeon performs the following steps:

1. The epidermis is removed with a single pass of the CO_2 laser, usually with a density overlap of 30%.
2. A second pass of the CO_2 laser is done uniformly across the entire face, usually with a density overlap of 20% to 30%.
3. A third pass of the CO_2 laser is done in areas still having visible photodamage or scarring, generally the glabella and nose, middle lower forehead, middle to lateral cheeks and upper lip, and lateral chin areas, usually with a density overlap of 20% to 30%.
4. The 3-mm spot of the CO_2 laser is used to vaporize or induce thermal necrosis in areas of distinct photodamage or selectively to tighten loose photodamaged tissue, such as the eyelids, lateral cheeks, and atrophic scars. When used to induce thermal necrosis, the handpiece is moved slowly across the shoulder of a deep wrinkle line, the sharp edges of a scar crater, along the elevated portions of a linear scar, or over any dermal or epidermal growth, such as rhinophyma, syringoma, or seborrheic keratosis. The intent is to cause some superficial brownish char that will subsequently be ablated with the erbium laser.
5. The Er:YAG laser is used in a uniform manner, as in step 2b for early photodamage, removing the superficial portion of the 50 to 70 μm of residual thermal damage left by the CO_2 laser, thereby enhancing the reepithelialization process. This requires two passes at 1.7 J/4-mm pulse.
6. The Er:YAG laser is used with a small, focused spot size to sculpt tissue previously treated with the 3-mm CO_2 spot to smooth the tissue as uniformly as possible by ablating the necrotic tissue.
7. The periphery is feathered with the Er:YAG laser using a defocused energy of 1.0 to 1.7 J/5- to 8-mm-diameter spot.

This treatment protocol maximizes the benefit that can be achieved with each laser (Figure 7-41). Further combination therapy can be performed in the same

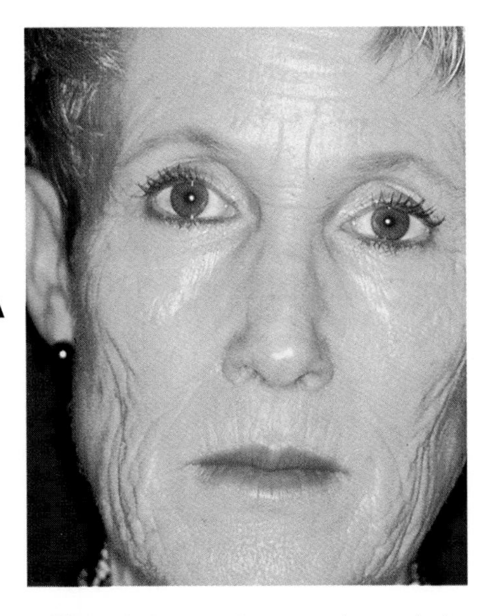
A

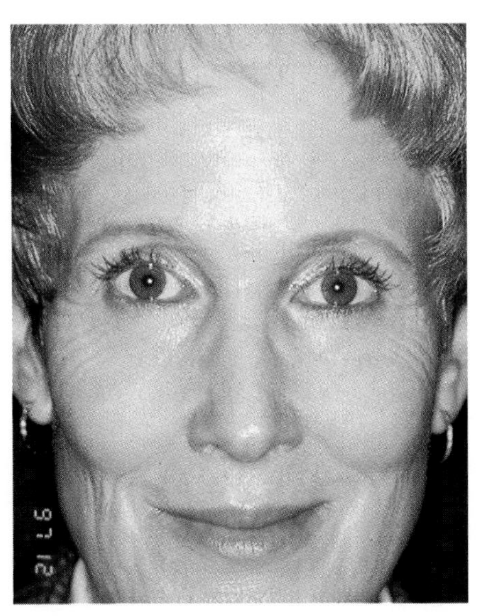
B

Figure 7-41 **A,** With more advanced photodamage, full treatment with CO_2 laser is performed (2-3 passes), then erbium laser is used to remove layer of thermal necrosis and selectively sculpt tissue. **B,** This technique reduces residual erythema, quickens healing, and results in enhanced clinical results, as seen 2 months postoperatively. CO_2 laser provides tissue tightening periorbitally and on cheeks, while erbium laser sculpts deep lines of upper lip, glabella, and forehead.

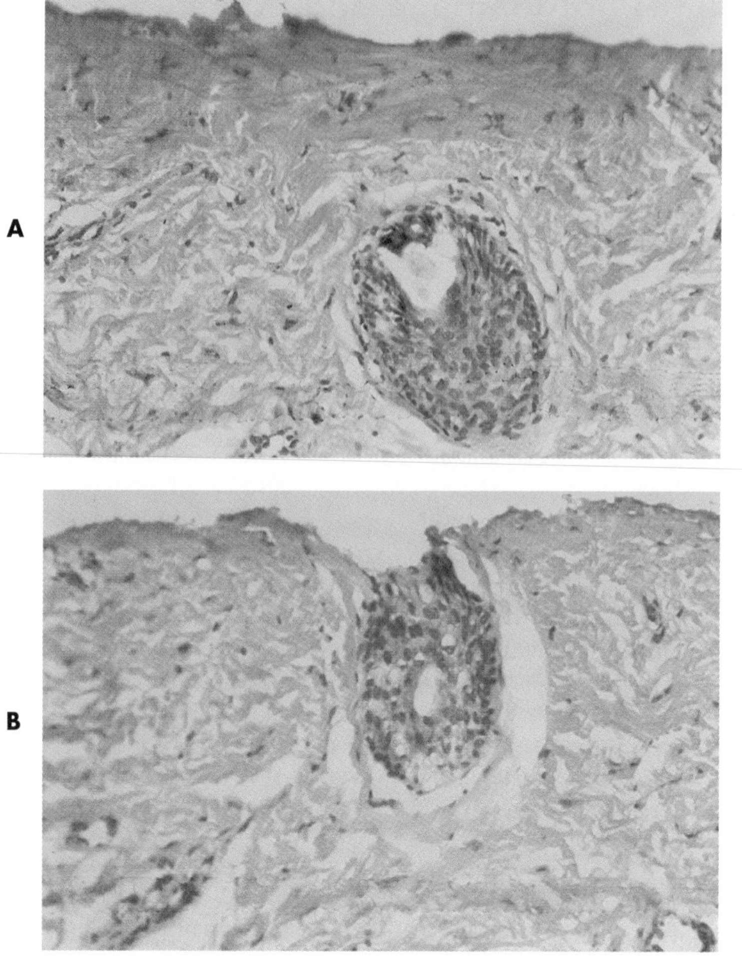

Figure 7-42 **A,** Two passes of CO_2 laser at 7 J/cm^2 leaves approximately 70 μm of residual thermal necrosis. **B,** Two passes of erbium laser at 10 J/cm^2 results in removal of approximately 50 μm of this necrotic tissue, resulting in faster wound healing.

treatment session. The 585-nm pulsed dye laser can be used to treat telangiectasias often found on the cheeks and nasal alae. One of the Q-switched lasers (neodymium:YAG, ruby, or alexandrite) can be used to remove pigmented brown shadows of the lower eyelids or extensions of seborrheic keratoses, lentigines, and other pigmented lesions in rete pegs into the dermis. Treatment of vascular lesions is usually performed before use of the resurfacing lasers, and the Q-switched lasers are best used immediately after resurfacing.

In one study, 10 patients had half their faces treated with two passes of the UltraPulse CO_2 laser and the other half treated with two passes of the UltraPulse laser plus two passes with the erbium laser to remove the residual thermal necrosis (Figure 7-42). Faster healing with less erythema was noted on the side with additional erbium laser treatment. Biopsy studies at 2 to 3 days, 1 week, and 4 to 8 weeks have shown that thermal necrosis is greatly reduced by adding the erbium laser treatment, speeding healing by 2 to 3 days without compromising new collagen production. In addition, inflammation is reduced at 1 week, and angiogenesis is relatively decreased at 1 to 8 weeks, reflecting the decreased erythema seen clinically (Figure 7-43). Necrotic tissue directly disregulates wound healing, induces proteases and inflammation, and is a major factor in all complications and adverse sequelae seen with resurfacing, including infection, scarring, and persistent erythema. Removal of this layer is advantageous in inducing enhanced healing and better clinical results.

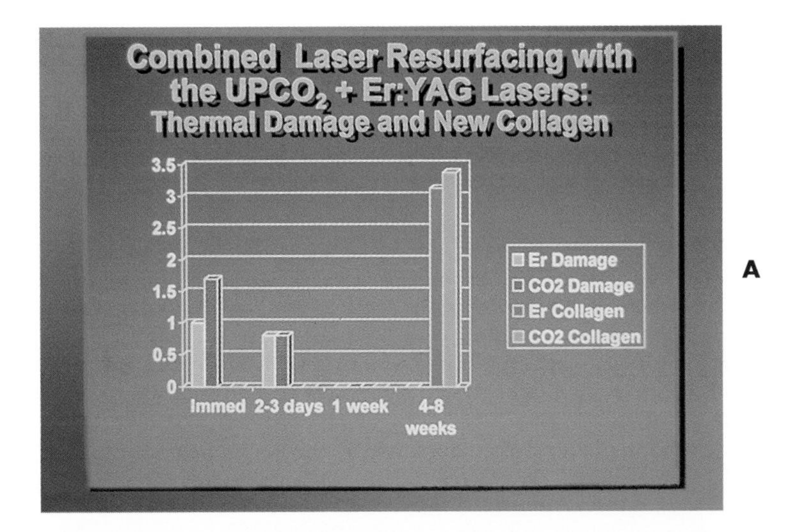

A

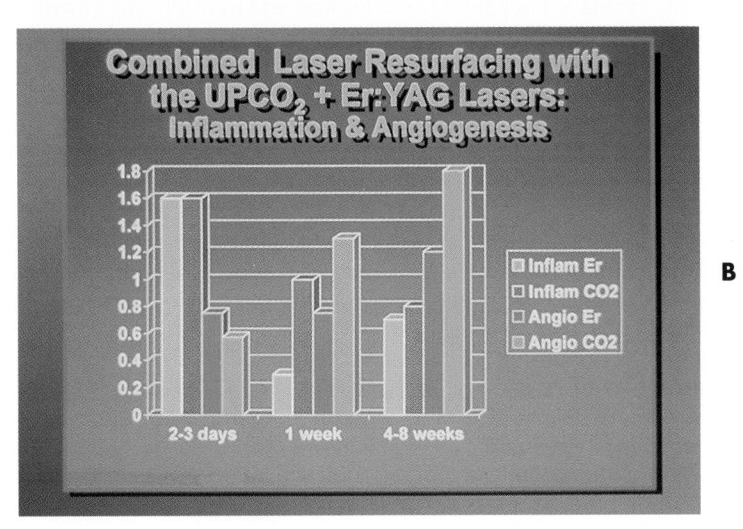

B

Figure 7-43 **A,** Initial thermal necrosis was shown to be reduced significantly by adding erbium laser passes after use of ultrapulsed CO_2 laser ($UPCO_2$), without compromising new collagen formation at 4 to 8 weeks. **B,** Inflammation was greatly reduced at 1 week postoperatively by removing thermal necrosis with erbium laser. Angiogenesis was also reduced at 1 to 8 weeks compared with use of $UPCO_2$ laser alone.

REFERENCES

1. Rice-Evans CA, Burdon RH, editors: *Free radical damage and its control,* New York, 1994, Elsevier.
2. Packer L, Fuchs J, editors: *Oxidative stress in dermatology,* New York, 1993, Dekker.
3. Fuchs J, editor: *Oxidative injury in dermatopathology,* Berlin, 1992, Springer-Verlag.
4. Scandalios JG, editor: *Molecular biology of free radical scavenging systems,* Cold Spring Harbor, 1992, Laboratory Press.
5. Sies H, editor: *Oxidative stress: oxidants and anti-oxidants,* London, 1991, Academic Press.
6. Carbonare MD, Pathak M: Skin photosensitizing agents and the role of reactive oxygen species in photoaging, *J Photochem Photobiol* 14:105, 1992.
7. Kligman LH, Gebre M: Biochemical changes in hairless mouse skin collagen after chronic exposure to ultraviolet-A radiation, *Photochem Photobiol* 54:233, 1991.
8. Hjalmarsson K, Marklund S, Engstrom A, Edlund T: Isolation and sequence of DNA coding human extracellular superoxide dismutase, *Proc Natl Acad Sci USA* 84:6340, 1987.
9. Schallreuter KU, Wood JM: Free radical reduction in the human epidermis, *Free Radic Biol Med* 6:519, 1989.

10. McCay P: Vitamin E: Interaction with free radicals and ascorbate, *Ann Rev Nutr* 5:323, 1985.
11. Niki E: Action of ascorbic acid as a scavenger of active and stable oxygen radicals, *Am J Clin Nutr* 54:1119S, 1991.
12. Frei B, England L, Ames B: Ascorbate in an outstanding antioxidant in human blood plasma, *Proc Natl Acad Sci USA* 86:6377, 1989.
13. Kagen VE, Serbinova EA, Packer L: Anti-oxidant effects of ubiquinones in microsomes and mitochondria are mediated by tocopherol recycling, *Biochem Biophys Res Comm* 169:851, 1990.
14. Kagen VE, Khans S, Swanson C et al: Anti-oxidant action of thioctic and dihydrolipoic acid, *Free Radic Biol Med* 9(suppl):15, 1990 (abstract).
15. Vile GF, Tyrrell RM: Oxidative stress resulting from ultraviolet A irradiation of human skin fibroblasts leads to a heme oxygenase-dependent increase in ferritin, *J Biol Chem* 268:14678, 1990.
16. Colvin RM, Pinnell SR: Topical vitamin C in aging, *Clin Dermatol* 14:227, 1996.
17. Murad S, Grove D, Lindberge KA et al: Regulation of collagen synthesis by ascorbic acid, *Proc Natl Acad Sci USA* 78:2879, 1981.
18. Phillips CL, Tajima S, Pinnell SR: Ascorbic acid and transforming growth factor $\beta 1$ (TGF-β) increase collagen biosynthesis via different mechanisms: coordinate regulation of pro$\alpha 1$ (I) and pro$\alpha 1$ (III) collagens, *Arch Biochem Biophys* 295:397, 1992.
19. Fuchs J, Huflejt ME, Rothfuss LM et al: Impairment of enzymic and noenzymic antioxidants in skin by UVB irradiation, *J Invest Dermatol* 93:769, 1989.
20. Pence BC, Naylor ME: Effects of single dose ultraviolet radiation in skin superoxide dismutase, catalase and xanthine oxidase in hairless mice, *J Invest Dermatol* 95:213, 1990.
21. Shindo Y, Witt E, Packer L: Anti-oxidant defense mechanisms on murine epidermis and dermis and their responses to ultraviolet light, *J Invest Dermatol* 100:260, 1993.
22. Miyachi Y, Imamura S, Niwa Y: Decreased skin superoxide dismutase activity by a single exposure of ultraviolet radiation is reduced by liposomal superoxide dismutase pretreatment, *J Invest Dermatol* 89:111, 1987.
23. Darr D, Combs S, Dunston S et al: Topical vitamin C protects porcine skin from ultraviolet radiation–induced damage, *Br J Dermatol* 127:247, 1992.
24. Iizawa O, Kato T, Tagami H et al: Long term follow-up study of changes in lipid peroxide levels and the activity of superoxide dismutase catalase and glutathione peroxidase in mouse skin after acute and chronic UV irradiation, *Arch Derm Res* 286:47, 1994.
25. Fuchs J, Huflejt ME, Rothfuss LM et al: Acute effects of near ultraviolet and visible light on the cutaneous antioxidant defense system, *Photochem Photobiol* 50:729, 1989.
26. Punnonen K, Puntala A, Ahotupa M: Effects of ultraviolet A and B irradiation on lipid peroxidation and activity of the anti-oxidant enzymes in keratinocytes in cultured human skin fibroblasts, *J Invest Dermatol* 100:692, 1993.
27. Moysan A, Marquis I, Gaboriau F et al: Ultraviolet A–induced lipid peroxidation and anti-oxidant defense system in cultured human skin fibroblasts, *J Invest Dermatol* 100:692, 1993.
28. Aronoff S: Catalase: kinetics of photo-oxidation, *Science* 150:72, 1965.
29. Fridovich I: Biologic effects of the superoxide radical, *Arch Biochem Biophys* 246:245, 1986.
30. Gilchrest BA: Skin aging and photoaging, *Dermatol Nurs* 2:79, 1990.
31. Warren R, Gartstein V, Kligman AM et al: Age, sunlight, and facial skin: a histologic and quantitative study, *J Am Acad of Dermatol* 25:751, 1991.
32. Frances C, Robert L: Elastin and elastic fibers in normal and pathologic skin, *Int J Dermatol* 23:166, 1984.
33. Daly CH, Odland GF: Age-related changes in the mechanical properties of human skin, *J Invest Dermatol* 73:84, 1979.
34. Escoffier C et al: Age-related mechanical properties of human skin: an in vivo study, *J Invest Dermatol* 93:353, 1989.
35. Nicol NJ, Fenske NA: Photodamage: cause, clinical manifestations and prevention, *Dermatol Nurs* 5:263, 1993.
36. Taylor CR, Stern RS, Leyden JJ et al: Photoaging/photodamage and photoprotection, *J Am Acad Dermatol* 22:1, 1990.
37. Weiss JS: Sun damage and photoaging, *Skin,* March/April 1996, p16.

38. Banfield WG, Brindley DC: Preliminary observations on senile elastosis using the electron microscope, *J Invest Dermatol* 41:9, 1963.
39. Smith JG, Davidson EA, Sams WM Jr et al: Alterations in human dermal connective tissue with age and chronic sun damage, *J Invest Dermatol* 39:347, 1962.
40. Felsher S: Observations on senile elastosis, *J Invest Dermatol* 37:163, 1961.
41. Uitto J: Collagen. In Fitzpatrick TB, Eisen AZ, Wolff K et al, editors: *Dermatology in general medicine,* vol 1, ed 4, New York, 1993, McGraw-Hill.
42. Bernstein EF, Chen YZ, Kopp JB et al: Long-term sun exposure alters the collagen of the papillary dermis: comparison of sun-protected and photoaged skin by Northern analysis, immunohistochemical staining, and con-focal laser scanning microscopy, *J Am Acad Dermatol* 34:209, 1996.
43. Lavker RM: Cutaneous aging: chronologic versus photoaging, In Gilchrest BA, editor: *Photoaging,* Cambridge, Mass, 1995, Blackwell.
44. Chen VL, Fleischmajer R, Schwartz E et al: Immunochemistry of elastotic material in sun-damaged skin, *J Invest Dermatol* 87:334, 1986.
45. Schwartz E, Cruickshank FA, Christensen CC et al: Collagen alterations in chronically sun-damaged human skin, *Photochem Photobiol* 53:841, 1993.
46. Oikarinen A, Kallioinen M: Biochemical and immunohistochemical study of collagen in sun-exposed and protected skin, *Photodermatology* 6:24, 1989.
47. Smith JG Jr, Davidson EA, Tindall JP et al: Hexosamine and hydroxyproline alterations in chronically sun-damaged skin, *Proc Soc Exp Biol Med* 108:533, 1961.
48. Peterson MJ, Hansen C, Craig S: Ultraviolet A irradiation stimulates collagenase production in cultured human fibroblasts, *J Invest Dermatol* 99:440, 1992.
49. Rimoldi D, Flessate DM, Samid D: Changes in gene expression by 193- and 248-nm excimer laser radiation in cultured human fibroblasts, *Radiat Res* 131:325, 1992.
50. Talwar HS, Griffiths CE, Fisher GJ et al: Reduced type I and type III procollagens in photodamaged adult human skin, *J Invest Dermatol* 105:285, 1995.
51. Yamauchi M, Prisayanh P, Haque Z, Woodley DT: Collagen cross-linking in sun-exposed and unexposed sites of aged human skin, *J Invest Dermatol* 97:938, 1991.
52. Schwartz E, Cruickshank FA, Christensen CC et al: Collagen alterations in chronically sun-damaged human skin, *Photochem Photobiol* 58:841, 1993.
53. Calderone DC, Fenske NA: The clinical spectrum of actinic elastosis, *J Am Acad Dermatol* 32:1016, 1995.
54. Birkedal-Hansen H, Moore WG, Bodden MK et al: Matrix metalloproteinases: a review, *Crit Rev Oral Biol Med* 4:197, 1993.
55. Matrisian LM, Hogan BL: Growth factor–regulated proteases and extracellular matrix remodeling during mammalian development, *Curr Top Dev Biol* 24:219, 1990.
56. Birkedal-Hansen H: Catabolism and turnover of collagens: collagenases, *Methods Enzymol* 144:140, 1987.
57. Denhardt DT, Feng B, Edwards DR et al: Tissue inhibitor of metalloproteinases (TIMP, aka EPA): structure, control of expression and biological functions, *Pharmacol Ther* 59:329, 1993.
58. Logan SK, Garabedian MJ, Campbell CE, Werb Z: Synergistic transciptional activation of the tissue inhibitor of metalloproteinases-1 promoter via functional interaction of AP-1 and Ets-1 transcription factors, *J Biol Chem* 271:774, 1996.
59. Borden P, Heller RA: Transcriptional control of matrix metalloproteinases and the tissue inhibitors of matrix metalloproteinases, *Crit Rev Eukaryot Gene Expr* 7:159, 1997.
60. Liu X, Wu H, Byrne M, Jeffrey J et al: A targeted mutation at the known collagenase cleavage site in mouse type I collagen impairs tissue remodeling, *J Cell Biol* 130:227, 1995.
61. Fisher GJ, Wang ZQ, Datta SC et al: Pathophysiology of premature skin aging induced by ultraviolet light, *N Engl J Med* 337:1419, 1997.
62. Barnhart BJ, Cox SH, Kraemer PM: Detachment variants of Chinese hamster cells: hyaluronic acid as a modulator of cell detachment, *Exp Cell Res* 119:327, 1979.
63. Lamberg SI, Yupsa SH, Hascall VC: Synthesis of hyaluronic acid is decreased and synthesis of proteoglycans is increased when cultured mouse epidermal cell differentiate, *J Invest Dermatol* 86:659, 1986.
64. Uzuka M, Nakajima K, Ohta S, Mori Y: The mechanism of estrogen-induced increase in hyaluronic acid biosynthesis, with special reference to estrogen receptor in the mouse skin, *Biochim Biophys Acta* 627:199, 1980.

65. Meyer LJ, Stern R: Age-dependent changes of hyaluronan in human skin, *J Invest Dermatol* 102:385, 1994.
66. Tammi R, Ripellino JA, Margolis RU, Tammi M: Localization of epidermal hyaluronic acid using the hyaluronate binding region of cartilage proteoglycan as a specific problem, *J Invest Dermatol* 90:412, 1988.
67. Moczar M, Robert L: Stimulation of cell proliferation by hyaluronidase during in vitro aging of human skin fibroblasts, *Exp Gerontol* 28:59, 1993.
68. Ghersetich I, Lotti T, Campanile G et al: Hyaluronic acid in cutaneous intrinsic aging, *Int J Dermatol* 33:119, 1994.
69. Manuskiatti W, Maibach HI: Hyaluronic acid and skin: wound healing and aging, *Int J Dermatol* 35:539, 1996.
70. Ghersetich I, Teofoli P, Benci M, Lotti T: Ultrastructural study of hyaluronic acid before and after the use of a pulsed electromagnetic field, electrorydesis, in the treatment of wrinkles, *Int J Dermatol* 33:661, 1994.
71. Fleischmajer R, Perlish JS, Bashey RI: *Aging of human dermis,* Basel, 1973, Karger.
72. Fleischmajer R, Perlish JS, Bashey RI: Human dermal glycosaminoglycans and aging, *Biochim Biophys Acta* 279:265, 1972.
73. Breen M, Weinstein HG, Blacik LJ et al: Microanalysis and characterization of glycosaminoglycans from human tissue via zone electrophoresis, New York, 1976, Academic Press.
74. Schachtschabel DO, Wever J: Age-related decline in the synthesis of glycosaminoglycans by cultured human fibroblasts (WI-38), *Mech Ageing Dev* 8:257, 1978.
75. Sluke G, Schachtschabel DO, Wever J: Age-related changes in the distribution pattern of glycosaminoglycans synthesized by cultured human diploid fibroblasts (WI-38), *Mech Ageing Dev* 16:19, 1981.
76. Willen MD, Sorrell JM, Lekan CC et al: Patterns of glycosaminoglycan/proteoglycan immunostaining in human skin during aging, *J Invest Dermatol* 96:968, 1991.
77. NIH Consensus Statement: Sunlight, ultraviolet radiation, and the skin, May 1989.
78. Miller DL, Weinstock MA: Non-melanoma skin cancer in the United States: incidence, *J Am Acad Dermatol* 30:774, 1994.
79. Griffiths EMG, Voorhees JJ: The tretinoin story, *Fitzpatrick's J Clin Dermatol* 3:14, 1995.
80. Rudolph R, Berg JV, Ehrlich HP: Wound contraction and scar contracture. In Cohen IK, Diegelmann RF, Lindblad WJ, editors: *Wound healing: biochemical and clinical aspects,* Philadelphia, 1992, Saunders.
81. Fisher GJ, Datta SC, Taluar HS et al: Molecular basis of sun-induced premature skin aging and retinoid antagonism, *Nature* 379:335, 1996.
82. Goldfarb MT, Ellis CN, Weiss JS et al: Topical tretinoin therapy: its use in photoaged skin, *J Am Acad Dermatol* 21:645, 1989.
83. Kligman AM, Graham CG: Histological changes in facial skin after daily application of tretinoin for 5 to 6 years, *J Dermatol Tx* 4:113, 1993.
84. Olsen EA, Katz HI, Levine N et al: Tretinoin emollient cream: a new therapy for photodamaged skin, *J Am Acad Dermatol* 26:215, 1992.
85. Weinstein GD, Nigra TP, Pochi PE et al: Topical tretinoin for treatment of photodamaged skin: a multicenter study, *Arch Dermatol* 127:659, 1991.
86. Weiss JS, Ellis CN, Headington JT et al: Topical tretinoin improves photoaged skin: a double-blind vehicle-controlled study, *JAMA* 259:527, 1988.
87. Griffiths CEM, Russman AN, Majmudar G et al: Restoration of collagen formation in photodamaged human skin by tretinoin (retinoic acid), *N Engl J Med* 329:530, 1993.
88. Kligman AM, Grove GL, Hirose R et al: Topical retinoic acid for photoaged skin, *J Am Acad Dermatol* 15:836, 1986.
89. Weiss JS, Ellis CN, Headington JT et al: Topical retinoic acid improves photoaged skin: a double-blind vehicle-controlled study, *J Am Acad Dermatol* 259:527, 1988.
90. Weiss JS, Ellis CN, Headington JT et al: Topical retinoic acid in the treatment of aging skin, *J Am Acad Dermatol* 19:169, 1988.
91. Kligman LH, Chen HD, Kligman AM: Topical retinoic acid enhances the repair of ultraviolet damaged dermal connective tissue, *Connect Tissue Res* 12:139, 1984.
92. Federspiel SJ, DiMari SJ, Howe AM et al: Extracellular matrix biosynthesis by cultured fetal rat lung epithelial cells. IV. Effects of chronic exposure to retinoic acid on growth differentiation, and collagen biosynthesis, *Lab Invest* 65:441, 1991.

93. Wlaschek M, Bolsen K, Herrmann G et al: UVA-induced autocrine stimulation of fibroblast-derived collagenase by IL-6: a possible mechanism in dermal photodamage? *J Invest Dermatol* 101:164, 1993.
94. Bauer EA, Seltzer JL, Eisen AZ: Retinoic acid inhibition of collagenase and gelatinase expression in human skin fibroblast cultures: evidence for a dual mechanism, *J Invest Dermatol* 81:162, 1983.
95. Ellis CN, Weiss JS, Hamilton TA et al: Sustained improvement with prolonged topical retinoic acid (retinoic acid) for photoaged skin, *J Am Acad Dermatol* 23:629, 1990.
96. Fisher GJ, Datta SC, Talwar HS et al: Molecular basis of sun-induced premature skin aging and retinoid antagonism, *Nature* 379:335, 1996.
97. Lundin F et al: Topical retinoic acid treatment of photoaged skin: its effects on hyaluronan distribution in epidermis and on hyaluronan and retinoic acid in suction blister fluid, *Acta Derm Venereol* 72:423, 1992.
98. Akiyama H, Saito M, Qiu G et al: Analytical studies on hyaluronic acid synthesis by normal human epidermal keratinocytes cultured in a serum-free medium, *Biol Pharm Bull* 17:361, 1994.
99. Tammi R, Ripellino JA, Margolis RU et al: Hyaluronic accumulation in human epidermis treated with retinoic acid in skin organ culture, *J Invest Dermatol* 92:326, 1989.
100. Tammi R, Tammi M: Influence of retinoic acid on the ultrastructure and hyaluronic acid synthesis of adult human epidermis in whole skin organ culture, *J Cell Physiol* 126:389, 1986.
101. Tammi R, Jansen CT, Tammi M: Effects of retinoic acid on adult human epidermis in whole skin organ culture, *Arch Dermatol Res* 277:276, 1985.
102. King IA: Increased epidermal hyaluronic acid synthesis caused by four retinoids, *Br J Dermatol* 110:607, 1984.
103. Rossi A, Bozzi M, Villano PA: Treatment of keloids and hypertrophic scars with retinoic acid, *Ann Ital Dermatol Clin Sper* 44:269, 1990.
104. Harris DWS, Beickley CC, Ostlere LS et al: Topical retinoic acid in the treatment of fine scarring, *Br J Dermatol* 125:81, 1991.
105. Elson ML: Treatment of striae distense with topical retinoic acid, *J Dermatol Surg Oncol* 16:3, 1990.
106. Kang S, Duell EA, Fisher GJ et al: Application of retinol to human skin in vivo induces epidermal hyperplasia and cellular retinoid binding proteins characteristic of retinoic acid but without measurable retinoic acid levels or irritation, *J Invest Dermatol* 105:549, 1995.
107. Kurlandsky SB, Xiao JH, Duell EA, Voorhees JJ et al: Biological activity of all-*trans* retinol requires metabolic conversion to all-*trans* retinoic acid and is mediated through activation of nuclear retinoid receptors in human keratinocytes, *J Biol Chem* 269:32821, 1994.
108. Stagnone JJ: Superficial peeling, *J Dermatol Surg Oncol* 15:924, 1989.
109. Ditre CM, Griffin TD, Murphy GF et al: The effects of alpha hydroxyacids (AHAs) on photoaged skin: a pilot clinical, histological and ultrastructural study, *J Am Acad Dermatol* 34:187, 1996.
110. Lavker RM, Kaidbey K, Leyden JJ: Effects of topical ammonium lactate on cutaneous atrophy from a potent topical corticosteroid, *J Am Acad Dermtol* 26:535, 1992.
111. Dunham WB, Zuckerhandl W, Reynolds R et al: Effect of intake of L-ascorbic acid on the incidence of dermal neoplasms induced in mice by ultraviolet light, *Proc Natl Acad Sci USA* 79:7532, 1982.
112. Black HS, Chant JT: Suppression of ultraviolet light–induced tumor formation by dietary anti-oxidants, *J Invest Dermatol* 65:412, 1975.
113. Packer L: Ultraviolet radiation (UVA, UVB) and skin anti-oxidants. In Rice-Evans CA, Burdon RH, editors: *Free radical damage and its control,* New York, 1994, Elsevier.
114. Roshchupkin DI, Pistsov MY, Potapenko AY: Inhibition of ultraviolet light–induced erythema by anti-oxidants, *Arch Derm Res* 266:91, 1979.
115. Potapenko AY, Abiev GA, Piquett F: Inhibition of erythema of skin photosensitized with 8-methoxypsoralen by α-tocopherol, *Bull Exp Biol Med* 89:611, 1980.
116. Trevithick JR, Xiong H, Lee S et al: Topical tocopherol acetate reduces post-UVB sunburn associated erythema, edema and skin sensitivity in hairless mice, *Arch Biochem Biophys* 296:575, 1992.

117. Bissett DL, Chatterjee R, Hannon DP: Protective effect of a topically applied antioxidant plus an anti-inflammatory agent against ultraviolet radiation–induced chronic skin damage in the hairless mouse, *J Soc Cosmet Chem* 43:85, 1992.
118. Norkus EP, Bryce RG, Bhagavan HN: Uptake and bioconversion of α-tocopherol acetate to α-tocopherol in skin and hairless mice, *Photochem Photobiol* 57:913, 1993.
119. Beijersbergen van Henegouwen GMJ, de Vries H, van den Brocke LT, Tunginger HE: RRR-tocopherols and their acetates as a possible scavenger of free radicals produced in the skin upon UVA exposure: an *in vivo* screening method, *Fat Sci Technol* 94:24, 1992.
120. Niki E, Yamamoto Y, Komuro E, Sato K: Membrane damage due to lipid oxidation, *Am J Clin Nutr* 53:201S, 1991.
121. Niki E, Kawakami A, Yamamoto Y et al: Oxidation of lipids. VIII. Synergistic inhibition of oxidation of phosphatidylcholine liposomes in aqueous dispersion by vitamin E and vitamin C, *Bull Chem Soc Jpn* 58:1971, 985.
122. Wefers H, Seis H: The protection by ascorbate and glutathione against microsomal lipid peroxidation is dependent on vitamin E, *Eur J Biochem* 174:353,1988.
123. Tappel AL: Will antioxidant nutrients slow the aging processes? *Geriatrics* 23:97, 1968.
124. Bast A, Haenen GRMM: Interplay between lipoic acid and glutathione in the protection against microsomal lipid peroxidation, *Biochim Biophys Acta* 963:358,1988.
125. Scholich H, Murphy ME, Sies H: Antioxidant activity of dihydrolipoaic against microsomal lipid peroxidation and its dependence on α-tocopherol, *Biochim Biophys Acta* 1001:256, 1989.
126. Fuchs J, Milbrandt R, Zimmer G: Dihydrolipoate inhibits reactive oxygen species mediated skin inflammation, *J Invest Dermatol* 94:526, 1990 (abstract).
127. Wayner DDM, Brown GW, Ingold KU, Locke S: Quantitative measurement of the total, peroxyl radical-trapping antioxidant capability of human blood plasma by controlled peroxidation, *FEBS Lett* 187:33, 1985.
128. Frei B, Stocker R, Ames BN: Antioxidant defense and lipid peroxidation in human blood plasma, *Proc Natl Acad Sci USA* 85:9748,1988.
129. Di Mascio P, Murphy ME, Sies H: Antioxidants' defense systems: the role of carotenoids, tocopherols, and thiols, *Am J Clin Nutr* 53:194S, 1991.
130. Darr D, Pinnell SR: Stabilized ascorbic acid compositions, US Patent No5,140,043, 1992.
131. Darr D, Dunstan S, Faust H et al: Effectiveness of antioxidants (vitamin C and E) with and without sunscreens as topical photoprotectants, *Acta Derm Venereol* 76:264, 1996.
132. Kipp DE, Schwarz RI: Effectiveness of isoascorbate versus ascorbate as an inducer of collagen synthesis in primary avian tendon cells, *Nutrition* 120:185, 1990.
133. Nakamura T, Pinnell SR, Streilein JW: Anti-oxidants can reverse the deleterious effects of ultraviolet (UVB) radiation on cutaneous immunity, *J Invest Dermatol* 104:600, 1995.
134. Darr D, Combs S, Pinnell SR: Ascorbic acid and collagen synthesis: rethinking a role for lipid peroxidation, *Arch Biochem Biophys* 307:299, 1994.
135. Phillips CL, Combs SB, Pinnell SR: Effects of ascorbic acid on proliferation and collagen synthesis in relation to the donor age of human dermal fibroblasts, *J Invest Dermatol* 103:228, 1994.
136. Phillips CL, Tajima S, Pinnell SR: Ascorbic acid and transforming growth factor-B1 increase collagen biosynthesis via different mechanisms; coordinate regulation of procol (I) and procol (III) collagens, *Arch Biochem Biophys* 295:397, 1992.
137. Pinnel SR, Murad S, Darr D: Induction of collagen synthesis by ascorbic acid: a possible mechanism, *Arch Dermatol* 123:1684, 1987.
138. Pinnell SR: Regulation of collagen biosynthesis by ascorbic acid: a review, *Yale J Biol Med* 58:553, 1985.
139. Bissett D, Chaterjee R, Hannon D: Photoprotective effect of superoxide scavenging antioxidants against ultraviolet radiation–induced chronic skin damage in the hairless mouse, *Photoderm Photoimmunol Photomed* 7:58, 1990.
140. Imai Y, Usui T, Matsuzaki T et al: The antiscorbutic activity of L-ascorbic acid phosphate given orally and percutaneously in guinea pigs, *Jpn J Pharmacol* 17:317, 1967.
141. Verlangieri AJ, Fay MJ, Bannon AW: Comparison of the anti-scorbutic activity of L-ascorbic acid and ester-C in the non-ascorbic synthesizing osteogenic disorder Shinogi (ODS) rat, *Life Sci* 48:9, 1991.
142. Wakamiya H, Suzuki E, Yamamoto I et al: Vitamin C activity of 2-0-alpha-D-glucopyranosyl-L-ascorbic acid in guinea pigs, *N Nutr Sci Vitaminol (Tokyo)* 38:235, 1992.

143. Perricone NV: The photoprotective and anti-inflammatory effects of topical ascorbyl palmitate, *J Geriatr Dermatol* 1:5, 1993.
144. Darr D, Dunstan S, Kamino H et al: Effectiveness of a combination of vitamin C and E in inhibiting UV damage in porcine skin, *J Invest Dermatol* 100:597, 1993 (abstract).
145. Epstein J: Effects of β-carotene on ultraviolet-induced cancer formation in the hairless mouse skin, *Photochem Photobiol* 25:211, 1977.
146. Pugliese PT, Lampley CB: Biochemical assessment of the anti-aging effects of cosmetic products, *J Appl Cosmet* 3:129, 1985.
147. Carroro C, Pathak MA: Studies on the nature of *in vitro* and *in vivo* photosensitization reaction by psoralen and porphyrins, *J Invest Dermatol* 90:267, 1988.
148. Peto R, Doll R, Buckley JD, Sporn MB: Can dietary beta-carotene reduce human cancer rates? *Nature (Lond)* 290:203, 1981.
149. Connett JE, Kuller LH, Kjelsberg MO et al: Relationship between carotenoids and cancer, *Cancer* 64:126, 1989.
150. Mathews-Roth MM: Carotenoids and cancer prevention: experimental and epidemiological studies, *Pure Appl Chem* 57:717, 1985.
151. Ogura R, Sugiyama M, Sakanashi T, Hidaka T: Role of oxygen in lipid peroxide of skin exposed to ultraviolet light. In Hayaishi O, Imamura S, Miyachi Y, editors: *The biological role of reactive oxygen species in skin,* New York, 1987, Elsevier.
152. Hamanaka H, Miyachi Y, Imamura S: Photoprotective effect of topically applied superoxide dismutase on sunburn reaction in comparison with sunscreen, *J Dermatol* 17:595, 1990.
153. Martin A: The use of antioxidants in healing, *Dermatol Surg* 22:156, 1996.
154. O'Donnell-Torney J, Nathan CF, Lanks K et al: Secretion of pyruvate: an antioxidant defense of mammalian cells, *J Exp Med* 165:500, 1987.
155. Shacter E: Serum-free medium for growth factor–dependent and –independent plasmocytomas and hybridomas, *J Immunol Meth* 99:259, 1987.
156. Niki E, Yamamoto Y, Komura E, Sato K: Membrane damage due to lipid oxidation, *Am J Clin Nutr* 53:201S, 1991.
157. Burke KE, Combs GF, Gross EG et al: The effects of topical and oral L-selenomethionine on pigmentation and skin cancer induced by ultraviolet irradiation, *Nutr Cancer* 17:123, 1992.
158. Mukhtar H, Katiyar SK, Agarwal R: Green tea on skin: anticarcinogenesis effects, *J Invest Dermatol* 102:3, 1994.
159. Clark SD, Kobayashi DK, Welgus HG: Regulation of the expression of tissue inhibitor of metalloproteinases and collagenase by retinoids and glucocorticoids in human fibroblasts, *J Clin Invest* 80:1280, 1987.
160. West MD: The cellular and molecular biology of skin aging, *Arch Dermatol* 130:87, 1994.
161. Kligman AM, Dogadkina D, Lavker RM: Effects of topical tretinoin on non-sun-exposed protected skin of the elderly, *J Am Acad Dermatol* 29:25, 1993.
162. Hung VC, Lee JY, Zitelli JA et al: Topical tretinoin and epithelial wound healing, *Arch Dermatol* 125:65, 1989.
163. Mandy SH: Tretinoin in the preoperative and postoperative management of dermabrasion, *J Am Acad Dermatol* 15:878, 1986.
164. Vagotis FL, Brundage SR: Histologic study of dermabrasion and chemical peel in an animal model after pretreatment with Retin-A, *Anesthetic Plast Surg* 19:243, 1995.
165. Popp C, Kligman AM, Stoudemayer TJ: Pretreatment of photoaged forearm skin with topical tretinoin accelerates healing of full-thickness wounds, *Br J Dermatol* 132:46, 1995.
166. Hevia O, Nemeth AJ, Taylor R: Tretinoin accelerates healing after trichloroacetic acid chemical peel, *Arch Dermatol* 127:678, 1991.
167. Effendy I, Kwangsukstith C, Lee JY, Maibach HI: Functional changes in human stratum corneum induced by topical glycolic acid: comparison with all-*trans* retinoic acid, *Acta Derm Venereol* 75:455, 1995.
168. Beasley D, Jones C, McDonald WS: Effect of pretreated skin on laser resurfacing, *Lasers Surg Med Suppl* 9:43, 1997.
169. Duke D, Grevelink JM: Care before and after laser skin resurfacing, *Dermatol Surg* 24:201, 1998.
170. Winton GR, Salasche SJ: Dermabrasion of the scalp as a treatment for actinic damage, *J Am Acad Dermatol* 14:661, 1986.

171. Glogau RG, Matarasso SL: Chemical peels: trichloroacetic acid and phenol, *Dermatol Clin* 13:263, 1995.
172. Stegman SJ, Tromovitch TA, Glogau RG: *Cosmetic dermatology surgery,* ed 2, Chicago, 1990,Year Book.
173. Duffy DM: Alpha hydroxy acids/trichloracetic acids risk/benefit strategies: a photographic review, *Dermatol Surg* 24:181, 1998.
174. Brody HJ: *Chemical peeling,* St Louis, 1992,Mosby.
175. Brody HJ: Histology and classification and wound healing. In Brody HJ, editor: *Chemical peeling,* St Louis, 1992, Mosby.
176. Matarasso SL, Glogau RG: Chemical face peels. In Thiers BT, editor: *Dermatologic Clinics,* Philadelphia, 1991, Saunders.
177. Roenigk HH Jr: Dermabrasion. In Roenigk RK, Roenigk HH, editors: *Dermatologic surgery: principles and practice,* New York, 1989, Dekker.
178. Benedetto AV, Griffin TD, Benedetto EA, Humenuik HM: Dermabrasion: therapy and prophylaxis of the photoaged face, *J Am Acad Dermatol* 27:439,1992.
179. Dover JS, Smoller BR, Stern RS et al: Low-fluence carbon dioxide laser irradiation of lentigines, *Arch Dermatol* 124:1219, 1988.
180. Kamat BR, Tang SV, Arndt KA et al: Low-fluence CO_2 laser irradiation: selected epidermal damage to human skin, *J Invest Dermatol* 85:274, 1985.
181. Wheeland RG: Revision of full-thickness skin grafts using the carbon dioxide laser, *J Dermatol Surg Oncol* 14:130, 1988.
182. Garrett AB, Dufresne RG, Ratz JL, Berlin AJ: Carbon dioxide laser treatment of pitted acne scarring, *J Dermatol Surg Oncol* 16:737, 1990.
183. Goldman L, Shumrick DA, Rockwell J: The laser in maxillofacial surgery: preliminary investigative surgery, *Arch Surg* 96:397, 1968.
184. David LM: Laser vermilion ablation for actinic cheilitis, *J Dermatol Surg Oncol* 11:605, 1985.
185. Brauner G, Schliftman A: Laser surgery in children, *J Dermatol Surg Oncol* 13:178, 1987.
186. David LM, Lask GP, Glassberg E et al: Laser ablation for cosmetic and medical treatment of facial actinic damage, *Cutis* 43:583, 1989.
187. Anderson RR, Parrish JA: Selective photothermolysis: precise microsurgery by selective absorption of pulsed radiation, *Science* 220:524, 1983.
188. Fitzpatrick RE et al: *Lasers Surg Med,* 1989 (abstract).
189. Fitzpatrick RE, Ruiz-Esparza J, Goldman MP: The clinical advantage of the superpulse carbon dioxide laser, *Lasers Surg Med Suppl* 2:52, 1990.
190. Fitzpatrick RE, Ruiz-Esparza, J, Goldman MP: The depth of thermal necrosis using the CO_2 laser: a comparison of the superpulsed mode and conventional mode, *J Dermatol Surg Oncol* 17:340, 1991.
191. Fitzpatrick RE: The UltraPulse CO_2 laser: selective photothermolysis of epidermal tumors, *Lasers Surg Med Suppl* 5:56, 1993.
192. Fitzpatrick RE, Goldman MP, Ruiz-Esparza JR: Clinical advantage of the CO_2 laser superpulsed mode: treatment of verruca vulgaris, seborrheic keratoses, lentigines and actinic cheilitis, *J Dermatol Surg Oncol* 20:449, 1994.
193. Fitzpatrick RE, Ruiz-Esparza J: The superpulsed CO_2 laser. In Roenigk RK, Roenigk H, editors: *New trends in dermatologic surgery,* London, 1993, Dunitz.
194. Green, HA, Burd E, Nishioka NS et al: Skin graft take and healing ablation of graft beds, *J Invest Dermatol* 92:436, 1989 (abstract).
195. Green HA, Burd E, Nishioka NS: Pulsed carbon dioxide laser ablation of burned skin: in vitro and in vivo analysis, *Lasers Surg Med* 10:476, 1990.
196. Green HA, Burd E, Nishioka NS, Bruggermann U et al: Mid-dermal wound healing: a comparison between dermatomal excision and pulsed carbon dioxide ablation, *Arch Dermatol* 128:639, 1992.
197. Smalley P: Personal communication, 1991.
198. Fitzpatrick RE, Tope WD, Goldman MP, Satur NM: Pulsed carbon dioxide laser, tricholoroacetic acid, Baker-Gordon phenol, and dermabrasion: a comparative clinical and histological study of cutaneous resurfacing in a porcine model, *Arch Dermatol* 132:469, 1996.
199. Weinstein C: Ultrapulse carbon dioxide laser removal of periocular wrinkles in association with laser blepharoplasty, *J Clin Laser Med Surg* 12:205, 1994.

200. Lowe NJ, Lask G, Griffin ME et al: Skin resurfacing with the UltraPulse carbon dioxide laser: observations on 100 patients, *Dermatol Surg* 21:1025, 1995.
201. Fitzpatrick RE, Goldman MP, Satur NM, Tope WD: Pulsed carbon dioxide laser resurfacing of photoaged skin, *Arch Dermatol* 132:395, 1996.
202. Arnold D, Slatkine M, Eliezer Z: Swiftlaser: a new technology for char-free ablation in rectal surgery, *J Clin Laser Med Surg* 11:309, 1993.
203. Krespi YP, Keidar A, Khosh MM et al: The efficacy of laser-assisted uvuloplasty in the management of obstructive sleep apnea and upper airway resistance syndrome, *Oper Tech Otolaryngol Head Neck Surg* 5:235, 1994.
204. Grevelink JM, Brennick JB: Hair transplantation facilitated by flashscanner-enhanced carbon dioxide laser, *Oper Tech in Otolaryngol Head Neck Surg* 5:278, 1994.
205. Chernoff WG, Shoenrock L: Cutaneous laser resurfacing, *Oper Tech Otolaryngol Head Neck Surg* 5:281, 1994.
206. Waldorf HA, Kauvar ANB, Geronemus RG: Skin resurfacing of fine to deep rhytides using char-free carbon dioxide laser in 47 patients, *Dermatol Surg* 21:940, 1995.
207. Lask G, Keller G, Lowe N, Gormley D: Laser skin resurfacing with the SilkTouch flashscanner for facial rhytides, *Dermatol Surg* 21:1021, 1995.
208. Alster TS: Comparison of two high-energy pulsed carbon dioxide lasers in the treatment of periorbital rhytides, *Dermatol Surg* 22:541, 1996.
209. Alster TS, Garg S: Treatment of facial rhytides with the UltraPulse high energy carbon dioxide laser, *Plast Reconstr Surg,* 1998 (in press).
210. Ho C, Nguyen Q, Lowe NJ et al: Laser resurfacing in pigmented skin, *Dermatol Surg* 21:1035, 1995.
211. Goldman MP, Fitzpatrick RE, Smith SS: Resurfacing complications and their management. In Coleman WP, Lawrence N, editors: *Laser resurfacing,* Baltimore, 1997, William & Wilkins.
212. Chernoff G, Shoenrock L, Cramer H et al: Cutaneous laser resurfacing, *Int J Aesthetic Rest Surg* 3:57, 1995.
213. Chernoff WG, Cramer H: Rejuvenation of the skin surface: laser exfoliation, *Facial Plast Surg* 12:135, 1996.
214. Dover JS: CO_2 laser resurfacing: why all the fuss? *Plast Reconstr Surg* 98:506, 1996 (editorial).
215. Goodman GJ: Facial resurfacing using a high-energy, short-pulsed carbon dioxide laser, *Aust J Dermatol* 37:125, 1996.
216. Trelles MA, Kaplan I, Rigau J, Buezo O: Periocular skin reshaping by CO_2 laser coagulation, *Aesthetic Plast Surg* 20:327, 1996.
217. Fulton JE Jr: Dermabrasion, chemabrasion, and laserabrasion: Historical perspectives, modern dermabrasion techniques, and future trends, *Dermatol Surg* 22:619, 1996.
218. Chernoff G, Slatkine M, Zair E, Mead D: SilkTouch: a new technology for skin resurfacing in aesthetic surgery, *J Clin Laser Med Surg* 13:97, 1995.
219. Walsh JJ, Deutsch TF: Pulsed CO_2 laser tissue ablation: measurement of the ablation rate, *Lasers Surg Med* 8:264, 1988.
220. Olbricht SM: Use of the carbon dioxide laser in dermatologic surgery: a clinical relevant update for 1993, *J Dermatol Surg Oncol* 93:364, 1993.
221. Fitzpatrick RE, Goldman MP: CO_2 laser surgery. In *Cutaneous laser surgery: the art and science of selective photothermolysis,* St Louis, 1994, Mosby.
222. Kauver ANB, Waldorf HA, Geronemus RG: A histopathological comparison of "char-free" carbon dioxide lasers, *Dermatol Surg* 22:343, 1996.
223. Cotton J, Hood AF, Gonin R et al: Histologic evaluation of preauricular and postauricular human skin after high-energy, short-pulse carbon dioxide laser, *Arch Dermatol* 132:425, 1996.
224. Stuzin JM, Baker TJ, Baker TM, Kligman AM: Histologic effects of the high energy pulsed CO_2 laser on photoaged facial skin, *Plast Reconstr Surg* 97:2036, 1997.
225. Alster TS: Histology of CO_2 resurfacing, *Semin Cutan Med Surg* •••-193, 1996.
226. Ross EV, Domankevitz Y, Skrobal M, Anderson RR: Effects of CO_2 laser pulse duration in ablation and residual thermal damage: implications for skin resurfacing, *Lasers Surg Med* 19:123, 1996.
227. Venugopalan V, Nishioka N, Mikic B: The effect of laser parameters on the zone of thermal injury produced by laser ablation of biological tissue, *ASME Biomech Eng* 116:62, 1994.

228. Gardner ES, Reinisch L, Stricklin GP et al: In vitro changes in non-facial human skin following laser resurfacing: a comparison study, *Lasers Surg Med* 19:379, 1996.
229. Schomacker K, Walsh J, Flott T, Deutsch T: Thermal damage produced by high-irradiance continuous wave CO_2 laser cutting of tissue, *Lasers Surg Med* 10:74, 1990.
230. McKenzie A: How far does thermal damage extend beneath the surface of CO_2 laser incisions? *Phys Med Biol* 28:905, 1983.
231. Walsh J, Flotte T, Anderson R, Deutsch T: Pulsed CO_2 laser tissue ablation: effects of tissue type and pulse duration on thermal damage, *Lasers Surg Med* 8:108, 1988.
232. Hobbs E, Bailin P, Wheeland R, Ratz J: Superpulsed lasers: minimizing thermal damage with short duration, high irradiance pulses, *J Dermatol Surg Oncol* 13:955, 1987.
233. Apfelberg DB: The UltraPulse carbon dioxide laser with computer pattern generator automatic scanner for facial cosmetic surgery and resurfacing, *Ann Plast Surg* 36:522, 1996.
234. Rubach BW, Schoenrock LD: Histological and clinical evaluation of facial resurfacing using a carbon dioxide laser with the computer pattern generator, *Arch Otolaryncol Head Neck Surg* 123:929, 1997.
235. Apfelberg DB: UltraPulse carbon dioxide laser with CPG scanner for full-face resurfacing for rhytids, photoaging, and acne scars, *Plast Reconstr Surg* 99:1817, 1997.
236. Apfelberg DB, Smoller B: UltraPulse carbon dioxide laser with CPG scanner for deepithelialization: clinical and histologic study, *Plast Reconstr Surg* 99:2089, 1997.
237. Hruza GJ, Fitzpatrick RE, Dover JS: Laser skin resurfacing. In Arndt KA, Olbricht SM, Dover JS, editors: *Cutaneous laser surgery,* Philadelphia, 1997, Lippincott-Raven.
238. Stuzin JM, Baker TJ, Baker TM, Kligman AM: Histologic effects of the high-energy pulsed CO_2 laser on photoaged facial skin, *Plast Reconstr Surg* 99:2036, 1997.
239. Rein R: Physical and surgical principles governing carbon dioxide laser surgery on the skin, *Dermatol Clin* 9:297, 1991.
240. Fitzpatrick RE, Smith SR, Sriprachya-anunt S: Depth of vaporization and the effect of pulse stacking with the UltraPulse CO_2 laser, *J Am Acad Dermatol,* 1998. (submitted for publication).
241. Nelson BR, Majmudar G, Griffiths CEM et al: Clinical improvement following dermabrasion of photoaged skin correlates with synthesis of collagen I, *Arch Dermatol* 130:1136, 1994.
242. Goldman MP, Fitzpatrick RE: New collagen, *J Clin Laser Med Sur.*
243. Flor PJ, Garrett RR: Phase transition in collagen and gelatin systems, *J Am Chem Soc* 80:4836, 1958.
244. Flor PJ, Spurr OK: Melting equilibrium for collagen fibers under stress: elasticity in the amorphous state, *J Am Chem Soc* 83:1308, 1960.
245. Flor PJ, Weaver ES: Helix coil transition in dilute aqueous collagen solutions, *J Am Chem Soc* 82:4518, 1959.
246. Stryer L: The stability of the collagen helix depends on cooperative interactions. In *Biochemistry,* ed 2, New York, 1981, Freeman.
247. Gross J: Thermal denaturation of collagen in the dispersed and solid state, *Science* 143:960, 1964 (abstract).
248. Bourne G, editor: *The biochemistry and physiology of bone,* New York, 1956, Academic Press.
249. Horn DJ, King NL, Kurth LB et al: Collagen crosslinks and their relationship to the thermal properties of calf tendons, *Arch Biochem Biophys* 28:21, 1980.
250. Gelman RA, Blackwell J, Kefalides NA et al: Thermal stability of basement membrane collagen, *Biochim Biophys Acta* 427:492, 1976.
251. Tanzer ML: Cross-linkage of collagen, *Science* 180:561, 1973.
252. Boedtker H, Doty P: The native and denatured states of soluble collagen, *J Am Chem Soc* 79:4267, 1956.
253. Boedtker H, Doty P: On the nature of the structural element of collagen, *J Am Chem Soc* 77:248, 1955 (editorial).
254. Sarkar SK, Hiyama Y, Niu CH et al: Molecular dynamics of collagen side chains in hard and soft tissues: a multicenter magnetic resonance study, *Biochemistry* 26:6793, 1987.
255. Mosler E, Foldhard W, Knorzer W et al: Stress-induced molecular arrangement in tendon collagen, *J Mol Biol* 182:589, 1985.
256. Gustavson KH: *The chemistry and reactivity of collagen,* New York, 1956, Academic Press.
257. Pearce JA, Thomsen S: Kinetic models of laser-tissue fusion processes, *Biomed Sci Instrum* 29:355, 1993.

258. Guthrie CR, Murray LW, Kopchok GE: Biochemical mechanisms of laser vascular tissue fusion, *J Invest Surg* 4:3, 1991.
259. Schmid TM, Linsenmayer TF: Denaturation-renaturation properties of two molecular forms of short-chain cartilage collagen, *Biochemistry* 23:553, 1984.
260. Tanaka S, Avigad G, Eikenberry EF et al: Isolation and partial characterization of collagen chains dimerized by sugar-derived cross-links, *J Biol Chem* 263:17650, 1988.
261. Lennox FG: Shrinkage of collagen, *Biochim Biophys Acta* 3:170, 1949.
262. Lloyd DJ, Garrod M: A contribution to the theory of the structure of protein fibres with special reference to the so-called thermal shrinkage of the collagen fibre, 1947.
263. Theis ER: Relation of swelling to shrinkage temperature of collagen, 1946.
264. Allain JC, Le Lous M, Cohen-Solal L et al: Isometric tensions developed during the hydrothermal swelling of rat skin, *Connect Tissue Res* 7:127, 1980.
265. Verzar F, Nagy IZ: Electronmicroscopic analysis of thermal collagen denaturation in rat tail tendons, *Gerontologia* 16:77, 1970.
266. Thomsen S: Pathologic analysis of photothermal and photomechanical effects of laser-tissue interactions, *Photochem Photobiol* 53:825, 1991.
267. Pearce JA: Thermodynamic principles of laser-tissue interaction, *Proc IEEE BME,* November 1990.
268. Sand BJ: Method for collagen treatment, US Patent No4,976,709, 1990.
269. Smelser GK, Polack FM, Ozanics V: Persistence of donor collagen in corneal transplants, *Exp Eye Res* 4:349, 1965.
270. Stringer HCW, Highton TC: The shrinkage temperature of skin collagen, *Aust J Dermatol* 5:230, 1960.
271. Vangsness CT Jr, Mitchell W III, Nimni M et al: Collagen shortening: an experimental approach with heat, *Clin Orthop Rel Res* 337:267, 1997.
272. Hayashi K, Thabit III, Massa KL et al: The effect of thermal heating on the length and histologic properties of the glenohumeral joint capsule, *Am J Sports Med* 25:107, 1997.
273. Ross EV, Naseef M, Skrobal JM et al: *In vivo* dermal collagen shrinkage and remodeling following CO_2 laser resurfacing, *Lasers Surg Med* 19(suppl 8):38, 1996.
274. Kirsch KM, Zelickson BD, Zachary CB et al: Ultrastructure of collagen thermally denatured by microsecond domain pulsed CO_2 laser. Paper presented at 17th Annual Meeting of American Society of Lasers in Medicine and Surgery, Phoenix, April 1997.
275. Brugmans MJP, Kemper J, Gijsbers GHM et al: Temperature response of biological materials to pulsed non-ablative CO_2 laser irradiation, *Lasers Surg Med* 11:587, 1991.
276. Polatnick J, La Tessa AJ, Katzin HM: Comparison of collagen preparations from beef cornea and sclera, *Biochim Biophys Acta* 26:365, 1957.
277. Lans LJ: Experimentelle Untersuchungen über Entstehung von Astigmatismus durch nicht-perforirende Corneawunden, *Graefes Arch Ophthalmol* 45:117, 1898.
278. Wray C: Case of 6 D of hypermetropic astigmatism cured by the cautery, *Trans Ophthalmol Soc UK* 34:109, 1914.
279. O'Connor R: Corneal cautery for high myopic astigmatism, *Am J Ophthalmol* 16:337, 1933.
280. Shaw EL, Gasset AR: Thermokeratoplasty (TKP) temperature profile, *Invest Ophthalmol* 13:181, 1974.
281. Gasset AR, Shaw EL, Kaufman HE et al: Thermokeratoplasty, *Trans Acad Ophthalmol Otol* 77:OP441, 1973.
282. Stringer H, Parr J: Shrinkage temperature of eye collagen, *Nature,* December 1964, p 1307.
283. Horn G, Spears KG, Lopez O et al: New refractive method for laser thermal keratoplasty with the Co:MgF_2 laser, *J Cataract Refract Surg* 16:611, 1990.
284. Parel JM, Ren Q, Simon G: Noncontact laser photothermal keratoplasty. I. Biophysical principles and laser beam delivery system, *J Refract Corneal Surg* 10:511, 1994.
285. Aquavella JV: Thermokeratoplasty, *Ophthal Surg* 5:39, 1974.
286. Aquavella JV, Buxton JN, Shaw EL: Thermokeratoplasty in the treatment of persistent corneal hydrops, *Arch Ophthalmol* 95:81, 1977.
287. Keates RH, Dingle J: Thermokeratoplasty for keratoconus, *Ophthal Surg* 6:89, 1975.
288. Fogle JA, Kenyon KR, Stark WJ: Damage to epithelial basement membrane by thermokeratoplasty, *Am J Ophthalmol* 83:392, 1977.
289. Aquavella JV, Smith RS, Shaw EL: Alterations in corneal morphology following thermokeratoplasty, *Arch Ophthalmol* 94:2082, 1976.

290. Arenstein JJ, Rodrigues MM, Laibson PR: Histopathologic changes after thermokeratoplasty for keratoconus, *Invest Ophthalmol Vis Sci* 16:32, 1977.
291. Itoi M: Computer photokeratometry changes following thermokeratoplasty. In Schachar RA, Levy NS, Schachar L, editors: *Refractive modulation of the cornea,* Denison, Texas, 1981, LAL.
292. Rowsey JJ, Gaylor JR, Dahlstrom R et al: Los Alamos keratoplasty techniques, *Contact Intraocular Lens Med J* 6:1, 1980.
293. Rowsey JJ, Doss JD: Preliminary report of Los Alamos keratoplasty techniques, *Ophthalmology* 88:755, 1981.
294. Neumann AC, Fyodorov S, Sanders DR; Radial thermokeratoplasty for the correction of hyperopia, *J Refract Corneal Surg* 6:404, 1990.
295. Neumann AC, Sanders D, Raanan M et al: Hyperopic thermokeratoplasty: clinical evaluation, *J Cataract Refract Surg* 17:830, 1991.
296. Neumann AC: Thermokeratoplasty for hyperopia, *Ophthalmol Clin North Am* 5:753, 1992.
297. Rowsey JJ: Electrosurgical keratoplasty: update and retraction, *Invest Ophthalmol Vis Sci* 28(suppl):224, 1987.
298. Feldman ST, Ellis W, Frucht-Pery J et al: Regression of effect following radial thermokeratoplasty in humans, *J Refract Corneal Surg* 5:288, 1989.
299. Thompson VM, Seiler T, Durrie DS et al: Holmium:YAG laser thermokeratoplasty for hyperopia and astigmatism: an overview, *J Refract Corneal Surg* 9:134,1993.
300. Mainstern MA: Ophthalmic applications of infrared lasers: thermal considerations, *Invest Ophthalmol Vis Sci* 18:414, 1979.
301. Beckman H, Fuller TA, Boyman R et al: Carbon dioxide laser surgery of the eye and adnexa, *Ophthalmology* 87:990, 1980.
302. Peyman GA, Larson B, Raichand M et al: Modification of rabbit corneal curvature with use of carbon dioxide laser burns, *Ophthal Surg* 11:325, 1980.
303. Householder J, Horwitz LS, Lowe K Murillo A: Laser induced thermal keratoplasty, *SPIE Proc* 1066:18, 1989.
304. McCally RL, Bargeron CB, Green WR et al: Stromal damage in rabbit corneas exposed to CO_2 laser radiation, *Exp Eye Res* 37:543, 1983.
305. Kanoda AN, Sorokin AS: Laser correction of hypermetropic refraction. In Fyodorov SN, editor: *Microsurgery of the eye: main aspects,* Moscow, 1987, MIR.
306. Spears KG, Horn G, Serafin J: Corneal refractive correction by laser thermal keratoplasty, *Proc SPIE* 1202:334, 1990.
307. Zhou Z, Ren QS, Simon G et al: Thermal modeling of laser photothermokeratoplasty (LPTK), *SPIE Proc* 1644:61, 1992.
308. Durrie DS, Seiler T, King MC et al: Application of the holmium:YAG laser for refractive surgery, *SPIE Proc* 1644:56, 1992.
309. Seiler T: Ho:YAG laser thermokeratoplasty for hyperopia, *Ophthalmol Clin North Am* 5:773, 1992.
310. Koch DD, Berry MJ, Vassiliadis A et al: Non-contact holmium:YAG laser thermal keratoplasty. In Salz JJ, editor: *Corneal laser surgery,* Philadelphia, 1994, Mosby.
311. Ariyasu RG, Sand B, Menefee R et al: Holmium laser thermal keratoplasty of 10 poorly sighted eyes, *J Refract Surg* 11:358, 1995.
312. Koch DD, Abarca A, Villarreal R et al: Hyperopic correction by non-contact holmium:YAG laser thermal keratoplasty: clinical study with two year follow-up, *Ophthalmology* 22:362, 1996.
313. Koch DD, Kohnen T, McDonnell PJ et al: Hyperopia correction by non-contact holmium:YAG laser thermal keratoplasty: U.S. Phase IIA clinical study with 1-year follow-up, *Ophthalmology,* 1998 (in press).
314. Moreira H, Campos M, Sawusch MR et al: Holmium laser thermokeratoplasty, *Ophthalmology* 100:752, 1993.
315. Seiler T, Matallana M, Bende T: Laser thermokeratoplasty by means of a pulsed holmium:YAG laser for hyperoptic correction, *Refract Corneal Surg* 6:335, 1990.
316. Koch DD: Histological changes and wound healing response following non-contact holmium:YAG laser thermal keratoplasty, *Trans Am Ophthalmol Soc* 94:745, 1996.
317. Koch DD, Kohnen T, Anderson JA et al: Histologic changes and wound healing response following 10-pulse non-contact holmium:YAG laser thermal keratoplasty, *J Refract Surg* 12:623, 1996.

318. Ren Q, Simon G, Parel JM: Non-contact laser photothermal keratoplasty. III. Histological study in animal eyes, *J Refract Corneal Surg* 10:529, 1994.
319. Farrell RA, Bargeron CB, McCally RL et al: Corneal effects produced by IR laser radiation: laser safety, eyesafe laser systems, and laser eye protection, *SPIE Proc* 1207:59, 1990.
320. Fing PT, Richards R, Iwamoto T et al: Heat shrinkage of extraocular muscle tendon, *Arch Ophthalmol* 105:716, 1987.
321. Hayashi K, Markel MD, Thabit G III et al: The effect of non-ablative laser energy on joint capsular properties: an in-vitro mechanical study using a rabbit model, *Am J Sports Med* 23:482, 1995.
322. Dillingham MF, Price JM, Fanton GS: Holmium laser surgery, *Orthopedics* 16:563, 1993.
323. Sherk HH: Current concepts review: the use of lasers in orthopaedic procedures, *J Bone Joint Surg* 75A:768, 1993.
324. Thabit G: Treatment of unidirectional and multidirectional glenohumeral instability by an arthroscopic holmium:YAG laser-assisted capsular shift procedure: a pilot study. In *Laser application in arthroscopy*, Neuchatel, Switzerland, 1994, International Musculoskeletal Laser Society.
325. Hayashi K, Thabit G III, Massa KL et al: The effect of thermal heating on the length and histologic properties of the glenohumeral joint capsule, *Am J Sports Med* 25:107, 1997.
326. Tang J, Godlewski G, Rouy S et al: Morphologic changes in collagen fibers after 830 nm diode laser welding, *Lasers Surg Med* 21:438, 1997.
327. Tang J, O'Calaghan D, Rouy S et al: Quantity change in collagen following 830 nm diode laser welding, *Proc SPIE* 2922:432, 1996.
328. Bass LS, Moazami N, Procsidio J et al: Changes in type I collagen following laser welding, *Lasers Surg Med* 12:500, 1992.
329. Bass LS, Treat MR, Dzakonski C, Trokel SL: Sutureless microvascular anastomosis using the THC:YAG laser: a preliminary report, *Microsurgery* 10:189, 1989.
330. Murray LW, Su L, Kopchok GE et al: Cross-linking of extracellular matrix proteins: a preliminary report on possible mechanism of argon laser welding, *Lasers Surg Med* 9:490, 1989.
331. Schober R, Ulrich F, Sander T et al: Laser-induced alteration of collagen substructure allows microsurgical tissue welding, *Science* 232:1421, 1986.
332. Oz MC, Bass LS, Popp HW et al: In vitro comparison of thulium-holmium-chromium:YAG and argon lasers for welding of biliary tissue, *Lasers Surg Med* 9:248, 1989.
333. Oz MC, Chuck RS, Johnson JP et al: Indocyanine green dye–enhanced welding with a diode laser, *Surg Forum* 40:316, 1989.
334. Anderson RR, Lemole GM Jr, Kaplan R et al: Molecular mechanisms of thermal tissue welding. Part 2, *Lasers Surg Med Suppl* 6:56, 1994 (abstract).
335. Lemole GM, Anderson RR, DeCoste S: Preliminary evaluation of collagen as a component in the thermally induced "weld," *Proc SPIE* 1422:116, 1991.
336. Solhpour S, Weldon E, Foster TE et al: Mechanism of thermal tissue "welding." Part I, *Lasers Surg Med Suppl* 6:56, 1994 (abstract).
337. White RA, Kopchok GE, White GH et al: Laser vascular anastomotic welding. In White RA, Grundfest WS, editors: *Lasers in cardiovascular disease*, Chicago, 1987,Year Book.
338. White RA, Kopchok G, Donayre C et al: Argon laser–welded arteriovenous anastomosis, *J Vasc Surg* 6:447, 1987.
339. White RA, Kopchok G, Donarye C et al: Comparison of laser-welded and sutured arteriotomies, *Arch Surg* 121:1133, 1996.
340. White RA, Abergel RP, Klein SR et al: Laser welding of venotomies, *Arch Surg* 121:905, 1986.
341. White RA, Kopchok G, Donayre CE et al: Mechanism of tissue fusion in argon laser welded vein-artery anastomosis, *Lasers Surg Med* 8:83, 1988.
342. Popp HW, Oz MC, Bass LS et al: Welding of gallbladder tissue using a pulsed 2.15 micron thulium-holmium-chromium:YAG laser, *Lasers Surg Med* 9:155, 1989.
343. Quigley MR, Bailes JE, Kwaan HC, Heiferman K: Microvascular laser-assisted anastomosis: results at one year, *Lasers Surg Med* 6:179, 1986 (abstract).
344. Quigley MR, Bailes JE, Kwaan HC et al: Microvascular anastomosis using the milliwatt CO_2 laser, *Lasers Surg Med* 5:357, 1985.

345. Abergel RP, Lyons RF, White RA et al: Skin closure by Nd:YAG laser welding, *J Am Acad Dermatol* 14:810, 1986.
346. Abergel RP, Lyons RF, Dwyer R et al: Use of lasers for closure of cutaneous wounds: experience with Nd:YAG, argon, and CO_2 lasers, *J Dermatol Surg Oncol* 12:1181, 1986.
347. Jain KK: Sutureless microvascular extra-intracranial anastomosis with Nd:YAG laser, *Lasers Surg Med* 3:311, 1984 (abstract).
348. Ashworth EM, Dalsing MC, Olson JF et al: Large-artery welding with a milliwatt carbon dioxide laser, *Arch Surg* 122:673, 1987.
349. Chuck RS, Oz MC, Delohery TM et al: Dye-enhanced laser tissue welding, *Lasers Surg Med* 9:471, 1989.
350. Pribil S, Powers SK: Carotid artery end-to-end anastomosis in the rat using the argon laser, *J Neurosurg* 63:771, 1985.
351. McCarthy WJ, Hartz RS, Yao JST et al: Vascular anastomoses with laser energy, *J Vasc Surg* 3:32, 1986.
352. Frazier OH, Painvin GA, Morris JR et al: Laser-assisted microvascular anastomoses: angiographic and anatomopathological studies on growing microvascular anastomoses: preliminary report, *Surgery* 97:585, 1985.
353. Sigel B, Dunn MR: The mechanism of blood vessel closure by high frequency electrocoagulation, *Surg Gynecol Obstet* 121:823, 1965.
354. Guthrie CR, Murray LW, Kopchok GE et al: Biochemical mechanisms of laser vascular tissue fusion, *J Invest Surg* 4:3, 1991.
355. Serure A, Wither EH, Thomsen S, Morris J: Comparison of carbon dioxide laser–assisted microvascular anastomosis and conventional microvascular sutured anastomosis, *Surg Forum* 34:634, 1983.
356. White RA, Kopchok G, Peng SK et al: Laser vascular welding: how does it work? *Ann Vasc Surg* 1:461, 1986.
357. Kopchok G, White RA, Grundfest WS et al: Thermal studies in in-vivo vascular tissue fusion by argon laser, *J Invest Surg* 1:5, 1988.
358. Kopchok WS, Grundfest WS, White RA et al: Argon laser vascular welding: the thermal component, *SPIE Lasers Med* 712:260, 1986.
359. Epstein M, Cooley CB: Electron microscopic study of laser dosimetry for microvascular tissue welding, *Lasers Surg Med* 6:202, 1986.
360. Weinstein C: Carbon dioxide laser resurfacing: Long-term follow-up in 2123 patients, *Clin Plast Surg* 25:109, 1998.
361. Fitzpatrick RE, Manuskiatti W, Goldman MP: Long-term effectiveness and side effects of carbon dioxide laser resurfacing for photoaged facial skin, *J Am Acad Dermatol,* 1998 (submitted for publication).
362. Burns JA: Personal communication, 1997.
363. Ross EV, Grossman MC, Duke D, Grevelink JM: Long-term results after CO_2 laser skin resurfacing: a comparison of scanned and pulsed systems, *J Am Acad Dermatol* 37:709, 1997.
364. Reed JT, Joseph AK, Bridenstine JB: Treatment of periorbital wrinkles: a comparison of the SilkTouch carbon dioxide laser with a medium-depth chemical peel, *Dermatol Surg* 23:643, 1997.
365. Abergel RP, Dahlman CM: The CO_2 laser approach to the treatment of acne scarring, *Cosmet Dermatol* 8:33, 1995.
366. Alster TS, West TB: Resurfacing of atrophic facial acne scars with a high-energy, pulsed carbon dioxide laser, *Dermatol Surg* 22:151, 1996.
367. Hruza JG: Skin resurfacing with lasers, *Fitzpatrick's J Clin Dermatol* 3:38, 1995.
368. Alamillos-Granados FJ, Naval-Gias L, Dean-Ferrer A et al: Carbon dioxide laser vermilionectomy for actinic cheilitis, *J Oral Maxillofac Surg* 51:118, 1993.
369. Stanley RJ, Roenigk RK: Actinic cheilitis: treatment with the carbon dioxide laser, *Mayo Clin Proc* 63:230, 1988.
370. Robinson JK: Actinic cheilitis: a prospective study comparing four treatment methods, *Arch Otolaryngol Head Neck Surg* 115:848, 1989.
371. Zelickson BD, Roenigk RK: Actinic cheilitis: treatment with the carbon dioxide laser, *Cancer* 65:1307, 1990.
372. Dufresne RJ, Garrett AB, Bailin PL et al: Carbon dioxide laser treatment of chronic actinic cheilitis, *J Am Acad Dermatol* 19:876, 1988.

373. Johnson TM, Sebastien TS, Lowe L et al: Carbon dioxide laser treatment of actinic cheilitis: clinicohistopathologic correlation to determine the optimal depth of destruction, *J Am Acad Dermatol* 27:737, 1992.
374. Ries WR, Duncavage JA, Ossoff RH: Carbon dioxide laser treatment of actinic cheilitis, *Mayo Clin Proc* 63:294, 1988.
375. Scheinberg RS: Carbon dioxide laser treatment of actinic cheilitis, *West J Med* 156:192, 1992.
376. Whitaker DC: Microscopically proven cure of actinic cheilitis by CO_2 laser, *Lasers Surg Med* 7:520, 1987.
377. Frankel DH: Carbon dioxide laser vermilionectomy for chronic actinic cheilitis, *Facial Plast Surg* 6:158, 1989.
378. Goldman MP, Fitzpatrick RE, Smith SS: Resurfacing complications and their management. In Coleman WP, Lawrence N, editors: *Laser resurfacing*, Baltimore, 1997, William & Wilkins.
379. Lowe NJ, Lask G, Griffin ME: Laser skin resurfacing: pre- and post-treatment guidelines, *Dermatol Surg* 21:1017, 1995.
380. Fitzpatrick RE, Goldman MP: Laser treatment of benign pigmented lesions using a 300 nanosecond pulse and 510 nm wavelength, *J Dermatol Surg Oncol* 19:341, 1993.
381. Goldberg D: Benign pigmented lesions of the skin: treatment with the Q-switched ruby laser, *J Dermatol Surg Oncol* 19:376, 1993.
382. Brauner GJ, Schliftman AB: Treatment of pigmented lesions of the skin with the alexandrite laser, *Lasers Surg Med* 4:72, 1992.
383. Monheit GD: The Jessner's + TCA peel: a medium-depth chemical peel, *J Dermatol Surg Oncol* 15:945, 1989.
384. Brody HJ, Hailey CW: Medium-depth chemical peeling of the skin: a variation of superficial chemosurgery, *J Dermatol Surg Oncol* 12:1268, 1986.
385. Taylor CR, Anderson RR: Ineffective treatment of refractory melasma and postinflammatory hyperpigmentation by Q-switched ruby laser, *J Dermatol Surg Oncol* 20:592, 1994.
386. Greenbaum SS, Krull EA, Watnich K: Comparison of CO_2 laser and electrosurgery in the treatment of rhinophyma, *J Am Acad Dermatol* 18:363, 1988.
387. Wheeland RG, Bailin PL, Ratz JL: Combined carbon dioxide laser excision and vaporization in the treatment of rhinophyma, *J Dermatol Surg Oncol* 13:172, 1987.
388. Apfelberg DB, Maser MR, Lash H et al: Superpulse CO_2 laser treatment of facial syringomata, *Lasers Surg Med* 7:533, 1987.
389. Wheeland RG, Bailin PL, Kronberg E: Carbon dioxide (CO_2) laser vaporization for the treatment of multiple trichoepithelioma, *J Dermatol Surg Oncol* 10:470, 1984.
390. Apfelberg DB, Maser MR, Lash H et al: Treatment of xanthelasma palpebrum with the carbon dioxide laser, *J Dermatol Surg Oncol* 13:149, 1987.
391. Wheeland RG, Bailin PL, Kantor GR et al: Treatment of adenoma sebaceum with carbon dioxide laser vaporization, *J Dermatol Surg Oncol* 11:861, 1985.
392. Ratz JL, Bailin PL, Wheeland RG: Carbon dioxide laser treatment of epidermal nevi, *J Dermatol Surg Oncol* 12:567, 1986.
393. Hohenleutner U, Landthaler M: Laser therapy of verrucous epidermal nevi, *Clin Exp Dermatol* 18:124, 1993.
394. Blitzer A, Brin MF, Keen MS et al: Botulinum toxin for the treatment of hyperfunctional lines of the face, *Arch Otolaryngol Head Neck Surg* 119:1018, 1993.
395. Carruthers JDA, Carruthers JA: Treatment of glabellar frown lines with *C. botulinum*-A exotoxin, *J Dermatol Surg Oncol* 18:17, 1992.
396. Garcia A, Fulton JE: Cosmetic denervation of the muscles of facial expression with botulinum toxin: a dose-response study, *Dermatol Surg* 22:39, 1996.
397. Keen M, Blitzer A, Aviv J et al: Botulinum toxin-A for hyperkinetic facial lines: results of a double-blind, placebo-controlled study, *Plast Reconstr Surg* 94:94, 1994.
398. Weinstein C, Ramirez OM, Pozner JN: Postoperative care following CO_2 laser resurfacing: avoiding pitfalls, *Plast Reconstr Surg* 100:1855, 1997.
399. Raz R, Miron D, Colodner R, Staler Z et al: A 1-year trial of nasal mupirocin in the prevention of recurrent staphylococcal nasal colonization and skin infection, *Arch Intern Med* 156:1109, 1996.
400. Sriprachya-anunt S, Fitzpatrick RE, Goldman MP et al: Infections complicating CO_2 laser resurfacing, *Dermatol Surg* 23:527, 1997.

401. Goldman MP, Fitzpatrick RE.
402. Russell SW, Dinehart SM, Davis I, Flock ST: Efficacy of corneal shields in protecting patients' eyes from laser irradiation, *Dermatol Surg* 22:613, 1996.
403. Fitzpatrick RE, Williams B, Goldman MP: Preoperative anesthesia and postoperative considerations in laser resurfacing, *Semin Cutan Med Surg* 15:170, 1996.
404. Dvork HF: Tumors: wounds that do not heal: similarities between tumor stroma generation and wound healing, *N Engl J Med* 315:1650, 1986.
405. Peacock EE Jr: Inflammation and the cellular response to injury. In Peacock EE Jr, editor: *Wound repair,* Philadelphia, 1984, Saunders.
406. Peacock EE Jr: Biological and pharmacological control of scar tissue. In Peacock EE Jr, editor: *Wound repair,* Philadelphia, 1984, Saunders.
407. Kanzler MH, Gorsulowsky DC, Swanson NA: Basic mechanisms in the healing cutaneous wound, *J Dermatol Surg Oncol* 12:1156, 1986.
408. Goslen JB: Wound healing for the dermatologic surgeon, *J Dermatol Surg Oncol* 14:959, 1988.
409. Stenn KS, Malhotra R: Epithelialization. In Cohen IK, Diegelmann RF, Lindblad WJ, editors: *Wound healing: biochemical and clinical aspects,* Philadelphia, 1992, Saunders.
410. Waldorf H, Fewkes J: Wound healing, *Adv Dermatol* 10:77, 1995
411. Bach R, Nemerson Y, Konigsberg W: Purification and characterization of bovine tissue factor, *J Biol Chem* 256:8324, 1981.
412. Leibovich SJ, Ross R: A macrophage-dependent factor that stimulates the proliferation of fibroblasts in vitro, *Am J Pathol* 84:501, 1976.
413. Leibovich SJ, Ross R: The role of the macrophage in wound repair: a study with hydrocortisone and antimacrophage serum, *Am J Pathol* 78:71, 1975.
414. Shavit ZB, Ray A, Goldman R: Complement and Fc receptor-mediated phagocytosis of normal and stimulated mouse peritoneal macrophages, *Eur J Immunol* 9:385, 1979.
415. Littman BH, Ruddy S: Production of the second component of complement by human monocytes: stimulation by antigen-activated lymphocytes or lymphokines, *J Exp Med* 145:1344, 1979.
416. Clark RAF: Cutaneous tissue repair: basic biologic considerations, *J Am Acad Dermatol* 13:701, 1985.
417. Clark RAF: Basics of cutaneous wound repair, *J Dermatol Surg Oncol* 19:693, 1993.
418. Krummel TM, Nelson JM, Diegelmann RF et al: Fetal response to injury in the rabbit, *J Pediatr Surg* 22:640, 1987.
419. DePalma RL, Krummel TM, Nelson JM et al: Fetal wound matrix is composed of proteoglycan rather than collagen, *Surg Forum* 38:626, 1987.
420. Longaker MT, Adzick NS, Hall JL et al: Studies in fetal wound healing. VII. Fetal wound healing may be modulated by hyaluronic acid stimulating activity in amniotic fluid, *J Pediatr Surg* 25:430, 1990.
421. Mast BA, Diegelmann RF, Krummel TM, Cohen IK: Hyaluronic acid modulates proliferation, collagen and protein synthesis of cultured fetal fibroblasts, *Matrix* 13:441, 1993.
422. Mast BA, Haynes JH, Krummel TM et al: In vivo degradation of fetal wound hyaluronic acid results in increased fibroplasia, collagen deposition, and neovascularization, *Plast Reconstr Surg* 89:503, 1992.
423. Hellstrom S, Laurent C: Hyaluronan and healing of tympanic membrane perforations: an experimental study, *Acta Otolaryngol Suppl (Stockh)* 442:54, 1987.
424. Bertheim U, Hellstrom S: The distribution of hyaluronan in human skin and mature, hypertrophic and keloid scars, *Br J Plast Surg* 47:483, 1994.
425. Passarini B, Tosti A, Fanti PA, Varotti C: [Effect of hyaluronic acid on the reparative process of non-healing ulcers: comparative study], *G Ital Dermatol Venereol* 117:XXVII, 1982.
426. Torregrossa F, Caroti A: [Clinical verification of the use of topical hyaluronic acid under non-adhesive gauze in the therapy of torpid ulcers], *G Ital Dermatol Venereol* 118:XLI, 1983.
427. Venturini D: [Clinical observations on the use of hyaluronic acid in dermatologic therapy], *G Ital Dermatol Venereol* 120:V, 1985.
428. Celleno L, Piperno S, Bracaglia R: [Clinico-experimental studies on the use of hyaluronic acid in skin healing processes: preliminary data], *G Ital Dermatol Venereol* 120:XLVII, 1985.

429. Retanda G: [Hyaluronic acid in the process of reparation of cutaneous ulcers: clinical experience], *G Ital Dermatol Venereol* 120:LXXI, 1985.
430. Abatangela G, Martelli M, Vecchia P: Healing of hyaluronic acid–enriched wounds: histological observations, *J Surg Res* 35:410, 1983.
431. Trabucchi E, Preis-Baruffaldi F, Baratti C, Montorsi W: Topical treatment of experimental skin lesions in rats: macroscopic, microscopic and scanning electron-microscopic evaluation of the healing process, *Int J Tissue React* 8:533, 1986.
432. King SR, Hickerson WL, Proctor KG: Beneficial actions of exogenous hyaluronic acid in wound healing, *Surgery* 109:76, 1991.
433. Laurent C, Hellstrom S, Fellenius E: Hyaluronan improves the healing of experimental tympanic membrane perforations: a comparison of preparations with different rheologic properties, *Arch Otolaryngol Head Neck Surg* 114:1435, 1988.
434. Doillon CJ, Dunn MG, Berg RA, Silver FH: Collagen deposition during wound repair, *Scanning Electron Microsc* 00:897, 1985.
435. Doillon CJ, Silver FH: Collagen-based wound dressing: effects of hyaluronic acid and fibronectin on wound healing, *Biomaterials* 7:3, 1986.
436. Burd DA, Greco RM, Regauer S et al: Hyaluronan and wound healing: a new perspective, *Br J Plast Surg* 44:579, 1991.
437. Borgognoni L, Reali UM, Santucci M: Low molecular weight hyaluronic acid induces angiogenesis and modulation of the cellular infiltrate in primary and secondary healing wounds, *Eur J Dermatol* 6:127, 1996.
438. Bailey AJ, Bazin S, Sims TJ et al: Characterization of the collagen of human hypertrophic and normal scars, *Biochim Biophys Acta* 21:404, 1974.
439. Oliver N, Baba M, Diegelmann R: Fibronectin gene transcription is enhanced in abnormal wound healing, *J Invest Dermatol* 99:579, 1992.
440. Skuta GL, Parrish RK II: Wound healing in glaucoma filtering surgery, *Surv Ophthalmol* 32:149, 1987.
441. Ross R, Raines EW, Bowen-Pope DR: The biology of platelet-derived growth factor, *Cell* 46:155, 1986.
442. Ross R: Fibroblast proliferation induced by blood cells, *Agents Actions Suppl* 7:81, 1980.
443. White A, Handler P, Smith EL: *Principles of biochemistry,* New York, 1978, McGraw-Hill.
444. Bijrkedal-Hansen H: Catabolism and turnover of collagens: collagenases, *Methods Enzymol* 144:140, 1987.
445. Liu X, Wu H, Byrne M et al: A targeted mutation at the known collagenase cleavage site in mouse type I collagen impairs tissue remodeling, *J Cell Biol* 130:227, 1995.
446. Matrisian LM, Hogan BL: Growth factor–regulated proteases and extracellular matrix remodeling during mammalian development, *Curr Top Dev Biol* 24:219, 1990.
447. Prockop D, Kivirikko K: Heritable diseases of collagen, *N Engl J Med* 311:376, 1984.
448. Mast BA: The skin. In Cohen IK, Diegelmann RF, Lindblad WJ, editors: *Wound healing: biochemical and clinical aspects,* Philadelphia, 1992, Saunders.
449. Lamberg SI, Stoolmiller AC: Glycosaminoglycans: a biochemical and clinical review, *J Invest Dermatol* 63:433, 1974.
450. VanLis JM, Kalsbeek GL: Glycosaminoglycans in human skin, *Br J Dermatol* 88:355, 1973.
451. Levensen SM, Geever EG, Crowley LV et al: The healing of rat skin wounds, *Ann Surg* 161:293, 1965.
452. Rudolph R: Contraction and the control of contraction, *World J Surg* 4:279, 1980.
453. Gabbiani G, Ryan GB, Majne G: Presence of modified fibroblasts in granulation tissue and their possible role in wound contraction, *Experientia* 27:549, 1971.
454. Majno G: Contraction of granulation tissue in vitro: similarity to smooth muscle, *Science* 173:543, 1971.
455. Rudolph R, Berg JV, Ehrlich HP: Wound contraction and scar contracture. In Cohen IK, Diegelmann RF, Linblad WJ, editors: *Wound healing: biochemical and clinical sspects,* Philadelphia, 1992, Saunders.
456. Schaffer CJ, Reinisch L, Polis SL et al: Comparisons of wound healing among excisional, laser-created, and standard thermal burns in porcine wounds of equal depth, *Wound Rep Reg* 5:52, 1997.
457. Fisher AA: Lasers and allergic contact dermatitis to topical antibiotics, with particular reference to bacitracin, *Cutis* 58:252, 1996.

458. Dooms-Goossens A, Degreef H: Contact allergy to petrolatums. II. Attempts to identify the nature of allergens, *Contact Dermatitis* 9:247, 1983.
459. Smack DP, Harrington AC, Dunn C et al: Infection and allergy incidence in ambulatory surgery patients using white petrolatum vs. bacitracin ointment, *JAMA* 276:972, 1996.
460. Hunter GR, Change FC: Outpatient burns: a prospective study, *J Trauma* 16:191, 1976.
461. Eaglstein WH, Mertz PM: "Inert" vehicles do affect wound healing, *J Invest Dermatol* 74:90, 1980.
462. Winter GD: Formation of scab and rate of epithelialization of superficial wounds in the skin of the domestic pig, *Nature* 193:293, 1962.
463. Hinman CC, Maibach H, Winter GD: Effect of air exposure and occlusion on experimental human skin wounds, *Nature* 200:377, 1963.
464. Rovee DY, Kurowsky CA, Lobun J et al: Effect of local wound environment on epidermal healing. In Maibach HL, Rovee DT, editors: *Epidermal wound healing,* Chicago, 1972, Year Book.
465. Geronemus RG, Robins P: The effect of two new dressings on epidermal wound healing, *J Dermatol Surg Oncol* 8:850, 1982.
466. Mandy S: A new primary wound dressing made of polyethylene oxide gel, *J Dermatol Surg Oncol* 9:153, 1983.
467. May SR: Physiology, immunology and clinical efficacy of an adherent polyurethane wound dressing: Op-Site. In Wise DL, editor: *Burn wound coverings,* vol 2, Boca Raton, Fla, 1984, CRC.
468. Eaglstein WH, Mertz PM: New methods for assessing epidermal wound healing: the effects of triamcinolone acetonide and polyethylene film occlusion, *J Invest Dermatol* 71:382, 1978.
469. Barnett A, Berkowitz RL, Mius R et al: Comparison of synthetic adhesive moisture vapor permeable and fine mesh gauze dressings for split-thickness skin graft donor sites, *Am J Surg* 145:379, 1983.
470. VanRijswijk L, Brown D, Friedman S et al: Multicenter clinical evaluation of hydrocolloid dressing for leg ulcers, *Cutis* 35:173, 1985.
471. Eaton AC: A controlled trial to evaluate and compare a sutureless skin closure technique (Op-Site skin closure) with conventional skin suturing and clipping in abdominal surgery, *Br J Surg* 67:857, 1980.
472. Kannon GA, Garrett AB: Moist wound healing with occlusive dressings: a clinical review, *Dermatol Surg* 21:583, 1995.
473. Eaglstein WH: Experiences with biosynthetic dressings, *J Am Acad Dermatol* 12:434, 1985.
474. Bolton LL, Johnson CL, Rijswijk LV: Occlusive dressings: therapeutic agents and effects on drug delivery, *Clin Dermatol* 9:573, 1992.
475. Winter GD: Epidermal regeneration studied in the domestic pig. In Maibach HL, Rovee DT, editors: *Epidermal wound healing,* Chicago, 1972, Year Book.
476. Alvarez OM, Mertz PM, Eaglstein WH: The effect of occlusive dressings on collagen synthesis and re-epithelialization in superficial wounds, *J Surg Res* 35:142, 1983.
477. Brown GL, Curtsinger L III, Brightwell JR et al: Enhancement of epidermal regeneration by biosynthetic epidermal growth factor, *J Exp Med* 163:1319, 1986.
478. Raab B: A new hydrophilic copolymer membrane for dermabrasion, *J Dermatol Surg Oncol* 17:323, 1991.
479. Wheeland RG: Wound healing and the newer surgical dressings. In Moschella SL, Hurley HJ et al, editors: *Dermatology,* Philadelphia, 1992, Saunders.
480. Afilalo M, Guttman A, Lloyd J: DuoDerm hydroactive dressing versus silver sulphadiazine/Bactigras in the emergency treatment of partial skin thickness burns, *Burns* 18:313, 1992.
481. Thomas S: Wound management: use of a calcium alginate dressing.
482. Passe ER, Blaine G: *Lancet* 2:651, 1948.
483. Oliver LC, Blaine G: *Br J Surg* 147:307, 1950.
484. Frantz VK: *Ann Surg* 127:1165, 1948.
485. Eaglstein WH, Davis SC, Mehle AL, Mertz PM: Optimal use of an occlusive dressing to enhance healing: effect of delayed application and early removal on wound healing, *Arch Dermatol* 124:392, 1988.
486. Mertz PM, Eaglstein WH: The effect of semi-occlusive dressing on the microbial population in superficial wounds, *Arch Surg* 119:287, 1984.

487. Geronemus RG, Mertz PM, Eaglstein WH: The effects of topical antimicrobial agents, *Arch Dermatol* 115:1311, 1979.
488. Linsky CB, Rovee DT, Dow T: Effect of dressing on wound inflammation and scar tissue. In Dineen P, Hildick-Smith G, editors: *The surgical wound,* Philadelphia, 1981, Lea & Febiger.
489. Marples RR: The effect of hydration on the bacterial flora of the skin. In Maibach HI, Hildick-Smith G, editors: *Skin bacteria and their role in infection,* New York, 1963, McGraw-Hill.
490. Buchan IA, Andrews JK, Lang SM: Laboratory investigation of the composition and properties of pig skin wound exudate under Op-Site, *Burns* 8:39, 1981.
491. Buchan IA, Andrews JK, Lang SM: Clinical and laboratory investigation of the composition and properties of human skin wound exudate under semi-permeable dressing, *Burns* 7:326, 1981.
492. Hutchison JJ, McGuckin M: Occlusive dressings: a microbiologic and clinical review, *Am J Infect Control* 18:257, 1990.
493. Handfield-Jones SE, Grattan CEH, Simpson RA et al: Comparison of a hydrocolloid dressing and paraffin gauze in the treatment of venous ulcers, *Br J Dermatol* 118:425, 1988.
494. Gilchrist B, Reed C: The bacteriology of chronic venous ulcers treated with occlusive hydrocolloid dressings, *Br J Dermatol* 121:337, 1989.
495. Leydon JL, Steward R, Kligman AM: Updated in vivo methods for evaluating topical antimicrobial agent on human skin, *J Invest Dermatol* 72:165, 1979.
496. Oliveria-Gandia M, Davis SC, Mertz PM: Can occlusive dressing composition influence proliferation of bacterial wound pathogens? *Wounds* 10:4, 1998.
497. Reynolds JEF: *The extra pharmacopocia,* ed 29, London, 1989, Pharmaceutical Press.
498. Ahmed K, Roberts ML, Mammion PT: Antimicrobial activity of glycerine-ichthammaol in otitis externa, *Clin Otolaryngol* 20:201, 1995.
499. Fitzpatrick RE, Geronemus RG, Grevelink JM et al: The incidence of adverse healing reactions occurring with UltraPulse CO_2 resurfacing during a multicenter study, *Lasers Surg Med Suppl* 8:34, 1996.
500. Yurt RW: Burns. In Mandell GL, Bennett JE, Dolin R, editors: *Mandell, Douglas and Bennett's Principles and practice of infectious diseases,* New York, 1995, Churchill Livingstone.
501. Phillips LG, Heggers JP, Robson MC et al: The effect of endogenous skin bacteria on burn wound infection, *Ann Plast Surg* 23:35, 1989.
502. Husain MT, Karim QN, Tajuri S: Analysis of infection in a burn ward, *Burns* 15:299, 1989.
503. Monheit GD: Facial resurfacing may trigger the herpes simplex virus, *Cosmetic Dermatol* 8:9, 1995.
504. Shalita A: Personal communication, 1997.
505. Roberts TL, Lettieri JT, Ellis LB: CO_2 laser resurfacing: recognizing and minimizing complications, *Aesth Surg Q* 16:141, 1996.
506. Ziering CL: Cutaneous laser resurfacing with the erbium:YAG laser and the char-free carbon dioxide laser: a clinical comparison of 100 patients, *Int J Aesthetic Rest Surg* 5:29, 1997.
507. Hibst R, Kaufmann R: Fundamentals of pulsed UV and mid-infrared laser skin ablation. In Steiner R, Kaufmann R, Landthaler M, Braun-Falco O, editors: *Lasers in dermatology,* Berlin, 1991, Springer-Verlag.
508. Kaufmann R, Hibst R: Pulsed UV and mid-infrared laser skin ablation: experimental and first clinical results. In Steiner R, Kaufmann R, Landthaler M, Braun-Falco O, editors: *Lasers in dermatology,* Berlin, 1991, Springer-Verlag.
509. Hohenleutner U, Hohenleutner S, Bäumler, Landthaler M: Fast and effective skin ablation with an Er:YAG laser: determination of ablation rates and thermal damage zones, *Lasers Surg Med* 20:242, 1997.
510. Kaufmann R, Hibst R: Pulsed 2.94 μm erbium:YAG laser skin ablation: experimental results and first clinical application, *Clin Exp Dermatol* 15:389, 1990.
511. Drnovšek-Olup B, Vedlin B: Use of Er:YAG laser for benign skin disorders, *Lasers Surg Med* 21:13, 1997.
512. Kaufmann R, Hibst R: Pulsed erbium:YAG laser ablation in cutaneous surgery, *Lasers Surg Med* 19:324, 1996.

513. Walsh JT, Deutsch TF: Er:YAG laser ablation of tissue: measurement of ablation rates, *Lasers Surg Med* 9:327, 1989.
514. McDaniel DH, Ash K, Lord J et al: The erbium:YAG laser: a review and preliminary report on resurfacing of the face, neck and hands, *Aesthetic Surg J* 17:157, 1997.
515. Teikemeier G, Goldberg DJ: Skin resurfacing with the erbium:YAG laser, *Dermatol Surg* 23:685, 1997.
516. Hibst R, Kaufmann R: Effects of Laser parameters on pulsed erbium:YAG laser skin ablation, *Lasers Med Sci* 6:391, 1991.
517. Kaufmann R, Hartmann A, Hibst R: Cutting and skin ablative properties of pulsed mid-infrared laser surgery, *J Dermatol Surg Oncol* 20:112, 1994.
518. Kaufmann R, Hibst R: Pulsed Er:YAG and 308 nmn UV-excimer laser: an in vitro and in vivo study of skin ablative effects, *Lasers Surg Med* 9:132, 1989.
519. Walsh JT, Flotte TJ, Deutsch TF: Er:YAG laser ablation tissue: effect of pulse duration and tissue type on thermal damage, *Lasers Surg Med* 9:314, 1989.
520. Kaufmann R, Hibst R: Vergleich verschildener Mittelin-frafot: Laser für die ablation der Hauset, *Lasermedizin* 11:19, 1995.
521. Walsh JT: Pulsed laser ablation of tissue: analysis of the removal process and tissue healing, PhD. Thesis, Cambridge, Mass, 1988, MIT Archives.
522. Wolbarsht ML: Laser surgery: CO_2 or HF.IEEE, *J Quantum Electronics* 20:1427, 1984.

CHAPTER eight

Photodynamic Therapy

Harvey Lui and Robert Bissonnette

The treatment of diseased tissue using highly reactive oxygen intermediates generated from exogenous photosensitizers and light is called photodynamic therapy (PDT). During PDT, photosensitizers are first administered through the topical, intravenous, or oral routes and then activated in situ by a specific wavelength of light that varies according to the photosensitizer being used (Table 8-1). With the approval of porfimer sodium (Photofrin, a first-generation systemic photosensitizer) by the U.S. Food and Drug Administration (FDA) in 1995, PDT is no longer considered a strictly experimental therapy, although this first U.S. approval of PDT only covers the treatment of esophageal carcinoma.

This chapter reviews the mechanism of action of PDT, the use of lasers versus other light sources, the range of available photosensitizers, and the clinical use of PDT in dermatology.

HISTORIC BACKGROUND

The sequential use of an exogenous sensitizer followed by light for medical therapy was practiced in ancient India and Egypt.[1] These civilizations both used plant-derived psoralens and natural sunlight to induce pigmentation. However, the first specific description of photodynamic drug activation was published at the beginning of the twentieth century by von Tappeiner. Studying the effect of the dye acridine on paramecia, von Tappeiner's medical student, Raab, observed that the killing efficiency of acridine was influenced by the amount of light entering the laboratory during the experiments.[1,2] In subsequent studies with eosin, another photosensitizing dye, von Tappeiner showed that oxygen was required and that PDT was effective for treating skin cancer.[3,4] Around the same time, hematoporphyrin and light were used on paramecia, mice, and guinea pigs. Meyer-Betz[5] was the first to demonstrate long-term cutaneous photosensitivity after injecting himself with hematoporphyrin.

In 1942, Auler and Banzer[6] used hematoporphyrin and a quartz lamp to treat tumors in animals and humans. During the 1960s, Lipson et al.[7] studied the tumor-localizing properties of a related and newly formulated drug called *hematoporphyrin derivative* (HPD). Lipson et al.[8] were also the first to use a xenon arc lamp to activate HPD in a patient with recurrent breast cancer. In the 1970s, Dougherty et al,[9,10] working initially with animals and later with patients, showed that complete responses and long-term cure of malignant skin tumors with PDT were possible using HPD and light. Extensive fundamental and clinical research using HPD and porfimer sodium (a purified commercial version of HPD) for a variety of malignancies was subsequently undertaken during the 1970s and 1980s. This work culminated in the regulatory approval of porfimer sodium in several countries in the 1990s, beginning first with Canada in 1993.

Despite these approvals and numerous published clinical studies of PDT for skin tumors,[11-16] the pivotal controlled studies necessary to achieve FDA clearance of PDT for dermatology had not yet taken place as of 1998. The prolonged photosensitivity

Table 8-1
Activation wavelengths most frequently used for PDT photosensitizers

Photosensitizer	Activation Wavelength(s) (nm)
Porfimer sodium (Photofrin)	628-635
Aminolevulinic acid (ALA)*	630-635
Benzoporphyrin derivative (BPD, Verteporfin)	690
Tin ethyl etiopurpurin (SnET2)	664
Metatetrahydroxyphenylchlorin (mTHPC)	652
Mono-l-aspartylchlorin e6 (NPe6)	675

*Protoporphyrin IX is the active photosensitizer derived from ALA.

associated with first-generation photosensitizers and the high 5-year cure rates obtained with other treatment modalities for nonmelanoma skin cancer may have been disincentives to performing these studies. Furthermore, data in the literature have been scarce on long-term (2-5 or more years) tumor response rates after PDT. The shorter photosensitivity associated with second-generation photosensitizers, the development of topical photosensitizers, and the recent focus on treating premalignant lesions[17] and inflammatory dermatoses[18,19] are recent advances that may ultimately expedite the official recognition of PDT in dermatology. It is interesting and also perhaps ironic to note that, as with HPD and porfimer sodium, many second-generation photosensitizers synthesized since the 1980s have first been evaluated in patients with skin tumors.[20-23]

MECHANISM OF ACTION

PDT is mediated by oxygen-dependent photochemical reactions. During PDT, tissue-bound photosensitizers are first excited by light from their ground state to a short-lived, higher-energy singlet state, followed by a transition to the reactive triplet state (Figure 8-1). From its triplet state the photosensitizer then can react with molecular oxygen to form reactive species, such as singlet oxygen (*type II reaction,* which predominates in PDT), or can react directly with a cellular substrate to form free radicals or radical ions (*type I reaction,* which predominates in 8-methoxypsoralen and ultraviolet light type A irradiation [PUVA]).[24] In support of a major role for oxygen, in vivo and in vitro experiments have shown decreased or abolished PDT effects under anoxic conditions[24,25] as well as when manual pressure is applied to tumor tissue during light treatment.[26] Tissue oxygen rather than photosensitizer concentration or light fluence can thus be the limiting factor for PDT under certain conditions. Significant tumor hypoxia with porfimer sodium has been observed in animal models using light fluences as low as 4.5 J/cm^2. It has been hypothesized that hypoxic tumor cells may be resistant to PDT, thereby leading to subsequent tumor recurrence.[27]

Varying the mode of light delivery during PDT by using lower irradiances (to allow for a lower rate of oxygen consumption) or by fractionating the total light dose into a series of shorter exposures (to allow for tissue reoxygenation between exposures) are two strategies that may enhance PDT effects by promoting adequate tissue oxygen levels. In mice and rats, higher therapeutic responses in transplanted tumors were achieved when the total light dose was divided into alternating 30-second periods of light exposure followed by darkness, versus a single uninterrupted exposure.[28] Similar results have been reported with light fractionation for aminolevulinic acid (ALA) mediated PDT of rat colonic mucosa.[29]

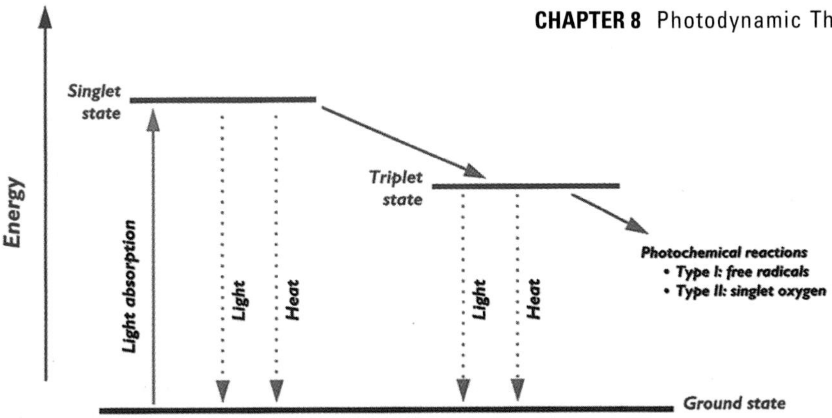

Figure 8-1 Schematic view of photosensitizer activation by light.

Cellular membranes, mitochondrial membranes, and the endoplasmic reticulum appear to be the principal targets for singlet oxygen leading to cellular damage and necrosis.[24,30,31] Apoptotic cell death has been observed in cell culture after PDT with ALA,[32] porfimer sodium,[33] tin ethyl etiopurpurin,[34] and aluminum phthalocyanine.[35] However, certain cell lines do not appear to undergo apoptosis after PDT[32,33] and the significance of programmed cell death in clinical PDT requires further study.

During PDT, treatment selectivity depends not only on limiting the area exposed to light, but also on preferential localization of photosensitizer to diseased versus normal tissue. Various factors can potentially influence this localization, including vascular permeability, presence of macrophages, lipoprotein binding, local pH, photosensitizer hydrophobicity, and lymphatic clearance.[36] Tissue effects are mediated through both vascular and target cell destruction, which in turn are respectively dependent on photosensitizer levels either in the circulation or in direct association with tumor cells.[24] Ischemic necrosis from vascular compromise seems to be the main mechanism of tumor destruction for most systemic drugs such as porfimer sodium.[37] Damage to tissue vasculature also accounts in part for local tissue hypoxia during light exposure. However, direct target cell damage may be predominant with certain systemic photosensitizers (e.g., aluminium phthalocyanine) or topical photosensitizers (e.g., ALA) when used to treat actinic keratoses.[37] Thus the primary site of PDT effect depends largely on the photosensitizer itself, its route of administration, and the disorder being treated.

LASERS AND OTHER LIGHT SOURCES FOR PDT

Although lasers are currently the most widely used PDT light sources, their use in PDT differs fundamentally from that in other cutaneous laser applications (Table 8-2). In PDT, lasers are used to drive photochemical reactions between exogenous sensitizers and oxygen, whereas the desired clinical effects of non-PDT lasers are the result of photothermal and for photomechanical interactions between laser light and chromophores already present in the skin. Selective photothermolysis is critically dependent on laser wavelength and pulse duration,[38] whereas in PDT, photosensitizer dose and total light fluence are perhaps the most important variables determining treatment efficacy. Although lasers or other high-intensity pulsed light sources are absolutely required for selective photothermolysis, PDT can be carried out with lasers as well as a variety of noncoherent broad-band light sources. The primary requirement for any PDT light source is that its emission spectrum include the activating wavelength(s) for the photosensitizer being used.

Lasers have become the standard source for PDT in medicine because (1) they can be efficiently coupled to flexible fiberoptics to allow access to internal tissues, and (2) their monochromaticity permits precise and efficient photosensitizer activation at

Table 8-2
Lasers applications in dermatology: photodynamic therapy versus selective photothermolysis

Photodynamic Therapy	Selective Photothermolysis
Photochemical reaction occurs.	Photothermal and/or photomechanical injury occurs.
Chromophore is a drug (photosensitizer).	Chromophore is present in situ.
Lasers are often useful, but not absolutely necessary.	Pulsed lasers or high-intensity pulsed noncoherent light sources are required.

one of its absorption peaks. Nevertheless, for an accessible organ such as the skin, fiberoptic light delivery is not necessarily an advantage except when implantable interstitial light-diffusing optical fibers are used for treating deep-seated tumors.[39] Another relative advantage of lasers is their ability to deliver high irradiances at specific wavelengths, thereby minimizing overall treatment times. However, this advantage is somewhat diminished when treating very large areas such as the entire trunk or body (e.g., for psoriasis) because of the drop in laser irradiance with increasing field size resulting from the inverse square law.

Tunable dye lasers have been used most often for PDT because their output wavelength can be adjusted or "tuned" to match a specific photosensitizer absorption peak. Coarse tuning of dye lasers is accomplished by physically changing the dye that passes through the lasing cavity, whereas more precise wavelength selection is carried out using optical components.[40] Dye lasers for PDT are typically tuned to wavelengths between 630 to 690 nm, with the dye laser being optically pumped by a second laser. The output mode of the dye laser used for treatment is determined by that of the pumping laser. Argon-pumping lasers will provide continuous-wave (CW) output, whereas the copper vapor, potassium titanyl phosphate (KTP), and excimer lasers will result in high-frequency pulsed light being produced by the tunable dye laser. Gold vapor lasers have also been used for PDT, but are much less versatile than tunable dye lasers because they can be operated only at 628 nm.

Whereas pulsed output is critical for achieving treatment selectivity with photothermal lasers, limited in vivo PDT experiments comparing the efficacy of pulsed and CW lasers have not shown any significant advantage for one laser mode over the other.[41-44] By delivering energy over short periods, pulsed lasers can generate high irradiances that are above the photodynamic saturation threshold of the sensitizer.[45] Using a mathematic model, Sterenborg and Vangemert[45] suggested that at irradiances several-fold higher than the photosensitizer saturation level, PDT effects depend only on the actual photosensitizer tissue concentration and not on the local irradiance.

Broad-band noncoherent light sources are typically smaller, easier to use, and less expensive to acquire and operate than lasers. These include arc lamps, incandescent bulbs (e.g., slide projectors), and fluorescent tubes. Additional advantages of these sources include the capability for exposing relatively large treatment fields and photosensitizer activation at multiple wavelengths for drugs that exhibit several absorption peaks. Light exposure can sometimes generate active photoproducts with absorption peaks that are different from the parent photosensitizer. If a broad-band source is used, some of these photoproducts could be activated to enhance the overall PDT effect.[46] The development of alternative noncoherent light sources that are inexpensive and portable will undoubtedly make PDT more practical for routine office use. Light-emitting diode (LED) arrays are portable, produce high irradiances (>100-200 mW/cm^2) within a narrow wave band (±10 nm), and represent a technology that is relatively less expensive than lasers.

For photosensitizers that exhibit multiple absorption peaks, the effective treatment depth of PDT is influenced by the tissue penetration of the activating wavelength of light used. For example, an ultraviolet (UV) or blue light source will induce a more superficial PDT effect than a red source, which operates at a longer wavelength.[47,48] For this reason, PDT photosensitizers with good absorption at longer wavelengths are desirable when treating tumors, although above 750 nm, PDT efficiency is limited because photon energy may be insufficient to drive photochemical reactions.[49] Conversely, shorter wavelengths may be preferable when deep PDT effects are either unnecessary or undesirable, as in actinic keratosis or psoriasis.

When evaluating studies of laser versus nonlaser light sources, it is important to realize that the reported fluences can be compared only in terms of their respective spectral irradiances.[50] For example, broad-band sources may include wavelengths that are either too short or too long for photosensitizer activation, resulting in wasted photons and overestimation of the effective fluence compared with lasers.

PHOTOSENSITIZERS

Porfimer Sodium

Porfimer sodium and its less purified parent, HPD, are prepared from hematoporphyrin and contain porphyrin dimers and oligomers as the photodynamically active compounds.[51] Although porfimer sodium exhibits its greatest absorption in the Soret band between 400 and 420 nm, light activation at the smaller 630-nm absorption peak is used clinically for tumor treatment because of its deeper tissue penetration. The drug is administered intravenously at a dose of 1 to 2 mg/kg of body weight, and light exposure is carried out 24 to 72 hours later. The main disadvantage of porfimer sodium, and also one of the most likely reasons why it has not been more widely used in dermatology, is that it predictably induces prolonged photosensitivity for 4 to 6 weeks and sometimes even several months.[52] In a study involving 180 patients, clinical photosensitivity was reported by 20% to 40% of patients after injection of porfimer sodium.[53] Photosensitivity appears to be dose dependent according to preliminary studies involving limited numbers of patients.[54,55]

The problems of prolonged generalized photosensitivity, limited light propagation into tissue at 630 nm, and the 1- to 3-day delay between drug infusion and light treatment associated with porfimer sodium have been addressed in part by second-generation photosensitizers. Other desirable photosensitizer attributes include a high quantum yield for singlet-oxygen generation, preferential drug localization to target tissues, rapid clearance from the circulation and normal tissues, minimal dark toxicity (i.e. no adverse drug effects in the absence of light), and low cost.

Aminolevulinic Acid

ALA is a naturally occurring molecule present in human cells and is produced by ALA synthetase, the major rate-limiting enzyme in heme biosynthesis. Although not actually a photosensitizer or porphyrin itself, ALA can be metabolized in vivo to *protoporphyrin IX,* a porphyrin intermediate with photodynamic activity. Administration of pharmacologic doses of ALA by either the oral, topical, or intravenous routes bypasses the rate-limiting step for porphyrinogenesis, thereby leading to protoporphyrin IX accumulation. The optimal wavelength for the in vivo photodynamic activation of protoporphyrin IX has recently been shown to be 635 nm in hamsters transplanted with amelanotic melanoma.[56]

ALA has been actively studied in dermatology and currently demonstrates the best topical efficacy of any PDT drug, largely because its smaller molecular size renders it more permeable across the skin than porphyrins. In clinical studies, topical ALA is used at concentrations of 5% to 20%. Localized photosensitivity occurs after topical ALA application, and patients must avoid direct sun exposure to treatment sites until after therapeutic light irradiation to avoid inadvertent porphyrin activation or photodegradation (photobleaching). No significant levels of porphyrin were detected in the urine, erythrocytes, or plasma after topical application of ALA for actinic keratoses.[57] Although the absence of systemic photosensitivity is a definite advantage of the topical route, percutaneous ALA penetration can be highly variable from one patient to another, particularly in nodular basal cell carcinomas (BCCs).[58]

Protoporphyrin IX can also accumulate in normal and diseased skin after oral ALA administration, which is not the case for most other photosensitizers.[59] Cutaneous photosensitivity after oral ALA ingestion has not been systematically studied but appears to last less than 24 hours.[60] A dose-dependent increase in serum transaminases and mild nausea have been described with the oral ALA.[61] Protoporphyrin IX fluorescence has been shown to accumulate in tumor cells after both oral[62] and intravenous[63] administration of ALA in patients with BCC.

Benzoporphyrin Derivative (Verteporfin)

Benzoporphyrin derivative (BPD) is administered intravenously but, unlike porfimer sodium, is a chemically well-defined photosensitizer that is synthesized from protoporphyrin and dimethyl acetylenedicarboxylate.[64] BPD exhibits an absorption peak at 690 nm, where photon penetration is deeper than at the 630- to 635-nm wavelengths used with porfimer sodium or ALA.[65] BPD is formulated in liposomes, which serves to enhance its delivery to target tissue and its clearance from normal tissue.[66] Because of BPD's pharmacokinetic profile, light treatment can be carried out on the day of drug infusion (porfimer sodium is usually activated 24 to 72 hours after drug administration), and normal skin photosensitivity is relatively short-lived.

The photosensitizing potential of systemic BPD has been evaluated by serial phototesting of normal skin using visible and UV-A light before and after drug administration. In 31 patients who were tested daily, the mean duration of measurable photosensitivity was 2.0 to 6.3 days, depending on the administered BPD dose.[21] Despite a low level of measurable light reactivity, no patients developed clinical photosensitivity reactions in this study. The relative BPD levels in BCCs versus the surrounding normal skin after intravenous BPD injection were monitored noninvasively using fluorescence spectroscopy before therapeutic light exposure. Analysis of the 690-nm BPD emission signal from the skin showed that the average ratio of BPD in BCC versus normal skin was approximately 5:1, suggesting a preferential affinity of BPD for skin tumors.[67]

Tin Ethyl Etiopurpurin

Tin ethyl etiopurpurin (SnET2) is structurally similar to chlorophyll and has an absorption peak at 664 nm. At this wavelength, photon penetration is intermediate between that used for porfimer sodium and BPD. Light treatment is given 1 day after intravenous drug infusion, and a mild clinical cutaneous photosensitivity, lasting less than a month, has been reported in 10% to 15% of the treated patients.[22] Phase I and II dose-finding trials have suggested efficacy for BCC and Kaposi sarcoma.[22,68]

Metatetrahydroxyphenylchlorin

Metatetraphyroxyphenylchlorin (mTHPC) has an absorption peak at 652 nm, is administered by intravenous infusion, and has been used for curative, palliative, or adjuvant treatments of head and neck cancers.[69,70] Photosensitivity for 3 to 10 days has been reported, but this has not been systematically evaluated.[71] The complete clinical response rate was 77% for 13 cutaneous squamous cell carcinomas (SCCs) in two immunosuppressed patients treated with mTHPC and light.[69]

Other Photosensitizers

Mono-l-*aspartylchlorin e6* (NPe6) is activated by 664-nm light and administered as an intravenous infusion.[23] Preliminary studies suggest that the clinical photosensitivity is shorter than with porfimer sodium.[72]

Tin-protoporphyrin is a metalloporphyrin that induces prolonged photosensitivity for 1 to 3 months after intravenous injection.[73] UV-A light treatments given 4 to 5 times a week for 3 weeks after a single tin-protoporphyrin injection have been shown to improve psoriasis, with a decrease in severity score from 7.9 to 3.6.[74] This improvement was maintained for at least 6 weeks longer according to the authors, although they did not perform severity score assessments after the end of the treatment period.

Topical mesotetraphenylporphinesulfonate (TPPS) can be activated with 645-nm light and has been successfully used for the treatment of BCC and cutaneous metastases of breast cancer.[75,76] Unfortunately however, TPPS has been associated with neurotoxicity.[76]

Finally, *porphycenes* are novel photosensitizers that can be activated by light as soon as 5 minutes after injection in animals,[77,78] but clinical data are not yet available. Although similar in structure and size to porphyrins, porphycenes may exhibit significant percutaneous uptake based on penetration studies in ex vivo human skin.[79]

TREATMENT CONSIDERATIONS

Before Treatment

Contraindications to PDT include pregnancy, lactation, allergy to the photosensitizer being used, porphyria, and a significant preexisting photosensitivity disorder such as systemic lupus erythematosus (SLE). Exacerbation of SLE has been reported after PDT.[80] The concurrent use of other photosensitizing medications is a concern for patients undergoing PDT. Because the risk of a phototoxic reaction after PDT may be higher when such medications are used, these patients should be warned that they must be particularly careful about sunlight and bright indoor light.

Written consent is advisable before performing PDT and should address the potential adverse effects (see later) as well as specific instructions for preventing phototoxic skin reactions. Although porfimer sodium is now commercially available, it must be emphasized that its use for any dermatologic condition is currently considered "off label." Precommercialization studies usually call for extensive baseline laboratory evaluation, including renal and hepatic function, but such testing is not mandatory outside the setting of a formal study unless indicated by specific clinical findings. The use of PDT agents in dermatology is essentially restricted to clinical studies until formal regulatory approval is achieved.

For systemic photosensitizers, the total patient drug dose is usually based on body weight, although evidence suggests that total body surface area may be more accurate, in which case height must also be recorded.[81] Topical photosensitizers are usually applied directly to the affected area of the skin and then covered with an opaque material until the time of light exposure.

During Treatment

After drug administration and before light exposure, a delay is necessary to allow for photosensitizer distribution and partitioning between target tissues and normal skin.

In addition, for ALA specifically, this delay also permits its enzymatic transformation to protoporphyrin IX in situ. The optimal waiting time between drug administration and light treatment is usually derived empirically from pharmacokinetic data, published studies, and prior clinical experience and varies widely from 1 hour (BPD) to 1 to 4 days (porfimer sodium) depending on the photosensitizer being used. For patients with multiple tumors or extensive skin disease, one advantage of drugs such as porfimer sodium that persist longer in target tissue is that multiple light treatments can be given over successive days without the need for repeated doses of photosensitizer.

The final step before light exposure involves delineation of the treatment field to be irradiated. After treatment, pain, erythema, edema, and occasionally necrosis are observed in normal peritumoral skin and can be minimized by using smaller exposure fields. The margin of normal skin to be included in the exposure field depends on the tumor being treated and should be equivalent to the margins used with surgery or radiotherapy. For cutaneous breast metastases the margin of normal skin should be at least 0.5 to 1 cm beyond the tumor, as assessed by clinical inspection and palpation.

As with any form of phototherapy, three important parameters govern light exposure: fluence or total light dose, light irradiance at the treatment site, and exposure time. These parameters are related as follows:

(EQ. 1)

$$\text{Exposure time (seconds)} = \frac{\text{Total light dose to be delivered (J/cm}^2\text{)} \times 1000}{\text{Irradiance at treatment site (mW/cm}^2\text{)}}$$

The PDT fluence to be used for treatment depends on the type and dose of photosensitizer and the specific condition being treated. Malignancies are usually treated at higher fluences than benign conditions. A degree of reciprocity exists between photosensitizer dose and light fluence, but the specific drug and light dose ranges over which this is valid are not clearly defined.[11,82] For example, because drug photobleaching (inactivation by light) occurs in addition to photodynamic drug activation during light exposure, disproportionately higher fluences may be necessary to achieve an equivalent PDT effect when lower systemic photosensitizer doses are used.[83] Ideally, photosensitizer doses should be as low as possible to minimize generalized skin photosensitivity, but not so low as to result in an inadequate PDT reaction or prohibitively long light-exposure times.

Irradiance can be measured directly by positioning a light meter detector at the treatment site (nonlaser sources) or can be calculated (equation 2) from measurements of the source's total light power output and the exposure spot diameter (laser sources). For lasers the total power output is measured at the output end of the fiberoptic, as follows:

(EQ. 2)

$$\text{Irradiance of laser (mW/cm}^2\text{)} = \frac{\text{Total power output from source (mW)} \times 4}{\pi \times [\text{Field diameter (cm)}]^2}$$

Typical PDT irradiances range between 50 and 150 mW/cm^2. For example, treatment of a 1 to 2 cm BCC with BPD-MA and 50 J/cm^2 from an LED with an irradiance of 100 mW/cm^2 would take 8 minutes and 20 seconds,[21] whereas the same tumor treated with 100 J/cm^2 of light from a slide projector with an irradiance of 40 mW/cm^2 would take 41 minutes and 40 seconds.[84] At very low irradiances, exposure times become excessively long, whereas at very high irradiances, there may be significant additive photothermal tissue effects. Such thermal effects have been shown to enhance tumor response to PDT in mice.[85]

After Treatment

When large tumors are treated, the issue of analgesia should be addressed because these patients often require narcotics to control post-PDT pain. Wound care is dictated by the type of lesion treated. Tumors undergoing necrosis will develop erosions or ulcerations, in which case they should be covered and kept moist. Otherwise, no other specific wound dressing is required. Patients can be reevaluated after 24 to 72 hours by which time the pain and edema will have peaked. Complete healing of treated sites generally occurs within 4 to 8 weeks after treatment. For tumors that demonstrate inadequate clearing after treatment, PDT has been repeated up to two or three times at intervals of 3 weeks[86] to 3 months.[16]

CLINICAL APPLICATIONS

Oncologic

Porfimer sodium and hematoporphyrin derivative

Although the bulk of clinical studies on porfimer sodium and HPD in dermatology have been devoted to skin cancer, it is very difficult to compare these studies to each other because of differences in drug and light doses, light sources, intervals between drug injection and light activation, and other treatment parameters.

Basal cell carcinomas respond to PDT with porfimer sodium and HPD, with complete responses ranging from 44% to 100%.[11-13,15,16,87-89] Because of a paucity of data on long-term follow-up of BCC treated by PDT, it is difficult to compare this modality with standard therapy. In one of the largest series published, the complete response rate was 88% for 151 BCCs in 37 patients treated with porfimer sodium at 1 mg/kg and light doses of 72 to 288 J/cm^2 from an argon-pumped dye laser.[16] Out of 18 lesions that showed a partial response, 11 were re-treated, and all showed a complete response with no recurrence. The recurrence rate was 16% after an average follow-up of 29 months. Almost all recurrences were located on the nose, and 89% of these were of the morphea type. The authors concluded that PDT using porfimer sodium according to their protocol is probably inadequate for morphea BCC although complete responses of extensive lesions have been reported.[90]

The cure rate for Bowen disease after PDT with porfimer sodium was close to 100% in two studies, one of which involved more than 700 lesions in two patients.[11,91] Complete responses of SCCs of the head and neck, including cutaneous tumors, have been reported with porfimer sodium, but the small number of reported cases precludes any meaningful conclusions about efficacy.[89,92,93]

The absorption of light by melanin makes cutaneous melanomas poor targets for PDT when wavelengths below 700 nm are used. However, recent studies using photosensitizers with an excitation peak of about 800 nm, such as phtalocyanine derivatives, have shown positive tumor response in animals transplanted with pigmented melanomas.[94] Partial and complete responses of Kaposi sarcoma to HPD and porfimer sodium have been described.[95-97] The use of HPD or porfimer sodium has also been reported in a few cases of mycosis fungoides,[10] perianal bowenoid papulosis,[98,99] and extramammary Paget's disease.[99]

HPD and porfimer sodium have been used to treat chest wall metastases of breast cancer[10,100] with complete responses achieved, although recurrences are frequent.[101] Recurrent chest wall disease can be controlled with repeated courses of PDT in certain patients.[102] It is much more preferable to consider PDT early in the course of local metastatic disease, because treatment of large tumors or inflammatory carcinoma results in significant morbidity, including severe pain, extensive necrosis, and slow wound healing.

Thus, although porfimer sodium seems to be an effective treatment for superficial cutaneous neoplasms such as BCC and Bowen disease, the prolonged photosensitivity seen after its administration and the paucity of studies describing long-term follow-up preclude its more widespread use in dermatology. Because many second-generation photosensitizers induce shorter periods of photosensitivity and have already shown promising early results in the treatment of BCC, porfimer sodium may never become the photosensitizer of choice for PDT of skin cancer.

Benzoporphyrin derivative

Twenty patients with 69 primary BCCs (Figure 8-2) or Bowen disease received 0.15 to 0.5 mg/kg of BPD and 50 to 150 J/cm^2 of 630-nm light from an argon dye laser in a dose-ranging study.[21] The overall complete response rate was 70% at 3 months across all drug and light doses used and ranged up to 100% at higher light or drug doses, with good to excellent cosmetic results. In the same study, 15 other patients were treated for

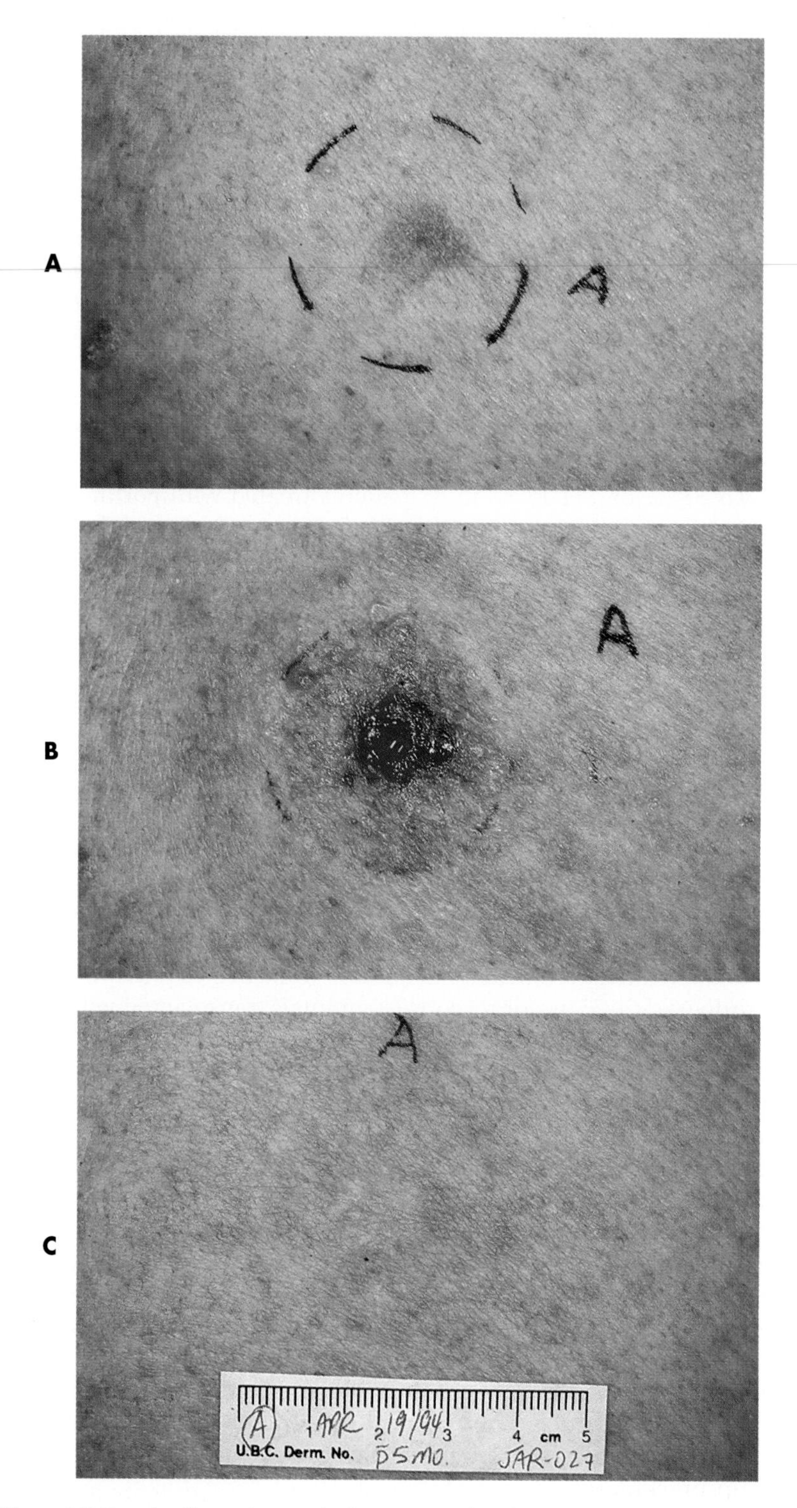

Figure 8-2 Basal cell carcinoma before (**A**) and 2 days (**B**) and 5 months (**C**) after PDT with 0.2 mg/kg of benzoporphyrin derivative (BPD) and 75 J/cm^2 of 690-nm light.

metastatic skin tumors, the majority of which arose from breast carcinoma (Figure 8-3). With the same drug-dose range and light doses of 25 to 150 J/cm², complete response was 47%. Cutaneous photosensitivity reactions were not observed in this study, making BPD a potentially useful drug for further clinical evaluation.

Aminolevulinic acid

PDT with topical ALA has shown potential efficacy in the treatment of superficial BCCs with complete responses in more than 85% to 90% of cases being reported by many

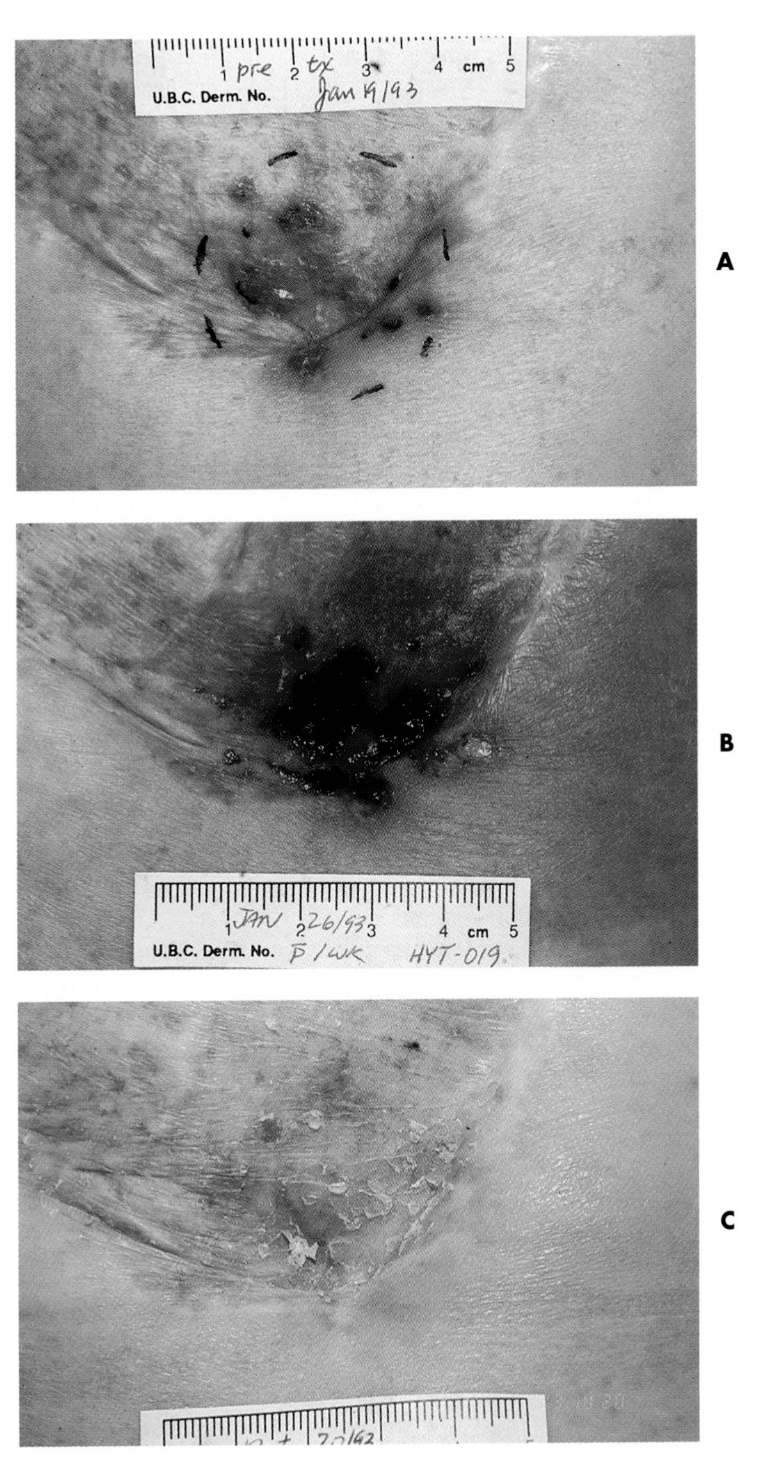

Figure 8-3 Metastatic breast cancer before (**A**) and 1 week (**B**) and 9 months (**C**) after PDT with 0.2 mg/kg of BPD and 150 J/cm² of 690-nm red light.

investigators.[20,86,103-108] It is important to emphasize that tumor response was primarily based on visual examination in most of these studies. The reported complete clinical response rates may possibly overestimate long-term response rates, as suggested by two separate studies in which response rates were 50% and 87% when histologic absence of tumor was used to define a complete response.[84,105] The overall complete response rates for nodular BCC range from 10% to 64% and are much lower than for superficial BCC.[86,103,105-108] The only study evaluating the histologic complete response rate of nodular BCCs showed that only 50% of lesions cleared after multiple (2-8) ALA-PDT treatments.[105] This poor response could be related to inadequate tumor penetration by ALA, as evidenced by a study showing an absence of homogenous protoporphyrin IX tumor fluorescence after up to 24 hours of topical ALA application to nodular BCCs.[109] Also in agreement with this explanation is the higher clearance rate observed in nodular BCCs with a depth of less than 2 mm compared with thicker tumors.[107] In a pharmacokinetic study in which tumors were not exposed to light, oral ALA appeared to induce a homogenous distribution of protoporphyrin IX in BCCs.[62]

Actinic keratoses, being superficial lesions, may be particularly well suited to ALA-PDT. Many clinical studies have shown good results in patients, with complete responses ranging from 59% to 100%.[17,20,103,105,106] Based on these encouraging results, a multicenter phase-III clinical trial has been initiated using ALA-PDT for actinic keratoses.

ALA-PDT has been used successfully for treating Bowen disease.[86,104-106,108,110] Cairnduff et al.[104] treated 36 lesions of Bowen disease in 14 patients with 20% ALA and a 630-nm copper vapor dye laser at fluences between 125 to 250 J/cm^2. The complete response was 97% at 2 months and fell to 89% after a median follow-up of 18 months. In the only controlled dermatologic PDT study published to date, 40 lesions of Bowen diseases were randomly assigned to receive either cryotherapy with liquid nitrogen (single freeze-thaw cycle) or PDT using a xenon arc lamp and a 630 ±30–nm bandpass filter 4 hours after an application of 20% ALA.[110] The complete response rate after a single treatment was significantly higher with PDT (15 of 20) compared with cryotherapy (10 of 20), with the additional advantage of no ulceration or infection in the PDT-treated arm; liquid nitrogen resulted in five cases of skin ulceration and two instances of skin infections. This study showed that ALA-PDT for Bowen disease is an effective treatment with demonstrated advantages over cryotherapy.

Although few studies have looked at ALA-PDT for invasive SCCs, the complete response for superficial lesions (less than 1 mm histologically) was 83% in a study of patients treated with 60 to 80 J/cm^2 of 630-nm light delivered from an argon dye laser 6 to 8 hours after topical application of 20% ALA.[105] Deeper SCCs do not appear to respond well to ALA-PDT,[20] as confirmed by a complete response of only 33% for tumors with depth of more than 1 mm.[105] In view of these preliminary results, ALA-PDT does not appear to be an appropriate treatment for invasive SCC.

Plaque and patch types of mycosis fungoides improved or cleared after PDT with topical ALA in studies involving two to six patients each.[86,103,111] Preferential synthesis of protoporphyrin IX in malignant T cells presumably accounts for the improvement.[112-114] It is hypothesized that activated and malignant lymphocytes manifest low intracellular iron levels because of increased metabolic demands. Because iron is required for heme synthesis from protoporphyrin IX, exogenous ALA leads to intracellular protoporphryin IX accumulation.

To improve the clinical response of thick tumors, various techniques have been used to enhance ALA penetration and protoporphyrin IX accumulation in target tissues. *Deferroxamine* increases protoporphyrin IX synthesis in cultured cells by chelating iron[115-117] and has been used topically in combination with ALA on BCC.[106] *DMSO* (dimethyl sulfoxide) and *EDTA* (ethylenediaminetetraacetic acid) can also increase intracellular protoporphyrin IX levels, by increasing ALA absorption and through iron chelation, respectively.[107] Pretreating the skin with DMSO and adding both DMSO and EDTA to ALA have been successfully used for the treatment of

BCC.[107] *Iontophoresis* can increase the delivery of ALA to the skin, as shown by in vivo protoporphyrin IX–fluorescence spectroscopy of normal volunteers.[118]

Nononcologic

The observation that PDT may selectively target activated lymphocytes[112-114,119] provides an intriguing rationale for using PDT as an immunomodulatory treatment for nonneoplastic disorders such as psoriasis. Complete clearing within psoriatic plaques has been reported in patients after a single treatment with 0.2 to 0.3 mg/kg of BPD and 75 J/cm² of 690-nm argon laser light[19] (Figure 8-4). Porfimer sodium has also been shown to improve psoriasis.[120-122] Protoporphyrin IX accumulates in psoriatic plaques after topical ALA application,[123] and preliminary reports have also suggested that topical ALA–PDT can improve psoriasis.[18,124] As with PUVA, multiple PDT treatment sessions may be required to achieve adequate responses consistently. Figure 8-5 shows clearing within the light-exposed portion of a psoriatic plaque after nine treatment sessions with 20% ALA followed by exposure to 20 J/cm² of red light from a filtered slide projector. The duration of clearing of psoriasis after treatment has not been systematically evaluated to date.

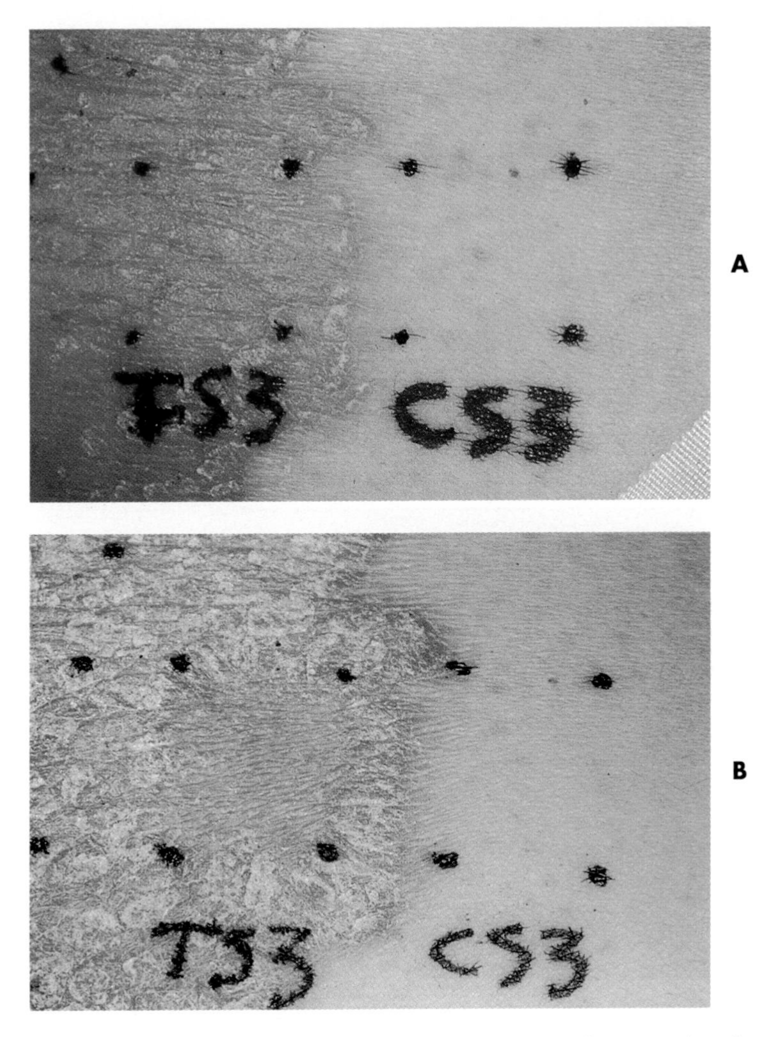

Figure 8-4 Psoriasis before (**A**) and 4 weeks (**B**) after PDT with 0.2 mg/kg of BPD and 75 J/cm² of 690-nm light. Only squares delineated by central black dots were exposed to light.

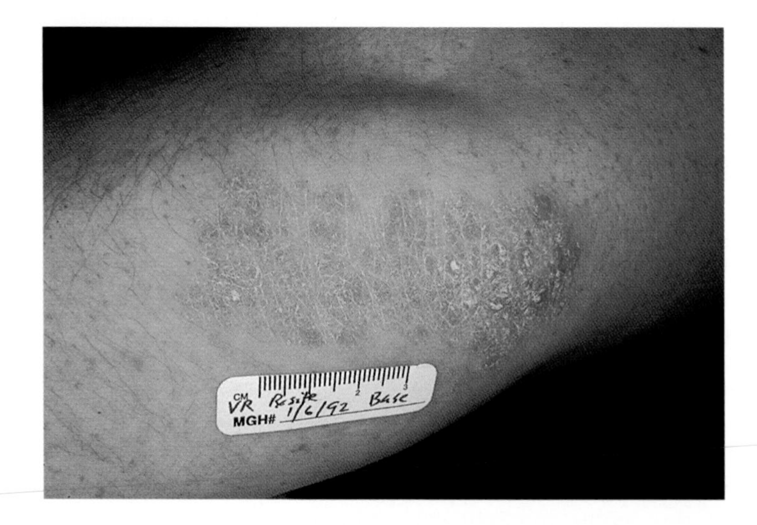

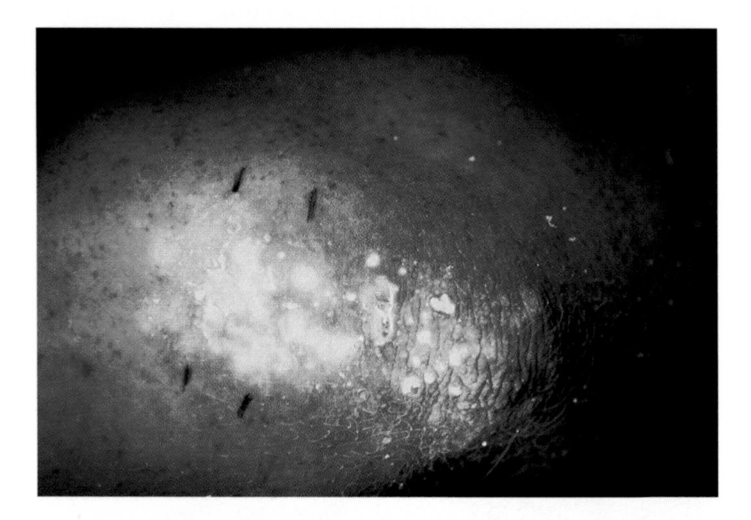

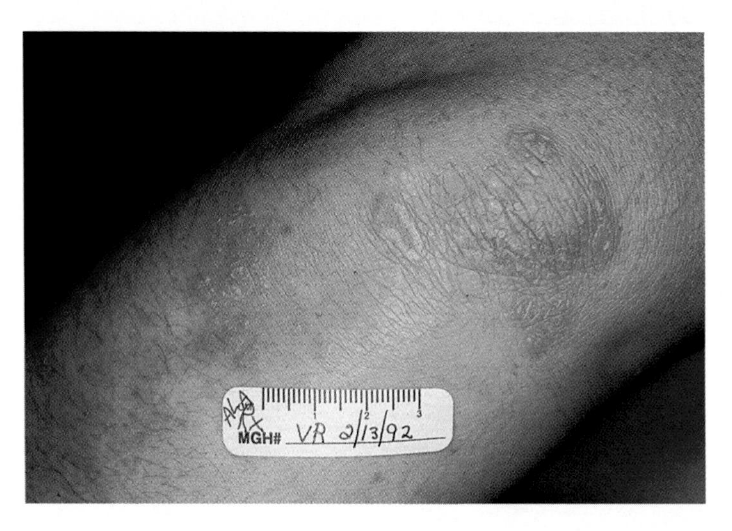

Figure 8-5 Psoriatic plaque treated nine times with 20% aminolevulinic acid (ALA) and 20 J/cm^2 of 630-nm red light. **A,** Before treatment; **B,** red fluorescence visualized by Wood's lamp; **C,** after treatment. Only central portion of plaque was treated with ALA and light, with lateral ends serving as drug-only and light-only controls.

ALA selectively photosensitizes pilosebaceous structures and may therefore be useful for hair disorders.[125] Topical ALA at a concentration 20% has been used as a depilatory agent.[126] Three hours after ALA application, wax-epilated or shaved skin was exposed to 100 to 200 J/cm² of 630-nm laser light. Hair regrowth was 50% after 3 months for sites treated with 200 J/cm², whereas 90% regrowth was observed at the control sites and the sites exposed to 100 J/cm². Postoperative hyperpigmentation was noted, but no scarring was reported. This preliminary study suggests that ALA-PDT could become a therapeutic alternative or adjunct to electolysis or long pulse laser surgery for removing unwanted hair.

The intense red fluorescence generated by PDT photosensitizers when irradiated with UV-A or blue light (see Figure 8-2, *B*) could be exploited *for photodiagnosis,*[59] as suggested by preliminary studies of skin cancers after oral or topical application of ALA.[127-130]

In a study of refractory common warts treated with 20% ALA and light exposure 5 to 6 hours later, only one of six patients achieved complete clearing.[131] This poor response may be related to inadequate percutaneous absorption, because selective lesional accumulation of protoporphyrin IX has been demonstrated after topical application of ALA to condylomas.[132] Porfimer sodium has also been used to successfully treat laryngeal viral papillomas.[133,134]

ADVERSE EFFECTS OF PDT

Skin photosensitivity remains one of the major potential side effects of PDT. Although all photosensitizers induce transient skin photosensitivity, certain agents (e.g., porfimer sodium) generate prolonged photosensitivity lasting at least 4 to 6 weeks.[135] Beginning immediately after drug administration, patients must avoid sunlight and bright artificial light, including operating rooms, medical and dental examination lamps, suntanning booths, and UV phototherapy units. A localized skin "burn" associated with pulse oximetry during general anesthesia was reported after porfimer sodium injection and was believed to result from the 660-nm red light emitted by the oximeter.[136]

Conventional chemical sunscreens provide minimal protection against this type of photosensitivity, which results from both visible and UV light. Animal studies suggest that opaque sunscreens such as titanium oxide or zinc oxide offer some protection if they are combined with a visible-light absorber such as iron oxide.[137] Low levels of ambient indoor lighting from incandescent or fluorescent sources are usually of no concern. In fact, these sources can theoretically shorten the duration of normal-skin photosensitivity by slowly inactivating any residual drug present in the skin through photobleaching.[138] The use of photosensitizers such as aluminum phthalocyanine, with weaker absorption in the visible spectrum, may be associated with a lower potential for inducing unwanted clinical photosensitivity.[139]

Skin edema, necrosis, and eschar formation (Figure 8-3, *B*) are expected after PDT treatment of neoplasms. Extensive edema lasting several days often occurs after PDT for tumors located on the face or extremities. A burning sensation or pain during light treatment also occurs frequently and can be controlled by local anesthetics if necessary,[16] whereas posttreatment pain is usually milder and responsive to oral analgesics. Large tumors, such as skin or chest wall metastases, can give rise to more intense pain in the first few days after PDT and may require narcotic agents.

Scarring, hyperpigmentation, and hypopigmentation are also possible after PDT, but the final cosmetic results of PDT are remarkably comparable to those of surgery for tumors.[107] A generalized Koebner phenomenon has been reported after treatment of actinic keratoses and SCCs in a patient with psoriasis treated with ALA-PDT.[140] We have observed a local Koebner reaction on light-exposed normal skin adjacent to a psoriatic plaque in a patient treated with 0.2 mg/kg of BPD and 75 J/cm² of 690-nm light from an argon dye laser (Figure 8-6).

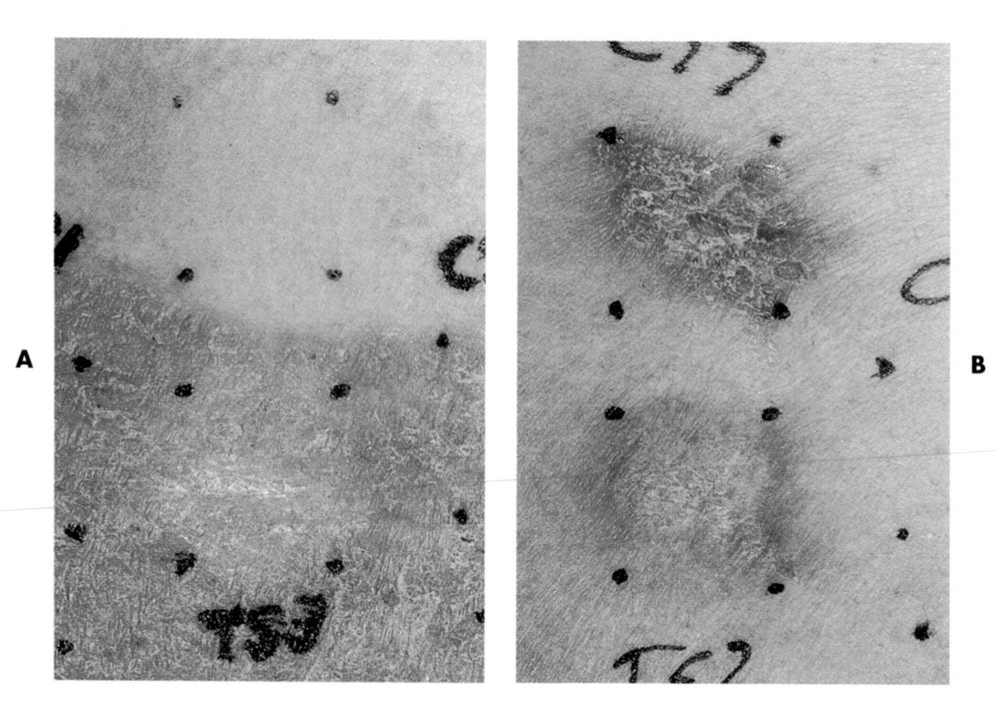

Figure 8-6 **A,** Psoriatic plaque and normal skin immediately after PDT with 0.2 mg/kg of BPD and 75 J/cm^2 of 690-nm red light. Only squares outlined by black dots were exposed to light. **B,** After 2 months, Koebner phenomenon is seen on normal skin (*CS3*, top).

SUMMARY

With the recent approval of porfimer sodium in many countries, including the United States, PDT has become an established novel therapeutic modality. Based on the current body of knowledge, PDT can be considered a reasonable option for the treatment of patients with multiple superficial cutaneous malignant tumors, such as occur in nevoid BCC syndrome. However, PDT is still at an early evaluation stage for nonneoplastic conditions.

Approval of topical and systemic photosensitizers for dermatologic indications is anticipated in the coming years and will undoubtedly create a demand for efficient and lower-cost light sources for office-based PDT. Although lasers remain good light sources for PDT of localized disease, such as superficial nonmelanoma skin cancer, they are expensive and cumbersome to use for conditions such as psoriasis, when it is necessary to expose relatively large body surfaces. As the range of indications for PDT broadens in concert with further clinical evaluation of second-generation photosensitizers, a concomitant need will arise for further refinements to existing light technologies.

REFERENCES

1. Daniell MD, Hill JS: A history of photodynamic therapy, *Aust NZ J Surg* 61:340, 1991.
2. Von Tappeiner H: Ueber die wirkung fluorescierenden stoffe auf infusiorien nach versuchen von O. Raab, *Munch Med Wochenschr* 47:5, 1900.
3. Von Tappeiner H, Jesionek A: Therapeutische versuche mit fluorescierenden stoffen, *Munch Med Wochenschr* 47:2042, 1903.
4. Von Tappeiner H, Jodlbauer A: Ueber wirkung der photodynamischen (fluorescierenden) stoffe auf protozoan und enzyme, *Dtsch Arch Klin Med* 80:427, 1904.
5. Meyer-Betz F: Untersuchungen uber die Biologische (photodynamische) wirkung des hamatoporphyrins und anderer derivative des Blut-und Gallenfarbstoffs, *Dtsch Arch Klin Med* 112:476, 1913.

6. Auler H, Banzer G: Untersuchungen über die rolle der porphyrine bei geschwulst-kranken menschen und tieren, *Z Krebsforsch* 53:65, 1942.
7. Lipson RL, Baldes EJ, Olsen AM: The use of a derivative of haematoporphyrin in tumour detection, *J Natl Cancer Inst* 26:1, 1961.
8. Lipson RL, Baldes EJ, Gray MJ: Hematoporphyrin derivative for detection and management of cancer, *Cancer* 20:2255, 1967.
9. Dougherty TJ, Grindey GB, Fiel R et al: Photoradiation therapy. II. Cure of animal tumors with hematoporphyrin and light, *J Natl Cancer Inst* 55:115, 1975.
10. Dougherty TJ, Kaufman JE, Goldfarb A et al: Photoradiation therapy for the treatment of malignant tumors, *Cancer Res* 38:2628, 1978.
11. Buchanan RB, Carruth JA, McKenzie AL, Williams SR: Photodynamic therapy in the treatment of malignant tumours of the skin and head and neck, *Eur J Surg Oncol* 15:400, 1989.
12. Dougherty TJ: Photoradiation therapy for cutaneous and subcutaneous malignancies, *J Invest Dermatol* 77:122, 1981.
13. Keller GS, Razum NJ, Doiron DR: Photodynamic therapy for nonmelanoma skin cancer, *Fac Plast Surg* 6:180, 1989.
14. McCaughan L: Lasers in photodynamic therapy, *Nurs Clin North Am* 25:725, 1990.
15. Waldow SM, Lobraico RV, Kohler IK et al: Photodynamic therapy for treatment of malignant cutaneous lesions, *Lasers Surg Med* 7:451, 1987.
16. Wilson BD, Mang TS, Stoll H et al: Photodynamic therapy for the treatment of basal cell carcinoma, *Arch Dermatol* 128:1597, 1992.
17. Jeffes EW, McCullough JL, Weinstein GD et al: Photodynamic therapy of actinic keratosis with topical 5-aminolevulinic acid, *Arch Dermatol* 133:727, 1997.
18. Boehncke WH, Sterry W, Kaufmann R: Treatment of psoriasis by topical photodynamic therapy with polychromatic light, *Lancet* 343:801, 1994.
19. Hruza L, Lui H, Hruza G et al: Response of psoriasis to photodynamic therapy using benzoporphyrin derivative monoacid ring A, *Lasers Surg Med Suppl* 7:43, 1995.
20. Kennedy JC, Pottier RH, Pross DC: Photodynamic therapy with endogenous protoporphyrin IX: basic principles and present clinical experience, *J Photochem Photobiol* 6B:143, 1990.
21. Lui H, Hruza L, McLean D et al: Photodynamic therapy of malignant skin tumors with BPD-verteporfin: a photosensitizer that does not induce prolonged cutaneous photosensitivity (submitted for publication).
22. Razum NJ, Snyder AB, Doiron DR: SnET2: clinical update, *SPIE Proc* 2675:43, 1996.
23. Allen R, Kessel D, Volz W, Tharratt RS: A phase 1 clinical trial of NPe6 in the treatment of superficial malignancy, *Lasers Med Sci* 7:218, 1992.
24. Henderson BW, Dougherty TJ: How does photodynamic therapy work? *Photochem Photobiol* 55:145, 1992.
25. Gomer CJ, Razum NJ: Acute skin response in albino mice following porphyrin photosensitization under oxic and anoxic conditions, *Photochem Photobiol* 40:435, 1984.
26. Anholt H, Peng Q, Moan J: Pressure against the tumor can reduce the efficiency of photochemotherapy, *Cancer Lett* 82:73, 1994.
27. Henderson BW, Fingar VH: Oxygen limitation of direct tumor cell kill during photodynamic treatment of a murine tumor model, *Photochem Photobiol* 49:299, 1989.
28. Foster TH: Effects of dose rate and dose fractionation in photodynamic therapy of solid tumors, *Lasers Surg Med Suppl* 7:39, 1995.
29. Messmann H, Mlkvy P, Buonaccorsi G et al: Improving the efficacy of photodynamic therapy on normal rat colon using 5-aminolaevulinic acid (ALA) sensitisation by light fractionation, *Lasers Surg Med Suppl* 7:40, 1995.
30. Nelson JS, Liaw LH, Orenstein A et al: Mechanism of tumor destruction following photodynamic therapy with hematoporphyrin derivative, chlorin, and phthalocyanine, *J Natl Cancer Inst* 80:1599, 1988.
31. Gomer CJ: Preclinical examination of first and second generation photosensitizers used in photodynamic therapy, *Photochem Photobiol* 54:1093, 1991.
32. Noodt BB, Berg K, Stokke T et al: Apoptosis and necrosis induced with light and 5-aminolaevulinic acid–derived protoporphyrin IX, *Br J Cancer* 74:22, 1996.
33. He XY, Sikes RA, Thomsen S et al: Photodynamic therapy with Photofrin II induces programmed cell death in carcinoma cell lines, *Photochem Photobiol* 59:468, 1994.

34. Luo Y, Chang CK, Kessel D: Rapid initiation of apoptosis by photodynamic therapy, *Photochem Photobiol* 63:528, 1996.
35. Agarwal ML, Clay ME, Harvey EJ et al: Photodynamic therapy induces rapid cell death by apoptosis in L5178Y mouse lymphoma cells, *Cancer Res* 51:5993, 1991.
36. Lin C-W: Selective localization of photosensitizers in tumors: a review of the phenomenon and possible mechanisms. In Kessel D, editor: *Photodynamic therapy of neoplastic disease,* vol 2, Boca Raton, Fla, 1990, CRC.
37. Margaron P, Madarnas P, Quellet R, Van Lier JE: Biological activities of phthalocyanines. XVII. Histopathologic evidence for different mechanisms of EMT-6 tumor necrosis induced by photodynamic therapy with disulfonated aluminum phthalocyanine or photofrin, *Anticancer Res* 16:613, 1996.
38. Anderson RR, Parrish JA: Selective photothermolysis: precise microsurgery by selective absorption of pulsed radiation, *Science* 220:524, 1983.
39. Lowdell CP, Ash DV, Driver I, Brown SB: Interstitial photodynamic therapy: clinical experience with diffusing fibres in the treatment of cutaneous and subcutaneous tumours, *Br J Cancer* 67:1398, 1993.
40. Hecht J: *Understanding lasers,* ed 2, New York, 1994, IEEE.
41. Ferrario A, Rucker N, Ryter SW et al: Direct comparison of in-vitro and in-vivo Photofrin-II mediated photosensitization using a pulsed KTP pumped dye laser and a continuous wave argon ion pumped dye laser, *Lasers Surg Med* 11:404, 1991.
42. Panjehpour M, Overholt BF, DeNovo RC et al: Comparative study between pulsed and continuous wave lasers for Photofrin photodynamic therapy, *Lasers Surg Med* 13:296, 1993.
43. Pope AJ, Masters JR, MacRobert AJ: The photodynamic effect of a pulsed dye laser on human bladder carcinoma cells in vitro, *Urol Res* 18:267, 1990.
44. Rausch PC, Rolfs F, Winkler MR et al: Pulsed versus continuous wave excitation mechanisms in photodynamic therapy of differently graded squamous cell carcinomas in tumor-implanted nude mice, *Eur Arch Otorhinolaryngol* 250:82, 1993.
45. Sterenborg H, Vangemert MJC: Photodynamic therapy with pulsed light sources: a theoretical analysis, *Phys Med Biol* 41:835, 1996.
46. Charlesworth P, Truscott TG: The use of 5-aminolevulinic acid (ALA) in photodynamic therapy (PDT), *J Photochem Photobiol* 18B:99, 1993.
47. Kwangsukstith C, Taylor CR, Anderson RR, Kollias B: Dosimetry of PDT with UVA radiation and red light on normal skin, *Photochem Photobiol* 63:65S, 1996.
48. Tsoukas MM, Lin GC, Lee MS et al: Predictive dosimetry for threshold phototoxicity in photodynamic therapy on normal skin: red wavelengths produce more extensive damage than blue at equal threshold doses, *J Invest Dermatol* 108:501, 1997.
49. Kochevar IE, Pathak MA, Parrish JA: Photophysics, photochemistry, photobiology. In Fitzpatrick TB, Eisen AZ, Wolff K et al, editors: *Dermatology in general medicine,* vol 1, New York, 1993, McGraw-Hill.
50. Stringer MR: Problems associated with the use of broad-band illumination sources for photodynamic therapy, *Phys Med Biol* 40:1733, 1995.
51. Kessel D: Photodynamic therapy of neoplastic disease, *Drugs Today* 32:385, 1996.
52. Wooten RS, Smith KC, Ahlquist DA et al: Prospective study of cutaneous phototoxicity after systemic hematoporphyrin derivative, *Lasers Surg Med* 8:294, 1988.
53. Dougherty TJ, Cooper MT, Mang TS: Cutaneous phototoxic occurrences in patients receiving Photofrin, *Lasers Surg Med* 10:485, 1990.
54. Dougherty TJ, Potter WR, Bellnier D: Photodynamic therapy for the treatment of cancer: current status and advances. In Kessel D, editor: *Photodynamic therapy of neoplastic disease,* vol 1, Boca Raton, Fla, 1990,CRC.
55. Lam S, Palcic B, McLean D et al: Detection of early lung cancer using low dose Photofrin II, *Chest* 97:333, 1990.
56. Szeimies RM, Abels C, Fritsch C et al: Wavelength dependency of photodynamic effects after sensitization with 5-aminolevulinic acid in vitro and in vivo, *J Invest Dermatol* 105:672, 1995.
57. Fritsch C, Verwohlt B, Bolsen K et al: Influence of topical photodynamic therapy with 5-aminolevulinic acid on porphyrin metabolism, *Arch Dermatol Res* 288:517, 1996.
58. Martin LK Jr, Black MC: Biomarker assessment of the effects of petroleum refinery contamination on channel catfish, *Ecotoxicol Environ Safety* 33:81, 1996.

59. Marcus SL, Sobel RS, Golub AL et al: Photodynamic therapy (PDT) and photodiagnosis using endogenous photosensitization induced by 5-aminolevulinic acid (ALA): current clinical and development status, *J Clin Laser Med Surg* 14:59, 1996.
60. Regula J, MacRobert AJ, Gorchein A et al: Photosensitisation and photodynamic therapy of oesophageal, duodenal, and colorectal tumours using 5 aminolaevulinic acid induced protoporphyrin IX: a pilot study, *Gut* 36:67, 1995.
61. Mlkvy P, Messmann H, Regula J et al: Sensitization and photodynamic therapy (PDT) of gastrointestinal tumors with 5-aminolaevulinic acid (ALA) induced protoporphyrin IX (PPIX): a pilot study, *Neoplasma* 42:109, 1995.
62. Tope WD, Kollias N, Martin A et al: Oral delta-aminolevulinic acid induces full-thickness protoporphyrin IX fluorescence in basal cell carcinoma, *Lasers Surg Med Suppl* 7:40, 1995.
63. Peng Q, Warloe T, Moan J et al: Distribution of 5-aminolevulinic acid–induced porphyrins in noduloulcerative basal cell carcinoma, *Photochem Photobiol* 62:906, 1995.
64. Richter AM, Kelly B, Chow J et al: Preliminary studies on a more effective phototoxic agent than hematoporphyrin, *J Natl Cancer Inst* 79:1327, 1987.
65. Levy JG: Photosensitizers in photodynamic therapy, *Semin Oncol* 21:4, 1994.
66. Richter AM, Waterfield E, Jain AK et al: Liposomal delivery of a photosensitizer, benzoporphyrin derivative monoacid ring A (BPD), to tumor tissue in a mouse tumor model, *Photochem Photobiol* 57:1000, 1993.
67. Lui H, Zeng H, McLean DI et al: In vivo fluorescence spectroscopy monitoring of BPD verteporfin concentration changes in skin tissue during photodynamic therapy of skin cancer, *J Dermatol Sci* 12:87, 1996.
68. Sommer CA, van Leengoed H, Conti CM et al: Photodynamic therapy (PDT) for cutaneous carcinomas using the second generation photosensitizer tin ethyl ethiopurpurin (SnET2), *Lasers Surg Med Suppl* 7:45, 1995.
69. Dilkes MG, Dejode ML, Rowntreetaylor A et al: M-THPC photodynamic therapy for head and neck cancer, *Lasers Med Sci* 11:23, 1996.
70. Poate TW, Dilkes MG, Kenyon GS: Use of photodynamic therapy for the treatment of squamous cell carcinoma of the soft palate, *Br J Oral Maxillofac Surg* 34:66, 1996.
71. Stables GI, Ash DV: Photodynamic therapy, *Cancer Treat Rev* 21:311, 1995.
72. Volz W, Allen R, Tharratt RS, Kessel D: Cutaneous phototoxicity of NPe6 in man, *Lasers Med Sci* 7:218, 1992.
73. Emtestam L, Angelin B, Berglund L et al: Photodynamic properties of Sn-protoporphyrin: clinical investigations and phototesting in human subjects, *Acta Derm Venereol* 73:26, 1993.
74. Emtestam L, Berglund L, Angelin B et al: Tin-protoporphyrin and long wave length ultraviolet light in treatment of psoriasis, *Lancet* 1:1231, 1989.
75. Santoro O, Bandieramonte G, Melloni E et al: Photodynamic therapy by topical meso-tetraphenylporphinesulfonate tetrasodium salt administration in superficial basal cell carcinomas, *Cancer Res* 50:4501, 1990.
76. Lapes M, Petera J, Jirsa M: Photodynamic therapy of cutaneous metastases of breast cancer after local application of meso-tetra-(para-sulphophenyl)-porphryin (TPPS4), *J Photochem Photobiol* 36B:205,1996.
77. Dellian M, Richert C, Gamarra F, Goetz AE: Photodynamic eradication of amelanotic melanoma of the hamster with fast acting photosensitizers, *Int J Cancer* 65:246, 1996.
78. Ortel B, Calzavarapinton PG, Szeimies RM, Hasan T: Perspectives in cutaneous photodynamic sensitization, *J Photochem Photobiol* 36B:209, 1996.
79. Karrer S, Abels C, Szeimies RM et al: Topical application of a first porphycene dye for photodynamic therapy: penetration studies in human perilesional skin and basal cell carcinoma, *Arch Dermatol Res* 289:132, 1997.
80. Abramson AL, Alvi A, Mullooly VM: Clinical exacerbation of systemic lupus erythematosus after photodynamic therapy of laryngotracheal papillomatosis, *Lasers Surg Med* 13:677, 1993.
81. McCaughan JS Jr, Miller C: Photosensitizer dosage: mg/kg or mg/m^2 of body surface? *SPIE Proc* 26:1993.
82. Fingar VH, Henderson BW: Drug and light dose dependence of photodynamic therapy: a study of tumor and normal tissue response, *Photochem Photobiol* 46:837, 1987.
83. Potter WR, Mang TS, Dougherty TJ: The theory of photodynamic therapy dosimetry: consequences of photo-destruction of sensitizer, *Photochem Photobiol* 46:97, 1987.

84. Lui H, Salasche S, Kollias N et al: Photodynamic therapy of nonmelanoma skin cancer with topical aminolevulinic acid: a clinical and histologic study, *Arch Dermatol* 131:737, 1995.
85. Waldow SM, Henderson BW, Dougherty TJ: Enhanced tumor control following sequential treatments of photodynamic therapy (PDT) and localized microwave hyperthermia in vivo, *Lasers Surg Med* 4:79, 1984.
86. Svanberg K, Andersson T, Killander D et al: Photodynamic therapy of nonmelanoma malignant tumours of the skin using topical delta-amino levulinic acid sensitization and laser irradiation, *Br J Dermatol* 130:743, 1994.
87. Tse DT, Kersten RC, Anderson RL: Hematoporphyrin derivative photoradiation therapy in managing nevoid basal-cell carcinoma syndrome: a preliminary report, *Arch Ophthalmol* 102:990, 1984.
88. Gregory RO, Goldman L: Application of photodynamic therapy in plastic surgery, *Lasers Surg Med* 6:62, 1986.
89. McCaughan JS Jr: Photodynamic therapy of skin and esophageal cancers, *Cancer Invest* 8:407, 1990.
90. Wilson BD, Mang T: Photodynamic therapy for cutaneous malignancies, *Clin Dermatol* 13:91, 1995.
91. Jones CM, Mang T, Cooper M et al: Photodynamic therapy in the treatment of Bowen's disease, *J Am Acad Dermatol* 27:979, 1992.
92. Gross DJ, Waner M, Schosser RH, Dinehart SM: Squamous cell carcinoma of the lower lip involving a large cutaneous surface: photodynamic therapy as an alternative therapy, *Arch Dermatol* 126:1148, 1990.
93. Wenig BL, Kurtzman DM, Grossweiner LI et al: Photodynamic therapy in the treatment of squamous cell carcinoma of the head and neck, *Arch Otolaryngol Head Neck Surg* 116:1267, 1990.
94. Michailov N, Peeva M, Angelov I et al: Fluence rate effects on photodynamic therapy of b16 pigmented melanoma, *J Photochem Photobiol* 37B:154, 1997.
95. Dougherty TJ, Oseroff AR, D WB et al: An update of Photofrin–photodynamic therapy (PDT) for cutaneous tumors, *Lasers Surg Med Suppl* 8:26, 1996.
96. Schweitzer VG, Visscher D: Photodynamic therapy for treatment of AIDS-related oral Kaposi's sarcoma, *Otolaryngol Head Neck Surg* 102:639, 1990.
97. Wilson BD, Bernstein Z, Sommer C et al: Photodynamic therapy for the treatment of Kaposi's sarcoma: a comparison study utilizing Photofrin and tin ethyl-etiopurpurin, *Lasers Surgery Med Suppl* 7:45, 1995.
98. Gahlen J, Stern J, Graschew G et al: Photodynamic therapy (PDT) for perianal bowenoid papulosis, *SPIE Proc* 2371:530, 1995.
99. Petrelli NJ, Cebollero JA, Rodriguez-Bigas M, Mang T: Photodynamic therapy in the management of neoplasms of the perianal skin, *Arch Surg* 127:1436, 1992.
100. Dougherty TJ, Lawrence G, Kaufman JH et al: Photoradiation in the treatment of recurrent breast carcinoma, *J Natl Cancer Inst* 62:231, 1979.
101. Sperduto PW, DeLaney TF, Thomas G et al: Photodynamic therapy for chest wall recurrence in breast cancer, *Int J Radiat Oncol Biol Phys* 21:441, 1991.
102. Schuh M, Nseyo UO, Potter WR et al: Photodynamic therapy for palliation of locally recurrent breast carcinoma, *J Clin Oncol* 5:1766, 1987.
103. Wolf P, Rieger E, Kerl H: Topical photodynamic therapy with endogenous porphyrins after application of 5-aminolevulinic acid: an alternative treatment modality for solar keratoses, superficial squamous cell carcinomas, and basal cell carcinomas? *J Am Acad Dermatol* 28:17, 1993.
104. Cairnduff F, Stringer MR, Hudson EJ et al: Superficial photodynamic therapy with topical 5-aminolaevulinic acid for superficial primary and secondary skin cancer, *Br J Cancer* 69:605, 1994.
105. Calzavara-Pinton PG: Repetitive photodynamic therapy with topical delta-aminolaevulinic acid as an appropriate approach to the routine treatment of superficial nonmelanoma skin tumours, *J Photochem Photobiol* 29B:53, 1995.
106. Fijan S, Honigsmann H, Ortel B: Photodynamic therapy of epithelial skin tumours using delta-aminolaevulinic acid and desferrioxamine, *Br J Dermatol* 133:282, 1995.
107. Warloe T, Heyerdahl H, Moan J et al: Photodynamic therapy with 5-aminolevulinic acid induced porphyrins and DMSO/EDTA for basal cell carcinoma, *SPIE Proc* 2371:226, 1995.

108. Wennberg AM, Lindholm LE, Alpsten M, Larko O: Treatment of superficial basal cell carcinomas using topically applied delta-aminolevulinic acid and a filtered xenon lamp, *Arch Dermatol Res* 288:561, 1996.
109. Martin A, Tope WD, Grevelink JM et al: Lack of selectivity of protoporphyrin IX fluorescence for basal cell carcinoma after topical application of 5-aminolevulinic acid: implications for photodynamic treatment, *Arch Dermatol Res* 287:665, 1995.
110. Morton CA, Whitehurst C, Moseley H et al: Comparison of photodynamic therapy with cryotherapy in the treatment of Bowen's disease, *Br J Dermatol* 135:766, 1996.
111. Oseroff AR et al: PDT with topical δ-aminolevulinic acid (ALA) for the treatment of patch and plaque stage cutaneous T-cell lymphoma, *Lasers Surg Med Suppl* 7:39, 1995.
112. Rittenhouse-Diakun K, Van Leengoed H, Morgan J et al: The role of transferrin receptor (CD71) in photodynamic therapy of activated and malignant lymphocytes using the heme precursor delta-aminolevulinic acid (ALA), *Photochem Photobiol* 61:523, 1995.
113. Boehncke WH, Ruck A, Naumann J et al: Comparison of sensitivity towards photodynamic therapy of cutaneous resident and infiltrating cell types in vitro, *Lasers Surg Med* 19:451, 1996.
114. Shanler SD, Wan W, Whitaker JE et al: Topical δ-aminolevulinic acid for photodynamic therapy of cutaneous carcinomas and cutaneous T cell lymphoma, *J Invest Dermatol* 101:406, 1993.
115. Berg K, Anholt H, Bech O, Moan J: The influence of iron chelators on the accumulation of protoporphyrin IX in 5-aminolaevulinic acid–treated cells, *Br J Cancer* 74:688, 1996.
116. Iinuma S, Farshi SS, Ortel B, Hasan T: A mechanistic study of cellular photodestruction with 5-aminolaevulinic acid–induced porphyrin, *Br J Cancer* 70:21, 1994.
117. Lim HW, Behar S, He D: Effect of porphyrin and irradiation on heme biosynthetic pathway in endothelial cells, *Photodermatol Photoimmunol Photomed* 10:17, 1994.
118. Rhodes LE, Tsoukas MM, Anderson RR, Kollias N: Iontophoretic delivery of ALA provides a quantitative model for ALA pharmacokinetics and PPIX phototoxicity in human skin, *J Invest Dermatol* 108:87, 1997.
119. Chowdhary RK, Ratkay LG, Neyndorff HC et al: The use of transcutaneous photodynamic therapy in the prevention of adjuvant-enhanced arthritis in MRL/lpr mice, *Clin Immunol Immunopathol* 72:255, 1994.
120. Berns MW, Rettenmaier M, McCullough J et al: Response of psoriasis to red laser light (630 nm) following systemic injection of hematoporphyrin derivative, *Lasers Surg Med* 4:73, 1984.
121. Pres H, Meffert H, Sonnichsen N: Photodynamic therapy of psoriasis palmaris et plantaris using a topically applied hematoporphyrin derivative and visible light, *Dermatol Monatsschr* 175:745, 1989.
122. Weinstein GD, McCullough JL, Nelson JS et al: Low dose Photofrin II photodynamic therapy of psoriasis, *Clin Res* 39:509A, 1991.
123. Stringer MR, Collins P, Robinson DJ et al: The accumulation of protoporphyrin IX in plaque psoriasis after topical application of 5-aminolevulinic acid indicates a potential for superficial photodynamic therapy, *J Invest Dermatol* 107:76, 1996.
124. Weinstein GD, McCulough JL, Jeffes EWB: Photodynamic therapy of psoriasis with topical 5-aminolevulinic acid and UVA, *Skin Pharmacol* 8:83, 1995.
125. Divaris DX, Kennedy JC, Pottier RH: Phototoxic damage to sebaceous glands and hair follicles of mice after systemic administration of 5-aminolevulinic acid correlates with localized protoporphyrin IX fluorescence, *Am J Pathol* 136:891, 1990.
126. Grossman M, Wimberly J, Dwyer P et al: PDT for hirsutism, *Lasers Surg Med Suppl* 7:44, 1995.
127. Lang S, Baumgartner R, Struck R et al: Photodynamic diagnosis and therapy of neoplasms of the facial skin after topical administration of 5-aminolevulinic acid, *Laryngorhinootologie* 74:85, 1995.
128. Svanberg K, Wang I, Rydell R et al: Fluorescence diagnostics of head and neck cancer utilizing oral administration of δ-amino levulinic acid, *SPIE Proc* 2371:129, 1995.
129. Wang I, Svanberg K, Andersson-Engels S et al: Photodynamic therapy of non-melanoma skin malignancies with topical δ-amino levulinic acid: diagnostic measurements, *SPIE Proc* 2371:243, 1995.
130. Leunig A, Rick K, Stepp H et al: Fluorescence photodetection of neoplastic lesions in the oral cavity following topical application of 5-aminolevulinic acid, *Laryngorhinootologie* 75:459, 1996.

131. Ammann R, Hunziker T, Braathen LR: Topical photodynamic therapy in verrucae: a pilot study, *Dermatology* 191:346, 1995.
132. Fehr MK, Chapman CF, Krasieva T et al: Selective photosensitizer distribution in vulvar condyloma acuminatum after topical application of 5-aminolevulinic acid, *Am J Obstet Gynecol* 174:951, 1996.
133. Abramson AL, Shikowitz MJ, Mullooly VM et al: Clinical effects of photodynamic therapy on recurrent laryngeal papillomas, *Arch Otolaryngol Head Neck Surg* 118:25, 1992.
134. Mullooly VM, Abramson AL, Shikowitz MJ: Dihematoporphyrin ether–induced photosensitivity in laryngeal papilloma patients, *Lasers Surg Med* 10:349, 1990.
135. Dougherty TJ, Marcus SL: Photodynamic therapy, *Eur J Cancer* 28A:1734,1992.
136. Farber NE, McNeely J, Rosner D: Skin burn associated with pulse oximetry during perioperative photodynamic therapy, *Anesthesiology* 84:983,1996.
137. Kaye ET, Levin JA, Blank IH et al: Efficiency of opaque photoprotective agents in the visible light range, *Arch Dermatol* 127:351, 1991.
138. Boyle DG, Potter WR: Photobleaching of Photofrin II as a means of eliminating skin photosensitivity, *Photochem Photobiol* 46:997, 1987.
139. Hopper C: The role of photodynamic therapy in the management of oral cancer and precancer, *Eur J Cancer B Oral Oncol* 32:71, 1996.
140. Stender IM, Wulf HC: Koebner reaction induced by photodynamic therapy using delta-aminolevulinic acid: a case report, *Acta Derm Venereol* 76:392, 1996.

CHAPTER nine

Laser Safety: Regulations, Standards, and Practice Guidelines

Penny J. Smalley and Mitchel P. Goldman

Over the past few years, use of lasers in dermatology, plastic surgery, cosmetic surgery, and aesthetics has become increasingly commonplace. The number of laser wavelengths, manufacturers available, and types of clinical applications have greatly increased. Along with this explosion in technology, more treatment options exist than ever before for physicians who want to employ lasers in their practices. Creative plans for financing a purchase, leases, rentals, and joint ventures provide greater opportunities for physicians to access the technology without making burdensome commitments of either financial or human resources.

An alarming result of this trend is a growing number of accidents, incidents, and untoward occurrences associated with laser use in practice settings outside the conventional hospital-based operating room. Standards, state and national regulations, and practice guidelines provide the basis for establishing and maintaining a laser-safe treatment environment for patients and a laser-safe working environment for personnel.

AMERICAN NATIONAL STANDARDS INSTITUTE: REVISED STANDARD Z136.3

The American National Standards Institute (ANSI) is a nonregulatory body that promulgates thousands of standards on a national level. This federation of manufacturers, trade associations, professional organizations, consumers, government and military agencies, research and educational facilities, and technical and scientific groups, through its nationwide activities and participation in international standards agencies, such as the International Organization for Standardization (ISO) and International Electrotechnical Commission (IEC), establishes and maintains national consensus standards.

ANSI Z136.3 is the Standard for the Safe Use of Lasers in Health Care Facilities and was revised in 1996. This document has become the accepted national benchmark for laser safety and as such forms the basis for guidelines used by the U.S. Occupational Safety and Health Administration (OSHA), Joint Commission for Accreditation of Healthcare Organizations (JCAHO), and most professional organizations' standards for practice. The courts often use this document to measure and evaluate safe practice in cases of litigation for malpractice. All laser users are expected to comply with the standard, regardless of the type of laser they are using, the clinical application, or the practice setting. This basic precept is reflected throughout the standard and is the key to appropriate policies and procedures for safety. On the first page of the document, under Section 1, the scope is described as follows:

> This standard includes engineering, procedural, and administrative controls necessary for the safety of patients and health care professionals. These controls are based upon: evaluation of potential hazards from laser radiation; unique problems related to operating rooms, outpatient clinics, mobile laser units, and private medical and dental offices; and exposure risks to patients and professional staff.[1]

Further, in Section 1 1.4, The Small Medical Clinic, the standard clearly discusses what is included in that mandate. It requires assurance that office-based practices have established safety procedures and training policies that are no less stringent than those in hospitals. These requirements include appointment of a *laser safety officer* (LSO), use of all appropriate control measures, provision of education and training for all staff, ensuring safe maintenance of equipment, and knowledge of all regulations, advisory guidelines, and professional standards for practice.

The individual named LSO has responsibilities as outlined in the standard (Section 1.3) for all health care facilities, including evaluating hazards, establishing and enforcing compliance with appropriate control measures, providing written policies and procedures, approving protective equipment, ensuring safety education and training, ensuring proper maintenance and service of equipment, monitoring medical surveillance, and complying with all regulatory, state, and local requirements (see Appendix F). The LSO must be available when lasers are in use and serves as the facility's point of contact for any investigation, audit, accreditation, or compliance review. The LSO must have adequate education to perform these duties and must be both authorized and responsible for monitoring and overseeing the laser environment. The presence of the LSO is considered one of the most important administrative control measures, and because of this, this officer should be an assertive and motivated person, able to function as the liaison among administration, staff, industry, and regulatory agencies. Classes are available throughout the United States for LSO education. However, no agency, organization, or examination can qualify, credential, or certify LSOs (or MLSOs), and each facility or practice must establish its own criteria for LSO education and maintain its own internal policies for certification.

The ANSI standards detail both direct and nonbeam hazards and recommend specific control measures for prevention of injury and accident. Section 4, Control Measures, states, "It is important to understand that regardless of the clinical setting, the presence of the patient creates the need for a set of unique control measures which must be dealt with in special ways." This further emphasizes the need for strict adherence to safe practice, both within and outside hospital boundaries.

Control measures include engineering, administrative, procedural, and protective equipment. *Engineering controls* refer to those safety features built into systems to prevent accidental emission of laser radiation. Some examples are guarded foot switch, key lock, housing interlocks, audible and visible emission indicators, beam stops, and aperture covers or shutters.

Administrative controls include appointment of the LSO, monitoring of the safety program by the laser committee; written policies, procedures, and documentation tools; mandatory education and training programs; and a reporting mechanism.

Procedural controls are perioperative activities or work practices expected of all personnel in a laser room defined by the facility's policies and procedures. These include monitoring controlled access; preparing a laser-safe operative site (nonflammable prep solutions and nonreflective, fire-retardant drapes); eliminating smoke from the surgical site intraoperatively; ensuring that only properly trained personnel are in the treatment room; setting up, checking, and testing the laser systems and accessory equipment; assisting the physician; operating the control panel; and providing patient advocacy.

Protective equipment controls are items designed to protect personnel from incidental or accidental laser emission. These include window barriers for all lasers with the potential to transmit through and strike personnel outside the room, signs, labels, protective eyewear, fire extinguishers, nonflammable drapes, anodized instruments, beam stops, skin protection, masks, in-line suction filters, and smoke evacuation systems.

OCCUPATIONAL SAFETY AND HEALTH ADMINISTRATION

Recently, health care facilities have experienced greater oversight and regulation from OSHA with regard to clinical areas and surgical technologies. Laser manufacturers and laser users should be aware of the stronger and more proactive positions taken at all levels of government in protecting health care worker safety, resulting from a new partnership with JCAHO and from increasing pressure from professional associations through a more organized approach to lobbying in Washington, DC, for clearer guidance in worker safety.[2]

Accident and incident reporting of occurrences not serious enough to be required by the Safe Medical Device Act is somewhat decentralized. No one agency, except through the *Medical Device Reports* of the U.S. Food and Drug Administration (FDA), provides a mechanism for such reports, and because of this, only a small percentage of these incidents/accidents are known and accessible by the public. Rockwell Laser, a private consulting firm based in Cincinnati, has a website (http://www.rli.com) for laser accident reporting and has accumulated a database of laser accident reports—as of April 1997, more than 330 cases, 63 of which are medically related.[3]

In March 1997 a new document was drafted by OSHA, *Guidelines for Healthcare Workers Exposed to Laser and Electrocautery Smoke*. This document details the hazards and control measures, both with equipment and work practices, necessary to manage this problem. The review process is still underway as of late 1998; OSHA will inform (has informed) the public when the document becomes available (that the document is available).

Currently, all OSHA audits are done under the umbrella of the *General Duty Clause*, which states that the employer has a duty to the employee to provide a risk-free workplace, proper safety equipment, and the education needed to promote safe work practices. Also, the employee has a duty to undertake the education, use the equipment, and work in such a way as to maintain safety. If any of these practices is not done, and there is an incident or accident investigation, the compliance officer may question any employee and require validation of their knowledge of the facility's safety policies and procedures.

Issues investigated by OSHA include employee exposure to harmful airborne contaminants, eye injuries from either failure to use protective eyewear or use of improper protective glasses, fires, burns, unrestricted/unsupervised operation of lasers in nonhospital practice settings, and noncompliance with 29CFR 1910.1030 (Blood-borne Pathogen Standard). Compliance with ANSI Z136.3 is expected, and if a facility is found deficient, it can be cited and fined.

If a laser safety audit is conducted by OSHA, the focus will be on reviewing administrative control measures, documentation, and the laser procedure manual, as well as interviewing personnel, rather than on actual content of policies and procedures. By looking at the process of safety management, a compliance officer can assess whether or not a facility has demonstrated that they have done the following:

1. Established written safety policies and procedures
2. Identified criteria for selection of protective equipment (ANSI Z136.3)
3. Implemented adequate education and training programs for all employees who may be exposed to the hazards
4. Performed and documented periodic safety audits
5. Ensured surveillance of the safety program

OSHA should be viewed as an advocate for safe practice who can offer education, assistance, advice, and resources to help the individual practice comply with standards and regulations. Everyone benefits, especially the patient, when laser users take advantage of these resources during the early phases of program planning, well before treating the first patient or making the decision to purchase or rent laser equipment.

EDUCATION AND TRAINING

Standards require education and training for everyone using or working with lasers (class 3b-4), including LSOs, clinicians, technicians, and all perioperative team members. Each facility or private practice is responsible for establishing its own criteria for this education, but it may consult the appendices in the ANSI Z136.3, affiliated hospitals or laser centers in the local area, private laser consultants, and well-recognized professional organizations (e.g., American Academy of Dermatology,[4] Association of Operating Room Nurses,[5] American Society for Lasers in Medicine and Surgery,[6] Laser Institute of America,[7]) for recommendations and guidance.

Educational criteria should have both didactic and practical components, be comprehensive in presenting laser science, and be laser wavelength and procedure specific. It should be taught by instructors with valid, longstanding credentials and without commercial bias. This is particularly important if the new laser user has no previous experience or training. The consumer must be informed and aware and avoid courses that advertised they will credential or certify, knowing that this is not possible and extremely misleading. A course certificate indicates attendance only and should not be accepted as proof of knowledge or competency.

It is essential to examine the program to be sure it includes all pertinent topics, including biophysics, tissue interactions, surgical and medical applications, techniques and dosimetry, case management, patient selection, indications and contraindications, safety standards, systems and instrumentation, infection control, and risk management. Some courses also include practice management and coding/marketing; although these topics are interesting, they are not essential to safe, appropriate, and effective laser practice.

Practical sessions must be an important component of training, and it is preferable that they be done in a wet laboratory, where physicians can learn on perfused tissues. Learning to use varying power densities, delivery systems, techniques, and fluences facilitates understanding of the principles of tissue relaxation, thermal damage control, hemostasis, and carbon-free surgical effects, which in turn results in positive patient outcomes and safety. So-called grocery labs, where the physician uses meat or vegetables as the tissue model, teach only operational techniques and very little about true laser-tissue interactions on living, perfused tissues.

Laboratory sessions should always be conducted on the same laser systems the physician is planning to use, because with so many different systems on the market, each with its own power parameters and delivery systems, the total effect on tissue is always different. If hands-on practical sessions are unavailable, preceptorship should be arranged through a credentialed practitioner who can instruct and demonstrate on the laser system to be employed.

Nursing and assistant staff education should also incorporate didactic and practical sessions. Classroom curriculum should not vary too much from that taken by the physician, but should stress perioperative safety and patient management. Practical experience includes demonstration and competency-based skills validation of the set-up, testing, calibration, operations, care, troubleshooting, and maintenance of the laser and all the delivery systems and accessory instrumentation (e.g., fibers, connectors, scopes, smoke evacuators).

Appendix D of the ANSI Z136.3 states, "Laser safety training for perioperative nursing and support personnel must be compatible with that taught to physicians.

A smoothly functioning laser team depends on this, and every effort must be made to eliminate the discrepancies in training materials."[1] Often, physician courses do not teach safety in the same depth taught to nurses, creating an information deficit that can lead to noncompliance. A course rarely includes a specific lecture on safety, and even when it does, it often focuses on eyewear and flammability concerns and does not include a discussion on standards, OSHA, documentation, or infection control. On the other side, nursing courses rarely discuss clinical applications and techniques in any great depth, making it difficult for nurses to prepare the instruments and assist during procedures. It is necessary for both physicians and perioperative personnel to seek training and education that include similar coverage of safety and appropriate techniques.

Further, the standards emphasize the need for appropriate instructor credentials, stating, "It is essential that the student relate to the training message given, and the perspective from which it is issued. Perioperative, clinical, and technical personnel should be educated by an individual who can relate to the appropriate experiences, [which are] presented in a manner and at a level that is applicable to the clinical or technical practice setting."[1] This indicates the importanceof having both physicians and nurses obtain their education from their professional peers, not from salesmen, service technicians, or physicists, in order to establish an appropriate framework and foundation on which to build a long-lasting laser safety program.

CAN NURSES PERFORM LASER PROCEDURES?

A new trend has begun to take hold in private clinics and office practices. Nurses, technicians, physician's assistants, and other nonmedical personnel are being hired to perform some of the less invasive and more time-consuming laser procedures, such as removal of port-wine stains, leg vein treatments, hair removal, and treatment of pigmented lesions. Because no nationally recognized credentialing criteria exist for such technical and clinical skills, many physicians have assumed that if they take responsibility and vouch for the training of their personnel, they can practice safely. This is not always true, and much more information should be acquired before initiating such a practice, especially if the employee is to be a registered professional nurse, with a license maintained by the individual's state board of nursing. If the employee is to be an unlicensed assistant, the determining factor is the provision for coverage under the physician's malpractice insurance carrier.

When the boards of nursing in each of the 50 states were surveyed as to their positions on this practice, only 15 (as of March 1997) had approved this within the stated scope of practice, and of those, nine specify that it must be done under supervision, only as a delegated medical act. Many state boards say without reservation that a nurse may not perform such procedures. Some have specific requirements for education, advanced practice training, or certification. Almost all require the individual facility to maintain written policies and procedures, as well as documentation of training.[8]

Both the physician/employer and the nurse/employee should carefully examine the following questions before commencing this practice:

1. Under whose license (malpractice insurance and liability) will the nurse practice?
2. What is the position of the state board of nursing?
3. If the state law does not sanction this practice, can it be appealed or changed?
4. What documentation is required?
5. What education and training are required, and where and how is it obtained?
6. Is this considered prescriptive authority, and who determines parameters?
7. Who does patient education and consultation and postoperative follow-up?
9. What supervision and control measures are necessary?

Nurses should understand that if they ignore the position of their state boards, then find themselves named in a legal action, they could risk losing their licensure. Insurance carriers should be educated on case-by-case basis, because they know so little about the technology and its application, and nurses performing these procedures have few precedents. Nurses may be very receptive; however, if they are not, they must understand that the physician's insurance may not provide needed coverage if they practice outside their known scope of practice. Nurses should never perform laser procedures without a physician's involvement or in a facility without input and supervision, because this is determined to be medical practice, not nursing practice.

PERIOPERATIVE SAFETY MEASURES

Hazards can be determined as either *beam hazards* (related to direct or reflected impact of the laser beam to tissue, such as eye damage, skin burn, or gas explosion), or *nonbeam* hazards (secondary hazards, such as plume, mechanical, electrical, or fire). After the hazards specific to each laser are known, control measures in the form of written policies and procedures are established to prevent each of the hazards. Everyone involved with operation and use of a laser should be familiar with the facility's safety procedures. The LSO should update the policies each year and whenever laser practices change through additional lasers, new delivery systems, new staff, new applications, or new local or national regulations or standards.

Each laser wavelength has certain hazards associated with it and requires its own specific safety procedures. Identifying hazards and implementing control measures are the most important responsibilities of the LSO but are also the concern and responsibility of everyone in a laser treatment room.

Procedural safety depends on controlling access to the room, using protective eyewear and proper intraoperative instrumentation, monitoring the controls and operations of the system, and ensuring effective interaction among laser team members and the patient, whenever the laser is activated.

Observers, company representatives, students, engineers or service technicians, family members, and the media must all adhere to safety policies and must be held accountable for compliance. It is helpful to have a written policy statement that can be given to anyone other than employed staff on entry into the laser treatment room and that describes expected behavior and safety procedures (e.g., use of eyewear, beam path obstruction, fiber placement, smoke evacuation). This not only prevents the need to address unsafe behaviors during a procedure or while a patient is in the room, but also complies with ANSI standards in Section 4.4.2.1, Laser Treatment Controlled Area, which outlines the following measures:

1. Posting of regulation "danger" signs
2. Supervision of room by trained laser personnel
3. Provision of protective equipment at room entrance (eyewear when laser in use)
4. Presence in room only of those authorized and appropriately trained
5. Addition of window barriers for lasers that can transmit through glass

Controlled access to a laser room prevents risk of injury resulting from distraction, unanticipated interruption, overcrowding, operations by untrained persons, transmission of the beam to areas outside the operative site, unprepared exposure to the beam, tripping and equipment hazards, and mechanical accidents (see Appendix L).

Laser keys should not be left in the console of the laser and should be secured elsewhere with access only by those who are authorized to operate the equipment. This is an OSHA regulation for all high-risk equipment, and noncompliance can lead to a citation and fine.

Beam Hazards

Fire

Fire and explosion hazards can occur whenever a laser beam is directed at a flammable substance or material. These materials can include hair preparations (styling sprays, mousse, gels) in the laser target site (hairline, neck, eyebrows), dry sponges, towels, alcohol-based prep solutions, methane gas (perianal area), oxygen, oil-based eye ointments, plastics, benzene, tape remover, hemostatic agents, skin degreasers (4% chlorhexidine gluconate [Hibiclens]), and iodofor-based prep solutions that have not dried thoroughly. To prevent these hazards, the operative site and the entire path of the laser beam must be kept free of all flammable materials. Safety equipment should include an open basin of water within reach of the laser operator, a fire extinguisher that is specific for electrical equipment and in good working order, a fire blanket of nonwoven materials, and only wet and/or nonflammable, nonreflective draping materials (Figure 9-1).

When cutaneous lesions are vaporized with a carbon dioxide (CO_2) laser in the continuous-wave (CW) mode, a layer of carbon often builds up on the skin. If this layer of debris is allowed to remain, the laser beam cannot penetrate to the tissue below and will continue to be absorbed by the carbon particles, causing superheating and spread of that heat to surrounding tissues. As the carbon reaches temperatures in excess of 1000° C, sparking can occur, which can result in fire, burn injury, and extensive tissue damage. The hazard is easily prevented by limiting the buildup of carbon and immediatly irrigating the tissue whenever carbon is observed on the tissue (see Appendix G).

Reflection of a laser beam from any surface can result in fire and burn injury to patient, physician, and staff. This can occur when the beam inadvertently strikes a metallic instrument, curved surface, or shiny material. Instruments used in the laser surgical site should be anodized; a black coating does not determine nonreflectivity. The surface of the metal must be sandblasted, etched, or in some way roughened so as to cause diffusion of the incident beam. Plastic accessories (e.g., mouth gags, eye shields, teeth guards) should never be used unless they have been thoroughly tested for safety with the intended laser wavelength and at surgical levels of power under simulated clinical conditions. Commercially available products should not be used before their safety is verified by the LSO, after carefully reading the testing specifications. Untested metal foil or foil drapes should never be used unless testing proves them safe and nonreflective. Wet cloth drapes should always be used to cover completely any exposed metal surface in the operative site.

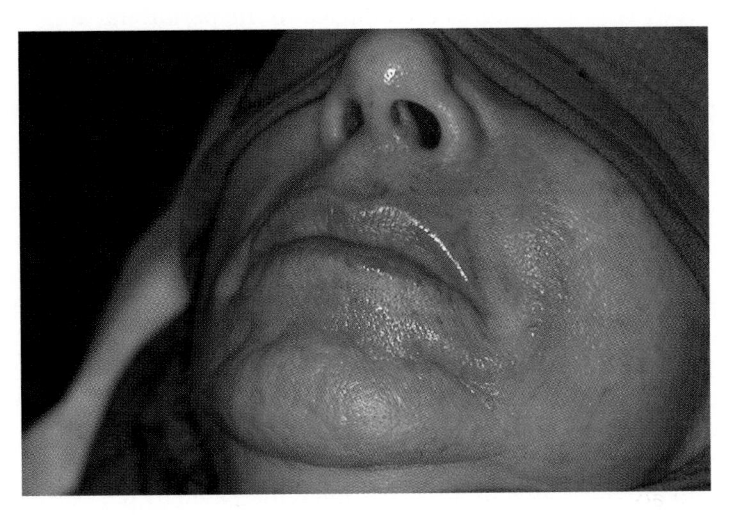

Figure 9-1 Only wet and/or nonflammable, nonreflective draping material is used to prevent fire hazards in the laser room.

Multiple reports of fire with use of the flashlamp-pumped pulsed dye laser (FLPDL) have been reported.[9-11] Heat buildup can occur when the laser energy is absorbed by a secondary chromophore (e.g., hair, melanin) or by combustible items within the surgical field to an oxygen-enriched atmosphere. This has occurred in a cotton fluff in a partially moistened eyepatch.[9] Another report occurred on moist gauze in an oxygen-enriched atmosphere.[10] Gauze will not ignite from FLPDL treatment unless it is bathed in at least 85% oxygen and hit with a laser energy of 9 J/cm^2.[11] Saline soaking prevented ignition. Hair will burn when an energy of 6 J/cm^2 is used in 100% oxygen. It will even burn when saturated with saline if an energy of 9 J/cm^2 is used. Four separate cases of eyebrow ignitions despite preoperative wetting of hair occurred when oxygen was delivered by a face mask.[12] That is caused by the leakage of oxygen by face masks of all sizes at concentrations of 63% to 100%. Flash fires can also occur 8 to 15 cm away from oxygen delivered through nasal prongs.[13] Only a laryngeal mask airway (LMA) will prevent oxygen leakage reproducibly (see Chapter 10).

Ocular

Ocular injuries are entirely preventable by using appropriate protective eyewear, enforcing a clear policy and procedure, and ensuring that all personnel have proper safety education. Class 4 lasers have the potential to cause eye injury, through short exposure to either the direct or the reflected beam, and should never be used without eye protection (see Appendix J).

Ordinary optical glass protects against all wavelengths shorter than 300 nm and greater than 2700 nm.[14] It is important for all eyewear to be marked with the wavelengths and optical densities provided at its wavelengths. In addition, eyewear should have side shields made of polycarbonate for CO_2 laser surgery and the appropriate absorbing material for lasers with wavelengths of 300 to 2700 nm.

CO_2 lasers emit at a long wavelength (10,600 nm) and are absorbed by water. Therefore the tear layer that covers the cornea can readily absorb a stray CO_2 beam and cause immediate but transient corneal burn injury. Fiberoptic lasers emitting at shorter wavelengths, such as the argon, potassium titanyl phosphate (KTP), neodymium:yttrium-aluminum-garnet (Nd:YAG), ruby, pulsed dye, and diode can transmit through that initial water barrier and through the human lens, which serves to refocus and strengthen the incoming energy while directing it at high-power densities, to the posterior segment, where permanent damage can occur to the retina, macula, or fovea. This permanent and disabling type of injury has occurred as a result of incorrect eyewear and policy.

Because many laser procedures are directed to the periorbital area, shielding the orbit is important. A study of six commercially available eye protectors found a difference in the thermal response curves and rates of warming for each.[15] *Plastic eye shields* showed significant thermal damage, with the CO_2 laser igniting a fire or burning through all of them. Commercial eye protectors such as Crouch corneal protectors (Storz, St. Louis), red and black sclera shields (Danker Laboratories, Sarasota, Fla.), or other eye shields sold with tanning beds or supplied by laser companies transmit about 7% to 10% of the light from the argon or FLPDL laser. The argon laser at a 10-sec pulse at 2 W burned through the Danker black shield. No burn-through occurred with either the argon or the FLPDL using other plastic shields.

Metallic eye shields offer protection from both transmitted light and heat. The Cox Stainless Ocular Laser Shield (OculoPlastik, Montreal, Quebec) has a brushed surface to reduce reflected laser energy (Figure 9-2). However, the thinness of this shield allows some heat to diffuse through. When exposed to 10 J/cm^2, the undersurface temperature increased by 1° C/sec, and it increased by 0.6° C/sec at a fluence of 5 J/cm^2.[15] The metallic eye shield from Stefanovsky (Willowick, Ohio) is a thicker, heavier shield and transmits no heat at the tested parameters. However, the

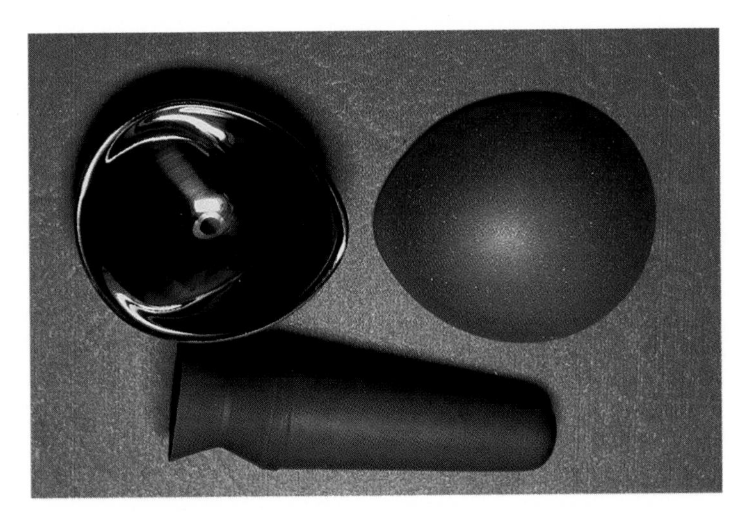

Figure 9-2 Eye shields offer protection from both transmitted light and heat. *Left,* Cox Stainless Ocular Laser Shield; *right,* Stefanovsky metallic eye shield; *bottom,* suction cup to place and remove eye shield.

Stefanovsky shield does reflect more light than the brushed surface of the Cox shield. This is important because even the brushed surface of the Cox eye shield reflects a significant degree of laser light (enough to produce a minor burn on the laser surgeon's hand during testing).

Reflections are most significant from flat, mirrorlike (*specular*) surfaces. Surface roughening is generally more effective than black (*ebonized*) surfacing to diffuse the laser beam. Combining a black surface with roughening provides increased protection, and adding a black polymer finish has been shown to offer the greatest protection.[16]

The ANSI requires that eyewear meet the following standards:

1. Permanent labels for both wavelength and optical density (recommended to be greater than 4.5, if the policy of determining the entire treatment room to be the nominal hazard area is established)
2. Side shield protection
3. Compliance with ANSI Z87 standard (impact resistance)
4. Compliance with manufacturer's standard for damage threshold testing
5. No front surface reflection
6. Proper comfort and fit
7. No cracks, scratches, or other physical damage to lens, frame, or straps
8. Examination and approval by the LSO

Clearly, prescription glasses (unless incorporated into laser-protective lenses), splash glasses or shields, fluid shields, contact lenses, tanning-booth goggles, and other untested, unlabeled eyewear are not approved and safety-tested eye protection and should not be worn by patients or staff during any laser procedure. **Eyewear should be examined before each use by each individual** and should *never* be worn if damaged or if the lenses look discolored. Abrasive cleaning methods and alcohol-based solutions and soaps can degrade the optical coating on the lenses and decrease the optical density, resulting in eye injury.

Protective eyewear is mandated by ANSI standards, OSHA, and all other regulations and guidelines. This applies to all laser procedures, including endoscopy and microscope systems, under all circumstances when using a class 3b or 4 laser.

Teeth

When working around the oral cavity, care should be taken to avoid exposing the teeth to a laser impact. Many patients have enamel veneers or dentures that can be

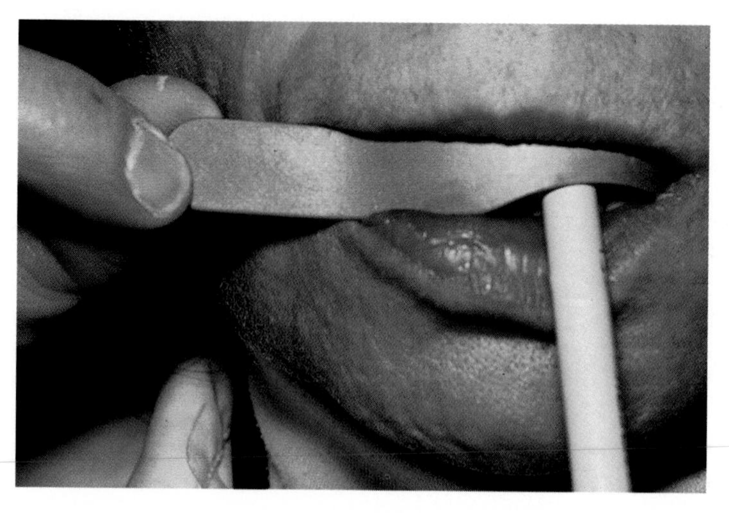

Figure 9-3 Covering teeth with specially designed protector can prevent such damage as cracking and discoloration to enamel veneers or dentures.

cracked or discolored if impacted by a high-energy laser. The teeth can be protected by covering them with water-soaked gauze or a specially designed protector (available from L.L. Lozeau, Ltée, 514-274-6577) (Figure 9-3).

Nonbeam Hazards

Electrical

Electrical safety precautions should be followed for the laser as for any other electrical system used in health care. Staff should examine the foot switch for integrity of the clamp and connecting cords before use and should perform a visual check of all power cords, fuses, circuit breakers, and plugs at each laser setup (see Appendix K).

Surgical smoke

Surgical smoke, its hazards, and its management have recently become a focus of government attention and debate and discussion within most professional organizations interested in air-quality issues in health care. Since 1996 an initiative has been underway to qualify and quantify the hazards and produce documents aimed at developing mandatory control measures.[17]

Research has proved that all surgical smoke, regardless of the energy source used to create it (e.g., laser, electrosurgical unit, harmonic scalpel), contains carbon (mu-

Box 9-1 Toxic chemical by-products resulting from pyrolysis of protein and lipids

Acetonitrile	Creosols	*p*-Aminohippuric acid (PAH)
Acetylene	Ethane	Phenol
Acrolein	Ethene	Propene
Acrylonitrile	Ethylene	Propylene
Alkyl benzenes	Formaldehyde	Pyridene
Benzene	Free radicals	Pyrrole
Butadiene	Hydrogen cyanide	Styrene
Butene	Isobutene	Toluene
Carbon monoxide	Methane	Xylene

From Ott D: *Endosc Surg* 1:230, 1993.

tagenic), blood, and blood-borne pathogens; viral particulates up to .01 μm in diameter; bacteria; and a variety of toxic gases, including benzene, formaldehyde, and acrolein.[18] Concern also surrounds the forceful ejection of tissue particulates resulting from microexplosions of the Q-switched Nd:YAG, ruby, or dye lasers. Tissue splatter may contain as equally harmful particles as tissue that has been disrupted with thermal energy (Box 9-1). Aerodigestive and respiratory ailments are often reported in personnel working in smoke-contaminated rooms without adequate evacuation and filtration.

Plume hazards, whether the result of lasers or other devices used to damage cells, such as electrosurgical instruments, ultrasonic scalpels, and argon beam coagulators, are the subject of widespread concern (see Appendix M). The potential for plume-related hazards has been known since 1986,[19] although a definitive study on the nature and extent of these hazards has not been completed. Research has shown that harmful particulates, including intact virions and viral deoxyribonucleic acid (DNA), are present in the plume during CO_2 laser tissue vaporization.[20] In addition, human immunodeficiency virus (HIV) proviral DNA has been found in laser smoke, although it was not able to replicate. This may be an effect of the laser in impairing HIV integrity.[21]

Laryngeal papillomatosis with human papillomavirus (HPV) DNA was contracted by a laser surgeon who treated anogenital papillomas despite wearing a standard surgical mask and using a smoke evacuator.[22] This occurrence may not be as rare as a single case report would suggest. A comparative study of members of the American Society of Laser Medicine and Surgery and the American Society of Dermatologic Surgery who use the CO_2 laser (570 respondents) found that 5.4% thought they had acquired warts secondary to exposure with a laser plume.[23] Four (0.7%) of the surgeons had nasopharyngeal warts. This is significantly higher than the usual percentage of nasopharyngeal warts in the general or clinic patient population. A study of nostrils, nasolabial folds, and conjunctiva of 11 operative personnel treating genital warts with the CO_2 laser found that one surgeon, who wore a standard mask, had a positive culture after a treatment session in the nasolabial fold, not in the nostril or conjunctiva.[24]

In addition to infectious and noxious particles present in the CO_2 laser plume, the aerodynamic size of the plume particles is also damaging to the lung. A sample of CO_2 laser plume generated by a focused beam of 6000 to 12,000 W/cm^2 (0.5-mm spot size at 15-30-W setting) used to vaporize endometrial implants gave off particles with a mean diameter of 0.31 μm (0.1-0.8 μm).[25] This size overlaps the size range of "lung-damaging dust" (0.5-5 μm).[26]

Carbon and toxic compounds such as formaldehyde and benzene can exist in the plume, although toxicity levels have not been established. The noxious odor and thick smoke can cause headache and nausea but may also cause emphysema, bronchiolitis, and congestive interstitial pneumonia.[19]

Much regulatory and advisory documentation exists to justify a policy for smoke evacuation with all smoke-producing procedures. The Association of Operating Room Nurses has recommended practices mandating evacuation of smoke caused by electrosurgical and laser devices. The American Academy of Dermatology has a position paper on universal precautions that recommends requiring the use of face masks, eye protectors, gloves, gowns, and shoe covers.[27]

ANSI standards state in Section 7.3.1: "Laser generated airborne contaminants (LGAC) contain blood and blood by-products. Laser users need to be aware of the potential for such products during any medical/surgical procedure and utilize control measures such as universal precautions, that are covered by the Blood-Borne Pathogen Standard (OSHA 29CFR 1910.1030)."[1] A note in the standard also states, "Electrosurgical devices and instrumentation are often used both separately and simultaneously with lasers. These devices have been found to produce the same type of airborne contaminants as produced by laser-tissue interactions, and should be evacuated from the surgical site."[1]

Of great importance in documentation of this problem is the *NIOSH Hazard Controls* letter published in September 1996 by the National Institute for Occupational Safety and Health and Centers for Disease Control and Prevention (NIOSH/CDC; see Appendix M).[28] This is the first time the government has issued a statement regarding surgical smoke, and it clearly identifies smoke from both laser and electrosurgery as a hazard requiring control measures in the form of both equipment and work practices. The letter also cites the OSHA Blood-borne Pathogens Standard and states, "Users shall also utilize control measures such as 'universal precautions.'"

Smoke evacuation systems are recommended for all external, plume-producing procedures. Risk of inhalation is reduced when proper collection technique is used at the point of impact. When the collection tube is held 1 cm from the point of impact, it is 98.6% effective, but when it is moved to 2 cm, effectiveness decreases to 50%[20] (Figure 9-4). Nurses or assistants should be alert when holding the plume collection device and never tape or clamp it to the drapes in an effort to keep it out of the way. Filtration levels vary with the manufacturer, but most filtration materials on the market claim to be effective to below 0.1 μm.

If the wall vacuum is used for smoke suction, a high-filtration in-line filter must be placed between the wall inlet and the suction canister to provide particulate filtration before smoke enters the wall system and clogs the central vacuum. The NIOSH letter states that this practice may decrease suction, and because wall suction was only meant for fluids (not gases or particulates) and with filters in place, it may not be effective for smoke removal. This filtration method is only useful when very little plume is expected over a short period. It may also be used to protect the wall suction if more than one suction line is set up and brought into the field or is used as a backup system should the smoke evacuator fail. In-line filters are rated for the number of minutes they will function and should be changed if longer suction time is required. They must be considered contaminated and disposed of properly after single use[28] (see Appendix M).

Laser masks can provide added protection only if worn properly. Plume cannot be filtered if it is drawn into gaps along the sides or under the nosepieces of tie-on masks. Laser masks should be worn during all external, plume-producing procedures. If the mask becomes damp, it should be changed, because its effectiveness is

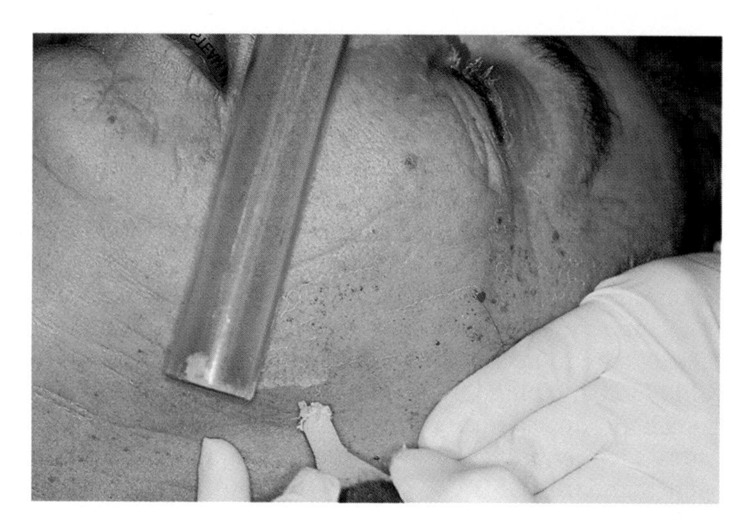

Figure 9-4 Risk of smoke inhalation is reduced when collection tube is properly held 1 cm from point of impact. Collection device should not be taped or clamped to drapes to keep it out of the way.

compromised. Both the CDC and NIOSH are investigating this potential hazard and have suggested that, if current face masks are found to be ineffective, operating room personnel may need to use respirators[29,30] (see Appendix M).

It is important to remember to handle laser masks, along with all materials, tubing, and filters used in the collection of plume, according to universal precautions and policies requiring gloves, gowning, masking, and disposal in red biohazard bags.

Plume collection is more difficult when working with lasers that generate intense pulses and cause tissue spatter or ejecta than when dealing with thermal tissue effects causing smoke. Modified handpiece cones or extended wands are available but they may not be completely effective. Some lasers can be fired through hydrogel materials (e.g., Vigilon) that have been applied directly to the skin over the target lesion without obstructing the physician's field of vision or altering color perception. This method is useful because it can contain the splatter and some particulates by acting as a barrier and preventing ejection into the air. This material should be considered contaminated and disposed of as a biohazard, just as all materials that have come in contact with blood and blood-borne pathogens.

SUMMARY

Safety hazards and control measures are not static. Policies and procedures should be reviewed and updated whenever a new laser is purchased or rented, a new application is initiated, a new delivery system is used, or a new regulation or standard is published. Annual in-service and safety updates keep physicians and staff informed, involved, and aware, helping to maintain a high degree of compliance and to minimize the risk for accident.

Of all safety hazards, *complacency* is by far the most dangerous. Accidents happen when we adopt the attitude, "I have been using lasers for years; we've never had a problem; and it won't happen here." Laser technology has given us new tools that can offer exciting and improved patient treatment options, but hazards should not be overlooked. It is the responsibility of every clinician and every perioperative staff member to ensure the safety of that care through appropriate, professional education and training, journals, conferences, networking with peers, and organizations. Most of all, safety depends on each person's daily commitment to compliance, to individual vigilance during every procedure, and ultimately, to good communication and teamwork.

REFERENCES

1. American National Standards Institute: *Z136.3: Standard for the Safe Use of Lasers in Health Care Facilities,* 1996, The Institute.
2. OSHA and JCAHO collaborate to promote health and safety for health care workers, *Internet News Release,* Aug 5, 1996, http://www.osha.gov and on http://www.jcaho.orgundernews/pressreleases/.
3. James Rockwell interview, Rockwell Laser Industries, Cincinnati, 1996.
4. Task Force on Professional Guidelines, American Academy of Dermatology: Report on credentialing and privileging. Part V, Section D. Specific components in credentials, *Laser Surg,* January 1988.
5. Association of Operating Room Nurses: Recommended practices for laser safety, Denver, 1990, The Association.
6. Safety Committee, American Society for Lasers in Medicine and Surgery, Wausau, Wis.
7. Laser Institute of America: *ANSI Z136.1-1993: Safe use of lasers,* Orlando, Fla, 1993, The Institute.
8. Technology Concepts International: Unpublished report for Candela Corp, Wayland, Mass, 1997.
9. Bean AK, Ceilley RI: Reducing fire risks of the flashlamp pumped 585-nm pulse dye laser, *J Dermatol Surg Oncol* 20:221, 1990.
10. Fretzin S, Beeson WH, Hanke CW: Ignition potential of the 585-nm pulsed-dye laser, *Dermatol Surg* 22:699, 1996.

11. Epstein RH, Brummett RR Jr, Lask GP: Incendiary potential of the flash-lamp pumped 585-nm tunable dye laser, *Anesth Analg* 71:171, 1990.
12. Epstein RH, Halmi BH: Oxygen leakage around the laryngeal mask airway during laser treatment of port-wine stains in children, *Anesth Analg* 78:486, 1994.
13. Waldorf HA, Kauvar ANB, Geronemus RG et al: Remote fire with the pulsed dye laser: Risk and prevention, *J Am Acad Dermatol* 34:503, 1996.
14. Sliney DH, Wolbarsht ML: *Safety with lasers and other optical sources,* New York, 1980, Plenum.
15. Ries WR, Clymer MA, Reinisch L: Laser safety features of eye shields, *Lasers Surg Med* 18:309, 1996.
16. Wood RL, Sliney DH, Basye RA: Laser reflections from surgical instruments, *Lasers Surg Med* 12:675, 1992.
17. Romig C, Smalley P: Regulation of surgical smoke plume, *AORN J* 65, April 1997.
18. Ulmer B: Air quality in the OR, *Surg Serv Manage* 3, March 1997.
19. Baggish M: The effects of laser smoke on the lungs of rats, *Am J Obstet Gynecol* 156:1260, 1987.
20. Garden JM: Papillomavirus in the vapor of carbon dioxide laser–treated verrucae, *JAMA* 259:8, 1988.
21. Baggish MS, Poiesz BJ, Joret D et al: Presence of human immunodeficiency virus DNA in laser smoke, *Lasers Surg Med* 11:197, 1991.
22. Hallmo P, Naess O: Laryngeal papillomatosis with human papillomavirus DNA contracted by a laser surgeon, *Eur Arch Otorhinolaryngol* 248:425, 1991.
23. Gloster HM Jr, Roenigk RK: Risk of acquiring human papillomavirus from the plume produced by the carbon dioxide laser in the treatment of warts, *J Am Acad Dermatol* 32:436, 1995.
24. Bergbrant I-M, Samuelsson L, Olofsson S et al: Polymerase chain reaction for monitoring human papillomavirus contamination of medical personnel during treatment of genital warts with CO_2 laser and electrocoagulation, *Acta Derm Venerol (Stockh)* 74:393, 1994.
25. Nezhat C, Winer WK, Nezhat F et al: Smoke from laser surgery: is there a health hazard? *Lasers Surg Med* 7:376, 1987.
26. Lapple CE: Characteristics of particles and particle dispersoids, *Stanford Res Inst J,* 3rd quarter, 1961.
27. American Academy of Dermatology, Dermatology Practice Administration: *Bloodborne pathogens,* Schaumburg, Ill, 1992, The Academy.
28. Centers for Disease Control and Prevention, US Department of Health and Human Services/National Institute for Occupational Safety and Health: *NIOSH hazard controls,* Pub No 96-128, September 1996.
29. Moss E: Presentation at National Institute for Occupational Safety and Health, International Laser Safety Conference, Cincinnati, December 1992.
30. Dolezal J: Requirements for surgical masks, *Schoch Lett* 43:1, 1993.

CHAPTER ten

Anesthesia for Cutaneous Laser Surgery

Richard E. Fitzpatrick, Mitchel P. Goldman, Danielle M. Reicher, Richard W. Cunningham, and Bradley G. Williams

CHILDREN

The use of anesthetics in children undergoing laser treatments of the skin remains a controversial issue.[1-7] Laser therapy in children with port-wine stains (PWSs) and other vascular lesions can be accomplished by use of a variety of anesthetic techniques. Some laser treatments can be accomplished without anesthetic agents of any type, depending on the location and extent of the lesion, as well as the age and cooperation of the patient.

Typically, hemangioma or PWS less than 1 to 2 cm in diameter can be treated without anesthesia. Lesions of this sort require less than 20 to 30 laser impacts, which can be generated in 20 to 30 seconds, using the repetitive 1-Hz mode of the SPTL-1A laser (Candela Laser Corporation, Wayland, Mass.). At times, talking with the patient, precooling the lesion, or intralesional or block anesthesia using 1% lidocaine with or without epinephrine or the use of a topical anesthetic agent such as EMLA cream (5% eutectic mixture of lidocaine and prilocaine) can be used. However, most treating physicians would probably agree that large lesions in young children are more effectively managed with the aid of general anesthesia or sedation.

The selection of anesthetic agents for these laser cases must be based on the following criteria[1,6]:

1. Patient's age and medical history, patient/family preference
2. Duration of procedure
3. Skill and experience of anesthesiologist in different technique options
4. Availability of appropriate monitoring equipment, medications, emergency equipment, and personnel
5. Prevention of ignition by limiting ambient oxygen concentration near the laser

PWSs have been shown to be derived from a progressive ectasia of the superficial vascular plexus (see Chapter 2). A new hypothesis on the etiology of PWSs stresses the importance of a near absence in innervation, particularly of the sympathetic type, that would modulate blood flow, possibly leading to defective maturation of the cutaneous sympathetic component and forming the basis for this progressive vascular ectasia.[8] In fact, histologic studies demonstrate that only 17% of PWSs in patients less than 20 years old had associated nerves, whereas control patients had 58% of superficial dermal vessels associated with nerves. The vessel-to-nerve ratio was 4.5; ±3.6 in patients with PWSs versus 0.9; ±0.3 in patients with normal skin ($p < 0.005$).[9]

This histologic observation may explain why patients do not notice a decrease in the pain of laser therapy with successive treatments. One would assume that as the lesion lightens (losing its target vascularity), less laser energy would be absorbed, leading to less pain. However, patients remark that as lesions lighten, successive treatments actually result in a slight increase in their perception of pain. This may be because treated PWSs reestablish a normal vessel growth pattern with normalization of vessel enervation.

The advantages of utilizing anesthesia are obvious. We believe that there is less long-term emotional trauma because fewer treatments, and usually no recall of treatment, occur. Treatments are fewer because the entire lesion can be treated in a methodical manner efficiently. Without anesthesia, patients usually can only tolerate a limited amount of treatment, thus necessitating additional treatment of an entire lesion. In addition, patient demands for rest periods and erratic patient movement serve to slow down the treatment session significantly. At times, erratic patient movement can result in excessive overlapping and double pulsing of laser impacts, with a possible adverse result (see Chapter 2). Finally, anesthesia serves to maintain a friendly rapport among the laser center staff, physician, patient, and family.

The disadvantage of anesthesia is the inherent risk of the anesthetic agent. An exhaustive list of each complication of anesthesia is beyond the scope of this chapter. The most significant complications include hypoxia from airway obstruction, bronchospasm, aspiration, hypoventilation, pulmonary edema, and laryngospasm. Allergic reactions to the anesthetic agent may also occur, with the rare possibility of malignant hyperthermia from inhalational anesthetic agents. Dysphoric and dystonic reactions, including emergence delirium, hallucinations, and flashbacks, may also occur with certain anesthetic agents (e.g., ketamine hydrochloride). In particular, with general anesthesia, children (especially those under 2 years of age) are at greater risk for hypoxia for a variety of reasons. These include the propensity for airway obstruction from their relatively large tongue, a small functional residual lung capacity, high oxygen consumption, possibility of undiagnosed arterial cardiac shunts, possible patency of foramen ovale, and frequent upper respiratory tract infections, which result in prolonged hyperreactivity of airways. The following represents a review of our experience utilizing anesthesia when treating hemangiomas and PWSs in children with the Candela flashlamp-pumped pulsed dye (FLPDL) laser.

Hypnosis "Talkathesia"

Some children and especially adolescents may do well with soothing verbal and tactile reinforcement during brief laser treatments. A supportive but not overprotective parent is important. This method uses *hypnosis* as an aid to developing a patient's self-control. The physician acts to coach the patient to relax and modify his or her own state of consciousness. One useful method is to have the patient concentrate on breathing. This simple maneuver is performed by having the patient take a slow, steady breath in to the count of "one-two-three" and a slow, steady breath out to the count of "one-two-three." We have found that timing the laser impact to a point in expiration appears to be less traumatic. A complete discussion on formal hypnotic techniques is beyond the scope of this chapter. The reader is referred to an excellent text on this subject.[10]

Topical Anesthesia

Lidocaine/prilocaine (EMLA)

EMLA cream (Astra Pharmaceutical Products, Inc., Westborough, Mass.) is a 5% eutectic mixture of two local anesthetics, lidocaine (107 mmol/L = 25 mg/L) and prilocaine (113 mmol/L = 25 mg/L), with Arlatone 289 (emulgent), Carbopol 934 (thickener), and distilled water in 1 ml cream. The pH is adjusted to 9.4 with sodium hydroxide. One gram of cream is applied to a 10-cm^2 area.

EMLA cream has been found to be nontoxic, with plasma levels in the circulation measured at 100 times lower than those associated with toxicity.[11,12] In 22 infants, ranging in age from 3 to 12 months, 2 ml of EMLA was applied to 15 cm^2 of skin surface for 4 hours. In each case the plasma concentration of lidocaine and prilocaine was below toxic levels.[11]

The only adverse sequelae reported in the literature include mild local reactions, such as pallor, erythema, or edema, observed in treated skin areas.[11,13-19] Cutaneous blanching is thought to be secondary to vasoconstriction, which raises the possibility of decreasing the efficacy of laser treatment. Decreased efficacy was not found in one clinical study,[20] nor have we noted a decreased efficacy in our patients treated with EMLA.

We recommend that EMLA cream be applied thickly under occlusion with a polyurethane dressing (Tegaderm) for 60 minutes (Figure 10-1). A maximum of 10 g should not be exceeded at any time in any patient. Below the age of 1 year the maximum application quantity is 2 g. A prospective double-blind randomized study assessing pain during laser treatment of PWS skin occluded with either EMLA or placebo showed that pain scores for EMLA-treated sites were significantly lower ($p < 0.0001$).[21]

A study with the argon laser compared injectable lidocaine hydrochloride to EMLA cream. Experimental subjects were adults with normal skin. The argon laser was used at a duration of 200 msec, beam diameter of 3 mm, and maximal intensity of 2.4 W. Interestingly, after 60 minutes of EMLA application, pain blockade was obtained in nine of 12 subjects, with total sensory blockade in the remaining three subjects. In addition, after a 60-minute application of EMLA, analgesia did not immediately occur after removal of the cream, but reached a maximum extent 15 minutes after cream removal. The analgesic efficiency of EMLA cream increased with longer application time (60-120 minutes), approaching an analgesic state similar to conventional lidocaine infiltration. Lack of anesthetic effect of the EMLA returned to baseline 90 minutes after removal of the cream.[22]

Unfortunately, our experience with EMLA cream has shown it to be variable at best. Whereas some patients will have excellent anesthesia with an almost imperceptible

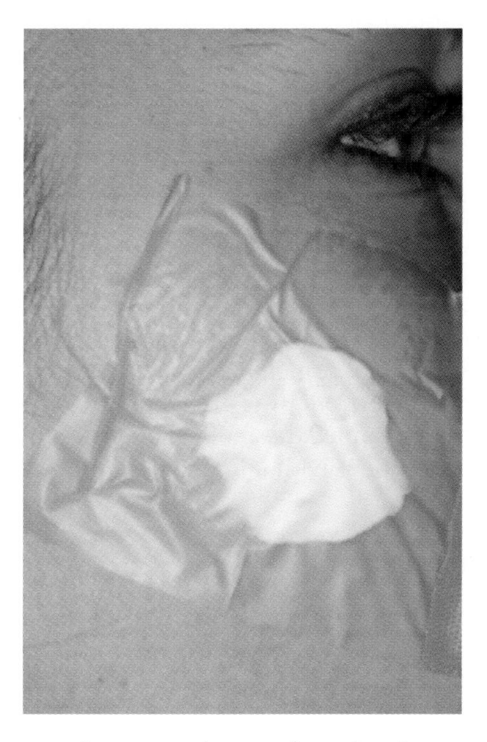

Figure 10-1 Appearance of EMLA under Tegaderm dressing. Note thickness of application.

reaction to laser pulses, the same patient on another day may have absolutely no response to the cream. Therefore our recommendation is to use EMLA for small lesions but not to rely on it for total, predictable anesthesia.

Lidocaine/tetracaine (LaserCaine)

Another topical anesthetic agent available is LaserCaine (Unit Dose Pharmacy and Packaging, Phoenix). This anesthetic cream is compounded for physician office use only.* LaserCaine Compound contains 1% lidocaine and 3% or 4% tetracaine in a proprietary formulation. It is available in 2- and 3-oz sizes in two strengths, Classic, 3% tetracaine, and Forte, 4% tetracaine. It is intended for use on intact skin.

Preliminary observations indicate that LaserCaine has a 30% to 50% faster onset than EMLA, produces little to minimal skin changes, and does not require the use of an occlusive dressing. It appears to have minimal toxicity. LaserCaine is rapidly metabolized in tissue through hydrolysis by serum cholinesterase. The half-life in serum is $1\frac{1}{2}$ to $2\frac{1}{2}$ minutes with a toxic blood level of 8 μg/ml, which is higher than the toxic level of lidocaine, 5 μg/ml. In addition, only 5% of tetracaine is present in the nonionized or active form at physiologic pH. However, patients with atypical plasma cholinesterase enzyme may be at increased risk for developing excessive plasma concentrations of local ester anesthetics because of absent or minimal hydrolysis.

Iontophoresis of Lidocaine

Iontophoresis describes the process of transporting charged ions across a membrane by means of an electric current. This technique can be used to deliver a large number of medications into and across the skin, including local anesthetics.[23] Anesthesia induced by iontophoretic delivery of lidocaine is most effective when treating lesions within the epidermis and upper dermis.[2] The procedure entails adding 1.5-ml lidocaine hydrochloride 4% with epinephrine 1:50,000 to the polymer gel medication delivery electrode for use with the iontophoretic delivery system. Anesthesia is achieved with a minimum current times the product of 20-mA minutes. The duration of anesthetic effect with this mixture lasts between 60 and 90 minutes.[24,25] Two studies evaluating three[26] and eleven[27] patients with PWSs were conducted to test the efficacy of iontophoresis. Patients demonstrated significant decreases in discomfort of pulsed dye laser impulses with this iontophoretic mixture. In addition, no detrimental effect on FLPDL ablation of PWSs occurred despite significant decreases in perfusion, as measured by laser-Doppler velocimetry of the PWS receiving iontophoresis with the lidocaine/epinephrine mixture.[27]

The average time of iontophoresis is approximately 12 minutes. This usually yields a duration of anesthesia of at least 30 minutes. The most common side effects to this treatment are prolonged erythema under the dispersive electrode and a burning sensation to underlying skin. A metallic taste has been noted by patients during some procedures when the electrode was placed on the face.[26]

Our experience, although limited, has not been as rewarding as that just cited.[26,27] However, in a cooperative patient with a limited lesion, this modality is useful.

Topical Cryothesia

We have found the application of ice bags to be effective in alleviating posttreatment tenderness and in minimizing treatment pain. However, laser operators should keep in mind that cooling of the vessels to be treated will result in the need for a higher

*Contact Linda Dixon, MD, at 602-443-4333 for more information. As of 1998, newer mixtures are being tested, and FDA clearance is being sought. Select data in this discussion through personal communication with L. Dixon, 1997.

fluence to achieve effective treatment. For this reason, we usually limit the pretreatment application to a few seconds and use ice immediately after treatment. The ice bag is then moved over previously treated areas during the course of treatment. We have not noted a decreased efficacy with this form of laser anesthesia.

General Anesthesia

As with any surgical procedure, general anesthesia involves a number of requirements of both the physician and the laser facility. Various federal and state requirements dictate the proper construction of the surgical suite. In summary, the facility must have a specific number of square feet built to a specific construction code or standard. Anesthesia machines with appropriate vaporizers must meet various government standards. Monitoring systems, both intraoperative and postoperative, are mandatory. Resuscitation equipment, including defibrillator, oxygen delivery, intubation equipment, and various intravenous drugs, should also be readily available. A strict record-keeping system of the monitoring environment and procedures, as prescribed by the U.S. Occupational Safety and Health Administration (OSHA) is also mandatory. Finally, additional specifically trained personnel are required. The physician is referred to the American Academy of Pediatrics (AAP) guidelines for the use of conscious sedation, deep sedation, and general anesthesia in pediatric patients for further information on this subject.[27] A complete discussion regarding these requirements is beyond the scope of this chapter.

Nitrous oxide

Nitrous oxide (N_2O_2) is a sweet-smelling, nonexplosive gas with low anesthetic potency. It must always be administered with at least 30% oxygen (O_2) to prevent hypoxia. Nitrous oxide also has good analgesic properties and thus is useful as the sole analgesic for brief procedures. Its safety and efficacy have been well documented in numerous studies.[28-33]

Anesthesia is usually given initially at a flow rate of 6 L/min N_2O_2 and 6 L/min O_2. After approximately 1 minute the O_2 and N_2O_2 flows are reduced to 3 L/min. Patients usually experience some lightheadedness and relaxation after approximately 2 to 3 minutes. Patients usually report a tingling sensation of the toes or fingers. We typically use "talkathesia" during N_2O_2 use to facilitate the anesthetic state. Nitrous oxide sedation is a helpful method for calming both children and adults and has been extremely safe in approximately 3000 pediatric procedures.[33]

Nitrous oxide is 35 times more soluble in blood than nitrogen. Therefore, at the end of the procedure, it is important to wash out all alveolar N_2O_2. To avoid diffusion hypoxia, we discontinue the N_2O_2 flow and ventilate the patient for 1 minute with 100% O_2 after the procedure has concluded.

Complications from N_2O_2 anesthesia use are limited. The most common adverse effect is nausea and vomiting, which has been stated to occur postoperatively in up to 15% of patients,[34] but the evidence is lower in our experience. An additional complication from N_2O_2 inhalation is fire. Gauze is capable of igniting when the FLPDL is used at 7 J/cm^2 in the presence of 100% O_2.[6] Hair has also been reported to ignite in room air only when struck repeatedly at this laser energy, and it is easily ignited in the setting of 100% O_2.[6] We have had one episode of ignition of a patient's eyebrow hair by the FLPDL during the use of nitrous oxide/oxygen. Therefore, wetting hair and gauze with saline and applying saline-soaked gauze to cover the exit ports of the nose inhalation piece are recommended (Figure 10-2).

Intravenous sedation

Preoperative preparation. A history is taken and physical examination is performed for each patient. The anesthetic plan is discussed with parent(s) or guardian, and informed consent is obtained. Families are alerted to the possibility of

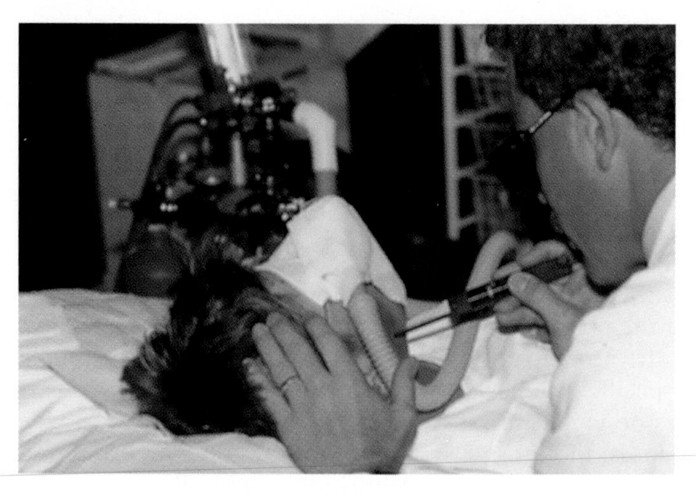

Figure 10-2 Saline-soaked 4 × 4 gauze is placed over the nitrous oxide mask exit ports and over flammable areas to prevent ignition.

unpleasant dreaming and emergence phenomena and are asked to report any such events so that future anesthesia can be modified as necessary.[35-40]

Routine laboratory tests are not required. Patients are given no solid food after bedtime. Clear liquids are allowed 4 to 6 hours before the procedure. This approach could probably be liberalized further based on recent studies.[41] In patients with acute, resolving, or recent respiratory infections the procedure is postponed until symptoms, especially nasal secretions and cough, resolve.[42]

Premedication. Typically no premedication is given for the first treatment. Subsequently, families are given the option of administering oral diazepam (Valium, 0.1-0.2 mg/kg) preoperatively if desired.

Induction/maintenance/emergence. The treatment room is prepared as follows. Oxygen E cylinder is checked and linked to a resuscitation bag. Suction equipment is assembled and readied with both a Yankauer suction and soft suction tip. Intravenous solution (IV) of lactated Ringer's with or without 5% glucose with microdrip system is prepared. Endotracheal tube and laryngoscope are readied. Medications are prepared, including ketamine, midazolam, fentanyl citrate hydrochloride, glycopyrrolate, atropine, succinylcholine chloride, droperidol, epinephrine, lidocaine, diphenhydramine hydrochloride, and others, as needed. Monitors include precordial stethoscope, temperature monitor, Criticare #506 (contains noninvasive blood pressure measurement, pulse oximetry, electrocardiography), and backup manual blood pressure cuff with sphygmomanometer. Ohmeda 9000 continuous/bolus infusion pump is readied with diluted ketamine solution, usually with milligrams of ketamine 3 to 6 times patient weight in kilograms in a final volume of 20 ml (Figure 10-3).

The patient and at least one family member are brought to the treatment room. Most patients allow IV placement with parental presence. Some patients are given an initial intramuscular (IM) dose of ketamine (Ketalar), 2 to 3 mg/kg of body weight with or without atropine, 0.02 mg/kg, as sedation for placing the IV catheter.

Once the IV 22-gauge catheter is secured, IV sedation is started. Initially, 0.01 mg/kg of glycopyrrolate (Robinul) is given, followed by small increments of midazolam (Versed) to induce amnesia and anxiolysis and prevent unpleasant dreaming and emergence phenomena from ketamine. Doses of midazolam vary with age, weight, and level of anxiety; for example, 0.25 mg for a 1-year-old versus 11 mg for a 10-year-old child. Ketamine is started, usually with a small bolus followed by an infusion. The typical initial bolus is usually up to about 1 to 3 mg/kg, sometimes in increments. This is followed by ketamine infusion titrated to effect. The dose range for infusion is typically between 50 and 200 μg/kg/min, with higher rates initially

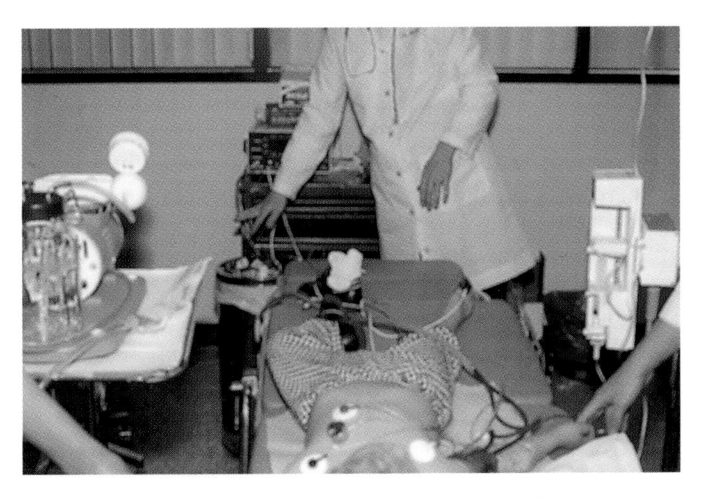

Figure 10-3 Typical laser operatory with monitoring, anesthesia, and emergency equipment readily available.

and lower rates as the procedure progresses. The infusion is stopped shortly before or at the conclusion of the procedure. The level of sedation varies among patients, with most patients calm and quiet on this regimen.

Some patients talk and move during the procedure. If patients move excessively or cry, the rate of ketamine infusion is increased or supplemented with other IV agents (usually, small doses of midazolam or fentanyl). Patients with a history of emesis periprocedurally are often given prophylactic droperidol (Inapsine), 0.1 to 0.25 ml IV. Some patients also receive IV diphenhydramine at the beginning of the procedure to help limit erythematous flaring around the lesion, which at times obscures the margins for treatment.

At the conclusion of the procedure, the patient is closely observed and monitored until consciousness resumes. In particular, the patient is closely monitored for any problems with emergence, such as vomiting, delirium, and coughing. Most patients do very well with the above regimen; they maintain stable vital signs, tolerate the procedure well, and awake calmly. One preschooler even commented, "Daddy, this time I didn't have any bad dreams." This child had undergone a similar treatment in the past without midazolam supplement. As with any technique, some problems are encountered, as follows:

Coughing during procedure
Coughing on emergence
Hiccups during procedure
Emesis during procedure
Emesis on emergence
Excitement on emergence
Irregular or decreased respiratory rate

Each of these events occurs infrequently (less than 4% of procedures), and most are mild. Coughing responses are the most worrisome reactions because of the concern for potential laryngospasm.[43,44] Occasional respiratory rate irregularity or slowing is extremely mild and responds well to adjustment of ketamine infusion and avoidance of other IV agents. Emesis is usually mild; vomitus is gently suctioned if necessary and droperidol occasionally given. Hiccups rarely occur secondary to midazolam or possibly ketamine use.[39,43,45]

The use of ketamine in small boluses and infusion usually permits adequate spontaneous ventilation so that supplemental O_2 is not routinely required. (Clearly, O_2 must always be available if needed, and oximetry is critical.) This is desirable in laser procedures where ignition is always a risk. This also allows avoidance of masks, which could restrict the field of the laser, because many of these lesions are on the face. The continuous infusion of ketamine helps limit the total dose of the drug and allows flexible and delicate titration during the procedure. The recommended dosage range is well documented.[46-52] Glycopyrrolate prevents the excessive secretions that ketamine typically causes, and midazolam promotes tranquility and amnesia.

Disadvantages exist with any technique. Although ketamine usually permits adequate or even increased ventilation, hypoventilation can occur.[40,44,53-56] Coughing and laryngospasm, although rare, may also occur.[39,43,44] Excessive salivation can usually be blocked with a drying agent; this is critical, because excess secretions may predispose to coughing and laryngospasm with ketamine.[39] Emergence phenomena can be a problem with ketamine, but in our series midazolam seems to control this problem adequately.[35,36,40,56] Midazolam itself can cause hypoventilation, hiccups, excessive sedation, emesis, and emergence delirium; careful dosing and vigilance are critical.[39]

Propofol anesthesia

Propofol (Diprivan) is an IV sedative-hypnotic agent that can be used for sedation or induction and maintenance of general anesthesia. It is only slightly soluble in water and is formulated as an emulsion containing the active agent 2,6-diisopropylphenol (10 mg/ml) along with soybean oil, egg lecithin, and glycerol. Propofol may be used as a single agent or in combination with other sedatives, narcotics, or inhaled anesthetics. Induction of anesthesia with propofol is smooth and rapid. Intermittent bolus injections or a continuous infusion can be used to maintain anesthesia.

Propofol sedation may offer advantages over the other sedative-hypnotics because of its short duration of effect, rapid recovery, and minimal side effects.[57] Propofol is highly lipid soluble, so after an induction dose, rapid blood-brain equilibration occurs, resulting in rapid loss of consciousness. After a single bolus, blood concentrations fall rapidly because of extensive tissue redistribution and rapid elimination. Metabolic clearance is the highest of any IV hypnotic, even with impairment of renal and hepatic function. Propofol blood concentration and depth of sedation may be maintained by intermittent bolus or continuous infusion.

Numerous dosage guidelines for propofol are provided in the literature.[58-62] A dosage range of 2 to 3 mg/kg for induction with an initial infusion of 100 to 300 μg/kg/min is common. If the infusion rate is titrated to match the level of anesthesia to the level of surgical stimulation, excessive drug level and prolonged recovery may be avoided. Dosage requirements decrease with age and debility as well as with adjuvant opiates and premedications. Maintenance of anesthesia should be administered by continuous infusion. Intermittent boluses will result in undesirable oscillations of the propofol blood concentrations and will vary the anesthetic depth. The infusion rate will have to be titrated to the level of desired central nervous system (CNS) depression and to the duration of the procedure.[58]

The major hemodynamic effect of propofol is arterial hypotension (up to 30%) with minimal change in heart rate. Both decreased systemic vascular resistance and direct myocardial depression have been implicated as important factors in producing hypotension after large bolus doses of propofol.[57] The cardiovascular effects are accentuated and may be significant in the presence of hypovolemia (excessive NPO status) and preexisting cardiovascular disease and in elderly patients. Most investigators seem to agree that the clinical significance of these changes in young, healthy, normovolemic patients is negligible.[63] Once again, dosage should be titrated for the individual patient and surgical procedure.

Propofol is a profound respiratory depressant. Ventilatory depression includes decrease in tidal volume and minute ventilation and depressed ventilatory response to hypoxemia[64] and hypercarbia. Apnea (20-30 seconds) may occur after a large bolus. In our experience with propofol sedation for cutaneous laser surgery, infusion rate titration has allowed spontaneous ventilation without supplemental oxygen. We have not experienced episodes of O_2 desaturation below 96%. The expertise and equipment necessary to monitor and maintain or secure the airway, including supplemental oxygen and ventilatory support, are implicit in the use of this drug.[65]

Several minor disadvantages accompany this technique. IV access must be established in small children over a series of treatments. Patient rapport, hypnosis, gentle technique with local anesthesia, and experience all play a part. With an uncooperative or very frightened child, low-dose IM ketamine, 2 to 3 mg/kg, with atropine, 0.02 mg/kg, is used as a preinduction sedative to facilitate establishment of IV access. Pain on injection of propofol into a vein in the dorsum of the hand is common (30%-45%). The incidence of pain is less (6%-12%) if injection is made into a large vein of the forearm or antecubital fossa.[61,65] Preceding injection with a dose of IV lidocaine, modified Bier block,[66] or addition of 1 mg/ml lidocaine to the propofol emulsion will significantly reduce the incidence of injection pain.

Studies suggest that propofol is not a malignant hyperthermia–triggering agent and appears to be a safe drug in malignant hyperthermia–susceptible patients.[67-69] Strict aseptic techniques must be maintained when handling propofol. It is a single-use product containing no antimicrobial preservatives. The emulsion is capable of supporting rapid growth of bacteria if contaminated. It is recommended that unused drug be discarded at the end of the procedure or at 6 hours, whichever occurs sooner.

Propofol has proved to be a reliable sedative agent. The most desirable features are rapid induction, lack of accumulation, which allows the drug to be given by infusion; and recovery characterized by rapid, clear emergence with minimal hangover effect and a low incidence of nausea and vomiting.[57] This technique has been well accepted by children and parents and facilitates a smooth course and turnover for our office procedures and recovery room.

Inhalation anesthesia

When general anesthesia has been selected as the anesthetic of choice, no single approach will be effective for all children in all situations. Of the various routes of induction (rectal, IV, IM, and inhalation), *halothane inhalation* is the most commonly used technique in pediatric anesthesia. Inhalation induction of anesthesia may be preferred for small infants and indicated for a child with an abnormal airway. Halothane offers a rapid, smooth induction and rapid recovery for brief procedures. Nausea and vomiting may occur, but recovery is usually uneventful. The other common potent agents isoflurane and enflurane produce a higher incidence of coughing, breath holding, and laryngospasm and require a longer period to achieve surgical anesthesia.[70] Two new potent agents, sevoflurane and desflurane, are in clinical trials. Both appear to have significant advantages over present agents.[71] A detailed discussion is beyond the scope of this book.

Summary

Some parents and children prefer general anesthesia. Many children strongly prefer the "mask" to the "shot." The choice of agent and technique should be based on the needs of the individual child[72] and the surgical requirements while balancing the risks and benefits of the various techniques.

A Survey of Laser Surgeons

Because of ongoing controversy in the use of inhalation anesthesia and IV sedation among physicians treating young children having capillary malformations and capillary hemangiomas, we mailed questionnaires to physicians in the United States known to be using the Candela FLPDL for treatment of these conditions. The questionnaire was designed to ascertain the frequency of various anesthesia usage, the protocol for use, age limits for various agents, and adverse sequelae encountered.

Twenty-two questionnaires were returned. The results of this questionnaire were combined with the published discussions of eight different treatment centers appearing in the June 1992 issue of *Pediatric Dermatology*.[7]

The number of pediatric patients treated per month in these 30 locations varied from two to 250. Included in this group were 10 private offices, four outpatient laser centers, and 16 university or children's hospitals. One hundred percent of the outpatient laser centers, 75% of the hospitals, and 50% of the private offices used either inhalation anesthesia or IV sedation in treatment of pediatric patients (Table 10-1). It should be noted that the majority of respondents use no anesthesia or topical and IM agents in children over the age of 9 years.

All inhalation anesthesia was performed in a hospital or surgery center operating room environment. Sophisticated monitoring equipment was used by all centers, and both inhalation anesthesia as well as IV sedation were administered by an anesthesiologist, usually a pediatric specialist, with the exception of one center, which used a nurse anesthetist for IV sedation. Of the centers responding to the question, only 40% used a separate anesthesia consent form, the majority having this consent as part of their surgical consent form.

The most common age group in which inhalation or IV sedation was used was the 4- to 9-year-old group. The second most common age group was 1 to 3 years old. The lower age limit for which each center would use either IV sedation or inhalation anesthesia varied from no limit to 9 years. However, 73% of those centers using inhalation anesthesia would do so in a 1-year-old infant, whereas 42% of those using IV sedation would do so (Table 10-2).

The only complications reported on the questionnaire and in the report from *Pediatric Dermatology*[7] were two cases of laryngospasm, both attributed to the increased airway reactivity induced by ketamine, and one case of nodal rhythm induced by inhalation anesthesia. The occurrence of these complications emphasizes the need for sophisticated monitoring equipment, complete resuscitative capabilities, and an anesthesiologist experienced in the management of pediatric cases.

Because early therapeutic intervention may be critical in the treatment of capillary hemangiomas and beneficial in treatment of capillary malformations (see Chapter 2), the question of the safety and appropriateness of IV sedation and general anesthesia in very young patients (often less than 6 months of age) becomes critical. To delay treatment in extensive and aggressively proliferating capillary hemangiomas may compromise the effectiveness of treatment and lead to cosmetic deformity (either transient or permanent) that could have been avoided by therapeutic intervention. Delay of treating capillary malformations may not be as critical, but early intervention is still advisable to maximize therapeutic response, particularly before age 4 years. Although small areas may be treated in young infants simply by restraining the child during treatment, this is impossible for extensive lesions. Few laser practitioners would advocate general or IV anesthesia for lesions that can be

Table 10-1
Availability of anesthesia with Candela vascular laser (SPTL) at 30 study locations

	Office-based Private Practice	Outpatient Laser Center	University or Children's Hospital	Total
No anesthesia	3	0	2	5
Inhalation anesthesia	2	3	10	15
IV sedation	3	1	2	6
Topical or IM sedation	2	0	2	4
Total	10	4	16	30

treated in toto with 10 to 50 laser pulses (treatment time 10-200 seconds). However, even this brief treatment session is psychologically difficult for most parents, medical personnel, and some patients.

Children under the age of 36 months allegedly do not have the neurologic capabilities to develop recall of an event of any type. This is corroborated by the total lack of recognition and fear in infants returning for treatment after previously leaving the office crying and bewildered. However, as patient age increases (over 9 months), treatment of even small lesions becomes problematic, especially in the age range of 2 to 4 years. Parents of a 2-year-old patient having a problematic capillary hemangioma 2 cm in diameter on the jaw line, who was treated in our office, allege that the child was diagnosed by a psychologist as having posttraumatic syndrome after undergoing four treatment sessions with the FLPDL using EMLA cream.

This points out the controversy of undertreatment of pain in children. Because very young children (under 2 years) are incapable of meaningful verbal communication, it is often difficult to interpret their cries and verbal efforts with understanding. When attempts at interpretation of memory and psychologic consequences are interposed, this becomes an even more difficult situation.

These factors, combined with the need for early treatment, may result in a difficult therapeutic situation. To be capable of an informed decision regarding proceeding with treatment with or without anesthesia, the relative risks must be evaluated. The most unacceptable risk, to be avoided with all diligence, is *anesthesia death.* A lethal risk from a nonlethal condition is simply not acceptable. Published death rates from anesthesia in pediatric cases range from 1:1000 to 1:2000 if premature infants are included.[73] If all children are considered, catastrophic anesthesia sequelae occur in around 1:10,000 cases, and serious complications occur in approximately 1:30,000.[74] However, most of these anesthesia cases involve surgeries performed in sick children, many of whom have serious and complex medical problems. The anesthesia risks involved with healthy children, using sophisticated monitoring systems, would be expected to be very different. In support of this concept, at NYU Hospital over 12 years, 50,000 anesthesia cases were administered for both serious and nonserious medical problems without a single anesthesia death.[7] In addition to this, no evidence indicates that anesthesia risk increases with the use of multiple sessions of administration. When consideration is given for the routine use of anesthesia in pediatric cases for needed but surgically minor cases (change of tracheotomy tube, insertion of pulmonary endotracheal tubes), the use of anesthesia in these cases seems much more reasonable.

In evaluation of the results of our questionnaire, the published articles, and informal discussion with colleagues, we conclude that some physicians are completely opposed to the use of general anesthesia in these cases for various reasons (they usually consider the need for treatment a low priority or consider the anesthesia risk too high), but that the majority of treating physicians support early intervention and

Table 10-2
Minimum age for use of anesthesia at 30 study locations

Age	Inhalation Anesthesia (%)	Intravenous Sedation (%)
No limit	20	0
≤6 mo	33	14
≤1 yr	20	28
≤3 yr	7	14
≤4 yr	20	28
≤9 yr	0	14

the use of general anesthesia or IV sedation in appropriate cases. The primary limiting factor appears to be access to anesthesia for the office-based private practitioner. In this instance, use of a hospital operating room or a licensed outpatient laser center is recommended. Of course, if the procedure can be done comfortably with no anesthesia, using topical medications or presurgery sedation, this is preferable.

ADULTS

As with children, many laser treatments in adults an be accomplished without anesthetic or with limited application of topical agents. However, full-face laser resurfacing with either the carbon dioxide (CO_2) or the newer erbium laser involves stimulation too intense for topical or local anesthesia alone.

Depending on the type of surgical procedure and degree of painful stimulation involved, a successful anesthetic may include alteration of consciousness, analgesia, depression or reflexes, and muscle relaxation. Facial laser resurfacing is a highly stimulating and painful procedure requiring significant analgesia and alteration of consciousness level for optimal results. For our purposes, muscular relaxation and loss of all reflexes is unnecessary and, in fact, undesirable.

There is rarely only one appropriate anesthetic approach for a given surgical procedure, and facial laser resurfacing is no exception. The use of IV sedation alone is inadequate, and when narcotic analgesics are added, they need to be administered in doses so large that airway maintenance and adequate ventilation become problematic. IV sedation in combination with facial field nerve blocks has been used in some practices, but we have found this technique unsatisfactory. The sensory innervation of the face is complex and in some areas overlapping, making it difficult to attain adequate analgesia. For complete and bilateral analgesia, one must block the forehead, periocular, nasal, medial and lateral face and cheeks, anterior areas of the ears, perioral areas, and jaw lines. The medial forehead is blocked through the supraorbital and supratrochlear nerves. Sensory blockade of the lateral face and cheek is a difficult block to perform and analgesia of the upper half of the ear is achieved through the mandibular nerve. The lower lip and chin are blocked through the mental nerve. The upper outer cheek and lateral forehead are anesthetized through the maxillary nerve, and the far lateral cheek and jaw line through the cervical plexus of each side. Even with perfect technique, the 14 separate nerve blocks required for facial analgesia may leave areas around the ear and lateral temporal region without adequate blockade (Figure 10-4).

General anesthesia with endotracheal (ET) intubation for full-face laser resurfacing is an acceptable technique and has certain advantages. It ensures airway control, is safe and quickly administered, and allows the administration of adequate narcotic analgesia without concern for respiratory depression. However, not all facilities are equipped to provide general anesthesia. Also the patient or physician may be reluctant to use general anesthesia for this procedure.

Advances in anesthetic airway management, specifically the development of the *laryngeal mask airway* (LMA), has extended some of the advantages of general anesthesia to the office-based practice. This technique allows facial laser resurfacing to be safely performed using IV and or inhaled agents while maintaining spontaneous ventilation with a degree of airway control previously attainable only with ET intubation. If necessary, the technique of IV anesthesia combined with the use of an LMA can provide safe and effective anesthesia for laser facial resurfacing without the need for an anesthesia machine (Figure 10-5).

The anesthetic goal is to render the patient insensitive to pain over the treated area, motionless during the procedure, and amnestic for the time spent in the operating suite. Specific pharmacologic agents are selected to meet these clinical objectives. Anxiolytics, hypnotics, dissociative agents, narcotics, and nonsteroidal

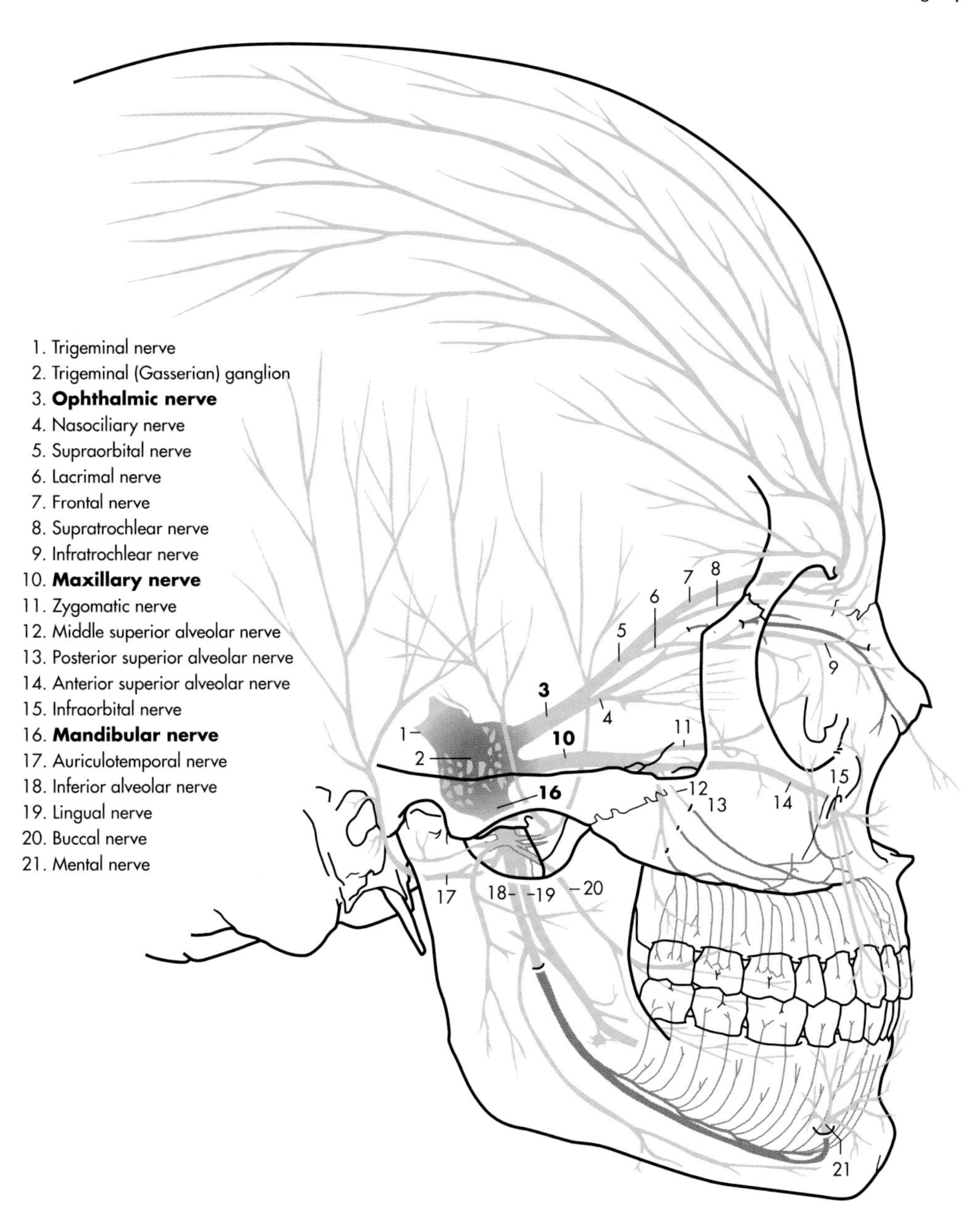

Figure 10-4 Nerve blocks required for facial analgesia. (Redrawn from Scott DB: *Techniques of regional anaesthesia,* East Norwalk, Conn, 1989, Appleton & Lange.

antiinflammatory drugs (NSAIDs), as well as inhaled anesthetics, all may play a role in meeting anesthetic goals.

Propofol (Diprivan) is the primary agent used and provides rapidly induced, easily maintained, and quickly terminated loss of consciousness. Analgesia is provided by fentanyl (Sublimaze) supplemented intermittently with ketamine (Ketalar). To counteract the potentially troublesome side effects of ketamine, as well as to provide sedation and amnesia, all patients receive midazolam (Versed) on initiation of IV access. Glycopyrrolate (Robinul) can be used as a drying agent to help keep the airway free of excess secretions. Using this regimen and limiting the total ketamine dose to about 1 mg/kg, our patients have had no problems with "bad dreams" or adverse psychic experiences.

After IV access has been secured, sedation is achieved with midazolam in a dose of 0.05 to 0.1 mg/kg. Glycopyrrolate 0.2 mg, and fentanyl, 50 to 100 μg are given,

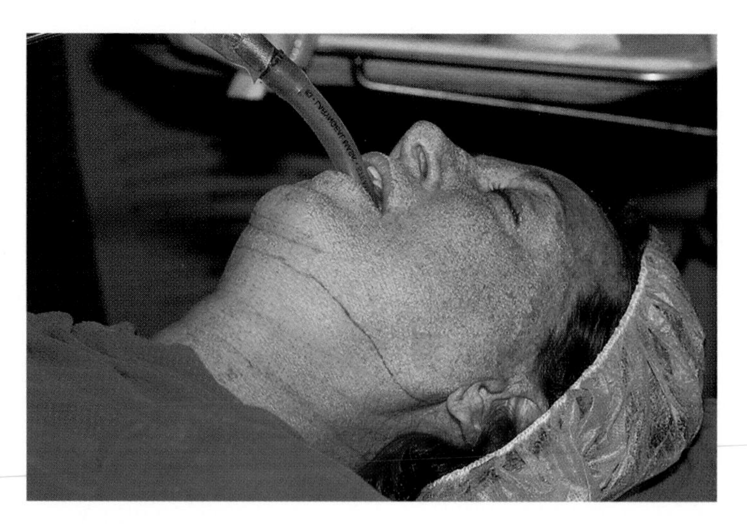

Figure 10-5 Laryngeal mask airway (LMA) in place during laser resurfacing.

followed by an initial dose of propofol, 1 to 2 mg/kg, to facilitate the placement of the LMA. With the LMA in proper position and the patient breathing spontaneously, propofol is administered in a continuous infusion using an IV infusion pump in a dose of 4 to 8 mg/kg/hr (Figure 10-5). Supplemental oxygen may be supplied from the circle system of an anesthetic machine or through tubing from an oxygen cylinder at 2 to 4 liters/min. If an anesthetic machine is being used, N_2O and anesthetic gases may also be used; however, their addition may lead to an increased incidence of postoperative nausea and vomiting. IV analgesia is provided as needed with small doses of ketamine, 10 to 20 mg, and/or fentanyl, 25 to 50 μg. At the conclusion of the laser resurfacing, the propofol infusion is discontinued, and the patient rapidly awakens. The LMA is removed when the patient is able to follow commands, usually within about 5 minutes. We monitor with continuous electrocardiography (ECG), pulse oximetry, blood pressure at 5-minute intervals, and continuous end-tidal CO_2 volume.

The requisite equipment for the technique consists of ECG, blood pressure monitor, functional suction apparatus, pulse oximeter, supplemental oxygen source, LAM and IV infusion pump. Capnography, although optional, is desirable to monitor the adequacy of ventilation. Prudence dictates that any facility administering narcotics or sedatives have appropriately trained medical personnel, a fully stocked resuscitation cart, intubation equipment (laryngoscope, blades, ET tubes), a method for delivering positive-pressure ventilation (Ambu bag or Jackson Rees circuit), and a charged and functional defibrillator. A recovery area staffed with qualified nursing personnel should have the capacity to monitor ECG, blood pressure, and pulse oximetry.

Concern over the safety of laser energy in proximity to oxygen and the patient's face is understandable. All modern inhaled anesthetics are nonflammable, and although CO_2 and N_2O_2 support combustion, neither is itself inflammable. It is imperative that flammable liquids and prep solutions that can yield flammable vapors not be used in the facial preparation. The LMA and its pilot tube used to inflate the pharyngeal cuff are both very resistant to damage from inadvertent laser strikes, but green O_2 tubing is easily damaged by a few laser pulses. However, the oxygen flowing through the tube will not ignite. ET and LMA tubes can be fully protected by wrapping them with saline-soaked gauze or towels. With proper procedures and caution that no combustible liquids are used near operative areas, laser resurfacing in the presence of oxygen and an anesthetic delivery system such as an ET or LMA is safe.

Is every patient a candidate for laser resurfacing in an office setting? Clearly not, but most patients can be accommodated. Patients with severe medical problems such as poorly controlled hypertension, congestive heart failure, or severe or easily triggered asthma, as well as those with orthopnea, morbid obesity, and other significant conditions are better treated in a hospital or outpatient surgery center setting. With proper preoperative screening, appropriate patient selection, and careful monitoring, the anesthetic techniques described can readily be adapted to meet the specific needs of practitioners and patients in a variety of clinical settings.

REFERENCES

1. Lowe NJ, Burgess P, Borden H: Flash pump dye laser fire during general anesthesia oxygenation: case report, *J Clin Laser Med Surg* 8:39, 1990.
2. Garden JM, Polla LL, Tan OT: The treatment of port-wine stains by the pulsed dye laser, *Arch Dermatol* 124:889, 1988.
3. Tan OT, Sherwood K, Gilchrest BA: Treatment of children with port-wine stains using the flashlamp-pulsed tunable dye laser, *N Engl J Med* 320:416, 1989.
4. Tan OT, Stafford TJ: Treatment of port-wine stains at 577 nm: clinical results, *Med Instru* 21:218, 1987.
5. Garden JM, Burton CS, Geronemus R: Dye-laser treatment of children with port-wine stains, *N Engl J Med* 321:901, 1989 (letter).
6. Epstein RH, Brummett RR, Lask GP: Incendiary potential of the flash-lamp pumped 585 nm tunable dye laser, *Anesth Analg* 71:171, 1990.
7. Rabinowitz LG, Esterly NB: Anesthesia and/or sedation for pulsed dye laser therapy: special symposium, *Pediatr Dermatol* 9:132, 1992.
8. Rosen S, Smoller BR: Port-wine stains: a new hypothesis, *J Am Acad Dermatol* 17:164, 1987.
9. Smoller BR, Rosen S: Port-wine stains: a disease of altered neural modulation of blood vessels? *Arch Dermatol* 132:177, 1986.
10. Spiegel H, Spiegel D: *Trance and treatment clinical uses of hypnosis,* New York, 1978, Basic.
11. Juhlin L, Hagglund G, Evers H: Absorption of lidocaine and prilocaine after application of a eutectic mixture of local anesthetics (EMLA) on normal and diseased skin, *Acta Derm Venerol* 69:18, 1989.
12. Engberg G, Danielson K, Henneberg S et al: Plasma concentrations of prilocaine and lidocaine and methaemoglobin formation of infants after epicutaneous application of a 5% lidocaine-prilocaine (EMLA), *Acta Anaesthesiol Scand* 31:624, 1987.
13. Hallen B, Olsson GL, Uppfeldt A: Pain-free venipuncture: effect of timing of application of local anaesthetic cream, *Anaesthesia* 39:969, 1984.
14. Moller C: A lignocaine-prilocaine cream reduces venipuncture pain, *Ups J Med Sci* 90:293, 1985.
15. Ohlsen L, Englesson S, Evers H: An anaesthetic lidocaine/prilocaine cream (EMLA) for epicutaneous application tested for cutting split skin grafts, *Scand J Plast Reconstr Surg* 19:201, 1985.
16. Rosdahl I, Edmar B, Gisslen H et al: Curettage of molluscum contagiosum in children: analgesia by topical application of a lidocaine/prilocaine cream (EMLA), *Acta Derm Venerol* 68:149, 1988.
17. Ehrenstrom-Reiz GM, Reiz SL: EMLA—a eutectic mixture of local anaesthetics for topical anaesthesia, *Acta Anaesthesiol Scand* 26:596, 1982.
18. Ehrenstrom-Reiz G, Reiz S, Stockmar O: Topical anaesthesia with EMLA, a new lidocaine-prilocaine cream and the Cresum technique for detection of minimal application time, *Acta Anaesthesiol Scand* 27:510, 1983.
19. Evers H, von Dardel O, Juhlim L et al: Dermal effects of composition based on the eutectic mixture of lignocaine and prilocaine (EMLA): studies in volunteers, *Br J Anaesth* 57:997, 1985.
20. Ashinoff R, Geronemus RG: Effect of the topical anesthetic EMLA on the efficacy of pulsed dye laser treatment of port-wine stains, *J Dermatol Surg Oncol* 16:1008, 1990.
21. Tan OT, Stafford TJ: EMLA for laser treatment of port-wine stains in children, *Lasers Surg Med* 12:543, 1992.
22. Arendt-Nielsen L, Bjerring P: Laser-induced pain for evaluation of local analgesia: a comparison of topical application (EMLA) and local injection (lidocaine), *Anesth Analg* 67:115, 1988.

23. Gangarosa LP, Park NH, Fong BC et al: Conductivity of the drugs used by iontophoresis, *J Pharm Sci* 67:1439, 1978.
24. Bezzant JL, Stephen RL, Petelenz TJ: Painless cauterization of spider veins with the use of iontophoretic local anesthesia, *J Am Acad Dermatol* 19:869, 1988.
25. Kennard CD, Whitaker DC: Iontophoresis of lidocaine for anesthesia during pulsed dye laser treatment of port-wine stains, *J Dermatol Surg Oncol* 18:287, 1992.
26. Maloney JM, Bezzant JL, Stephen RL et al: Iontophoretic administration of lidocaine anesthesia in office practice: an appraisal, *J Dermatol Surg Oncol* 18:937, 1992.
27. Committee on Drugs, Section on Anesthesiology, American Academy of Pediatrics: Guidelines for elective use of contra sedation, deep sedation, and general anesthesia in pediatric patients, *Pediatrics* 75:317, 1985.
28. Ruben H: Nitrous oxide analgesia in dentistry: its use during 15 years in Denmark, *Br Dent J* 132:195, 1972.
29. Langa H: *Relative analgesia in dental practice,* Philadelphia, 1976, Saunders.
30. Langa H: Nitrous oxide–oxygen analgesia for modern dentistry, *Dent Dig* 66:126, 1960.
31. Allen GD: Nitrous oxide–oxygen sedation machines and devices, *J Am Dent Assoc* 88:611, 1974.
32. Stuebner EA: Nitrous oxide—analgesia or anesthesia? *Dent Clin North Am* 17:235, 1973.
33. Griffin GC, Campbell VD, Jones R: Nitrous oxide–oxygen sedation for minor surgery, *JAMA* 245: 2411, 1981.
34. American Medical Association: *AMA drug evaluations: nitrous oxide,* Chicago, 1983.
35. Mattila MAK, Larni HM, Nummi SE et al: Effect of diazepam on emergence from ketamine anaesthesia, *Anaesthesia* 28:20, 1979.
36. Cartwright PD, Pingel SM: Midazolam and diazepam in ketamine anaesthesia, *Anaesthesia* 39:439, 1984.
37. Miller RD, editor: *Anesthesia,* ed 2, New York, 1986, Churchill Livingstone.
38. Gregory GA et al: *Pediatric anesthesia,* New York, 1983, Churchill Livingstone.
39. *Physicians' desk reference 1993,* ed 47, Montvale, NJ, 1993, Medical Economics.
40. Brown TCK, Cole WHJ, Murray GH: Ketamine: a new anaesthetic agent, *Aust NZ Surg* 39:305, 1970.
41. Schreiner MS, Triebwasser A, Keon TP: Ingestion of liquids compared with preoperative fasting in pediatric outpatients, *Anesthesiology* 72:593, 1990.
42. Cohen MM, Cameron CB: Should you cancel the operation when a child has an upper respiratory tract infection? *Anesth Analg* 72:282, 1991.
43. Dundee JW, Wyatt GM: Dissociative anaesthesia. In Dundee JW, editor: *Intravenous anaesthesia,* Boston, 1964, Little Brown.
44. Coppel DL, Dundee JW: Ketamine anaesthesia for cardiac catheterization, *Anaesthesia* 27:25, 1972.
45. Bailey PL, Pace NL, Ashburn MA et al: Frequent hypoxemia and apnea after sedation with midazolam and fentanyl, *Anesthesiology* 73:826, 1990.
46. Scarborough DA, Bisaccia E, Swensen RD: Anesthesia for outpatient dermatologic cosmetic surgery: midazolam–low-dosage ketamine anesthesia, *J Dermatol Surg Oncol* 15:658, 1989.
47. Pandit SK, Kothary SP, Kumar SM: Low dose intravenous infusion technique with ketamine, *Anaesthesia* 35:669, 1980.
48. Lilburn JK, Dundee JW, Moore J: Ketamine infusions, *Anaesthesia* 33:315, 1978.
49. Sher MH: Slow dose ketamine—a new technique, *Anaesth Intens Care* 8:359, 1980.
50. White PF: Use of continuous infusion versus intermittent bolus administration of fentanyl or ketamine during outpatient anesthesia, *Anesthesiology* 59:294, 1983.
51. Jastak JT, Goretta C: Ketamine HCl as a continuous-drip anesthetic for outpatients, *Anesth Analg* 52:341, 1973.
52. Ackerly JA: Ketamine anesthesia in burn patients. In *Anesthesiology Forum,* vol IV: Ketamine anesthesia in open heart and burn patients. Presented in part at the Ketalar Roundtable, New Orleans, Oct 13, 1984; printed by Parke-Davis, Morris Plains, New Jersey.
53. Virtue RW, Alanis JM, Mori M et al: An anesthetic agent: 2-orthochlorophenyl, 2-methylamino cyclohexanone HCl (CI-581), *Anesthesiology* 28:823, 1967.
54. Wilson RD, Traber DL, McCoy NR: Cardiopulmonary effects of CI-581: the new dissociative anesthetic, *South Med J* 61:692, 1968.

55. Kelly RW, Wilson RD, Traber DL et al: Effects of two new dissociative anesthetic agents, ketamine and CL-1848C, on the respiratory response to carbon dioxide, *Anesth Analg* 50:262, 1971.
56. Corssen G, Domino EF: Dissociative anesthesia: further pharmacologic studies and first clinical experience with the phencyclidine derivative CI-581, *Anesth Analg* 45:29, 1966.
57. Van Hemelrijck J, Gonzales JM, White PF: Pharmacology of intravenous anesthetic agents. In Rogers MC et al, editor: *Principles and practice of anesthesiology,* St Louis, 1993, Mosby.
58. Stanski DR, Shafer SL: New intravenous anesthetics (no. 274). Presented at 41st Annual Refresher Course Lectures and Clinical Update Program, Park Ridge, Ill, 1990, American Society of Anesthesiologists.
59. Fragen RJ, editor: *Drug infusions in anesthesiology,* New York, 1991, Raven.
60. Bloomfield EL, Masaryk TJ, Caplan A et al: Intravenous sedatives for MR imaging of the brain and spine in children: pentobarbital versus propofol, *Radiology* 186:93, 1993.
61. Cauldwell CB, Fisher DM: Sedating pediatric patients: is propofol a panacea? *Radiology* 186:9, 1993.
62. Patel DK, Keeling PA, Newman BG: Induction dose of propofol in children, *Anaesthesia* 43:949, 1988.
63. Apfelbaum JL: Outpatient anesthesia for adult patients (no. 412). Presented at 43rd Annual Refresher Course Lectures, Park Ridge, Ill, 1992, ASA Inc.
64. Blouin RT, Seifert HA, Conrad PF et al: Propofol significantly depresses hypoxic ventilatory drive during conscious sedation, *Anesthesiology* 77, 1992.
65. Valtonen M, Iisalo E, Kanto J et al: Propofol as an induction agent in children: pain on injection and pharmacokinetics, *Acta Anaesthesiol Scand* 33:152, 1989.
66. Holak E, Mangar D: Modified Bier block abolishes local pain associated with propofol injection, *Anesthesiology* 75, 1991.
67. Raff M, Harrison GG: The screening of propofol in MHS swine, *Anesth Analg* 68:750, 1989.
68. Denborough M, Hopkinson KC: Propofol and malignant hyperpyrexia, *Lancet* 1:191, 1988.
69. Verburg MP, DeGrood PMRM: Safety of propofol in malignant hyperthermia: preliminary results, *Anaesthesia* 43(suppl):121, 1988.
70. Steward DJ: Anesthesia for pediatric outpatients. In White PF, editor: *Outpatient anesthesia,* New York, 1990, Churchill Livingstone.
71. Eger EI: New inhalational anesthetic agents (no. 245). Presented at 43rd Annual Refresher Course Lectures, Park Ridge, Ill, 1992, American Society of Anesthesiologists.
72. Hannallah RS: Anesthesia for pediatric outpatients (no. 133). Presented at 43rd Annual Refresher Course Lectures, 1992, Park Ridge, Ill, American Society of Anesthesiologists.
73. Stafford TJ, Crocker D: Role of anesthesia in laser therapy. In Tan OT, editor: *Management and treatment of benign cutaneous vascular lesions,* Philadelphia, 1992, Lea & Febiger.
74. *Anesthesia Patient Safety Foundation Newsletter* 5:4, 1990-1991.

Afterword: A Look Ahead

John A Parrish

The present understanding of possible effects of lasers on tissue and the rapidly developing laser and optical technologic capabilities could lead to a wide range of possibilities that will greatly benefit health care during the twenty-first century. The intention is to develop procedures that are faster, less invasive, and less expensive. Long, inpatient procedures may become brief, outpatient procedures; currently impossible procedures may become possible.

In the 1970s and 1980s the major barrier to the advancement of laser medicine was intellectual: there was limited understanding of the nature of laser-tissue interactions, especially those interactions resulting from pulsed lasers. We did not understand laser-tissue interactions well enough to introduce applications of lasers that went much beyond "shoot and see what happens." The host response was even less well studied, especially those aspects of the biologic responses possibly unique to laser-induced injury.

Our understanding of laser-tissue interaction is still incomplete. However, intellectual barriers are no longer the major limiting factor. In the last two decades, basic research has led to a significant increase in understanding and quantifying the nature of the effects of lasers on various biologic materials. We are beginning to be able to predict and manipulate laser effects on tissue to design new therapeutics and diagnostics. We have learned how to vary wavelength, pulse duration, and energy to maximize desired effects and minimize collateral damage. It is possible to modify the biologic host response to laser injury by the use of wavelength interactions, heat, and other biologic or physical factors.

Perhaps the most interesting and most useful cognitive advance is the increased recognition and understanding of the laser-tissue interactions caused by *pulsed lasers*. In the future these may become increasingly useful in developing therapeutics and diagnostics. Pulsed lasers are still used primarily in medicine for their thermal effects to coagulate, seal, cut, and ablate tissue. They can also lead to plasma-mediated and photoacoustic changes in tissue. Microsurgery with controlled thermal injury (selective photothermolysis) has been used primarily to treat skin lesions to date. Recently, however, pulsed lasers have new applications in the gastrointestinal and urinary tracts using plasma to cut tissue, to break stones or other hard objects, and as a probe of photoacoustic effects. Various nonlinear effects, including multiphoton photochemistry, have been demonstrated in vivo and can lead to new photoproducts and new biologic host responses. Combinations of photophysical mechanisms and perturbations specific to high peak power may add to therapeutic and diagnostic capabilities of light. Short pulses of optical radiation are extremely powerful as spectroscopic tools. Further basic and applied research may allow us to better utilize these effects to create new laser-based applications.

Another important area of increased learning relates to the use of *exogenous chromophores*. Hundreds of known compounds can act as photosensitizers in living systems and may be used to target, manipulate, confine, and control laser effects. The use of exogenous chromophores is a classic field within photobiology; however, the molecular engineering of cell-selective phototoxic compounds and the sudden growth of basic work in multiphoton photochemical reactions are direct results of research stimulated by laser medicine. A large variety of specific photochemical mechanisms are possible and require further study. Although conventional noncoherent light sources are often the most practical sources for the treatment of cancer with photoactive drugs and light, in many clinical situations the unique properties of lasers combine with optical delivery systems to give unique advantages that make the treatment possible. Photodynamic therapy (or photochemotherapy) of nonmalignant processes is an active field of research and an underutilized opportunity.

In addition to these intellectual advances, there have been many technical advances. Laser technology itself has become much more sophisticated over the past two decades. This gives us more options in the laser parameters we apply. Solid-state lasers and diode lasers are creating new opportunities for smaller, more reliable, and less expensive equipment with more wavelength options. There are now a variety of techniques to alter wavelength and pulse duration, either within or outside the laser cavity.

The field of *optically based remote sensing,* developed largely by the military and communications industry, is now being fruitfully exploited to develop laser-based optical diagnostics in tissue. Fiberoptics technology is improving; coherent optical fiber bundles can transmit ultraviolet and infrared radiation into tissues. As this technology advances, we may be able to use it to enhance our capabilities in laser medicine. We also borrow information constantly from the materials-processing sciences to better understand laser-tissue interactions.

Much remains to be done, and a variety of expertise is required. We must consider lasers as one component of committed medical and surgical systems. Sophisticated, high-power, controllable optical delivery systems remain a problem in the development of laser medicine. There has been a steady advance in fiberoptics and endoscopes, and we are now able to consider committed systems and cooperative engineering efforts using fiberoptics, endoscopes, and laser diagnostics combined with ultrasonic, radiologic, or other feedback techniques. The opportunities are enormous, but the challenge to bring together a wide range of expertise is also very great.

Laser medicine has come up against another limiting factor, a barrier that may prove to be a more difficult to define and to overcome. It is a "people" or organizational barrier, caused mainly by competing priorities of the academic, industrial, government agency–based contributors required for progress in laser medicine. The self-interests of the parties involved are understandable and defensible, but they may prevent the pooling of resources and cooperation needed to make rapid advances in laser medicine. This is a *psychosocial barrier.* Although we have much to learn, we can already imagine what can be done with existing knowledge and technology and often cannot muster the expertise and resources in one place to do it.

It is imperative that academic and industrial efforts be integrated. Government laboratories can also be powerful players because of their enormous technologic and intellectual resources. The government-industry-academia triad could use laser and optical technology to improve medical care greatly, but it is unlikely that sufficient cooperative efforts can be organized. The challenge is not technologic only, but also political, managerial, and financial. Our ability to achieve a working collaboration among government, industry, and academia to capture and sustain the immense opportunities now apparent in laser photomedicine will ultimately determine success in terms of improved medical care.

Dermatology has played an important role in laser medicine. Skin is an obvious, highly accessible target organ for diagnostic and therapeutic uses of lasers. Dermatologist investigators and physicians have contributed fundamental new knowledge, concepts, and ideas useful in other organ systems. The well-informed practicing dermatologist using lasers with skill and good judgment can help solidify the image and substance of laser medicine and dermatology. In doing so, he or she can also take better care of patients. This book is meant to further those goals.

Appendices

Laser Organizations

American Academy of Dermatology
930 North Meacham Rd.
Schamburg, IL 60173-6016
(847) 330-0230

American Board of Laser Surgery
John Fisher, MD, President
417 Palm Tree Dr.
Bradenton, FL 34210
(941) 756-2316

American College of Surgeons
633 N. St. Clair St.
Chicago, IL 60611-3211
(312) 202-5000
FAX: (312) 202-5001

American Society for Laser Medicine and Surgery
2404 Stewart Square
Wausau, WI 54401
(715) 845-9283
FAX: (715) 848-2493

Association of Operating Room Nurses
10170 E. Mississippi Ave.
Denver, CO 80231
(303) 755-6300
FAX: (312) 750-3212

Gynecologic Laser Society
6900 Grove Rd.
Thorofare, NJ 08086
(609) 848-1000, ext. 208
FAX: (609) 848-5274

International College of Pediatric Laser Surgery
399 North York Rd.
Warminster, PA 18974
(215) 443-8209

International Society of Cosmetic Laser Surgeons
930 North Meacham Rd.
Schamburg, IL 60173-6016
(847) 330-9830
FAX: (847) 330-1135

International Society for Lasers in Surgery and Medicine
Narong Nimsakul, MD, President
Institute of Modern Medicine
420 Sukhotai Mansion, Sawankalok Rd.
Bangkok, 10300, Thailand

Laser Institute of America
12424 Research Parkway, #125
Orlando, FL 32826
(407) 380-1553
FAX: (407) 380-5588
Secretariat for the ANSI Z136.3 standards

Laser Nursing Magazine
Mary Ann Liebert, Inc.
2 Madison Ave.
Larchmont, NY 10538
(914) 834-3100
FAX: (914) 934-3771

Medical Laser Industry Report
One Technology Park Dr.
Westford, MA 01886
FAX: (978) 692-0700

U.S. Occupational Safety and Health Administration (OSHA)
Bureau of National Affairs
1231 25th St. NW
Washington, DC 20037
(202) 452-4200
FAX: (202) 452-4610

Procedures for Obtaining Laser Surgery Privileges

I. Purpose To delineate criteria for surgeons wanting to obtain laser surgery privileges.

II. Scope Medical staff with current surgical privileges.

III. Responsibility The laser committee will review all applications and make recommendations to the credentials committee.

IV. Policy All laser privilege applications will be submitted to, and reviewed by, the laser committee. Laser surgery is considered an alternative for conventional surgery, and the physician must have current surgical privileges. Laser applications must be specific to the wavelength laser to be used. Final approval of privileges will be granted by the executive committee.

V. Procedures

A. Applications
   1. Obtain application packet from the medical staff office.
   2. Submit proof of current staff privileges.
   3. Documentation for attendance at a training program must include the course brochure, syllabus, or certificate, and content must include:
      a. Minimum 12 hours, category 1, CME credit
      b. Didactics covering biophysics, safety, tissue interactions of specific wavelength requested, indications, case management, and laboratory experience with both inanimate and appropriate animate tissue models, designed to demonstrate proper surgical techniques and understanding of laser dosimetry
   4. Residency training must be verified by a letter from the director and must be equivalent in substance to training course as stated above
   5. Five documented laser cases using the same wavelength from another facility may be substituted for the training criteria stated above

B. Conditional privileges may be granted by the laser committee, based on review of the application, and will cover completion of five proctored cases, followed by a written summary from the proctor verifying safe and appropriate surgical application.

C. If the physician has current privileges but requests an additional wavelength, the application process must be completed for the new wavelength. Documentation must include proof of didactics relating to the physics, safety, and tissue responses specific to the new wavelength, and tissue laboratories designed to demonstrate safe and appropriate surgical applications of that laser.

D. Physicians must complete an equipment orientation, given by the laser safety officer for each new laser before first clinical use.

E. Completed applications will be reviewed by department heads. Department heads will forward them to the laser committee for evaluation and recommendations. The chair of the laser committee will forward applications to the executive committee for final comment and approval.
F. Physicians will be notified in writing of privilege approvals. Should the application be denied, the physician may initiate an appeal through the laser committee.
G. Copies of privileges will be on file in the department of surgery, the operating room, and with the laser safety officer.
H. Privileges will be reviewed every 2 years. Renewal will be granted if the physician has documented:
   1. Eight cases completed with no negative outcomes
   2. Attendance at an approved refresher course
   3. Preceptorship as defined by the laser committee

Laser Skills Checklist

_______ 1. Has read policies and procedures
2. Has attended in-service:
_______ a. Lecture
_______ b. Hands-on
_______ 3. Knows where to obtain key
_______ 4. Knows how to move and position laser
_______ 5. Follows safety rules for room setup
_______ 6. Knows how to assemble accessories and delivery systems for laser
_______ 7. Performs laser test and fiber calibration test, and accurately assesses beam profile
_______ 8. Properly positions foot switch
_______ 9. Can perform daily maintenance procedures
10. Operates control panel properly:
_______ a. Power settings
_______ b. Time exposures
_______ c. Emergency off
_______ d. Standby/ready
_______ 11. Completes all documentation forms
_______ 12. Knows proper methods of cleaning and storage for all accessories
_______ 13. Has passed employee eye examination
_______ 14. Demonstrates knowledge of safe handling of equipment and ability to monitor safety of the environment

Recommended Perioperative Practices Related to the Use of Lasers in Medicine and Surgery*

INTRODUCTION

As part of a continued commitment to provide quality care to patients undergoing laser procedures, the nurses of the American Society for Laser Medicine and Surgery recommend these perioperative practices for patients undergoing laser procedures, including the assessment and nursing diagnosis of patient problems, and the planning, implementation, and evaluation of nursing care.

The American Society for Laser Medicine and Surgery is a dynamic, professional association dedicated to the exploration and application of laser technology to biology, medicine, and surgery. The goal is to ensure the optimum in quality patient care during laser treatment. It is the responsibility of the nursing section of the Society to formulate recommended perioperative practices for reference by clinical nurses and allied health care providers, to be used as guidelines assisting in the establishment of safe, effective laser programs in hospitals and other health care settings.

The recommended perioperative practices provide a broad set of guidelines to assess and evaluate the quality of nursing care in the environment where lasers are in operation. They are not intended as mandated criteria or requirements. As the scope of laser application advances, these recommended perioperative practices will be appropriately updated and revised.

DEFINITION

Nurses who work with lasers and care for patients undergoing laser therapy will derive from the nursing process techniques assessment skills, nursing diagnosis, planning criteria, implementation, and evaluation of outcomes for their clients with need for medical or surgical intervention. They will utilize an experienced knowledge base of many specialties, including but not limited to ophthalmology, otorhinolaryngology, oncology, plastic surgery, dermatology, general surgery, thoracic surgery, pulmonary medicine, gastroenterology, urology, gynecology, neurosurgery, orthopedics, podiatry, and vascular surgery. Nursing practice with respect to laser technology is multifaceted and also requires knowledge in aseptic techniques, technologic expertise, administrative proficiency, and research methodology. In addition, the following laser training and experiences are recommended:

1. The trainee shall review the pertinent literature and audiovisual aids concerning specific needs and assessment, nursing diagnosis, planning, and implementation of care for patients undergoing laser therapy. This should be incorporated in a course or

*These revised standards represent the knowledge that is available to the Board of Directors of the American Society for Laser Medicine and Surgery, Inc., as of Nov. 11, 1990.

seminar that includes laser physics, tissue interaction, safety standards, clinical applications, instrumentation, and nursing interventions. A hands-on demonstration and experience should define safe practices and appropriate use. A minimum of 6 to 8 hours should be required for the above activities with at least 2 hours devoted to the actual hands-on training. The number of participants at each hands-on station should be kept to a minimum to ensure adequate hands-on experience.
2. Ideally, personnel responsible for handling the laser should be supervised by a qualified instructor during two or three procedures to ensure proper laser and instrumentation setup, safety compliance, and laser system operation. An evaluation should follow to note the trainee's competency.
3. Since laser technology is dynamic, laser systems, accessories, instrumentation, and procedure techniques can change. Continuing education is recommended on a regular basis (e.g., via publications) or at least annually (e.g., via seminars) to maintain an acceptable knowledge base and skill level.

RECOMMENDED PRACTICE I

The nurse shall utilize the nursing process to assess the needs of patients undergoing medical or surgical laser therapy. The assessment shall be documented and communicated to appropriate persons.

Interpretation

The nurse shall identify needs of patients based on:
1. Physical and emotional needs of patients and significant others
2. Knowledge of laser procedures to be performed
3. Principles of laser safety
4. Predicted outcomes and potential consequences of the procedure(s) performed

RECOMMENDED PRACTICE II

The nurse shall develop and implement an appropriate plan of patient care and evaluate patient outcomes.

Interpretation

The nurse shall identify appropriate goals for each patient to include but not be limited to:
1. Meeting educational needs
2. Providing for physical safety
3. Offering emotional support
4. Ensuring continuity of care
5. Ensuring patients' rights

The goals shall be addressed in order of priority for individual patient care. Nursing care given shall be evaluated and outcomes documented.

RECOMMENDED PRACTICE III

The nurse shall be responsible for prompt, complete, and accurate recording of pertinent clinical data.

Interpretation

Data should be recorded according to the policies of each institution. U.S. Food and Drug Administration (FDA) regulations or institutional review board (IRB) requirements shall be observed when investigative protocols requiring approval are used.

RECOMMENDED PRACTICE IV

Nursing staff working with lasers shall be appropriately qualified to ensure safe operation of laser systems.

Interpretation

Nursing staff shall demonstrate a level of competency that ensures optimal technical skills and theoretical understanding of laser technology. Reference the American National Standards Institute (ANSI) Z136.3 "Recommended Practices for Lasers in Health Care Facilities" and the standards of the American Society for Laser Medicine and Surgery, "Standards for Training and Practice for Nurses in the Use of Lasers in Medicine and Surgery."

RECOMMENDED PRACTICE V

Nurses responsible for laser systems shall participate in the development of the standards of practice related to the maintenance and operation of laser systems.

Interpretation

Nurses should work within the organizational structure of their institution to participate in the establishment of written policies and procedures that ensure maintenance and safe operation of laser systems and accessory equipment.

RECOMMENDED PRACTICE VI

Nurses should develop quality-monitoring criteria to evaluate nursing practice.

Interpretation

Quality-monitoring criteria are necessary to evaluate outcomes of patient care. Additionally, failure to meet criteria thresholds should provide guidelines to document need for change in intervention processes or need for education to maintain quality patient care.

RECOMMENDED PRACTICE VII

Laser treatment areas shall be designated to ensure a safe environment for patients and personnel who care for them.

Interpretation

The nurse shall ensure that established safety guidelines are followed in the laser treatment environment. Recommended guidelines are ANSI Z136.3 "Recommended Practices for Lasers in Health Care Facilities" and the Association of Operating Room Nurses (AORN) "Recommended Practices."

RECOMMENDED PRACTICE VIII

Performance expectation related to management and maintenance of laser systems shall be established for nurse and support staff.

Interpretation

Performance expectation with regard to activities such as scheduling laser use, transporting lasers, maintaining fibers and optics, and routine laser maintenance should be clearly defined to ensure efficient and safe use of the laser.

RECOMMENDED PRACTICE IX

Lasers and laser equipment shall be appropriately maintained.

Interpretation

All laser equipment used shall be routinely inspected for reliable and safe performance. A preventive maintenance schedule shall be established and inspections documented. All laser and accessory equipment shall be kept in a constant state of readiness.

Laser Program

LASER PROGRAM DIRECTOR JOB DESCRIPTION

SCOPE

This position is at the __________ level, and will report directly to __________.

SALARY

This is a salaried position, with a range of ( ) to be determined on the basis of experience and credentials.

QUALIFICATIONS

1. Registered nurse, nurse practitioner, physician assistant, or medical physician with current state licensure
2. Three years management experience
3. Three years operating room experience
4. One year clinical laser experience
5. Applicant must be self-directed, experienced in communications, flexible, and able to work well with hospital administration, medical and nursing staffs, and members of the laser industry. Candidates with adult education skills are preferred.

RESPONSIBILITIES

1. Laser Program Director (LPD) will schedule, coordinate, and co-chair all laser committee meetings.
2. LPD will supervise clinical laser activity and function as the liaison among staff, biomedical personnel, physicians, and administration.
3. LPD will compile monthly quality assurance and utilization data and report to committee.
4. LPD will participate in designated national laser organizations and conferences as the representative for the laser center.
5. LPD will facilitate physician and nursing access to continuing education programs and provide current, updated information to the committee and to staff.
6. LPD will participate in the development and implementation of laser center marketing activities.
7. LPD will receive and evaluate requests for lasers and accessory instrumentation and make recommendations for purchases to the laser committee.
8. LPD will maintain credentials and nurse certification records, providing current information to the OR in case of question regarding use of lasers.
9. LPD will establish and maintain nursing certification criteria for staff operating lasers.
10. LPD will attend all designated hospital committees as representative of the laser center.

11. LPD will hire, supervise, evaluate, and terminate assigned personnel, according to hospital policy on personnel management.
12. LPD will review, update, and recommend laser policies, procedures, quality assurance, and documentation tools, in keeping with evolving national and state laser regulations.
13. LPD will assume responsibility for daily operational activities of the laser center.

TEN-POINT LASER PROGRAM REVIEW

1. Organizational structure
    a. Laser committee membership/leadership
    b. Meetings have regular or preset agenda
    c. Has the committee dealt effectively with problems?
2. Staffing
    a. Laser safety officer (LSO) position established and defined
    b. LSO effective in dealing with problems/concerns
    c. Expansion of position and/or alteration of duties needed
3. Equipment
    a. Timely repairs and periodic maintenance
    b. Additional lasers or instrumentation needed
    c. Smoke evacuation up to date or additional needed
    d. Safety equipment in good repair or additional needed
4. Policies and procedures
    a. Annual review of current policies and procedures
    b. Updates complete
5. Quality assurance
    a. Documentation reviewed
    b. Incidents reported
    c. Statistics
    d. Problems identified/action taken
6. Continuing education
    a. Medical staff: new wavelengths and procedures
    b. Nursing staff: annual updates and ongoing in-service programs
    c. Additional staff to be trained
    d. Meetings and professional organization activities
7. Recredentials
    a. Policy established
    b. Implementation
8. Marketing
    a. Strategies
    b. Physician based/community based
    c. Telemarketing
    d. Measurement and data collection
9. Expansion
    a. New procedures
    b. New physicians recruited
    c. Clinical research
10. Further program review
    a. Monthly laser committee meeting reports
    b. Quarterly/annual review

Suggested Agenda Topics for Laser Use Committee

1. Education and training of professional staff
2. Biomedical engineer's role in equipment maintenance
3. Evaluation and acquisition of lasers and instrumentation
4. Laser safety controls (policies and procedures)
5. Marketing strategies
6. Budget/charges
7. Development of reference library
8. Review of clinical literature; report of new applications
9. Quality assurance
10. Credentials
11. Incident report reviews
12. Medical records audits
13. Patient education materials
14. In-service education
15. Research
16. Job descriptions
17. Case presentations (grand rounds)
18. Documentation methods

Laser Safety Officer Responsibilities

As a manager, the laser safety officer:

1. Writes, reviews, and updates all policies and procedures.
2. Participates actively in equipment evaluation procedures.
3. Co-chairs the laser use committee.
4. Performs documentation audits.
5. Monitors and reports on quality assurance of the program.
6. Establishes and maintains a resource center.
7. Contributes to creation of patient education materials and makes physician office visits for direct marketing.
8. Joins professional organizations and keeps the laser team current with new technology and applications.
9. Reviews and updates all aspects of the program, with respect to new standards and regulations.
10. Directs continuing education programs, staff orientation, and physician in-service activities.
11. Contributes to clinical research projects.

As a clinical expert, the laser safety officer:

1. Supervises daily operations.
2. Conducts in-service and continuing education programs.
3. Monitors quality assurance and incident reporting.
4. Contributes to the laser use committee activities.
5. Functions as a liaison among physicians, nursing staff, vendors, and hospital administration.
6. Joins and participates in professional organizations to maintain and expand clinical expertise.
7. Supervises equipment evaluation procedures.
8. Encourages and supports the laser team.

From Laser Resources and Consulting Services, 1990.

Flammability Hazards

PURPOSE: To prevent the risk of incidents involving laser ignition of materials, tissues, or other substances.

POLICY: All procedures regarding safe application of laser energy will be adhered to during clinical use, demonstrations, service, practice laboratories, and evaluations.

PROCEDURES:

1. The laser operator will know the location of the nearest fire extinguisher appropriate for control of fire involving electrical equipment.
2. A basin of water will be open and positioned within the operator's reach.
3. Nonreflective instruments will be used in the operative field. No plastic instruments will be allowed.
4. If nonreflective instruments are not available, specular surfaces will be draped with wet sponges.
5. No alcohol or alcohol-containing preparations or solutions will be used in or near the laser impact site.
6. Wet cloth towels will be used to drape the site and surrounding tissues that may be exposed to a direct or reflected laser impact.
7. The anus will be packed with a wet sponge during perianal laser procedures to prevent ignition of methane gas.
8. No disposable, dry, or paper materials will be placed in the operative site or near the path of the beam.
9. Carbon sparking resulting from carbonization of tissue will be controlled by means of irrigation or other appropriate surgical means.
10. The laser will be placed in standby mode whenever it is not directly aimed at the intended target.

APPROVED:

DATE: DATE REVIEWED:

From Laser Resources and Consulting Services, 1990.

Laser Safety for Fiberoptic Delivery Systems

1. Only laser-trained personnel will operate the laser and its delivery systems.
2. All policies and procedures will be followed whenever a laser is used.
3. Lasers will be positioned in the procedure room and checked before use.
4. Appropriate eye-safety filters will be used with endoscopes and microscopes.
5. Windows that access the laser room will be covered completely with shades, blinds, towels, or other appropriate filters, as necessary.
6. Position laser, fibers, smoke evacuation unit, foot pedals, hoses, and cords for safe traffic patterns in the room.
7. Examine the fiber for breaks or damage of the distal tip, the proximal connector, and along the catheter sheath.
8. Calibrate the fiber according to the manufacturer's directions.
9. Always use appropriate coaxial cooling with a fiber.
10. *Never* fire the laser unless you can see the distal tip of the fiber at least 1 inch beyond the end of the endoscope.
11. Never fire the laser unless you see the aiming beam.
12. Monitor the patient, the equipment, and the environment throughout the laser procedure.
13. Monitor the fiber for:
    a. Distortion of the beam
    b. Decreased power transmission
    c. Accumulation of debris on the tip
    d. Proper handling at all times
14. Never place the fiber directly on paper drapes or in water for cooling. Wait until tip is cool.
15. Never use alcohol in the operative field. Fibers may be rinsed in hydrogen peroxide or saline intraoperatively.
16. Always put the laser in standby when not aimed at target.
17. Dispose of fiber or repolish according to manufacturer's directions after use. *Do not reuse disposable fibers.*

From Laser Resources and Consulting Services, 1990.

Test Firing the Carbon Dioxide Laser

PURPOSE: To determine the operational status, beam alignment, and beam geometry of the CO_2 laser before use.

POLICY: The CO_2 laser will be test-fired on the day it is to be used before a scheduled laser procedure. It will also be tested if it is moved from room to room or used for in-service demonstrations or other nonsurgical uses.

PROCEDURES:

1. Set up a room according to controlled access procedures.
2. Drape Mayo stand with wet cloth towels (no metal exposed).
3. Follow all ocular, flammability, electrical, and other appropriate safety precautions throughout test.
4. Place wet tongue depressor on wet towel surface. Be sure target is placed at the same angle as the laser delivery system (microscope, handpiece, etc.).
5. Set laser, with single short-time exposure.
6. Fire onto the wet tongue depressor. Never fire if you do not see the helium-neon beam.
7. Examine test spot for alignment and proper geometry.
8. Fire once in all modes on control panel: continuous wave, superpulse, all time exposures, single, and repeat.
9. Turn off laser, or place in standby mode if it is to be used right away. *Do not leave laser controls while it is in operate mode.*
10. Document test results on log sheet.

APPROVED:

DATE: DATE REVIEWED:

From Laser Resources and Consulting Services, 1990.

Ocular Safety

PURPOSE: To prevent ocular injuries to patients receiving laser treatment or to personnel working in the laser room.
POLICY: All personnel will adhere to eye protection procedures during all laser applications. Service personnel, biomedical technicians, and those involved in demonstrations and equipment evaluations will follow all ocular safety procedures whenever a laser is in operation in this facility.
PROCEDURES:

1. Appropriate eyewear will be worn by everyone in the room while a laser is in operation. Exceptions are:
   a. Operator of a CO_2 laser attached to a microscope
   b. Operator of a properly filtered endoscope
2. Personnel will wear comfortable and properly fitted eyewear labeled with wavelength (in nanometers) and optical density. CO_2 eyewear is not labeled.
3. All goggles must have side shields to protect from peripheral impact.
4. Contact lens wearers must wear appropriate goggles.
5. Eyewear will be examined before use for defects in the optical coating. If scratched or cracked, goggles must not be worn during a procedure.
6. All personnel will wear appropriate safety eyewear during all endoscopic, video, and ophthalmic procedures.
7. Patients receiving local or regional anesthesia will wear appropriately labeled eyewear while the laser is in use.
8. Patients receiving general anesthesia will have wet cloth towels placed across the eyes or will be fitted with properly labeled eyewear or eye shields.
9. The laser safety officer will inspect all safety eyewear monthly and replace defective goggles, filters, and lenses.

APPROVED:

DATE: DATE REVIEWED:

From Laser Resources and Consulting Services, 1990.

Electrical Hazards

PURPOSE: To prevent electrical accidents involving laser equipment.
POLICY: All personnel handling, operating, or providing maintenance, service, or modifications of laser equipment will comply with electrical safety procedures.
PROCEDURES:

1. Personnel will review hospital policy regarding the use and handling of electrical equipment.
2. Biomedical engineering will inspect all laser equipment for electrical leakage and label at the time of inspection according to hospital policy.
3. Laser equipment being brought into the facility for purposes of evaluation, demonstration, or seminars must be inspected and labeled before delivery to or operation in a patient care area.
4. Dedicated outlets will be designated for any laser requiring greater than a 110-V source.
5. No extension cords will be used on laser equipment.
6. Daily visual inspection of circuit breakers, fuses, and foot switch cord connectors will be completed by the designated laser operator before activating the laser.
7. Defects or damage to any electrical component of the laser will be repaired before clinical use.
8. Water or solutions must not be hung or placed on or near the laser.

APPROVED:

DATE: DATE REVIEWED:

From Laser Resources and Consulting Services, 1990.

Controlled Access to the Laser Room

PURPOSE: To define the area in which controls must be applied and to describe the control measures necessary to maintain a safe treatment environment for patients and a safe working environment for personnel.

POLICY: Lasers will be operated only in areas where traffic flow and compliance with all safety procedures can be controlled and monitored.

PROCEDURES:

1. Regulation "Danger" laser signs will be prominently posted at eye level on all doors that access a room where a laser will be operated. These signs will state the wavelength and class of laser to be used.
2. Safety goggles of the appropriate wavelength will be placed with each door sign posted.
3. Glass windows will be covered with ______________ (an appropriate covering) whenever a fiber-optic laser (Nd:YAG, KTP, PDPL, FLPDL, argon) is to be operated. Coverings will remain in place while the laser is operational.
4. Laser keys will be kept in ______________ (designated area) and signed out only by those authorized to do so.
5. All procedures will be followed during service calls, demonstrations, and evaluations as well as during clinical procedures.

APPROVED:

DATE: DATE REVIEWED:

From Laser Resources and Consulting Services, 1990.

Smoke Hazards

LASER PLUME MANAGEMENT

PURPOSE: To remove laser plume contaminants effectively from the laser impact site to reduce the risk of transmission of potentially hazardous particulates to personnel in the laser room.

POLICY: A laser plume management system, appropriate to the laser wavelength and clinical application, will be employed whenever a laser is in use.

PROCEDURES:

1. Position smoke evacuator or recirculation unit for closed procedures in room whenever a laser case is anticipated.
2. Check the operation of the system before the beginning of the case.
3. Install a clean filter on the system if it has been used ________ (times used), or for contaminated cases (e.g., HIV, herpes, condyloma).
4. Follow standard hospital procedures for handling of biohazardous materials.
5. In-line filters with 0.3-μm filtration will be placed between wall suction and the fluid canister for:
   a. Suction lines not connected to evacuator
   b. Cases producing minimal plume
   c. Evacuator failures before or during procedure
6. Distal collection port of the smoke evacuation system must be no more than 2 cm from impact site.
7. Laser masks (minimum 0.3-μm filtration) must be worn by everyone in the laser room for CO_2 lasers. Standard barrier masks must be worn by everyone in the room when Q-switched lasers are in use.
8. All tubing, connectors, adaptors, and wands will be changed ________ (no. of times).

APPROVED:

DATE: DATE REVIEWED:

From Laser Resources and Consulting Services, 1990.

CONTROL OF SMOKE FROM LASER AND ELECTROSURGICAL PROCEDURES

HAZARD

During surgical procedures using a laser or electrosurgical unit, the thermal destruction of tissue creates a smoke by-product. Research studies have confirmed that this smoke plume can contain toxic gases and vapors such as benzene, hydrogen cyanide, and formaldehyde, bioaerosols, dead and live cellular material (including blood fragments), and viruses. At high concentrations the smoke causes ocular and upper respiratory tract irritation in health care personnel and creates visual problems for the surgeon. The smoke has unpleasant odors and has been shown to have mutagenic potential.

CONTROLS

NIOSH research has shown that airborne contaminants generated by these surgical devices can be effectively controlled. Two methods of control are recommended: ventilation and work practices.

Ventilation

Recommended ventilation techniques include a combination of general room and local exhaust ventilation (LEV). General room ventilation is not by itself sufficient to capture contaminants generated at the source. The two major LEV approaches used to reduce surgical smoke levels for health care personnel are portable smoke evacuators and room suction systems.

Smoke evacuators contain a suction unit (vacuum pump), filter, hose, and inlet nozzle. The smoke evacuator should have high efficiency in airborne particle reduction and should be used in accordance with the manufacturer's recommendations to achieve maximum efficiency. A capture velocity of about 100 to 150 feet per minute at the inlet nozzle is generally recommended. It is also important to choose a filter that is effective in collecting the contaminants. A high-efficiency particulate air (HEPA) filter or equivalent is recommended for trapping particulates. Various filtering and cleaning processes can remove or inactivate airborne gases and vapors. The various filters and absorbers used in smoke evacuators require monitoring and replacement on a regular basis and are considered a possible biohazard requiring proper disposal.

Room suction systems pull at a much slower rate and are designed primarily to capture liquids rather than particulates or gases. If these systems are used to capture generated smoke, users must install appropriate filters in the line and ensure that the line is cleared and that filters are disposed of properly. In general, smoke evacuators are more effective than room suction systems to control the generated smoke from nonendoscopic laser and electrosurgical procedures.

Work Practices

The smoke evacuator or room suction hose nozzle inlet must be kept within 2 inches of the surgical site to capture effectively airborne contaminants generated by these surgical devices. The smoke evacuator should be ON (activated) at all times when airborne particles are produced during all surgical or other procedures. At the completion of the procedure, all tubing, filters, and absorbers must be considered infectious waste and be disposed of appropriately. New filters and tubing should be installed on the smoke evacuator for each procedure. Although many commercial smoke evacuator systems are available, all these LEV systems must be regularly inspected and maintained to prevent possible leaks. Users also must use control measures such as *universal precautions,* as required by the U.S. Occupational Safety and Health Administration (OSHA) Blood-Borne Pathogen Standard.

FOR MORE INFORMATION

To obtain information about controlling this hazard, or for information on other occupational health and safety issues, call NIOSH at (800) 35-NIOSH/(800) 356-4674.

The following reports on this topic are available free on request from NIOSH:

- Evaluation of a smoke evacuator used for laser surgery, *Lasers Surg Med* 9:276, 1989.
- NIOSH Health Hazard Evaluation and Technical Assistance Reports, HETA 85-, 126-1932 (1988) and HETA 88-, 101-2008 (1990).

NIOSH is the Federal agency responsible for conducting research and making recommendations for *preventing* work-related illness and injuries. *Hazard Controls* are based on research studies that show reduced worker exposure to hazardous agents or activities.

Acknowledgments

The principal contributor to this *Hazard Controls* is C. Eugene Moss, Division of Surveillance, Hazard Evaluations and Field Studies. Assistance was provided by the Education and Information Division, NIOSH.

From Centers for Disease Control and Prevention, U.S. Department of Health and Human Services/National Institute for Occupational Safety and Health: *NIOSH hazard controls,* Pub No 96-128, September 1996.

Vascular Lesions Support Groups

Arteriovenous Malformation Support Group
107 Bella Vista Way
San Francisco, CA 94127
(415) 344-8012

Association of Birth Defect Children, Inc.
5400 Diplomat Circle, Suite 270
Orlando, FL 32810

Disfigurement Guidance Centre
PO Box 7
Cupar Fife KY1S 4PF
Scotland, United Kingdom
Ph#: 01334839084
FAX: 01334839105

Hereditary Hemorrhagic Telangiectasia Foundation International, Inc.
PO Box 8087
New Haven, CT 06530

Klippel-Trenaunay Support Group
4610 Wooddale Avenue
Edema, MN 55424
(612) 925-2596

Let's Face It
PO Box 711
Concord, MA 01742-0711
(508) 371-3186

The National Vascular Malformations Center, Inc.
8320 Nightingale St.
Dearborn Heights, MI 48127
(313) 274-1243

The Sturge-Weber Foundation
Karen L. Ball, President
PO Box 460931
Aurora, CO 80046
(303) 690-9735

Index

Q

R